Pulmonary Medicine

Editor: Lily Hartman

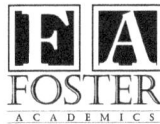

FA
FOSTER
ACADEMICS

www.fosteracademics.com

www.fosteracademics.com

FA
FOSTER
ACADEMICS

Cataloging-in-Publication Data

Pulmonary medicine / edited by Lily Hartman.
 p. cm.
Includes bibliographical references and index.
ISBN 978-1-63242-797-7
1. Lungs--Diseases. 2. Respiratory organs--Diseases. 3. Respiratory infections. I. Hartman, Lily.
RC756 .P85 2019
616.24--dc23

Foster Academics,
118-35 Queens Blvd., Suite 400,
Forest Hills, NY 11375, USA

ISBN 978-1-63242-797-7 (Hardback)

Contents

Permissions

List of Contributors

Index

Preface

Every book is a source of knowledge and this one is no exception. The idea that led to the conceptualization of this book was the fact that the world is advancing rapidly; which makes it crucial to document the progress in every field. I am aware that a lot of data is already available, yet, there is a lot more to learn. Hence, I accepted the responsibility of editing this book and contributing my knowledge to the community.

The field of medicine associated with the diseases related to the respiratory tract is known as pulmonology. It is a branch of internal medicine. It includes the management of the patients who require constant life support and mechanical ventilation. Doctors who have specialized in the field of chest conditions like asthma, pneumonia, tuberculosis, etc. are called pulmonologists. Some of the common respiratory diseases which come under pulmonology include sinusitis, tonsillitis, severe acute respiratory syndrome and lung cancer. Interventional pulmonology is a sub-field of pulmonary medicine which deals with the use of procedures like bronchoscopy and pleuroscopy. This book elucidates the concepts and innovative models around prospective developments with respect to pulmonary medicine. It studies, analyzes and upholds the pillars of pulmonary medicine and its utmost significance in modern times. This book includes contributions of doctors and experts which will provide innovative insights into this field.

While editing this book, I had multiple visions for it. Then I finally narrowed down to make every chapter a sole standing text explaining a particular topic, so that they can be used independently. However, the umbrella subject sinews them into a common theme. This makes the book a unique platform of knowledge.

I would like to give the major credit of this book to the experts from every corner of the world, who took the time to share their expertise with us. Also, I owe the completion of this book to the never-ending support of my family, who supported me throughout the project.

Editor

Outcomes of lung transplantation in adults with bronchiectasis

Jodie Birch[1], Syba S. Sunny[2], Katy L. M. Hester[1,2], Gareth Parry[4], F. Kate Gould[3], John H. Dark[4], Stephen C. Clark[4], Gerard Meachery[4], James Lordan[4], Andrew J. Fisher[1,4], Paul A. Corris[1,4] and Anthony De Soyza[1,2]*

Abstract

Background: Lung transplantation is a well-established treatment for end-stage non-cystic fibrosis bronchiectasis (BR), though information regarding outcomes of transplantation remains limited. Our results of lung transplantation for Br are reported here.

Methods: A retrospective review of case notes and transplantation databases was conducted for patients that had underwent lung transplantation for bronchiectasis at the Freeman Hospital between 1990 and 2013.

Results: Fourty two BR patients underwent lung transplantation, the majority (39) having bilateral sequential lung transplantation. Mean age at transplantation was 47.1 years. Pre-transplantation osteoporosis was a significant non-pulmonary morbidity (48%). Polymicrobial infection was common, with *Pseudomonas aeruginosa* infection frequently but not universally observed (67%). Forced expiratory volume in 1 second (% predicted) improved from a pre-transplantation mean of 0.71 L (22% predicted) to 2.56 L (79 % predicted) at 1-year post-transplantation. Our survival results were 74% at 1 year, 64% at 3 years, 61% at 5 years and 48% at 10 years. Sepsis was a common cause of early post-transplantation deaths.

Conclusions: Lung transplantation for end-stage BR is a useful therapeutic option, with good survival and lung function outcomes. Survival values were similar to other bilateral lung transplants at our centre. Pre-transplantation *Pseudomonas* infection is common.

Keywords: Transplantation, Bronchiectasis, Pseudomonas

Background

Bronchiectasis is an abnormal dilation of the bronchi and bronchioles that results in chronic cough, sputum production and recurrent infections. Bronchiectasis can lead to progressive loss of lung function, resulting in chronic morbidity and premature mortality [1]. Bronchiectasis not due to cystic fibrosis (often referred to as non-cystic fibrosis bronchiectasis; thereafter BR) has diverse causes, though post-infectious and idiopathic bronchiectasis are the most common [2, 3].

BR has been identified as a cause of increasing morbidity and mortality in the U.S. and Europe [4–6]. As Bronchiectasis is increasingly encountered (or recognised) there is a greater need to understand the benefits and risks of lung transplantation for this indication. Lung transplantation is an intensive therapeutic intervention that can be performed for the treatment of end-stage BR [7, 8]. However, the recent guidelines from the British Thoracic Society (BTS) specifically note scarce data on the results of lung transplantation for bronchiectasis [2]. This knowledge gap results in uncertainty for clinicians in managing patients with more severe bronchiectasis.

A number of studies have assessed the association between pathogenic microorganisms and prognosis in adult BR. Persistent *Pseudomonas aeruginosa* infection is seen in approximately 30-40% of BR patients and it is linked with a poorer quality of life and increased mortality [9, 10]. Furthermore, it predicts a more severe disease phenotype with increased hospitalisation rates and is associated with poorer lung function and accelerated

* Correspondence: Anthony.de-soyza@newcastle.ac.uk
[1]Institute of Cellular Medicine, Newcastle University, M2060 Leech Building, The Medical School, Framlington Place, Newcastle upon Tyne NE2 4HH, UK
[2]Sir William Leech Centre for lung research, The Freeman Hospital, High Heaton, Newcastle upon Tyne Hospitals NHS Foundation Trust, Newcastle upon Tyne NE7 7DN, UK
Full list of author information is available at the end of the article

functional decline in BR patients [9–12]. In some settings, *Pseudomonas* infection post-transplantation has been linked with increased rates of allograft dysfunction/obliterative bronchiolitis [13]. In contrast, information regarding the prognostic effects of pre-transplantation *Pseudomonas* status on both early and long-term outcomes of lung transplantation for BR remains limited.

In view of the above, we aimed to assess the survival outcomes of patients transplanted for BR at our centre. Additionally, we aimed to investigate a range of pre-transplant factors including pre-transplantation microbiology and their relationship to post-transplantation outcomes.

Methods

Our primary outcome of interest was post-transplant survival in those transplanted for BR. Other aims were to describe the demographic profiles of patients transplanted and the post-transplant outcomes in patients with BR as compared to other lung transplant indications

Case finding and definitions

A retrospective analysis of the pulmonary transplantation databases and case notes was performed for all BR patients who underwent pulmonary transplantation at our institution from 1990 to 2013. All adult recipients with bronchiectasis as a primary diagnosis were assessed and their case notes and microbiological results reviewed. In general, the exclusion of cystic fibrosis was through genetic testing by UK Health service genetic laboratories and/or sweat tests in line with more recent guidelines. Immunological work up included assessment of serum immunoglobulins although additional tests were performed upon consultation with immunologists if clinical suspicion of immunodeficiency was made.[2] As a control group we included all lung transplants for any other indication across the same time cohort. Data where available were extracted to define the Bronchiectasis severity index scores [4], the FACED scores [14] and the eFACED scores [15].

Peri-transplantation management

Induction therapy changed over the time cohort but has included intravenous methylprednisolone and in earlier patients included anti-thymocyte globulin [16]. A 3-day induction protocol with intravenous methylprednisone (2 mg/kg) was used in the majority of patients. Post-transplantation immunosuppression comprised of cyclosporine, prednisolone and azathioprine for all patients [16]. Prophylactic antibiotics were given to the recipient in accordance with the most recent sensitivities derived from sputum cultures as per our CF protocol [16]. Aztreonam (2 g) 8 hourly for 2-7 days was used if the isolate was multiply resistant. Multiple antibiotic

synergy testing has been incorporated since 2001 into our microbiological work up using previously described methods [17, 18].

Operative interventions

Bilateral single sequential lung transplantations (BSLTx) were performed via clamshell incisions as per our CF lung transplant protocol [16]. The donor bronchial stump was kept as short as possible to avoid ischaemic injury. Cardiopulmonary bypass was used in all cases with aprotinin used as standard. Heart-lung transplantation was performed *via* sternotomy with tracheal anastomosis and bicaval anastomosis.

Surveillance associated complications

Surveillance transbronchial biopsies and bronchoalveolar lavage (BAL) were routinely performed at 1 week, 1 month, 3 months, 6 months and one year post-transplant and at times of deterioration [16]. Acute vascular rejection grade A2 or greater were recorded. Major complications of transbronchial biopsy were recorded as present if there was requirement for chest drain insertion, biopsy associated bleeding with requirement for invasive ventilation or death following a procedure [16].

Obliterative bronchiolitis

Pulmonary function tests were performed according to accepted guidelines. The data were collected prior to the use of chronic allograft dysfunction in clinical practice [19] so Bronchiolitis obliterans syndrome terminology was used. We used "Freedom from BOS" as previously [20] to define patients who failed to demonstrate a fall in FEV_1 to the threshold used for BOS 1 or higher. The best consecutive FEV_1 attained as directed by the guidelines was used to set thresholds for BOS 1 (FEV_1 66-80% of best recorded post-transplantation FEV_1) BOS 2 (FEV_1 51-65%) and BOS 3 (FEV_1 <50%). BOS 0-p (potential for BOS development) was also recorded.

Survival analysis and causes of death recording

Survival data are routinely collected as part of the national transplant surveillance programme. StatView software V. 4.5 was used to conduct actuarial survival analysis within our cohort. Causes of post-transplantation mortality were recorded from patient notes where available. Sepsis related deaths were recorded where a pathogen was identified clinically as causal to the recipient's death or where a clinical diagnosis of infection was made and alternate diagnoses were excluded.

Microbiology

Peri-transplantation microbiology from sputum and/or BAL of the recipient lung on the day of transplantation was recorded from patient notes and the microbiology database. In most cases sputum was collected with infrequent need for BAL at transplant. Pre-transplantation sputum microbiology results e.g. from referring centres or at our transplant assessment visits were also recorded from patient notes. The presence/absence of bacterial infection was based on qualitative microbial culture. No quantitative cultures were undertaken. Pulsed field gel electrophoresis assessment of microbiological clonality was not routinely conducted. Post-transplantation BAL data from routine surveillance BAL undertaken at 1 year was cross-checked between the computerised pathology reporting system and from paper records.

Systemic disease

Pre-transplantation cardiac dysfunction, body mass index (BMI) and osteoporosis rates from Dual-energy X-ray absorptiometry (DEXA) scans were captured. Post-transplantation renal function was determined by serial serum creatinine levels that were recorded pre--transplantation and at 1 year, 5 years and 10 years post-transplantation.

Results

The total number of lung transplantation procedures performed for all indications at data capture (1990-2013) was 752, with 42 lung transplantations performed for BR (6% of the total lung transplant population). There were 39 patients that underwent BSLTx from cadaveric donors, one patient had single lung transplantation (SLTx) and two patients had heart-lung transplantation. Lung transplantation commenced at this institution in 1987 with the first transplantation for BR performed in 1990. The assessment protocol has evolved in this time period and hence full datasets are not available for all parameters.

There were 25 patients transplanted for BR between 1990 and 2000 from a total of 260 lung transplants performed (9.6%). Significantly fewer were transplanted between 2001 and 2011; 17 from a total of 429 (4.0%; Chi-square test, p<0.001). Thus, lung transplantation for BR was less frequent in the second 10-year time cohort compared to the first 10 years of transplantation. All recipients were adults (age >17 years), with a mean age at transplantation of 47.1 years (range; 22.6-62 years). There were 13 female patients (31%) and 29 male patients (69%) transplanted. For the control cohort (all sequential single lung transplants performed for any other indication) the mean age was 42 years with 42% female and 58% male (the majority of these other indications were cystic fibrosis and COPD without bronchiectasis).

Bronchiectasis aetiology

Bronchiectasis aetiology was categorised in 29 of 42 patients, with post-infectious (9 patients), idiopathic (6 patients) and COPD-associated (5 patients) accounting for the majority of cases (31%, 21% and 17% of cases, respectively).

Bronchiectasis associated with Kartagener's syndrome was noted in 14% of cases (4 patients) and Young's syndrome in 10% of cases (3 patients). Neonatal ventilatory trauma and X-linked agammaglobulinaemia led to secondary bronchiectasis in single cases. In the remaining cases the presumptive aetiologies were idiopathic or post infectious but insufficient details were available to conclusively exclude other aetiologies.

Bronchiectasis severity scores

Full data sets were not available in all transplant recipients. We were able to calculate the BSI, FACED and eFACED scores in 34 patients. According to the BSI, 33 had severe bronchiectasis (score 9 or greater) and one had moderate severity (BSI score 7). In contrast whilst 18 were deemed to have severe bronchiectasis 16 were deemed to have moderate bronchiectasis according to FACED. Using eFACED scores, 28 were deemed to have moderate bronchiectasis and 8 were deemed to have severe bronchiectasis.

Pre-transplantation morbidity

Pulmonary disease

The mean pre-transplantation FEV_1 at lung transplant assessment was 0.71l ± 0.27 (22 % predicted) (n = 37). From 36 patients where full data was available, 32 were in respiratory failure (89 %) and on long-term oxygen therapy. Of these, one patient was on long-term non-invasive ventilation (NIV).

Pre-transplantation arterial blood gas values taken at assessment were available for 35 patients. The mean PO2 was 8.3 ± 2.8kPa and mean pCO2 was 6.9 ± 1.2kPa (30/35 patients on oxygen therapy). Six minute walk test mean distance walked was 280.8 metres (range; 60-640 metres), with lowest arterial oxygen saturation recorded at a mean of 75.4% (range; 49-91%) (n = 36).

Data regarding other co-morbidities were available for 31 of 42 patients. Of these, we noted 12 patients (39%) with a co-existent diagnosis of asthma pre-transplantation. There were 10 patients (32%) with COPD. Five were felt to have COPD as an aetiology and five patients had another diagnosis felt to be the primary cause of the bronchiectasis but also had COPD listed as a comorbidity. A history of previous pneumothorax was reported by 4 patients (13%). We noted 3 patients (10%) with echocardiographic evidence of pulmonary hypertension and 2 patients (6%) with clinical features of allergic bronchopulmonary aspergillosis.

Non-Pulmonary disease

Osteoporosis was a significant non-pulmonary pre-transplantation morbidity affecting 14 patients (48%) (n = 29). 3 patients had documented pre-transplantation diabetes (10%, n=31). Pre-transplantation echocardiogram results were available for 33 patients. Of these patients, 18 (55%) had an abnormal result, with some patients having multiple abnormalities. Right ventricular dilation was noted in 13 cases, right ventricular atrophy in 4 cases, left ventricular dilatation noted in 2 cases and pulmonary hypertension noted in 1 case. Pre-transplantation ischaemic heart disease affected 2 patients (6%) and Wolff-Parkinson-White syndrome affected one patient. At assessment the pre-transplantation mean BMI was 25.4 kg/m2 (± 4.8) (range; 16-31.9 kg/m2) (n = 25).

Survival and causes of death

The survival figures for the whole cohort were 74% survival at 1 year, 64% at 3 years, 61% at 5 years and 48% at 10 years (Fig. 1).,The calculated 50% survival was at 9.3 years. We compared our Kaplan-Meier survival rates for the BR cohort with that of BSLTx for all other transplantation indications at our centre (Fig. 1). There was no significant difference in survival between the BR and non-BR transplantation cohorts (log rank testing; Mantel-Cox, p = 0.23).

At data capture, 14 of 42 BR lung transplant recipients were alive (33%). Data allowing determination of cause of death was available in 13 cases (Table 1). Death caused by sepsis was noted in 5 cases (staphylococcal infection was identified as a cause of death in two cases and cytomegalovirus in one case). In the remaining two cases, a sepsis syndrome was identified although no specific pathogen was isolated. Therefore 38% of all recorded BR transplantation recipient deaths were due to sepsis where data were available. Of the sepsis-related deaths, 3 occurred early post-transplantation. None of these occurred in patients with known immunodeficiency related bronchiectasis. Multi-organ failure occurring within the first month following transplantation was the cause of death in 2 cases. Later causes of death included respiratory failure or obliterative bronchiolitis, which was recorded in 4 cases. Other identified causes of death include malignancy (n = 1, post transplantation lymphoproliferative disease) and cerebrovascular accident (n = 1).

Pulmonary function post-transplantation

Mean pre-transplantation FEV_1 was 0.71l ± 0.27 (22% predicted) (n = 37), which improved to 2.56l ± 1.02 (79 % predicted; n=31) at 1 year post-transplantation. The mean FEV_1 at 5 years post-transplantation was 2.3l ± 0.95 (74 % predicted) (n = 18) and 2.36l ± 0.72 (78% predicted) (n = 9) at 10 years post-transplantation (p <0.001 at each time point compared with pre-transplantation values; paired t-test).

The prevalence of severe airflow limitation as BOS 3 was 18% at 1 year and 25% at 5 years. Where data were available at 10 years post-transplantation, no patients were at stage BOS 3 (n=9).

Renal disease

Mean serum creatinine for patients at pre-transplantation assessment was 83.2 mg/dl (± 17.4) (range; 53-118 mg/dl) (n = 39). By 1-year post-transplantation, creatinine levels worsened for all patients, rising to a mean of 166.8 mg/dl (± 60.2) (range 73-281 mg/dl) (n = 29) (p <0.001; paired t-test). Of those patients still alive at data capture, no patients had however required haemodialysis or had

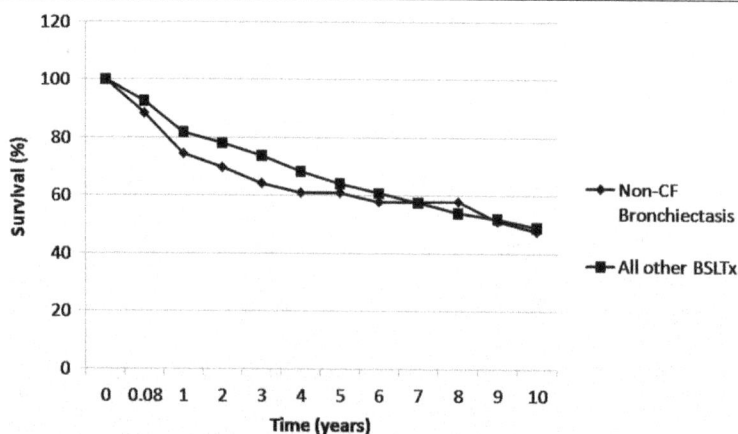

Fig. 1 Actuarial survival of patients with non-CF bronchiectasis (BR) at the Freeman Hospital Lung Transplant Programme (n=42) compared with all other bilateral sequential single lung transplants (BSLTx) performed at our centre (n=409). No significant difference in survival was found between the cohorts (log-rank testing; Mantel-Cox, p = 0.23).

Table 1 Causes of death in non-CF bronchiectasis recipients transplanted at the Freeman Hospital

Cause of death	No of patients (%)
Infection	5 (38)
Staphylococcus	2 (15)
Cytomegalovirus	1 (8)
Unknown	2 (15)
Respiratory failure	2 (15)
Obliterative bronchiolitis	2 (15)
Multi-organ failure	2 (15)
Malignancy	1 (8)
Cerebrovascular accident	1 (8)
Total No of deaths	13 (100)

Transplant Programme. Causes of death in recipients were recorded from case notes. Data are expressed as percentage of deaths observed in this cohort where data detailing cause of death were available. Data was available for 13 patients, however 28 patients from the cohort were deceased. Percentages have been rounded up or down to the first decimal place

undergone renal transplantation following lung transplantation ($n = 14$).

Surveillance biopsies

Acute vascular rejection (grade A2 or greater, as defined by the International Society for Heart Lung Transplantation (ISHLT)) [21] was noted in 2 patients from available transbronchial biopsy results at 3 months and 6 months post-transplantation ($n = 14$). Of all patients alive at data capture, none had experienced significant morbidity (e.g. invasive mechanical ventilation or blood transfusion) or mortality following standard transbronchial biopsy procedures at the unit.

Microbiology

Peri-transplantation microbiological cultures, including those at or before transplantation assessment, immediately pre-operatively and at 1 year post-transplantation were carried out. Polymicrobial infections in individual recipients were common (Fig. 2). We noted 67% of patients (where data were available, $n = 36$) had documented history of infection with *P. aeruginosa* before transplantation assessment. At transplant assessment, 62% of patients were infected with *P. aeruginosa* ($n = 34$) and at time of transplantation 45% of patients were infected with *P. aeruginosa* ($n = 37$). None of the patients in this cohort had infection with pan-resistant *P. aeruginosa*, however 45% of patients were recorded as having previous infection with multi-resistant *P. aeruginosa* ($n = 20$).

Other organisms commonly isolated pre-transplantation include a mixture of probable commensals and pathogens: *Candida* was noted in 44% of patients, *Aspergillus* spp. in 30%, *Haemophilus influenzae* infection in 28%, *Streptococcus pneumoniae* in 19%, *Stenotrophomonas* spp. infection in 17%, *methicillin resistant Staphylococcus aureus* (MRSA) infection in 14%, *Moraxella catarrhalis* in 14% and *Alcaligenes* spp. infection in 3% ($n = 36$).

Prior to transplantation 24 patients (69%) of 35 patients with available data, were taking nebulised antibiotics. Only 4 patients were receiving azithromycin pre-transplantation,

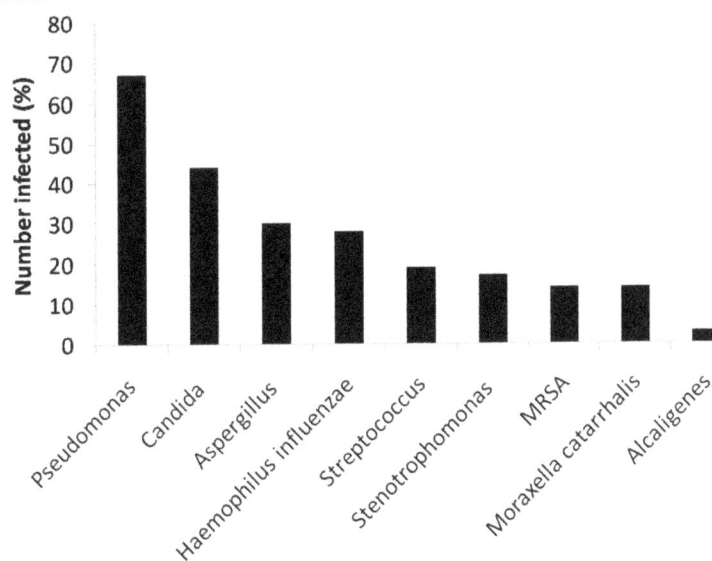

Fig. 2 Microbial infections prior to transplantation. Percentage of the cohort (where data were available) infected with each pathogen is noted. The majority of patients had more than one pathogen isolated from the same individual's sputa in the year before transplantation. MRSA, methicillin resistant S aureus.

perhaps reflecting the more recent widespread use of macrolides in inflammatory lung disease.

Post-transplantation lavage

Microbiology results for BAL specimens collected at 1 year post-transplantation were retrieved for 29 patients of the 31 recipients alive at 1 year. Most did not grow respiratory pathogens in their BAL (18 patients, 62%). The most commonly isolated pathogen was *P. aeruginosa* in 6 patients (21%), all of whom had persistent *P. aeruginosa* infection prior to transplantation. Other organisms isolated included *Candida* species (3 patients; 10%), *Staphylococcus aureus* (2 patients; 7%), *Aspergillus fumigatus* (1 patient; 3%) and *Paecilomyces lilacinus* (1 patient).

Discussion

Despite exciting new therapeutic pipelines in BR, a rising mortality rate and increasing hospitalisation rates for BR suggests there are significant unmet medical needs [6, 9]. Lung transplantation is one option for managing severe end stage BR. Lung transplantation for BR accounts for 6% of all lung transplantations performed at our centre, a distribution similar to that of the International Society for Heart Lung Transplantation (ISHLT) registry [21, 22]. We noted excellent post-transplant outcomes with greater than 50% survival at 5 years. Our outcomes were comparable to lung transplant outcomes for other indications at our centre. Our approach has predominantly been with BSLTx, which has been argued as the procedure of choice for this group of patients [21, 22]. Notably BR has been calculated to have a better cost effectiveness outcome following lung transplantation as compared to COPD, the commonest indication for lung transplantation [23]. The combined UK transplant experience also suggested that BR has one of the best post-transplant outcomes [24].

In view of this, the low rates of lung transplantation for BR need to be considered. They may be due to a number of factors including concerns about the risk benefit ratio of lung transplantation in BR. The prevalence of BR peaks in older patients who may be perceived beyond the optimal window for lung transplantation. Furthermore the lack of a validated prognostic scoring systems for BR in contrast to those for COPD may prevent timely referral for lung transplantation [25]. The role of either of the recently published indices, Bronchiectasis severity index (BSI) [4] or FACED score [14] in guiding transplant referrals remains to be defined. We noted that the majority of patients were classified as severe bronchiectasis using BSI but not with FACED. Further studies are needed to define the role of these scores in helping prompt referral for transplant assessment. These latter scores

underrepresent those with severe disease until the age is beyond 70 years due to the weighting of the scores.

As highlighted in recent BR guidelines very few studies have examined lung transplantation in detail. The survival in our series was similar to the survival figures previously reported by our institution for CF patients [16].

The most recent case series of 34 patients from Germany reported good outcomes for bronchiectasis with one-year Kaplan-Meier survival for patients with bronchiectasis being 85% and 5-year survival being 73%. These outcomes were comparable to the overall lung transplant cohort. Notably however the mean age group was much younger at 40 years. In those with pre-transplant Pseudomonas infection poorer outcomes and higher rates of BOS were reported from the Hannover group [26]. The UK wide experience spanning 5 centres with 123 BR patients listed for transplantation was noted in a study of all lung transplant indications published in 2009 [24]. Unfortunately, little in depth data beyond survival in BR were available but the study demonstrated only 54 BR patients listed survived on the waiting list to transplantation (48%). Of those transplanted the median waiting time on the list was nearly 1 year with a median post-transplantation survival of 3000 days. Notably the BR post-transplantation survival was the best of 5 major indications for lung transplantations. Despite this apparently good outcome it seems unlikely that the BR cohort were less sick than the other indications studied; along with interstitial lung disease, BR had the highest "on-list" pre-transplantation mortality rates (59/123 died on the waiting list). This correlates well with our observed high rates of respiratory failure and secondary pulmonary hypertension in our cohort.

The ISHLT registry data show that the major causes of mortality in the first year following lung transplantation for any indication are graft failure and infection. We noted a large range of pathogens with potential to complicate the early postoperative period. Our immediate pre-transplantation rate of *Pseudomonas* infection was 45%, which is broadly similar to a prior Spanish series of 17 patients where 64% of patients had *Pseudomonas* infection pre-transplantation [27]. These contrast with our experience in CF, where the majority of patients had *Pseudomonas* pre-transplantation [16].

BR transplant recipients could be predicted to suffer high rates of infection or, in the event of over-cautious immunosuppression, high rates of acute rejection. Firstly we observed an early septic death rate of 7%, which appears similar to that observed elsewhere for other non-septic lung transplantation [16]. Whilst there were high rates of multi-resistance in those with *Pseudomonas* infection, none were pan-resistant. Furthermore, the septic deaths were unrelated to *Pseudomonas* infection *per se*. The prior literature denotes that *Pseudomonas* infection is seen in those with more severe bronchiectasis, which has led other authors to conclude that it is a marker of more severe lung disease. It is plausible that a non-significant trend towards more deaths in the *Pseudomonas* group herein reflects more severe disease. Alternatively, as suggested by Rademacher and colleagues in the Hannover series, Pseudomonas may be driving poorer outcomes [26].

The previously noted UK wide BR transplant data set of 54 patients is likely to include many of the 37 BR patients transplanted at Papworth Hospital, reported in a case series in 2005 [28]. In this cohort, 32 were defined as "bronchiectasis alone" and the remaining 5 had an antibody deficiency that required immunoglobulin replacement therapy. In this latter case series the observed actuarial survival was similar in the 2 groups (81% at 12 months in the bronchiectasis group and 80% in the antibody deficiency group). The post-operative complication rates were acceptable with infection episodes per 100 patient-days for bronchiectasis alone being 0.90 vs. 0.53 and rejection episodes per 100 patient-days being 0.59 vs. 0.24. Whilst we did not quantify rejection rates in this manner, our rates of symptomatic or surveillance rejection were not detected.

Whilst this is the largest single centre study of lung transplantation in bronchiectasis to date limitations of our study should be acknowledged. These include missing data points: whilst there were 28 deaths we could only report data on 13 of these cases reflecting that many of the deaths occurred late transplant and occurred at the referring centre and not transplant centre. The newer definition of chronic lung allograft dysfunction (CLAD) [19] was not used in our study awaiting ISHLT guidelines on the implementation of CLAD. The study is limited by the sample size that are inherent in the single centre retrospective design. Furthermore there have been changes in both our peri transplant protocols reflecting novel immunosuppressants and anti-viral agents used over the study period. Additionally the majority of the transplants performed are sequential single lung transplants so we cannot define the differences between heart-lung transplantation and our preferred operative type. Larger multicentre studies, with multivariate analyses, that define pre-transplant characteristics that are associated with increased risks of early deaths would be helpful. Nevertheless our study highlights important findings that have not been reported before. Important areas to be considered for future studies will be an assessment of rejection rates and frequency of and prognostic implications of clonal *Pseudomonas* strains [29].

Conclusions

Transplantation for BR has excellent outcomes yet poor on-list survival [24]. In our experience the numbers of transplants for this indication may be declining for reasons unknown. Physicians should consider transplantation as an option in those with severe bronchiectasis.

Abbreviations
BR: non-cystic fibrosis bronchiectasisxzBSLTxBilateral single sequential lung transplantationsBALbroncho-alveolar lavageBOSbronchiolitis obliterans syndromeBMIbody mass indexDEXADual-energy X-ray absorptiometrySLTx-single lung transplantationNIVnon-invasive ventilationBSIbronchiectasis severity index.

Acknowledgments
The authors would like to acknowledge the clinical and administrative staff of the transplant unit.

Funding
Sources of funding: JB was supported by NIHR/MRC PhD studentship

Author's contributions
JB collected, analysed and interpreted patient data and was a major contributor in writing the manuscript. SSS contributed to data collection and analysis and to manuscript writing. KLH contributed to data collection, analysis and manuscript writing. GP conducted survival analysis and contributed to the manuscript. FKG collected and analysed microbiology data. JHD SCC GM JL AJF PAC ADS designed the study, interpreted data and contributed to manuscript writing. All authors have seen and approved the final manuscript

Competing interests
The authors declare that they have no competing interests.

Author details
[1]Institute of Cellular Medicine, Newcastle University, M2060 Leech Building, The Medical School, Framlington Place, Newcastle upon Tyne NE2 4HH, UK. [2]Sir William Leech Centre for lung research, The Freeman Hospital, High Heaton, Newcastle upon Tyne Hospitals NHS Foundation Trust, Newcastle upon Tyne NE7 7DN, UK. [3]Department of Medical Microbiology, The Freeman Hospital, High Heaton, Newcastle upon Tyne Hospitals NHS Foundation Trust, Newcastle upon Tyne NE7 7DN, UK. [4]Institute of Transplantation, The Freeman Hospital, High Heaton, Newcastle upon Tyne Hospitals NHS Foundation Trust, Newcastle upon Tyne NE7 7DN, UK.

References
1. O'Donnell AE. Bronchiectasis. Chest. 2008;134(4):815–23.
2. Pasteur MC, Bilton D, Hill AT. British Thoracic Society guideline for non-CF bronchiectasis. Thorax. 65(Suppl 1):i1–58.
3. Pasteur MC, et al. An investigation into causative factors in patients with bronchiectasis. Am J Respir Crit Care Med. 2000;162(4 Pt 1):1277–84.
4. Chalmers JD, et al. The bronchiectasis severity index. An international derivation and validation study. Am J Respir Crit Care Med. 2014;189(5):576–85.
5. Roberts HJ, Hubbard R. Trends in bronchiectasis mortality in England and Wales. Respir Med. 2010;104(7):981–5.
6. Seitz AE, et al. Trends in bronchiectasis among medicare beneficiaries in the United States, 2000 to 2007. Chest. 2012;142(2):432–9.
7. Neves PC, et al. Non-cystic fibrosis bronchiectasis. Interact Cardiovasc Thorac Surg. 2011;13(6):619–25.
8. Rademacher J, Welte T. Bronchiectasis–diagnosis and treatment. Dtsch Arztebl Int. 2011;108(48):809–15.
9. Loebinger MR, et al. Mortality in bronchiectasis: a long-term study assessing the factors influencing survival. Eur Respir J. 2009;34(4):843–9.
10. Wilson CB, et al. Effect of sputum bacteriology on the quality of life of patients with bronchiectasis. Eur Respir J. 1997;10(8):1754–60.

11. King PT, et al. Microbiologic follow-up study in adult bronchiectasis. Respir Med. 2007;101(8):1633–8.

12. Martinez-Garcia MA, et al. Factors associated with lung function decline in adult patients with stable non-cystic fibrosis bronchiectasis. Chest. 2007; 132(5):1565–72.

13. Botha P, et al. Pseudomonas aeruginosa colonization of the allograft after lung transplantation and the risk of bronchiolitis obliterans syndrome. Transplantation. 2008;85(5):771–4.

14. Martinez-Garcia MA, et al. Multidimensional approach to non-cystic fibrosis bronchiectasis: the FACED score. Eur Respir J. 2014;43(5):1357–67.

15. Martinez-Garcia MA, et al. Predicting high risk of exacerbations in bronchiectasis: the E-FACED score. Int J Chron Obstruct Pulmon Dis. 2017;12:275–84.

16. Meachery G, et al. Outcomes of lung transplantation for cystic fibrosis in a large UK cohort. Thorax. 2008;63(8):725–31.

17. Aaron SD, et al. Multiple combination bactericidal antibiotic testing for patients with cystic fibrosis infected with Burkholderia cepacia. Am J Respir Crit Care Med. 2000;161(4 Pt 1):1206–12.

18. Lang BJ, et al. Multiple combination bactericidal antibiotic testing for patients with cystic fibrosis infected with multiresistant strains of Pseudomonas aeruginosa. Am J Respir Crit Care Med. 2000;162(6):2241–5.

19. Verleden GM, et al. A new classification system for chronic lung allograft dysfunction. J Heart Lung Transplant. 2014;33(2):127–33.

20. Quattrucci S, et al. Lung transplantation for cystic fibrosis: 6-year follow-up. J Cyst Fibros. 2005;4(2):107–14.

21. Christie JD, et al. The Registry of the International Society for Heart and Lung Transplantation: Twenty-eighth Adult Lung and Heart-Lung Transplant Report–2011. J Heart Lung Transplant. 2011;30(10):1104–22.

22. Rao JN, et al. Bilateral lung transplant: the procedure of choice for end-stage septic lung disease. Transplant Proc. 2001;33(1-2):1622–3.

23. Groen H, et al. Cost-effectiveness of lung transplantation in relation to type of end-stage pulmonary disease. Am J Transplant. 2004;4(7):1155–62.

24. Titman A, et al. Disease-specific survival benefit of lung transplantation in adults: a national cohort study. Am J Transplant. 2009;9(7):1640–9.

25. Celli BR, et al. The body-mass index, airflow obstruction, dyspnea, and exercise capacity index in chronic obstructive pulmonary disease. N Engl J Med. 2004;350(10):1005–12.

26. Rademacher J, et al. Lung transplantation for non-cystic fibrosis bronchiectasis. Respir Med. 2016;115:60–5.

27. de Pablo A, et al. Lung transplant therapy for suppurative diseases. Arch Bronconeumol. 2005;41(5):255–9.

28. Nathan JA, et al. The outcomes of lung transplantation in patients with bronchiectasis and antibody deficiency. J Heart Lung Transplant. 2005; 24(10):1517–21.

29. De Soyza A, et al. Molecular epidemiological analysis suggests cross-infection with Pseudomonas aeruginosa is rare in non-cystic fibrosis bronchiectasis. Eur Respir J. 2014;43(3):900–3.

2

Obliterative bronchiolitis associated with rheumatoid arthritis: analysis of a single-center case series

Erica Lin[1], Andrew H. Limper[2] and Teng Moua[2*]

Abstract

Background: Rheumatoid arthritis (RA) is a systemic autoimmune condition characterized by erosive inflammation of the joints. One rare pulmonary manifestation is obliterative bronchiolitis (OB), a small airways disease characterized by the destruction of bronchiolar epithelium and airflow obstruction.

Methods: We retrospectively reviewed the clinical data of patients with rheumatoid arthritis-associated obliterative bronchiolitis (RA-OB). Presenting clinical features, longitudinal pulmonary function testing, radiologic findings, and independent predictors of all-cause mortality were assessed.

Results: Forty one patients fulfilled criteria for diagnosis of RA-OB. There was notable female predominance (92.7%) with a mean age of 57 ± 15 years. Dyspnea was the most common presenting clinical symptom. Median FEV1 was 40% (IQR 31–52.5) at presentation, with a mean decline of − 1.5% over a follow-up period of thirty-three months. Associated radiologic findings included mosaic attenuation and pulmonary nodules. A majority of patients (78%) received directed therapy including long-acting inhalers, systemic corticosteroids or other immunosuppressive agents, and macrolide antibiotics. All-cause mortality was 27% over a median follow-up of sixty-two months (IQR 32–113). No distinguishable predictors of survival at presentation were found.

Conclusions: RA-OB appears to have a stable clinical course in the majority of patients despite persistent symptoms and severe obstruction based on presenting FEV1.

Keywords: Rheumatoid arthritis, Obliterative bronchiolitis, Small airways disease

Background

Rheumatoid arthritis (RA) is a systemic autoimmune condition characterized primarily by erosive inflammation of the joints affecting approximately 1% of the world's population [1]. It is often associated with high morbidity due to extra-articular manifestations. Pulmonary manifestations of rheumatoid arthritis include airways disease, interstitial lung disease, parenchymal nodules, pleural disease, and pulmonary vasculitis [1–3]. These pulmonary findings can present early in the disease course [4] and account for up to 10% of rheumatoid arthritis-associated deaths [5, 6].

Obliterative bronchiolitis (OB, synonymous with constrictive bronchiolitis) is a rare small airways disease characterized by the destruction of bronchiolar epithelium and subsequent progressive airflow obstruction [7]. It has been found in a wide range of clinical settings. While obliterative bronchiolitis after transplantation has been well-described [8, 9], its presentation in non-transplant patients is still poorly understood and continues to be a source of interest [10]. Outside of organ transplantation, obliterative bronchiolitis is most commonly associated with connective tissue diseases, such as rheumatoid arthritis [8, 9]. Unfortunately, due to its rarity, there is still a paucity of literature regarding the clinical course of rheumatoid arthritis-associated obliterative bronchiolitis (RA-OB). It has been previously described as variable, in that some patients have periods of prolonged stability while others have a more rapid decline with respiratory failure and death [7].

* Correspondence: moua.teng@mayo.edu
[2]Division of Pulmonary and Critical Care Medicine, Mayo Clinic, 200 First St. SW, Rochester, MN 55905, USA
Full list of author information is available at the end of the article

Therefore, its longitudinal progression should be further evaluated for appropriate management and counseling of patients.

The majority of published studies represent individual case reports or case series, often characterizing the suspected association with penicillamine therapy used for management of RA [11–17]. One concern in assessing the functional history of such patients is the contribution of FEV1 decline from smoking. In a large case series that described both rheumatoid arthritis-associated follicular and obliterative bronchiolitis in fifteen biopsy-proven cases, a third had history of tobacco use [18]. The largest published retrospective study on RA-OB to date included over half with radiologic evidence of emphysema, perhaps confounding the severity of pulmonary function testing [19]. The purpose of this study was to characterize the clinical course and overall prognosis of patients with suspected RA-OB in the absence of radiologic emphysema.

Methods

Study population

Institutional Review Board approval was obtained (IRB #16–009418). The electronic medical record was searched to identify patients with RA-OB using key terms "rheumatoid arthritis" and "bronchiolitis." Consecutive patients with suspected RA-OB evaluated at our institution from 1/1/2000 to 12/31/2015 were reviewed. Rheumatoid arthritis was defined according to criteria established by the American College of Rheumatology [20], confirmed with formal Rheumatology consultation. Obliterative bronchiolitis was defined using the following criteria: 1) presence of active compatible respiratory symptoms including dyspnea or cough plus 2) abnormal pattern on pulmonary function testing (PFT) in the absence of radiologic emphysema or 3) evidence of small airways disease on high-resolution computed tomography (CT) of the chest such as mosaicism or air trapping or centrilobular nodules or 4) histopathologic features on lung biopsy consistent with OB, when available in 5) the absence of an alternative diagnosis that could account for the findings. Indeed, there is not a standardized definition of RA-OB. The above-mentioned definition is based off findings by Hertz et al. [8]. Final diagnoses were made by multidisciplinary review at the time of clinical presentation. In order to select patients with obstructive airways disease attributed to suspected OB alone, patients were excluded if there was concomitant emphysema on imaging. Presenting clinical features, longitudinal PFTs, radiologic findings, therapeutic interventions, and all-cause mortality were collected from the electronic medical record. PFTs were performed in our laboratory using Medical Graphics equipment through standardized protocols by an experienced technician [21]. Collated PFT findings included percent predicted total lung capacity (TLC%), forced vital capacity (FVC%), forced expiratory volume in the first second (FEV1%), and diffusing capacity for carbon monoxide (DLCO%). Airflow obstruction was defined as FEV1 to FVC ratio less than the lower limit of normal (LLN), with staging of obstructive disease based on GOLD criteria for FEV1 [22]. Bronchodilator response was defined as spirometric findings of FEV1 improvement greater than 12% and g200 mL from baseline spirometry. High-resolution CT images were obtained using a scanning protocol in which 10–20 mm images were reconstructed using a high-spatial-resolution algorithm. Along with air-trapping or mosaicism, radiologist assessed presence of other rheumatoid-related pulmonary processes such as suspected rheumatoid lung nodules, lung fibrosis or fibrotic disease, pleural effusion, and non-traction related bronchiectasis, were collated. Biopsies were obtained by either surgical or transbronchial approach and reviewed by an experienced thoracic pathologist at the time of biopsy.

Statistical analysis

Statistical analysis was performed using JMP Software (Version 10.0, SAS Corporation 2012). Quantitative variables were expressed as mean ± standard deviation or median and interquartile range, and qualitative variables as counts and percentage. Comparison of PFT at diagnosis and last available follow-up was assessed using Wilcoxon signed-rank test. Independent predictors of all-cause mortality were assessed using univariable Cox proportional hazards regression. Analysis was performed with statistical significance defined as two-tailed p values < 0.05.

Results

Eighty-nine patients were found using the aforementioned key search terms. Upon review of the cases, forty-eight were excluded: eighteen had obliterative bronchiolitis secondary to other etiologies, seventeen had an incomplete diagnosis of obliterative bronchiolitis not meeting study criteria, eight did not have obliterative bronchiolitis, three were excluded for radiologic emphysema, and two did not have rheumatoid arthritis. After exclusion of non-qualifying patients, forty-one fulfilled the criteria for diagnosis of RA-OB. In most patients, the clinical, physiologic and radiologic findings precluded the need for confirmatory histopathologic diagnosis.

Demographic characteristics are presented in Table 1. There was notable female predominance (93%F:7%M) with a mean age of 57 ± 15 years (range, 22 to 84) at the time of diagnosis. Six were smokers without radiologic evidence of emphysema. Patients had a diagnosis of RA on average fourteen years before the diagnosis of RA-OB. Four patients were diagnosed with small airways disease either concomitantly or during the same year of their RA diagnosis. One patient had an overlap syndrome with RA

Table 1 Demographics and Clinical Presentation (N = 41)

Age at diagnosis (mean ± SD)	57 ± 15
Sex	
Male, N (%)	3 (7.3)
Female, N (%)	38 (92.7)
Positive tobacco use, N (%)	6 (14.6)
Pack year history (median (IQR))	13.5 (6.1-37.5)
Duration of RA prior to diagnosis, years (mean ± SD)	14 ± 12
Use of penicillamine, N (%)	4 (9.8)
Use of gold salts, N (%)	8 (19.5)
Non-pulmonary, extra-articular symptoms at diagnosis, N (%)	10 (24.4)
Active joint symptoms at diagnosis, N (%)	16 (39.0)
Sjögren's syndrome	7 (17)
Respiratory symptoms at diagnosis	
Dyspnea, N (%)	38 (92.7)
Cough, N (%)	13 (31.7)
Chest Pain, N (%)	8 (19.5)
Radiologic findings of OB at diagnosis (N=39)	
Mosaic attenuation, N (%)	20 (51.3)
Centrilobular nodules, N (%)	3 (7.7)
Radiologic findings of other RA-related pulmonary disease (N=39)	
Pulmonary nodules, N (%)	21 (53.8)
Fibrosis, N (%)	12 (30.8)
Pleural effusion, N (%)	2 (5.1)
Bronchiectasis, N (%)	19 (48.7)
Patients biopsied, N (%) (one patient had both wedge and transbronchial)	11 (26.8)
Wedge biopsy, N (%)	5 (41.7)
Transbronchial biopsy, N (%)	7 (58.3)
Unique biopsies consistent with OB diagnosis, N (%)	7 (58.3) (5 wedge, 2 TBB)

Abbreviations: *IQR* interquartile range, *RA* rheumatoid arthritis, *OB* obliterate bronchiolitis, *TBB* transbronchial biopsy

and systemic lupus erythematosus (SLE). During the study period, patients received a wide range of therapeutic agents. Ten percent were previously on D-penicillamine. Twenty-four percent had non-pulmonary extra-articular manifestations. Specifically, 17% had secondary Sjögren's syndrome. In addition to obliterative bronchiolitis, the majority had other rheumatoid arthritis-associated pulmonary disease, most commonly pulmonary nodules and/or bronchiectasis.

Dyspnea was the primary respiratory symptom, present in nearly all patients (92.7%). Thirty-nine percent had active joint symptoms at the time of diagnosis. Eleven underwent histologic assessment, consisting of surgical or transbronchial biopsy. Fifty percent of histopathologic slides were confirmatory, the rest were non-diagnostic with the majority showing non-specific chronic inflammation. Interestingly, all five surgical biopsies resulted in confirmatory histopathologic findings. In comparison, only two of the seven transbronchial biopsies resulted in confirmatory findings. This included one patient who underwent both wedge and transbronchial biopsies. Chest CT was obtained in 95% of patients, which revealed mosaic attenuation in 51.3%. Expiratory views were performed in 72% of CT studies. Physiologic studies were obtained at diagnosis and at last available follow-up (Table 2). Eighty-five percent had evidence of obstruction at initial assessment. There appeared to be no statistically significant absolute change in TLC%, FEV1%, FVC%, and DLCO% obtained at diagnosis and last available follow-up (median duration between PFTs of 33 months (IQR 14.6–51.7)). Mean percent change per year was also calculated in those with available follow-up study for each PFT parameter. Mean FEV1% change per year was − 0.4% with a mean increase in TLC% of 1.5% per year.

Thirty-two patients received directed medical therapy for RA-OB including long-acting inhalers (bronchodilators and inhaled corticosteroids), systemic corticosteroids or other immunosuppressive agents, and macrolide antibiotics (Table 3). Five patients were on supplemental oxygenation, and one underwent lung transplantation. Patients were followed for median duration of 61.7 months (IQR 32.1–113.1). All-cause mortality was 27% over the follow-up timeline. Clinical variables were assessed for their contribution to all-cause mortality (Table 4). No distinguishable predictors of survival at presentation were found on Cox regression analysis.

Discussion

To our knowledge, this study represents the largest case series to date of patients with rheumatoid arthritis-associated obliterative bronchiolitis. The syndrome occurs primarily in middle-aged women after more than a decade of rheumatoid arthritis. The majority presented with dyspnea and radiologic findings of mosaic attenuation and centrilobular nodules. Serial pulmonary function testing demonstrated severe (median FEV1 40%) but stable obstructive disease over time. Seventy-eight percent received directed therapy including long-acting inhalers, systemic corticosteroids or other immunosuppressive agents, and macrolide antibiotics. All-cause mortality was 27% over a median follow-up of five years, without any distinguishable predictors of survival at presentation on Cox regression analysis.

Obliterative bronchiolitis has been described in the literature as a manifestation of underlying rheumatologic disease or secondary to its therapeutic agents. Geddes et al.

Table 2 Pulmonary Function Testing (PFTs)

	PFTs at diagnosis (N = 40)	Last PFTs (N = 25)	Total mean change from first to last PFT, % predicted (N = 25)	Mean % change per year	P-value¶
Obstruction, N (%)	34 (85.0)	21 (84.0)			
TLC% (median (IQR))	106 (88.0–115.0)	112 (105.0–123.0)	4.8	1.5 (N = 15)	0.46
RV/TLC% (median (IQR))	158 (144.0–181.5)	152 (146.3–166.8)	− 6.6	− 1.7 (N = 14)	0.07
FVC% (median (IQR))	66 (53.0–75.0)	61 (54.5–74.5)	− 1.9	− 0.5 (N = 25)	0.42
FEV1% (median (IQR))	40 (31.0–52.5)	41 (29.5–48.0)	−1.5	−0.4 (N = 25)	0.43
DLCO% (median (IQR))	69 (57.5–78.0)	64 (57.0–76.8)	−2.3	−0.6 (N = 18)	0.34
Duration between first and last available PFT, months (median (IQR) and mean (SD))	33(14.6–51.7), 42 (40)				

Abbreviations: *TLC%* percent of predicted total lung capacity, *RV/TLC%* percent of predicted residual volume over total lung capacity, *FVC%* percent of predicted forced vital capacity, *FEV1%* percent of predicted forced expiratory volume in the first second
¶Wilcoxon signed rank test for comparing two related samples

first described several cases in 1977 [11]. During their initial reports, the syndrome appeared to be more prevalent in patients on D-penicillamine therapy, raising the possibility of drug-induced bronchiolopathy [12, 13, 16]. However, patients treated with D-penicillamine for other conditions, such as Wilson's disease, did not develop similar airway findings [12, 16]. In our study, only 10% were previously on D-penicillamine.

The majority of our patients were female. This has also been observed in other studies [16, 23] and may reflect the female predominance associated with rheumatoid arthritis. Interestingly, Fernandez Perez et al. noted that male gender was an independent predictor of mortality in connective tissue disease-associated obliterative bronchiolitis [24]. Our study did not show a similar relationship between gender and mortality.

The mean interval between diagnosis of rheumatoid arthritis and obliterative bronchiolitis was fourteen years. This duration is longer than the five to ten years found in other studies [18, 19]. The diagnosis of RA-OB may be delayed in patients due to lack of recognition by local providers and thus reflect referral bias in a tertiary care center. It may also be confounded by earlier diagnosis of rheumatoid arthritis. Similar to other studies [16, 18, 19],

Table 3 Treatment and Outcome

Directed therapy (N = 32, 78.0%)	
Long-acting inhaler, N (%)	27 (84.4)
Systemic corticosteroids, N (%)	10 (31.3)
Macrolides, N (%)	18 (56.3)
Oxygen supplementation at rest	
Less than or equal to 3 L O2, N (%)	4 (12.5)
Greater than 3 L, N (%)	1 (3.1)
Transplantation, N (%)	1 (3.1)
Mortality, N (%)	11 (26.8)
Time from OB diagnosis to death, months (mean ± SD)	54 ± 53

we found that initial clinical presentation of airways disease was non-specific with predominant symptoms of dyspnea and cough. Less than 40% had active joint symptoms at diagnosis, similar to findings by Devoussoux et al. [19]. A quarter of patients had non-pulmonary and extra-articular manifestations, most commonly secondary Sjögren's. Geli et al. reviewed the CT findings of patients with primary Sjögren's and noted that 65% had bronchiolar abnormalities [25]. This incidence may be a reflection of the association between bronchiolopathies and generalized connective tissue disorders. It is unclear whether secondary Sjögren's affects the development or clinical course of obliterative bronchiolitis in patients with RA. Further studies to evaluate the relationship between obliterative bronchiolitis and primary versus secondary Sjögren's syndrome are needed.

While our study did not evaluate chest radiographs, prior studies reported radiologic findings such as hyperinflation and hyperlucency [18, 19]. We found that half of our patients had characteristic findings of mosaic attenuation with expiratory air trapping on CT [18]. We suspect the frequency of mosaic attenuation may be under-estimated as expiratory images were not routinely obtained on chest CT at presentation(only 72% had specific expiratory images). We note that Devouassoux et al. found a high prevalence of emphysema on CT in patients with RA-OB, even in nine non-smokers [19]. We specifically excluded those with radiologic evidence of emphysema given concern for confounding of PFT severity and long-term survival by this finding. This may have resulted in a more biased subset of individuals, not reflecting the possible co-existence of small airways disease and emphysema in non-smokers. In general, patients with rheumatoid arthritis often have several or multiple radiologic abnormalities on high-resolution chest CT. Remy-Jardin and colleagues found the most common abnormalities were bronchiectasis and bronchiolectasis [26], as airways disease is often the earliest manifestation of RA

Table 4 Univariable Cox regression predictors of all-cause mortality

Characteristics	HR (95% CI)	P-value
Age at diagnosis, years	0.99 (0.94–1.05)	0.78
Gender, female	0.93 (0.15–17.6)	0.94
Duration of RA prior to diagnosis, years	0.98 (0.94–1.03)	0.58
Active joint symptoms at diagnosis	1.87 (0.24–11.42)	0.51
Mosaic attenuation at diagnosis	0.59 (0.12–2.17)	0.44
Lung fibrosis at diagnosis	2.12 (0.58–7.76)	0.24
Bronchiectasis at diagnosis	1.02 (0.28–3.69)	0.97
Baseline PFTs at diagnosis		
TLC%	0.99 (0.95–1.04)	0.76
RV/TLC%	1.01 (0.98–1.03)	0.51
FVC%	0.94 (0.87–1.03)	0.19
FEV1%	0.99 (0.91–1.07)	0.96
Positive bronchodilator response	3.41 (0.73–17.7)	0.11
Macrolide therapy	1.73 (0.40–7.44)	0.44

Abbreviations: *TLC%* percent of predicted total lung capacity, *RV/TLC%* percent of predicted residual volume over total lung capacity, *FVC%* percent of predicted forced vital capacity, *FEV1%* percent of predicted forced expiratory volume in the first second, *RA* rheumatoid arthritis

in the lung [3]. In contrast, Tanaka et al. reported a higher prevalence of interstitial findings, such as ground glass opacities or reticulation. This discrepancy may be the result of referral bias, as many of the patients included in this study were first evaluated in an interstitial lung disease clinic [27]. In our series, the most common radiologic finding was pulmonary nodules, followed by bronchiolar abnormalities. The predominance of bronchiectasis is consistent with RA with or without obliterative bronchiolitis. In advanced cases of obliterative bronchiolitis, there may be wall thickening in both small and large airways. Interestingly, only 30% of our patients had evidence of fibrosis. This lower percentage may be a reflection of gender differences, as rheumatoid arthritis-associated pulmonary fibrosis is more common in males than females [3]. None of these additional findings on their own contributed to an increased risk of mortality, as assessed by univariate Cox regression analysis, likely due to the limited sample size and number of events (deaths) in our series.

Diagnosis of obliterative bronchiolitis may be confirmed with biopsy, either surgical or transbronchial. In our study, all surgical biopsies resulted in confirmatory histopathologic findings, compared to only two of seven transbronchial biopsies. This included one patient with both wedge and transbronchial biopsies. In our small sample size, the diagnostic yield of surgical biopsy was superior to transbronchial biopsy. Further studies to better understand the diagnostic yield of each modality are needed. While the diagnosis of RA-OB may be obtained clinically,

in patients with suspected but indeterminate findings requiring histopathologic confirmation, we recommend surgical biopsy for greater yield, if feasible and safe.

In our study, pulmonary function tests were typically consistent with an obstructive pattern. There was a minority of patients with non-specific, restrictive, or normal findings. Diffusing capacity was relatively maintained in comparison to other airway or parenchymal diseases such as chronic obstructive pulmonary disease (COPD) or interstitial lung disease (ILD) associated with RA. While other studies have noted that FEV1 was significantly lower in patients previously on D-penicillamine [19], we did not find evidence of worsening pulmonary impairment in patients on this agent. Fernandez Perez et al. investigated the longitudinal progression of pulmonary function testing in patients with connective tissue disease associated-obliterative bronchiolitis [24]. While their study did not distinguish between underlying rheumatoid arthritis versus other connective tissue diseases, they discovered that the rate of FEV1 change was minimal during their three-year follow-up, regardless of therapy [24]. Similarly, our study cohort had minimal change in FEV1, suggesting the clinical and functional course of RA-OB may stabilize for a period of time in some.

Given the paucity of literature regarding this syndrome, current evidence for therapy is limited. Case reports mention corticosteroids [16] and other immunosuppressive agents including azathioprine [14], cyclophosphamide [23], and etanercept [28] as possible therapeutic agents directed at small airways disease. Case series have demonstrated that macrolides improve or slow the progression of respiratory impairment in RA-OB [18], which is also evident for other bronchiolar diseases [29]. Unfortunately, large randomized trials for RA-OB are lacking due to disease rarity. Our observational data reveal that medical therapy often included a combination of long-acting inhalers, systemic corticosteroids or other immunosuppressive agents, and macrolide antibiotics. Despite these options, treatment of obliterative bronchiolitis does not appear to reverse disease. It is unclear if FEV1 stabilization in our cohort was a result of natural clinical course or directed therapy. We found that all-cause mortality was 27% over a median follow-up of five years. While the severity of disease based on clinical symptoms and functional findings on PFTs was poor, there again appeared to be a fairly stable clinical course in the majority with gradual deterioration on a time scale of years. This is in contrast to other studies that highlight obliterative bronchiolitis as severe or advancing with immediate decline over months [11–14]. It remains unclear why there is such heterogeneity in disease course.

Our study has several limitations. This is a single center study assessing patients diagnosed and managed over a number of years, reflecting local practices and their evolution over time. Patients referred to tertiary care centers may have more advanced or refractory disease, and thus may not be fully representative of the general disease population. Patients also had physiologic studies measured at varied intervals over time which make accurate assessment of rates of decline less reliable over the study interval. Because of the lack of standardized therapy, we were unable to make inferences about the efficacy of any particular treatment regimen on pulmonary function testing or clinical course. Lastly, as a retrospective study, exact circumstances involved in decision making are difficult to determine, particularly causal effects of management. Despite being one of the larger retrospective studies to date, the absolute number of patients still limited statistical analyses, including multivariable comparisons.

Conclusions

Rheumatoid arthritis-associated obliterative bronchiolitis appears to have a fairly stable clinical course despite persistent symptoms and severe airflow obstruction. While diagnosis may be obtained clinically using supporting radiographic evidence, in patients with suspected disease requiring histopathologic confirmation, we recommend performing surgical biopsy for greater yield, if feasible and safe. Interestingly, serial pulmonary function testing showed only mild deterioration in FEV1 over time. There were no distinguishable predictors at presentation to frame the likelihood of therapeutic response or more rapid clinical decline. Characterizing this longitudinal progression though has valuable implication in the appropriate counseling of patients and future design of clinical trials.

Funding
This research received no grant from any funding agency in the public, commercial or non-profit sectors.

Authors' contributions
EL contributed to the literature search, data collection, data analysis, and data interpretation. AL contributed substantially to the literature search and study design. TM also contributed substantially to the literature search, study design, data analysis, and data interpretation. All authors participated in writing and revising the manuscript. All authors read and approved the final manuscript.

Competing interests
All authors declare that they have no competing interests.

Author details
[1]Department of Internal Medicine, 200 First St. SW, Rochester, MN 55905, USA. [2]Division of Pulmonary and Critical Care Medicine, Mayo Clinic, 200 First St. SW, Rochester, MN 55905, USA.

References

1. Brown KK. Rheumatoid lung disease. Proc Am Thorac Soc. 2007;4(5):443–8.
2. Anaya JM, Diethelm L, Ortiz LA, Gutierrez M, Citera G, Welsh RA, Espinoza LR. Pulmonary involvement in rheumatoid arthritis. Semin Arthritis Rheum. 1995;24(4):242–54.
3. Lynch DA. Lung disease related to collagen vascular disease. J Thorac Imaging. 2009;24(4):299–309.
4. Metafratzi ZM, Georgiadis AN, Ioannidou CV, Alamanos Y, Vassiliou MP, Zikou AK, Raptis G, Drosos AA, Efremidis SC. Pulmonary involvement in patients with early rheumatoid arthritis. Scand J Rheumatol. 2007;36(5):338–44.
5. Sihvonen S, Korpela M, Laippala P, Mustonen J, Pasternack A. Death rates and causes of death in patients with rheumatoid arthritis: a population-based study. Scand J Rheumatol. 2004;33(4):221–7.
6. Suzuki A, Ohosone Y, Obana M, Mita S, Matsuoka Y, Irimajiri S, Fukuda J. Cause of death in 81 autopsied patients with rheumatoid arthritis. J Rheumatol. 1994;21(1):33–6.
7. Lynch JP 3rd, Weigt SS, DerHovanessian A, Fishbein MC, Gutierrez A, Belperio JA. Obliterative (constrictive) bronchiolitis. Seminars in respiratory and critical care medicine. 2012;33(5):509–32.
8. Barker AF, Bergeron A, Rom WN, Hertz MI. Obliterative bronchiolitis. N Engl J Med. 2014;370(19):1820–8.
9. Schlesinger C, Veeraraghavan S, Koss MN. Constrictive (obliterative) bronchiolitis. Curr Opin Pulm Med. 1998;4(5):288–93.
10. Parambil JG, Yi ES, Ryu JH. Obstructive bronchiolar disease identified by CT in the non-transplant population: analysis of 29 consecutive cases. Respirology (Carlton, Vic). 2009;14(3):443–8.
11. Geddes DM, Corrin B, Brewerton DA, Davies RJ, Turner-Warwick M. Progressive airway obliteration in adults and its association with rheumatoid disease. Q J Med. 1977;46(184):427–44.
12. Epler GR, Snider GL, Gaensler EA, Cathcart ES, FitzGerald MX, Carrington CB. Bronchiolitis and bronchitis in connective tissue disease. A possible relationship to the use of penicillamine. Jama. 1979;242(6):528–32.
13. Murphy KC, Atkins CJ, Offer RC, Hogg JC, Stein HB. Obliterative bronchiolitis in two rheumatoid arthritis patients treated with penicillamine. Arthritis Rheum. 1981;24(3):557–60.
14. Penny WJ, Knight RK, Rees AM, Thomas AL, Smith AP. Obliterative bronchiolitis in rheumatoid arthritis. Ann Rheum Dis. 1982;41(5):469–72.
15. Lahdensuo A, Mattila J, Vilppula A. Bronchiolitis in rheumatoid arthritis. Chest. 1984;85(5):705–8.
16. Yam LY, Wong R. Bronchiolitis obliterans and rheumatoid arthritis. Report of a case in a Chinese patient on d-penicillamine and review of the literature. Ann Acad Med Singap. 1993;22(3):365–8.
17. Schwarz MI, Lynch DA, Tuder R. Bronchiolitis obliterans: the lone manifestation of rheumatoid arthritis? Eur Respir J. 1994;7(4):817–20.
18. Hayakawa H, Sato A, Imokawa S, Toyoshima M, Chida K, Iwata M. Bronchiolar disease in rheumatoid arthritis. Am J Respir Crit Care Med. 1996;154(5):1531–6.
19. Devouassoux G, Cottin V, Liote H, Marchand E, Frachon I, Schuller A, Bejui-Thivolet F, Cordier JF. Characterisation of severe obliterative bronchiolitis in rheumatoid arthritis. Eur Respir J. 2009;33(5):1053–61.
20. Arnett FC, Edworthy SM, Bloch DA, McShane DJ, Fries JF, Cooper NS, Healey LA, Kaplan SR, Liang MH, Luthra HS, et al. The American rheumatism association 1987 revised criteria for the classification of rheumatoid arthritis. Arthritis Rheum. 1988;31(3):315–24.
21. Miller MR, Hankinson J, Brusasco V, Burgos F, Casaburi R, Coates A, Crapo R, Enright P, van der Grinten CP, Gustafsson P, et al. Standardisation of spirometry. Eur Respir J. 2005;26(2):319–38.
22. Vogelmeier CF, Criner GJ, Martinez FJ, Anzueto A, Barnes PJ, Bourbeau J, Celli BR, Chen R, Decramer M, Fabbri LM, et al. Global strategy for the diagnosis, management, and prevention of chronic obstructive lung disease 2017 report. GOLD executive summary. Am J Respir Crit Care Med. 2017;195(5):557–82.
23. van de Laar MA, Westermann CJ, Wagenaar SS, Dinant HJ. Beneficial effect of intravenous cyclophosphamide and oral prednisone on D-penicillamine-associated bronchiolitis obliterans. Arthritis Rheum. 1985;28(1):93–7.
24. Fernandez Perez ER, Krishnamoorthy M, Brown KK, Huie TJ, Fischer A, Solomon JJ, Meehan RT, Olson AL, Achcar RD, Swigris JJ. FEV1 over time in patients with connective tissue disease-related bronchiolitis. Respir Med. 2013;107(6):883–9.
25. Franquet T, Gimenez A, Monill JM, Diaz C, Geli C. Primary Sjogren's syndrome and associated lung disease: CT findings in 50 patients. AJR Am J Roentgenol. 1997;169(3):655–8.
26. Remy-Jardin M, Remy J, Cortet B, Mauri F, Delcambre B. Lung changes in rheumatoid arthritis: CT findings. Radiology. 1994;193(2):375–82.

27. Tanaka N, Kim JS, Newell JD, Brown KK, Cool CD, Meehan R, Emoto T, Matsumoto T, Lynch DA. Rheumatoid arthritis-related lung diseases: CT findings. Radiology. 2004;232(1):81–91.

28. Cortot AB, Cottin V, Miossec P, Fauchon E, Thivolet-Bejui F, Cordier JF. Improvement of refractory rheumatoid arthritis-associated constrictive bronchiolitis with etanercept. Respir Med. 2005;99(4):511–4.

29. Yadav H, Peters SG, Keogh KA, Hogan WJ, Erwin PJ, West CP, Kennedy CC. Azithromycin for the treatment of Obliterative bronchiolitis after hematopoietic stem cell transplantation: a systematic review and meta-analysis. Biology of blood and marrow transplantation : journal of the American Society for Blood and Marrow Transplantation. 2016;22(12):2264–9.

3

Cross-sectional and longitudinal analyses of the association between lung function and exercise capacity in healthy Norwegian men

Amir Farkhooy[1,2]*(iD), Johan Bodegård[3], Jan Erik Erikssen[4], Christer Janson[2], Hans Hedenström[1], Knut Stavem[5,6,7] and Andrei Malinovschi[1]

Abstract

Background: It is widely accepted that exercise capacity in healthy individuals is limited by the cardiac function, while the respiratory system is considered oversized. Although there is physiological, age-related decline in both lung function and physical capacity, the association between decline in lung function and decline in exercise capacity is little studied. Therefore, we examined the longitudinal association between lung function indices and exercise capacity, assessed by the total amount of work performed on a standardized incremental test, in a cohort of middle-aged men.

Methods: A total of 745 men between 40 and 59 years were examined using spirometry and standardized bicycle exercise ECG test within "The Oslo Ischemia Study," at two time points: once during 1972–1975, and again, approximately 16 years later, during 1989–1990. The subjects exercise capacity was assessed as physical fitness i.e. the total bicycle work (in Joules) at all workloads divided by bodyweight (in kg).

Results: Higher FEV_1, FVC and PEF values related to higher physical fitness at both baseline and follow-up (all p values < 0.05). Higher explanatory values were found at follow-up than baseline for FEV_1 ($r^2 = 0.16$ vs. $r^2 = 0.03$), FVC ($r^2 = 0.14$ vs. $r^2 = 0.03$) and PEF ($r^2 = 0.13$ vs. $r^2 = 0.02$). No significant correlations were found between decline in physical fitness and declines in FEV_1, FVC or PEF.

Conclusions: A weak association between lung function indices and exercise capacity, assessed through physical fitness, was found in middle-aged, healthy men. This association was strengthened with increasing age, suggesting a larger role for lung function in limiting exercise capacity among elderly subjects. However, decline in physical fitness over time was not related to decline in lung function.

Background

The amount of oxygen consumed during exercise is dictated by the quantity of oxygenated blood distributed by the heart and the working muscle's ability to take up the oxygen within that blood [1]. Thus, it is generally accepted that exercise capacity in healthy individuals is principally limited by maximum cardiac output [2, 3]. In contrast, the respiratory system is considered oversized in both respiratory volume and diffusing capacity, and is therefore believed not to be the limiting factor of maximum exercise capacity in healthy, non-endurance athletes [4]. Impaired lung function restricts the exercise capacity in patients with pulmonary disease [5, 6]. Although there is a physiological decline in lung function parameters with age [7], the association between age-related decline of lung function and decline in exercise capacity is little studied [8].

In healthy aging, there is a steady deterioration of the dynamic lung volumes. Both forced expiratory volume in

* Correspondence: amir.farkhooy@medsci.uu.se
[1]Department of Medical Sciences, Clinical Physiology, Uppsala University Hospital, SE-751 85 Uppsala, Sweden
[2]Department of Medical Sciences: Respiratory, Allergy and Sleep Research, Uppsala University, Uppsala, Sweden
Full list of author information is available at the end of the article

one second (FEV$_1$) and forced vital capacity (FVC) decline with age, and the flow-volume curve may change shape and become more similar to the curve in patients with chronic obstructive lung disease (COPD) [9, 10]. Normal aging of the lung can mimic the development of COPD in more ways than one [11]. The age-related loss of elastic tissue in the lung parenchyma exposes the airways to dynamic collapse during expiration causing a "pseudo-obstruction" that may be indistinguishable from true obstruction when only FEV$_1$ is studied. In addition, with age, both the residual volume and the closing volume increase and alveolar walls disappear, producing a situation that has been termed "senile emphysema" [12]. The prevalence of dyspnoea increases with age in people not suspected of having lung disease, and physiological decline in lung function is believed to plays a role in the limitation of physical function in natural aging [13]. However, most studies investigating the relationship between declining lung function parameters and reduced maximum exercise capacity have been performed on elderly populations and/or with a cross-sectional study design [14–16].

To our knowledge, the impact of normal age-related decrease in lung function parameters on maximum exercise capacity in healthy middle-aged and young people has not previously been examined in a longitudinal study. Therefore, we wanted to investigate whether lung function indices were associated with maximum exercise capacity, assessed through physical fitness, in middle-aged, healthy subjects. Further, we sought to explore the relationship between age-related decline of lung function parameters and decrease of exercise capacity over time.

Methods

Subjects

The present analysis is based on data from a cardiovascular observational study, "The Oslo Ischemia Study," in which men aged 40–59 years were recruited from five companies/governmental institutions in Oslo during the years 1972–1975. Of the 2341 apparently healthy men who were eligible and invited, 2014 men (86%) consented to participate. The participants had to be free from known or suspected heart disease, hypertension, diabetes mellitus, malignancy, advanced pulmonary, renal, or liver disease and should have no locomotor activity limitation. Further details about selection procedures and exclusion criteria have been presented elsewhere [17, 18]. The subjects underwent a clinical examination survey including questionnaires, assessment of cardiovascular risk factors, chest x-ray, dynamic spirometry and symptom-limited exercise test. The survey was repeated in 1989–1990 [19].

Of the 2014 subjects enrolled at the baseline survey, 391 were excluded due to lack of spirometry or unsatisfactory quality of the lung function test (as outlined below). Furthermore, 605 subjects were excluded as their lung function values at the baseline survey differed from the predicted normal values, as described in greater detail below. The survey was repeated in 1989–1990, and a total of 273 subjects did not participate in the follow-up survey or were not included (a total of 12 subjects did not perform either exercise test or lung function testing). The remaining 745 subjects, with lung function and exercise capacity data from both surveys, were included in the current study (Fig. 1).

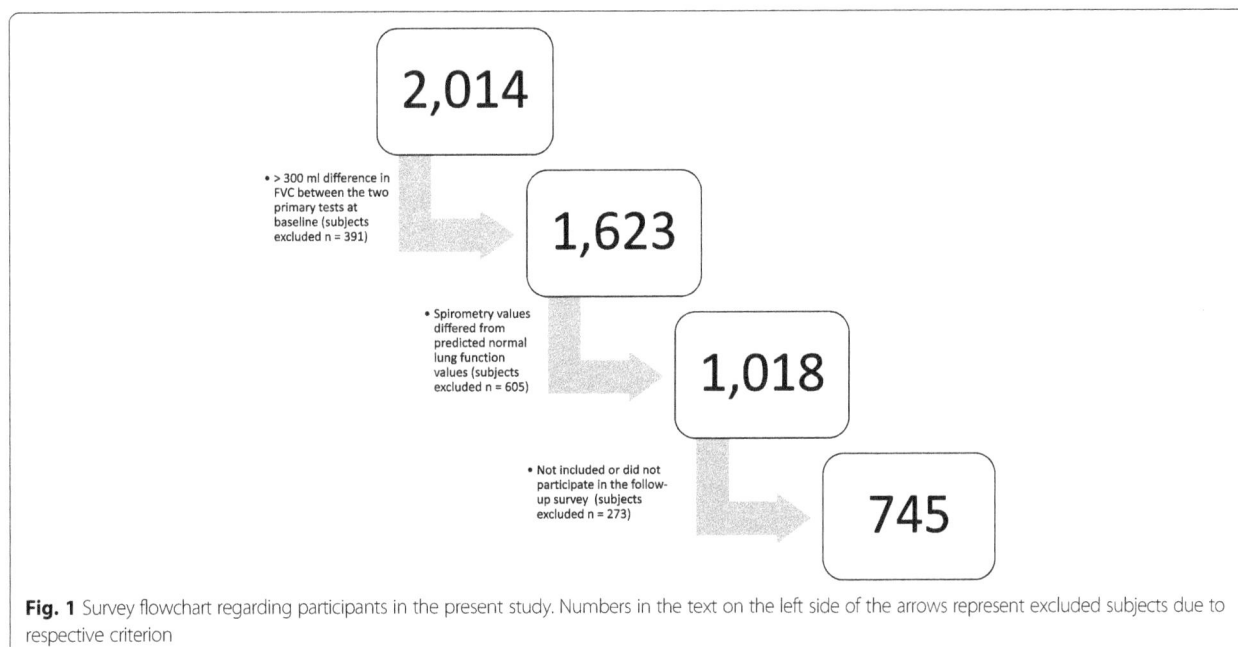

2,014

• > 300 ml difference in FVC between the two primary tests at baseline (subjects excluded n = 391)

1,623

• Spirometry values differed from predicted normal lung function values (subjects excluded n = 605)

1,018

• Not included or did not participate in the follow-up survey (subjects excluded n = 273)

745

Fig. 1 Survey flowchart regarding participants in the present study. Numbers in the text on the left side of the arrows represent excluded subjects due to respective criterion

In 1972, no institutional or regional review board existed in Norway. Hence, no formal institutional approval for the investigation protocol could be obtained. However, the survey protocol was circulated among prominent physicians at two hospitals in Oslo, who commented on the protocol at an ad hoc meeting. All subjects gave their verbal informed consent before inclusion both at baseline and follow-up survey. Both study protocols underwent ethical assessments retrospectively and were approved by the regional committee for medical and health research ethics in Norway (REK nr. 188/89). Nevertheless, written consent were gathered for the surviving cohort at 2007.

Spirometry

At the baseline examination, FVC and FEV_1 were measured with a calibrated Bernstein spirometer, using a standardized procedure [20]. After one trial test, FVC and FEV_1 values were recorded from two successive maximum expiratory manoeuvres, corrected for body temperature and ambient pressure and saturated with water vapour, based on daily room temperature measurements and an assumption of atmospheric pressure of 760 mmHg. Originally, only the mean FEV_1 and FVC values were recorded. To obtain the maximum of the two tests, the original spirograms and recorded values for both manoeuvres were retrieved in 2001 [21]. In order to increase the reliability of the data, as the original dataset was obtained before criteria for standardization were available, only subjects with < 0.3 L difference between the two FVC tests ($n = 1625$) were included, as previously described [22]. Additionally, in order to limit the present analyses to healthy individuals, only subjects with normal lung function values, defined as a FEV_1/FVC ratio ≥ 0.7 and a FEV_1 value greater than or equal to 80% of predicted, according to Norwegian reference values [23], were included in the current analysis. During the follow-up examination, a Vitalograph spirometer was used, with a similar protocol for the procedure. Peak expiratory flow (PEF) measurements were performed with a Wright's peak flow meter, noting the mean value of the last two out of at least three tests.

Exercise test

All participants performed a standardized bicycle exercise ECG test and were examined by the same physician, as previously described elsewhere [24]. The initial workload was 100 W for 6 min and then increased by 50 W every 6 min. The exercise test was continued until a heart rate of at least 90% of maximum predicted heart rate was reached, unless specific symptoms or signs necessitated premature termination. If an individual seemed physically fit despite reaching 90% of maximum predicted heart rate + 10 beats per minute at the end of one load, he was encouraged to continue as long as possible at the next load, i.e., at most an additional 6 min at a higher load. Exercise testing was repeated within 2 weeks in 130 of the participants and showed high reproducibility for heart rates and working capacity between the two tests, within ±5% in 90% of the men, and within ±10% in all of them [19, 25]. Exercise capacity, measured through physical fitness, was defined as the total bicycle work per unit of weight and calculated as the sum of work (in Joules) at all workloads divided by bodyweight (in kg).

Anthropometric data

Height and weight were recorded at both the baseline and the follow-up visits.

Questionnaire data

The subjects' smoking habits (smoker/non-smoker) and exercise routines were recorded at the baseline visits. The subjects were divided into three groups based on their self-reported physical activity, as follows: 1) no existing exercise habits, 2) non-exhausting activity once in a while, and 3) routinely undertaking physical activity, from medium exhaustion at least five times per week up to competitive sports.

Statistical analysis

Statistics were generated using computer software programs (STATA 12.1, StataCorp, College Station, TX, USA). Means ± standard deviations (SDs) were used to present descriptive statistics. A simple linear regression model was used to analyse the correlation between lung function parameters and variables relating to physical fitness. Only absolute values (L, L/min or kJ/kg) were used in all association analysis. These relations were tested for consistency at the baseline visit in a multiple linear regression model that included besides lung function parameters, age, height, exercise habits and current smoking, which are known as determinants of lung function and/or exercise capacity. A similar model at the follow-up visit included age (defined as age at start-up + 16 years, the median-follow-up time) and height, in addition to the lung function parameters. The longitudinal analysis on the change in lung function and physical fitness over time was done by means of simple linear regression.

The residuals in the regression models were checked for non-normality using plots versus fitted values and the dependent variables and appeared as normally distributed. A p value < 0.05, using two-sided tests, was considered statistically significant.

Results

Population characteristics

Subject's characteristics for the whole group at inclusion are presented in Table 1. Lung function parameters at baseline and follow-up surveys are presented in Table 2. There was a significant decrease of lung function indices, in absolute values, and of physical fitness, between the baseline and follow-up surveys (Table 2).

Physical fitness in relation to spirometry indices at baseline visit

A significant association of higher degree of self-reported physical activity, FEV_1, FVC and PEF with higher objectively assessed physical fitness was found, as was a significant association of decreasing physical fitness with higher age (Fig. 2) and current smoking. The strongest correlation with physical fitness was found for subjects' self-reported physical activities, followed by age. All three lung function parameters showed significant correlation with physical fitness (Fig. 2, Table 3).

The relation with the three different lung function parameters was consistent also in multiple regression models after adjusting for age, height, weight, physical activity, and smoking (Table 3). FEV_1 and FVC remained significantly related to physical fitness in a regression model containing all three lung function parameters, even after adjusting for age, height, physical activity and smoking (data not shown).

Physical fitness in relation to spirometry indices at follow-up visit

In the follow-up survey, the strongest correlation with physical fitness was found for subject age, followed by FEV_1 (Fig. 2). Significant associations of higher FEV_1,

FVC and PEF with higher physical fitness were found (Fig. 2, Table 4), as was as a significant association of lower physical fitness with higher age (Fig. 2).

Age and FEV_1 had a higher explanatory value for a subject's physical fitness at follow-up than at baseline (Fig. 2).

The relations with FEV_1, FVC and PEF (all $p < 0.001$) were consistent also in multiple regression models after adjusting for age and height (Table 4). A similar model, where all three lung function parameters were inserted concomitantly, yielded PEF as the sole lung function parameter associated with physical fitness (p < 0.001), while no significant relations were found with FEV_1 ($p = 0.21$) or FVC (p = 0.21).

Decline in physical fitness in relation to decline in lung function or lung function at baseline

No significant correlation was found between decline in physical fitness and decline in FEV_1 ($p = 0.12$), decline in FVC ($p = 0.80$), or decline in PEF ($p = 0.78$) when a simple linear regression model was used. A similar linear regression model with decline of physical fitness as outcome yielded neither baseline FEV_1 ($p = 0.22$) nor baseline FVC ($p = 0.36$) as significant predictors. On the other hand, a significant negative correlation was found between decline in physical fitness and baseline PEF ($r^2 = 0.01$, $p = 0.02$).

Discussion

In the present study, we found that lung function indices obtained through dynamic spirometry (i.e., FEV_1, FVC and PEF) were associated with exercise capacity, assessed through objectively measured physical fitness, in middle-aged, healthy men. This association was seen in cross-sectional analyses at both baseline and follow-up, approximately 16 years later, and, in fact, the relation to lung function seemed to increase over time. However, decline in physical fitness over time was not related to decline in lung function.

Numerous studies have explored the physiological changes in the respiratory system during aging [11, 26], but the relationship between physiological decline in lung function and declining exercise capacity has not been fully understood. Other studies investigating the impact of aging and exercise capacity have had a cross-sectional study design [27] and/or predominantly examined the relationship between cardiac function and exercise capacity [28]. To our knowledge, this is the first longitudinal study investigating the relationship between spirometric parameters and exercise capacity in healthy, middle-aged subjects.

As expected, our study subjects displayed physiological decline of lung function parameters over time. The decline of physical fitness by almost 50% constitutes a higher reduction in exercise capacity over time than in

Table 1 Subject characteristics at the baseline survey

	At baseline
Number of subjects	745
Age (years)	48.5 ± 5.3
Current smoker	245 (34.1%)
Height (cm)	176.4 ± 6.0
Weight (kg)	76.6 ± 9.3
BMI (kg/m^2)	24.6 ± 2.6
Systolic BP (mmHg)	128.8 ± 16.7
Diastolic BP (mmHg)	86.4 ± 10.1
MAP (mmHg)	100.7 ± 11.8
Self-reported physical activity	
No physical activity routine	77 (10.3%)
Low physical activity routine	548 (73.6%)
High physical activity routine	120 (16.1%)

Legend: Values presented as mean (SD) or N (%). *BMI* body mass index, *BP* blood pressure, *MAP* mean arterial pressure

Table 2 Lung function and physical fitness at baseline and follow-up, $n = 745$

	Baseline visit		Follow-up visit		p value*
	Absolute values	% predicted	Absolute values	% predicted	
FEV$_1$ (L)	3.8 ± 0.5	95.0 ± 9.8	3.5 ± 0.7	97.5 ± 16.3	< 0.001
FVC (L)	4.7 ± 0.7	95.6 ± 10.1	4.4 ± 0.7	92.8 ± 11.1	< 0.001
PEF (L/min)	558.4 ± 65.5	92.3 ± 10.2	544.7 ± 72.4	90.5 ± 12.0	< 0.001
Physical fitness (kJ/kg)	2.1 ± 0.8	–	1.02 ± 0.6	–	< 0.001

Legend: Values presented as mean ± SD. *FEV$_1$* forced expiratory volume in 1 s; *FVC* forced vital capacity, *PEF* peak expiratory flow. * p value for paired t-test for absolute values

other similar studies [29]. We hypothesize that this is due to the exercise testing protocol used in the survey. Modern protocols uses 1–2-min incremental intervals, while we used 6-min intervals, a protocol more similar to steady-state exercise testing. This was the protocol of choice at the time of the baseline study. On the other hand, exercise capacity was presented as the cumulative workload divided by weight in the present study. Hence, an increase in weight over time would lead to lower calculated exercise capacity. This does differ from similar studies using treadmill exercise tests, in which body-weight is not considered in calculating peak exercise capacity (in those protocols, exercise capacity is often converted to metabolic equivalent or is expressed as percent predicted for subject age). Another explanation might be development of cardiovascular or muscular limitations over time which were not quantified.

All lung function indices included in the study correlated significantly with physical fitness both at baseline and in the follow-up survey. All three investigated parameters, i.e., FEV$_1$, FVC and PEF, behaved in the same manner, although they reflect different aspects. FEV$_1$ is more closely related to airway obstruction, FVC to lung volumes and PEF to obstruction and muscular strength [30]. Given that the healthy respiratory system is oversized, one would expect to observe a relationship between lung function parameters and exercise capacity only when the dimensions of the respiratory system are reduced below a threshold value which represents the lower limit of normal lung function. However, there was a relationship between exercise capacity and lung function even at baseline, when the subjects were presumed healthy and had a normal lung function. The notion that lung function influences exercise capacity in healthy individuals is supported by previous animal study of Kirkton et al. [31], as they demonstrated that relatively larger lungs are required for increased endurance capacity in rats. Moreover, this relationship was strengthened at the follow-up survey, which was reflected in larger variation in lung function values at follow-up, with decreased values in some of the subjects. This may partly be related to a loss of lung elastic recoil in aging, which is associated with a reduction in the expiratory boundary of the maximal flow-volume envelope [32].

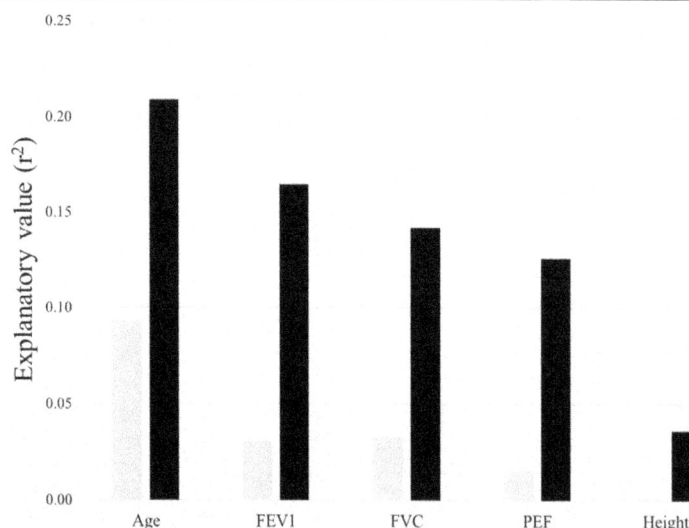

Fig. 2 Comparison between surveys of explanatory values for physical fitness. Legend: Explanatory value (expressed in r² value from a simple linear regression model) of each of the investigated parameters for physical fitness at baseline (grey) and follow-up (black)

Table 3 Regression coefficients (95% CI) of lung function for physical fitness at baseline ($n = 745$)

	Unadjusted	Adjusted[a]
FEV_1 (per L)	0.26 (0.16, 0.37)	0.19 (0.08, 0.31)
FVC (per L)	0.22 (0.13, 0.31)	0.18 (0.08, 0.29)
PEF (per 100 L/min)	0.16 (0.07, 0.25)	0.09 (0.04, 0.17)

Legend: [a] adjusted for age, height, current smoking and physical activity habits

We could not find any association between decline in exercise capacity and decline in lung function. This might be attributed to the changes in exercise capacity being larger than the changes in lung function, and therefore the cardiovascular and muscular limitation of function over time may become more important for determination of physical fitness. The lack of association could also be referred to the fact that the pulmonary capacity is moving from a state of "overcapacity" in younger age to a weak limiting factor at older age. In such a situation, the decline in lung function is not expected to be associated with the decline in exercise capacity. Moreover, the design of our study with a rigorous selection of individuals with only normal spirometry values may also have limited the magnitude of changes in lung function. Furthermore, two different spirometry equipment were used between the surveys which could have an implication of the obtained results. However, we believe that exclusion of subjects with spirometry values below the normal range helped to ensure the accuracy of our original data gathered in the 1970s.

It could be discussed if there is a causal relation between loss of lung function and loss of physical fitness and the direction of this relation. One might contemplate that physiological decline in lung function with ageing may result in impaired physical fitness. However it could also be argued that decreased physical activity may result in accelerated loss in lung function, as suggested by a recent hypothesis article by Hopkinson and Polkey [33]. However, most of these studies cited in the article had primarily used questionnaire data on physical activity and there were no objective measures of physical fitness.

A strength of our study is the large number of participants and a follow-up period extending over 15 years. Some limitations of the study should be mentioned. The

study included only male subjects, and spirometry was performed according to earlier and less rigorous standards than those used nowadays. Furthermore, we lack data on physical activity and smoking habits on follow-up survey, which could not be adjusted for at the follow-up visit, and therefore the adjusted models at baseline and follow-up visit differ. An additional limitation of the study is the use of a different protocol than those currently used for assessing exercise capacity, and a lack of normal values for physical fitness from other populations. The selection of subjects with normal lung function may be regarded as a strength, as we probably excluded subjects with possible respiratory disease. However, this may have contributed to a lower variability of the lung function variables in the baseline analysis. We did not have access to information regarding any comorbidities in the form of cardiovascular or neuromuscular limitations which might have developed during the follow-up period. The information regarding comorbidity could explain the relatively large decline in physical fitness between the surveys, which may have masked an effect of declining lung function. The information on physical activity at baseline was self-reported and this information is known to be inferior to objective measurements [34].

Conclusions

In this study, lung function was significantly associated with physical fitness in healthy, middle-aged men both at baseline and follow-up surveys. Furthermore, our data suggests an increasing association between FEV_1 and physical fitness with age, indicating that natural decline in lung functions may play a more essential role in the limitation of physical function in elderly. This finding might contribute to the understanding of the physiology of exercise and determinants of exercise capacity.

Abbreviations
COPD: Chronic obstructive lung disease; FEV_1: Forced expiratory volume in one second); FVC: Forced vital capacity; PEF: Peak expiratory flow

Acknowledgements
The authors thank all participators of the study for their time and effort.

Funding
This study was not funded by any private or governmental institutions.

Table 4 Regression coefficients (95% CI) of lung function for physical fitness at follow-up ($n = 745$)

	Unadjusted	Adjusted[a]
FEV_1 (per L)	0.38 (0.32, 0.44)	0.25 (0.18, 0.32)
FVC (per L)	0.30 (0.25, 0.35)	0.20 (0.14, 0.27)
PEF (per 100 L/min)	0.28 (0.23, 0.33)	0.17 (0.12, 0.22)

Legend: [a] adjusted for age and height

Authors' contributions
The manuscript has been read and approved by all named authors and there were no other persons who satisfied the criteria for authorship but are not listed. AF contributed to the study design, analysis and interpretation of data, and writing the first draft of the manuscript. JB, JEE, CJ and HH contributed to study design and interpretation of data. KS and AM were the principal investigators, guarantors of the manuscript and contributed to the study design and analysis and interpretation of data.

Competing interests
The authors declare that they have no competing interests.

Author details
[1]Department of Medical Sciences, Clinical Physiology, Uppsala University Hospital, SE-751 85 Uppsala, Sweden. [2]Department of Medical Sciences: Respiratory, Allergy and Sleep Research, Uppsala University, Uppsala, Sweden. [3]Department of Cardiology, Oslo University Hospital, Ullevaal, Norway. [4]Faculty of Medicine, University of Oslo, Oslo, Norway. [5]Institute of Clinical Medicine, University of Oslo, Lørenskog, Norway. [6]Department of Pulmonary Medicine, Medical Division, Akershus University Hospital, Lørenskog, Norway. [7]Health Services Research Unit, Akershus University Hospital, Lørenskog, Norway.

References
1. Wagner PD. Determinants of maximal oxygen transport and utilization. Annu Rev Physiol. 1996;58:21–50.
2. McGuire DK, Levine BD, Williamson JW, Snell PG, Blomqvist CG, Saltin B, et al. A 30-year follow-up of the Dallas bedrest and training study: I. Effect of age on the cardiovascular response to exercise. Circulation. 2001;104(12): 1350–7.
3. Bassett DR Jr, Howley ET. Limiting factors for maximum oxygen uptake and determinants of endurance performance. Med Sci Sports Exerc. 2000;32(1): 70–84.
4. Dempsey JA, McKenzie DC, Haverkamp HC, Eldridge MW. Update in the understanding of respiratory limitations to exercise performance in fit, active adults. Chest. 2008;134(3):613–22.
5. Farkhooy A, Janson C, Arnardottir RH, Malinovschi A, Emtner M, Hedenstrom H. Impaired carbon monoxide diffusing capacity is the strongest predictor of exercise intolerance in COPD. COPD. 2013;10(2):180–5.
6. Chin RC, Guenette JA, Cheng S, Raghavan N, Amornputtisathaporn N, Cortes-Telles A, et al. Does the respiratory system limit exercise in mild chronic obstructive pulmonary disease? Am J Respir Crit Care Med. 2013; 187(12):1315–23.
7. Fletcher C, Peto R. The natural history of chronic airflow obstruction. Br Med J. 1977;1(6077):1645–8.
8. Babb TG, Long KA, Rodarte JR. The relationship between maximal expiratory flow and increases of maximal exercise capacity with exercise training. Am J Respir Crit Care Med. 1997;156(1):116–21.
9. Hardie JA, Buist AS, Vollmer WM, Ellingsen I, Bakke PS, Morkve O. Risk of over-diagnosis of COPD in asymptomatic elderly never-smokers. Eur Respir J. 2002;20(5):1117–22.
10. Guenard H, Marthan R. Pulmonary gas exchange in elderly subjects. Eur Respir J. 1996;9(12):2573–7.
11. Janssens JP, Pache JC, Nicod LP. Physiological changes in respiratory function associated with ageing. Eur Respir J. 1999;13(1):197–205.
12. Langhammer A, Johnsen R, Holmen J, Gulsvik A, Bjermer L. Cigarette smoking gives more respiratory symptoms among women than among men. The Nord-Trondelag health study (HUNT). J Epidemiol Community Health. 2000;54(12):917–22.
13. Roman MA, Rossiter HB, Casaburi R. Exercise, ageing and the lung. Eur Respir J. 2016;48(5):1471–86.
14. Hassel E, Stensvold D, Halvorsen T, Wisloff U, Langhammer A, Steinshamn S. Association between pulmonary function and peak oxygen uptake in elderly: the generation 100 study. Respir Res. 2015;16:156.
15. Johnson BD, Badr MS, Dempsey JA. Impact of the aging pulmonary system on the response to exercise. Clin Chest Med. 1994;15(2):229–46.
16. Weiss CO, Hoenig HH, Varadhan R, Simonsick EM, Fried LP. Relationships of cardiac, pulmonary, and muscle reserves and frailty to exercise capacity in older women. J Gerontol A Biol Sci Med Sci. 2010;65(3):287–94.
17. Sandvik L, Erikssen J, Thaulow E, Erikssen G, Mundal R, Rodahl K. Physical fitness as a predictor of mortality among healthy, middle-aged Norwegian men. N Engl J Med. 1993;328(8):533–7.
18. Mundal R, Kjeldsen SE, Sandvik L, Erikssen G, Thaulow E, Erikssen J. Exercise blood pressure predicts mortality from myocardial infarction. Hypertension. 1996;27(3 Pt 1):324–9.
19. Bodegard J, Erikssen G, Bjornholt JV, Gjesdal K, Liestol K, Erikssen J. Reasons for terminating an exercise test provide independent prognostic information: 2014 apparently healthy men followed for 26 years. Eur Heart J. 2005;26(14):1394–401.
20. Rose GA, Blackburn H. Cardiovascular survey methods. Monogr Ser World Health Organ. 1968;56:1–188.
21. Stavem K, Aaser E, Sandvik L, Bjornholt JV, Erikssen G, Thaulow E, et al. Lung function, smoking and mortality in a 26-year follow-up of healthy middle-aged males. Eur Respir J. 2005;25(4):618–25.
22. Stavem K, Sandvik L, Erikssen J. Breathlessness, phlegm and mortality: 26 years of follow-up in healthy middle-aged Norwegian men. J Intern Med. 2006;260(4):332–42.
23. Langhammer A, Johnsen R, Gulsvik A, Holmen TL, Bjermer L. Forced spirometry reference values for Norwegian adults: the bronchial obstruction in Nord-Trondelag study. Eur Respir J. 2001;18(5):770–9.
24. Erikssen J, Enge I, Forfang K, Storstein O. False positive diagnostic tests and coronary angiographic findings in 105 presumably healthy males. Circulation. 1976;54(3):371–6.
25. Sandvik L, Erikssen J, Ellestad M, Erikssen G, Thaulow E, Mundal R, et al. Heart rate increase and maximal heart rate during exercise as predictors of cardiovascular mortality: a 16-year follow-up study of 1960 healthy men. Coron Artery Dis. 1995;6(8):667–79.
26. DeLorey DS, Babb TG. Progressive mechanical ventilatory constraints with aging. Am J Respir Crit Care Med. 1999;160(1):169–77.
27. Soer R, Brouwer S, Geertzen JH, van der Schans CP, Groothoff JW, Reneman MF. Decline of functional capacity in healthy aging workers. Arch Phys Med Rehabil. 2012;93(12):2326–32.
28. Mendonca GV, Pezarat-Correia P, Vaz JR, Silva L, Heffernan KS. Impact of aging on endurance and neuromuscular physical performance: the role of vascular senescence. Sports Med. 2017;47(4):583–98.
29. Myers J, Prakash M, Froelicher V, Do D, Partington S, Atwood JE. Exercise capacity and mortality among men referred for exercise testing. N Engl J Med. 2002;346(11):793–801.
30. Miller MR, Crapo R, Hankinson J, Brusasco V, Burgos F, Casaburi R, et al. General considerations for lung function testing. Eur Respir J. 2005;26(1):153–61.
31. Kirkton SD, Howlett RA, Gonzalez NC, Giuliano PG, Britton SL, Koch LG, et al. Continued artificial selection for running endurance in rats is associated with improved lung function. J Appl Physiol (1985). 2009;106(6):1810–8.
32. McClaran SR, Babcock MA, Pegelow DF, Reddan WG, Dempsey JA. Longitudinal effects of aging on lung function at rest and exercise in healthy active fit elderly adults. J Appl Physiol (1985). 1995;78(5):1957–68.
33. Hopkinson NS, Polkey MI. Does physical inactivity cause chronic obstructive pulmonary disease? Clin Sci (Lond). 2010;118(9):565–72.
34. Gimeno-Santos E, Frei A, Dobbels F, Rudell K, Puhan MA, Garcia-Aymerich J, et al. Validity of instruments to measure physical activity may be questionable due to a lack of conceptual frameworks: a systematic review. Health Qual Life Outcomes. 2011;9:86.

4

Pulmonary sequestration in adults: a retrospective review of resected and unresected cases

Mohammad Alsumrain*[iD] and Jay H. Ryu

Abstract

Background: Pulmonary sequestration (PS) is a form of congenital pulmonary malformation that is generally diagnosed in childhood or adolescence and usually resected when diagnosed. We aim to identify the clinical presentation and course of patients diagnosed to have PS during adulthood.

Methods: Using a computer-assisted search of Mayo clinic medical records, we identified adult patients with PS diagnosed between 1997 and 2016. Clinical and radiological data were collected including postoperative course for those who underwent surgical resection.

Results: We identified 32 adult patients with PS; median age at diagnosis was 42 years (IQR 28–53); 17 patients (53%) were men. The median sequestration size was 6.6 cm (IQR 4.4–9.3). The type of sequestration was intralobar in 81% and extralobar in 19%. The most common location was left lower lobe posteromedially (56%). Forty-seven percent of the patients presented with no relevant symptoms. The most common radiographic finding was mass/consolidation in 61% and the most common feeding artery origin was the thoracic aorta (54%). Surgical resection was performed in 18 patients (56%) and postoperative complication was reported in 5 patients (28%). There was no surgical mortality. Median duration of follow-up after diagnosis for unresected cases, most of whom were asymptomatic, was 19 months (IQR 4–26) with no complications related to the PS reported.

Conclusions: Nearly one-half of adult patients with PS present with no relevant symptoms. The decision regarding surgical resection needs to weigh various factors including clinical manifestations related to PS, risk of surgical complications, comorbidities, and individual patient preferences.

Keywords: Pulmonary sequestration

Background

Pulmonary sequestration (PS) is a congenital lung malformation that consists of a nonfunctioning lung tissue with no apparent communication with the tracheobronchial tree [1]. The blood supply to PS is through aberrant vessels from systemic circulation, most commonly the descending thoracic aorta. The term sequestration is derived from the Latin verb *sequestare,* which means 'to separate' and it was first introduced as a medical term by Pryce in 1964 [2, 3]. PS is rare, representing about 1 to 6% of all congenital lung anomalies and may go undetected during the prenatal period and early childhood years [4].

The PS is divided into two types, intralobar sequestration (ILS) which is the more common type, where the lesion lies within pleural layer surrounding the lobar lung and extralobar sequestration (ELS) which has its own pleural covering, maintaining complete anatomic separation from adjacent normal lung [5].

Most patients with ILS present in adolescence or early adulthood with recurrent pneumonias in the affected lobe [4]. Patients with PS can be asymptomatic and the diagnosis achieved incidentally. Other presenting symptoms may include cough, hemoptysis, chest pain and dyspnea [6, 7]. ELS rarely becomes infected because it is

* Correspondence: alsumrain@yahoo.com
Division of Pulmonary and Critical Care Medicine, Gonda 18 South, Mayo Clinic, 200 First St. SW, Rochester, MN 55905, USA

separated from the tracheobronchial tree by its own pleural investment [4].

There are multiple radiologic manifestations of PS on computed tomography (CT) which include mass, consolidation with or without cysts, bronchiectasis and cavitary lesions [4, 7]. Hyperlucency can be seen in ILS due to the entrance of air from the collateral drift from normal lung resulting in air trapping [4]. The arterial supply to PS is most commonly from the thoracic aorta as described for 74% of cases reported by Savic et al. in a review of 540 published cases [8]. The supplying artery may also arise from the abdominal aorta, celiac artery, splenic artery or even a coronary artery [4]. Most ILS drains to pulmonary veins while venous drainage for most ELS is to the azygos or hemiazygos vein or to the inferior vena cava [4, 8].

Most of the data pertaining to PS are from the pediatrics literature. Occasionally, PS may be diagnosed for the first time in adulthood [6, 9, 10]. Due to paucity of published data, natural history and optimal management of PS diagnosed in adults remain unclear. Furthermore, the outcome of adult patients with unresected PS is not known. Thus, we aimed to explore the clinical presentation and course of adult patients with PS including those who do not undergo surgical resection.

Methods

Using a computer-assisted search of Mayo clinic medical records, we identified 32 adults (age 18 or greater) who were first diagnosed to have PS between 1997 and 2016. Mayo Clinic Institutional Review Board approval was obtained (#17–002077). The diagnosis was confirmed in all resected cases by histopathologic examination and the non-resected cases were diagnosed by imaging characteristics including the presence of anomalous systemic arterial supply identified by thoracic radiologists. Among the resected cases we didn't encounter hybrid lesion of congenital pulmonary airway malformation (congenital cystic adenomatoid malformation) and PS.

Available medical records and imaging studies were reviewed to confirm the diagnosis of PS. Clinical and radiological data were collected including postoperative course in those who underwent surgical resection and the clinical course of those who did not undergo surgical resection.

Statistical methods

Data were presented as median and interquartile range (IQR) for continuous variables and counts and percentages for categorical variables. For comparisons Mann-Whitney U test was used for continuous variables and Fischer exact test for categorical variables. Two-side p-value < 0.05 was considered statistically significant.

Table 1 Type and location of pulmonary sequestration ($n = 32$)

Characteristic	Number of patients (%)
Type of sequestration	
Intralobar	26 (81)
Extralobar	6 (19)
Location	
Left lower lobe	18 (56)
Posteromedial	18 (56)
Right lower lobe	14 (44)
Posteromedial	13 (41)
Anterior	1 (3)

Results

We identified 32 adult patients with PS whose median age was 42 years (IQR 28–53); 17 patients (53%) were men. The median sequestration size was 6.6 cm (IQR 4.4–9.3). The type of sequestration was intralobar in 81% and extralobar in 19%. The most common location was left lower lobe posteromedially (56%) (Table 1). The most common presenting symptom was cough (34%); however, 15 (47%) had no relevant symptoms (Table 2). Other presenting symptoms included dyspnea, thoracic pain, and hemoptysis. Recurrent respiratory infections were a presenting complaint in 16% of the patients. Asymptomatic patients had PS detected incidentally on chest imaging studies.

The most common radiologic finding was mass/consolidation in 61% followed by hyperlucency in 42%; cystic changes were noted in 23% (Table 3) (Fig. 1). Dilated bronchi were seen in 15% and mixed radiologic features were in 34% of the patients. The most common feeding artery origin was the thoracic aorta (54%); others include abdominal aorta (23%), celiac (11%) and inferior phrenic/left gastric (4%). The origin of the feeding artery was not specifically identified in 2 cases (8%) both of which were resected.

Surgical resection was performed in 18 patients (56%). The most common indication for surgery was recurrent respiratory infections in 12 (66%) followed by

Table 2 Presenting symptoms ($n = 32$)

Characteristic	Number of patients (%)
Cough	11 (34)
Chest/back pain	5 (16)
Dyspnea	5 (16)
Fever	5 (16)
Recurrent respiratory infections	5 (16)
Hemoptysis	3 (9)
Right upper abdominal pain	2 (6)
Asymptomatic	15 (47)

Note: one patient may have more than one symptom

Table 3 Radiologic manifestations (n = 26)

Radiologic manifestations[a]	Number of patients (%)
Mass/consolidative	16 (61)
Hyperlucency	11 (42)
Cystic changes	6 (23)
Dilated bronchi	4 (15)
Mixed features	9 (34)
Feeding artery	
Thoracic Aorta	14 (54)
Abdominal Aorta	6 (23)
Celiac	3 (11)
Inferior phrenic/left gastric	1 (4)
Not determined[b]	2 (8)
Venous drainage	
Pulmonary veins	8 (30)
Azygos vein	2 (8)
Hemiazygos vein	1 (4)
Left atrium	2 (8)
Not determined	13 (50)

[a]CT available for current review in 26 patients
[b]These two patients underwent surgery resection of pulmonary sequestration but exact origin of the feeding artery was not identified on CT

hemoptysis and pleural effusion in one patient each (Table 4). Four remaining patients underwent surgery for an asymptomatic lung lesion suspected to be PS. Sub-lobar resection was done in 13 (8 ILS, 5 ELS) of 18 (72%) and the remaining five patients underwent lobectomies (all ILS). Postoperative complications were reported in 5 patients (28%; 4 ILS, 1 ELS) and included chylous leak, intraoperative mild bleeding, chronic chest pain, arm numbness and pneumonia. Two of these 5 patients who experienced postoperative complications had been asymptomatic in regard to their lung lesion preoperatively.

There was no significant difference in age, gender or sequestration size between surgical and non-surgical patients. However, surgical patients were more often symptomatic at presentation compared to non-surgical (78% vs 29%, $P = 0.011$) (Table 5). There was no surgical mortality (in-hospital).

Follow-up data after diagnosis were available in 9 unresected cases and 17 resected cases; the median duration of follow-up was 19 months (IQR 4–26) and 2.5 months (IQR 1–143), respectively, with no complications related to the sequestration reported during follow up.

Discussion

In this retrospective review of 32 cases of PS diagnosed in adults over a 20-year period in a tertiary care center,

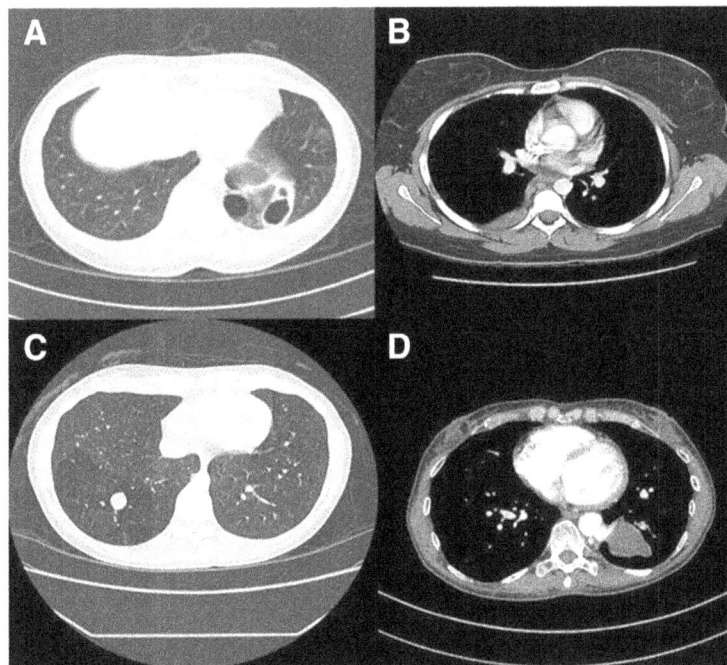

Fig. 1 a: Pulmonary sequestration (intralobar) presenting as a multi-cystic lesion in the postero-basal segment of the left lower lobe. **b**: Pulmonary sequestration (extralobar) presenting as extra-pulmonary mass in the right paravertebral region. **c**: Pulmonary sequestration (intralobar) presenting as an area of hyperlucency and dilated bronchus filled with mucus in the right lower lobe. **d**: Left lower lobe sequestration (intralobar) presenting as a mass in the left lower lobe with feeding artery from descending aorta

Table 4 Surgical management data (n = 18)

	Number of patients (%)
Indication for surgery	
Recurrent pulmonary infections	12 (66)
Hemoptysis	1 (6)
Pleural effusion	1 (6)
Asymptomatic lung lesions	4 (22)
Type of resection	
Thoracotomy	
Lobectomy	1 (6)
Segmentectomy/sequestrectomy	3 (17)
Wedge resection	2 (11)
VATS	
Lobectomy	4 (22)
Segmentectomy/sequestrectomy	6 (33)
Wedge resection	2 (11)

VATS Video-assisted thoracoscopy (VATS)

we found that 56% of the patients underwent surgical resection. The patients who underwent surgery were more likely to be symptomatic compared to those who did not. Surgical resection of PS was associated with a postoperative complications rate of 28%. The median follow up duration was 19 months for the non-surgical group, and no complications related to the sequestration were reported during the follow up period.

Nearly one-half of the adult patients diagnosed with PS manifested no relevant symptoms. It has been generally believed that most patients should have their PS resected even if they are asymptomatic due to concerns regarding eventual complication, mainly infection of PS. However, this issue remains debatable since data regarding the long-term clinical course and outcome of those with unresected PS are sparse, particularly in the adult population. Our study cohort included adults in their third to seventh decades of life without symptoms referable to the presence of PS and no relevant symptoms or events occurred during follow-up of patients with unresected PS.

Petersen et al. reviewed the literature for patients above the age of 40 with ILS and found 15 cases including two patients from their own medical center [6]. Most of these adult patients underwent surgical resection of their ILS. The largest study in the literature on PS is from China where Wei et al. reported 2625 cases of PS including 132 adult patients. However, their report does not describe how many of their adult PS patients underwent surgical resection, associated surgical outcome, nor clinical course of patients who did not undergo surgical resection [7]. In a study by Makhija et al., 102 older patients (age 4 to 80 years) with congenital cystic lung disease undergoing surgical management were reported and included 20 with PS (20%); postsurgical complication rate of 9.8% for the entire cohort was reported [5].

Berna et al. studied 26 adult patients with ILS all of whom underwent surgical resection [11]. Hemoptysis or recurrent infection was present in 54%. All 26 patients underwent surgical resection of their PS including 20 patients (77%) who underwent lobectomies. Postoperative complication rate was 25% and included pleural empyema, hemoptysis, prolonged air leak, arrhythmia, and fistulae. All patients were alive and well at long-term follow-up (mean 36.5 months).

In our cohort, 56% of patients underwent surgical resection for various indications; the most common indication was recurrent respiratory infection although it was often difficult to prove the relationship between those infections and the sequestration. None of our patients had experienced massive hemoptysis and only three patients (9%) described mild hemoptysis.

The surgical resection of sequestration carries the risk of complications; the surgical complication rate in our cohort was 28% which included chylous leak, intraoperative mild bleeding, chronic chest pain, arm numbness

Table 5 Comparison of surgical vs non-surgical patients

Characteristics	Surgical (n = 18)	Nonsurgical (n = 14)	P-value
Age, median (IQR)	41 (27–50)	43 (33–68)	0.218
Sex, n (%)			0.087
Male	7 (39)	10 (71)	
Female	11 (61)	4 (29)	
Sequestration Size, median (IQR)	6.5 (4–7)	6 (3.4–8.9)	0.778
Type of sequestration, n (%)			0.196
Intralobar	13 (72)	13 (93)	
Extralobar	5 (28)	1 (7)	
Presenting symptoms, n (%)			0.011
Asymptomatic	4 (22)	10 (71)	
Symptomatic	14 (78)	4 (29)	

and pneumonia. No surgical mortality occurred. These results are similar to those reported by Berna et al [11].

There are limitations to this study. The retrospective nature of this study limited the extent of data that could be retrieved including preceding symptoms and the exact relationship to the PS. The number of study subjects was modest due to the rarity of PS encountered in the adult population. Nonetheless, our data provide additional insight beyond what is currently available in the literature regarding the clinical course of PS in adults, particularly those who choose not to undergo surgical resection.

Conclusions

Nearly one-half of adult patients with pulmonary sequestration present with no relevant symptoms. The decision regarding surgical resection needs to weigh various factors including clinical manifestations related to PS, risk of surgical complications, comorbidities, and individual patient preferences.

Abbreviations
CT: Computed tomography; ELS: Extralobar sequestration; ILS: Intralobar sequestration; IQR: Interquartile range; PS: Pulmonary sequestration

Authors' contributions
MA contributed to data abstraction and analysis and manuscript writing. JHR contributed to the conceptualization and design of the study and manuscript writing. MA and JHR are guarantors of this work. All authors read and approved the final manuscript.

Competing interests
Authors declare no competing interests related to this study.

References
1. Liechty KW, Flake AW. Pulmonary vascular malformations. Semin Pediatr Surg. 2008;17(1):9–16.
2. Corbett HJ, Humphrey GME. Pulmonary sequestration. Paediatr Respir Rev. 2004;5(1):59–68.
3. Pryce DM. Lower accessory pulmonary artery with intralobar sequestration of lung; a report of seven cases. J Pathol Bacteriol. 1946;58(3):457–67.
4. Walker CM, Wu CC, Gilman MD, Godwin JD, 2nd, Shepard J-AO, Abbott GF: The imaging spectrum of bronchopulmonary sequestration. Curr Probl Diagn Radiol 2014, 43(3):100–114.
5. Makhija Z, Moir CR, Allen MS, Cassivi SD, Deschamps C, Nichols FC 3rd, Wigle DA, Shen KR. Surgical management of congenital cystic lung malformations in older patients. Ann Thorac Surg. 2011;91(5):1568–73. discussion 1573
6. Petersen G, Martin U, Singhal A, Criner GJ. Intralobar sequestration in the middle-aged and elderly adult: recognition and radiographic evaluation. Journal of Thoracic & Cardiovascular Surgery. 2003;126(6):2086–90.
7. Wei Y, Li F. Pulmonary sequestration: a retrospective analysis of 2625 cases in China. Eur J Cardiothorac Surg. 2011;40(1):e39–42.
8. Savic B, Birtel FJ, Tholen W, Funke HD, Knoche R. Lung sequestration: report of seven cases and review of 540 published cases. Thorax. 1979;34(1):96–101.
9. Hirai S, Hamanaka Y, Mitsui N, Uegami S, Matsuura Y. Surgical treatment of infected intralobar pulmonary sequestration: a collective review of patients older than 50 years reported in the literature. Annals of Thoracic & Cardiovascular Surgery. 2007;13(5):331–4.
10. Montjoy C, Hadique S, Graeber G, Ghamande S. Intralobar bronchopulmonary sequestra in adults over age 50: case series and review. W V Med J. 2012;108(5):8–13.
11. Berna P, Cazes A, Bagan P, Riquet M. Intralobar sequestration in adult patients. Interactive Cardiovascular & Thoracic Surgery. 2011;12(6):970–2.

5

Heparin-binding protein in sputum as a marker of pulmonary inflammation, lung function, and bacterial load in children with cystic fibrosis

Gisela Hovold[1], Victoria Palmcrantz[2], Fredrik Kahn[1], Arne Egesten[3] and Lisa I. Påhlman[1]* ⓘ

Abstract

Background: Cystic fibrosis (CF) is associated with bacterial pulmonary infections and neutrophil-dominated inflammation in the airways. The aim of this study was to evaluate the neutrophil-derived protein Heparin-binding protein (HBP) as a potential sputum marker of airway inflammation and bacterial load.

Methods: Nineteen CF patients, aged 6–18 years, were prospectively followed for 6 months with sputum sampling at every visit to the CF clinic. A total of 41 sputum samples were collected. Sputum-HBP was analysed with ELISA, neutrophil elastase activity with a chromogenic assay, and total bacterial load with RT-PCR of the 16 s rDNA gene. Data were compared to lung function parameters and airway symptoms.

Results: HBP and elastase correlated to a decrease in FEV_1%predicted compared to the patients' individual baseline pulmonary function (ΔFEV_1), but not to bacterial load. Area under the receiver operating characteristic curve values for the detection of > 10% decrease in ΔFEV_1 were 0.80 for HBP, 0.78 for elastase, and 0.54 for bacterial load.

Conclusions: Sputum HBP is a promising marker of airway inflammation and pulmonary function in children with CF.

Keywords: Cystic fibrosis, Sputum, Inflammation, Airway infection, Lung function, Children

Background

Cystic fibrosis (CF) is associated with persistent bacterial infection and neutrophil-dominated inflammation in the respiratory tract [1]. Several bacterial species cause airway infection in CF, for example *Staphylococcus aureus*, Non-typable *Haemophilus influenzae* (NtHi), *Burkholderia cepacia complex*, and *Pseudomonas aeruginosa*, and it is well described that exacerbations contribute to the progressive lung destruction and pulmonary function decline that is a hallmark of CF [2, 3]. Many bacterial species show increasing resistance to antibiotics, and there is therefore a need for robust biomarkers to monitor airway inflammation and infection. Such biomarkers could prevent unnecessary use of antibiotics that promote development of bacterial resistance.

Heparin-binding protein (HBP) is stored in the secretory and azurophilic granules of neutrophils, and is released upon cell activation [4]. HBP is a multi-functional pro-inflammatory mediator that for example activates immune cells, has broad antibacterial activity, and induces vascular leakage [5, 6]. Plasma HBP has been described as a promising predictor of the progression into severe sepsis and septic shock [7]. HBP levels also increase in cerebrospinal fluid during bacterial meningitis [8] and in urine during urinary tract infection [9], suggesting its use as a biomarker indicating bacterial infection. Recently, HBP was described as a useful biomarker in broncho-alveolar lavage fluid for the detection of pulmonary infection in lung transplant recipients [10].

The aim of the present study was to evaluate if HBP levels in sputum from children with CF can be used as a

* Correspondence: Lisa.Pahlman@med.lu.se
[1]Department of Clinical Sciences Lund, Division of Infection Medicine, BMC B14, Lund University, Skåne University Hospital, Tornavägen 10, SE-22184 Lund, Sweden
Full list of author information is available at the end of the article

biomarker for pulmonary inflammation and bacterial load. Neutrophil elastase was analysed for comparison and as a marker reflecting neutrophil load in the airways.

Methods

Study population

CF patients, 6 to 18 years of age, at the paediatric CF centre of Skåne University Hospital in Lund, were eligible for inclusion in the study. Patients under shared care with other clinics were excluded. At each visit to the clinic, the subjects donated an expectorated or induced sputum sample to the study, and their lung function was evaluated with spirometry. Sputum was induced by administering individually tailored hypertonic saline (median 5%, range 3–7%), followed by airway clearance techniques such as positive expiratory pressure (PEP) and forced expiration technique (FET). Sputum was collected during or directly after airway clearance. The procedure was supervised by a physiotherapist. Forced expiratory volume in one second in % of predicted (FEV1%predicted) and forced expiratory flow between 25 and 75% of expired forced vital capacity in % of predicted (FEF%predicted) were determined from predicted values according to Zapletal [11]. A mean of the two best values of FEV_1%predicted or FEF%predicted from the previous year were used as baseline to calculate the change in FEV_1%predicted (ΔFEV_1) or change in FEF%predicted (ΔFEF), respectively, at the time of sampling. At start of *iv* antibiotic treatment, a blood sample was also donated to the study.

Sputum cultures were analysed at the department of Medical Microbiology, Laboratory medicine, Skåne University Hospital, according to approved conventional methods in the routine laboratory [12]. Information about pulmonary symptoms such as dyspnoea, cough, fever, increased mucus, or change in sputum colour, was extracted from the medical journal. The sample collection was performed from January to June 2015.

A written informed consent was obtained from all participants and/or their guardian. The study was approved by the Medical Ethic Committee (Institutional Review Board) of Lund University (reference number 2011/434).

Sample preparation

All sputum samples were taken care of within two hours of sampling. One aliquot of the sample was mixed with an equal volume of Saliva Preservation Solution (Norgen Biotek Corporation, Canada) and frozen at – 80 °C until further processing. The remaining portion of the sample was homogenized by mixing sputum 1:1 (*w/v*) with 0.1% dithiothreitol (DTT) in PBS. The samples were incubated at 37 °C for 20 min with intermittent mixing, followed by centrifugation at 3000 rpm for 10 min. The cell-free supernatants were collected and stored at – 80 °C until further analyses.

Blood samples were centrifuged at 3000 rpm for 10 min. Plasma was collected and stored at – 80 °C until analyses. All plasma samples were centrifuged and frozen within one hour from sampling.

Quantification of HBP

HBP concentrations were analysed with ELISA as previously described [4]. All samples were assayed in duplicates.

Neutrophil elastase activity

Ten µl of liquefied sputum sample was mixed with 90 µl of HEPES buffer (0.1 M HEPES, 0.5 M NaCl; pH 7.5), supplemented with 5 mM EDTA, 2 µg/ml of E64 (Sigma, St. Louis, MO) and 1 µg/ml of Pepstatin A (Sigma-Aldrich, St. Louis, MO) in a 96-wells plate. Neutrophil elastase (Sigma-Aldrich) in 2-fold dilutions from a 2 U/ml stem solution was used as a standard. Fifty µl of the chromogenic substrate N-methoxysuccinyl-Ala-Ala-Pro-Val p-nitroanilide (Sigma-Aldrich) was added to each well to a final concentration of 0.5 mM. The plates were incubated at 37 °C and the absorbance at 415 nm was determined every 10 min to measure enzyme kinetics. All samples were analysed in duplicates.

Nucleic acid extraction and real-time PCR

Sputum samples were homogenized with DTT as described above. DNA extraction was performed with a Sputum DNA isolation kit (cat. #46200, Norgen Biotek Corporation) according to the manufacturer's protocol.

Total bacterial load was quantified with real-time PCR of 16 s rDNA, using the following primer pair: forward: TGCCAGCAGCCGCGGTAA, reverse: AGGCCCGGG AACGTATTCAC. One µl of DNA template was added to 19 µl master mix containing SYBR® Green (cat. #172–5121, Bio-Rad, Hercules, CA), sterile water, and the forward and reverse primers. Expression was analyzed using the iTaq™ Universal SYBR® Green Supermix (Bio-Rad). Known amounts of *Staphylococcus aureus* DNA in 10-fold dilutions were analyzed in parallel and used as a standard. Amplification was performed at 54 °C for 35 cycles in an iCycler Thermal Cycler (Bio-Rad, Hercules, CA) and DNA concentrations were calculated from the standard curve.

Statistics

Statistical calculations were done using the GraphPad Prism 7 software (GraphPad Software, San Diego, CA) and R (R Core Team 2017, R Foundation for Statistical Computing, Vienna, Austria) using R Studio (RStudio, Inc., Boston, MA) with installed packages nlme, mgcv, r2glmm, geepack and MuMln (https://cran.r-project.org/ web/packages/r2glmm/index.html) [13, 14] (https:// cran.r-project.org/web/packages/MuMIn/index.html).

Comparisons between unpaired groups were made with the non-parametric Mann-Whitney U test, and with Wilcoxon matched-pairs signed rank test for paired observations. Correlations were done with Spearman rank coefficient. Cut-off values for the calculation of sensitivity, specificity and predictive values were chosen based on receiver operator characteristics data.

To account for possible dependency due to repeated measurements from the same patient, we used mixed model with random effects and generalised estimating equation (GEE) models with subjects as the random components. The linear relationship between biomarkers and lung function was confirmed using a mixed additive model with random effects. To assess the relative importance of each variable in the mixed model, a semi-partial r-square was calculated according to Jaeger et al. [15]. Two-tailed $P < 0.05$ and 95% confidence intervals (CIs) that did not overlap 1.0 were regarded as statistically significant.

Results

Patient characteristics

A total of 22 patients suffering from CF (aged 6–18 years) were eligible and enrolled in the study. The study participants had a median age of 9 years, and male sex was the dominating gender (Table 1). The participants were followed with consecutive sputum sampling during a six months period, from January to June 2015. Three patients were unable to donate a sputum sample during the study period and were therefore excluded (Fig. 1). The remaining 19 patients donated a total of 50 sputum samples. Nine sputum samples were excluded as no lung function evaluation had been performed at the time of sampling. This left 41 sputum samples from 17 patients, with a median of 2 samples per patient (range 1–4 samples). 83% of sputum samples were induced with sodium chloride. Samples collected from the same patient were obtained with a median of 37 days apart (range 7–176 days). Another 6 samples were excluded from DNA analyses, as they contained small volumes of sputum that only allowed HBP and elastase measurements.

Staphylococcus aureus and *Pseudomonas aeruginosa* were the most commonly found bacterial species in sputum cultures (32 and 24%, respectively). Thirty-six % of sputum samples were collected during on-going symptoms from the respiratory tract (dyspnoea, cough, fever, increased mucus, or change in sputum colour). Nine samples were collected at start of intravenous antibiotic treatment. Six of these treatments were initiated to eradicate *P. aeruginosa* and the remaining to treat exacerbations.

HBP, elastase and bacterial load in sputum

Sputum concentrations of HBP and elastase, but not bacterial load, were significantly increased in samples

Table 1 Patient characteristics

Median age (IQR)[a]	9 (8–11)
Male gender; % (*n*)	71 (12)
CFTR mutation; % (*n*)	
- ΔF508/ΔF508	59 (10)
- Others	41 (7)
Pancreas insufficiency; % (*n*)	100 (17)
No of samples/patient; median (IQR)	2 (2–3)
Induced sputum; % (*n*)	83 (34)
Pseudomonas colonization[b]; % (*n*)	
- Never infected	24 (4)
- Free of infection	6 (1)
- Intermittent infection	53 (9)
- Chronic infection	18 (3)
Sputum culture growth; % (*n*)	
- *Staphylococcus aureus*	34 (12)
- *Pseudomonas aeruginosa*	26 (10)
- *Haemophilus influenzae*	14 (5)
- *Burkholderia cepacia*	6 (2)
- Negative culture	6 (2)

[a]IQR = Interquartile range
[b]Pseudomonas aeruginosa (PA) colonization according to Leeds criteria: Never infected, Free of infection (no PA growth during the previous 12 months), Intermittent infection (PA growth in 50% or less of cultures), or Chronic infection (PA growth in > 50% of cultures)

collected in the presence of respiratory symptoms (Fig. 2). To account for the possibility of bias due to repeated measures from the same patient, logistic regression with general estimating equation (GEE) models was performed using the logarithmic values of HBP, elastase

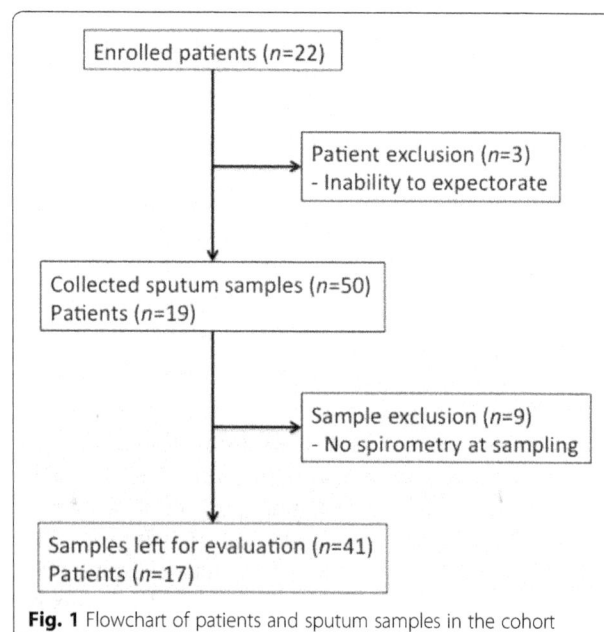

Fig. 1 Flowchart of patients and sputum samples in the cohort

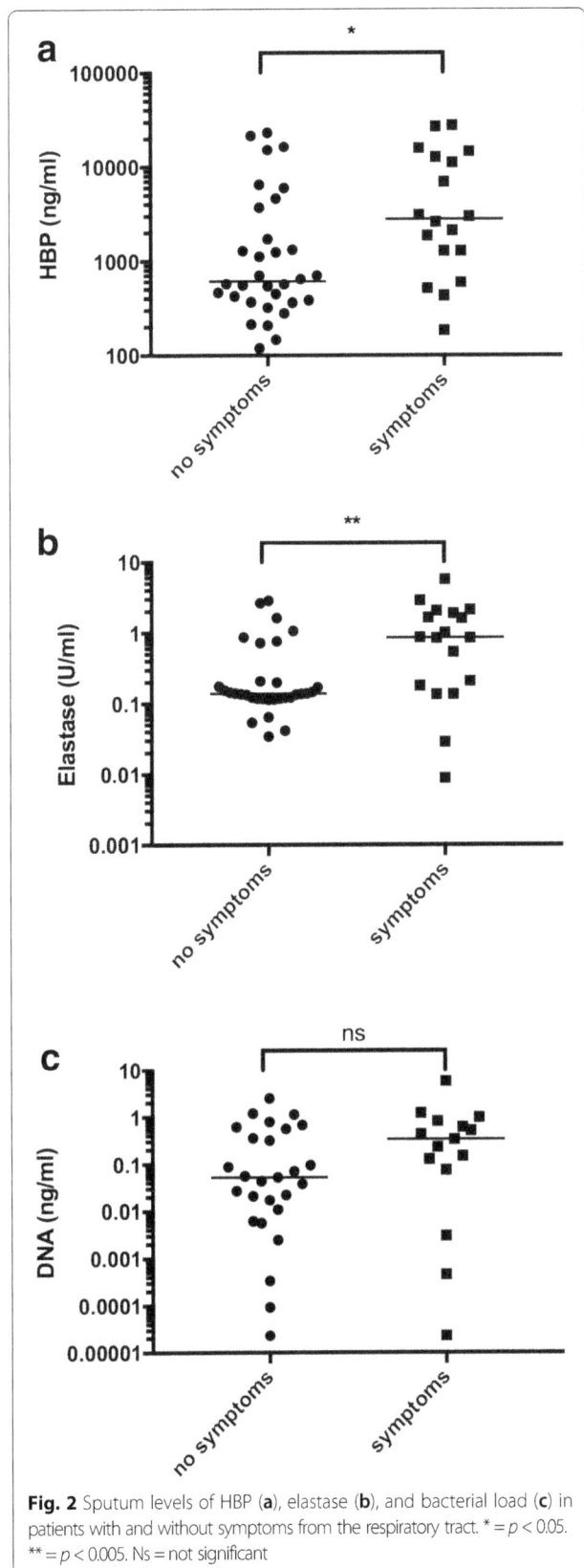

Fig. 2 Sputum levels of HBP (**a**), elastase (**b**), and bacterial load (**c**) in patients with and without symptoms from the respiratory tract. $* = p < 0.05$. $** = p < 0.005$. Ns = not significant

and bacterial DNA as continuous variables. Using GEE analyses, the odds ratios (ORs) for the prediction of respiratory symptoms were 1.4829 (95% CI 1.02766–2.140) for log(HBP), 1.705 (95% CI 1.082–2.69) for log(Elastase), and 1.124 (95% CI 0.972–1.30) for log(bacterial load).

Six participants had a sputum sample taken at start of antibiotic therapy, and a follow-up sample taken within one month. Median values decreased after therapy for all markers, but only HBP reached statistical significance (Fig. 3). Neither levels of HBP nor elastase differed between induced and naturally expectorated sputum ($p = 0.09$ for HBP and $p = 0.2$ for elastase).

Next, HBP, elastase and bacterial DNA were correlated to FEV_1%predicted at the time of sampling, and to the change in FEV_1%predicted compared to baseline levels (ΔFEV_1). A mean of the patient's two best FEV_1%predicted values from the previous year was used as baseline, and the change in lung function was expressed in percent. Both HBP and elastase correlated more strongly to ΔFEV_1 than FEV_1%predicted, whereas no convincing correlation was found between total bacterial load in sputum and either FEV_1%predicted or ΔFEV_1 (Fig. 4). To account for repeated measurements from the same patient, the correlations between biomarkers and ΔFEV_1 were validated both in a mixed model with patients as random effects, as well as using GEE. The mixed model with random effects estimated log(HBP) to − 2.5 (− 4.63 − − 0.379, $p = 0.0229$) and a semi-partial R-square of 0.122 (0.005–0.344). The estimate for log(elastase) was − 3.17 (− 5.41− − 0.933, $p = 0.0075$) with a semi-partial R-square of 0.161 (0.016–0.389), and for log(bacterial load) the estimate was 0.11 (− 1.23–1.44, $p = 0.8705$) with a semi-partial R-square of 0.001 (0–0.142). Importantly, GEE gave point estimates for the prediction of a decrease in ΔFEV_1 in agreement with the mixed models, but only HBP remained statistically significant. The estimates from the GEE were − 2.57 ($p = 0.023$) for log(HBP), − 2.96 ($p = 0.086$) for log(Elastase), and − 0.0538 ($p = 0.93$) for log(bacterial load).

No correlation was detected between HBP and bacterial DNA ($r = 0.09$, $p = 0.56$) or between elastase and bacterial DNA ($r = 0.24$, $p = 0.13$), whereas HBP and elastase correlated well ($r = 0.85$, $p < 0.001$). No differences in sputum HBP or elastase were found between the different groups of *Pseudomonas* colonisation according to Leeds criteria (data not shown).

In order to reflect involvement of small airway disease [16], sputum HBP levels were also correlated to FEF25/75 in % of predicted values (FEF%predicted), and to a change in FEF%predicted compared to baseline levels (ΔFEF%). HBP showed a weaker, but not statistically different correlation to both FEF%predicted ($r = − 0.27$, $p = 0.09$) compared to FEV_1%predicted ($p = 0.43$), and to ΔFEF% ($r = − 0.17$, $p = 0.30$) compared to ΔFEV_1, ($p = 0.09$).

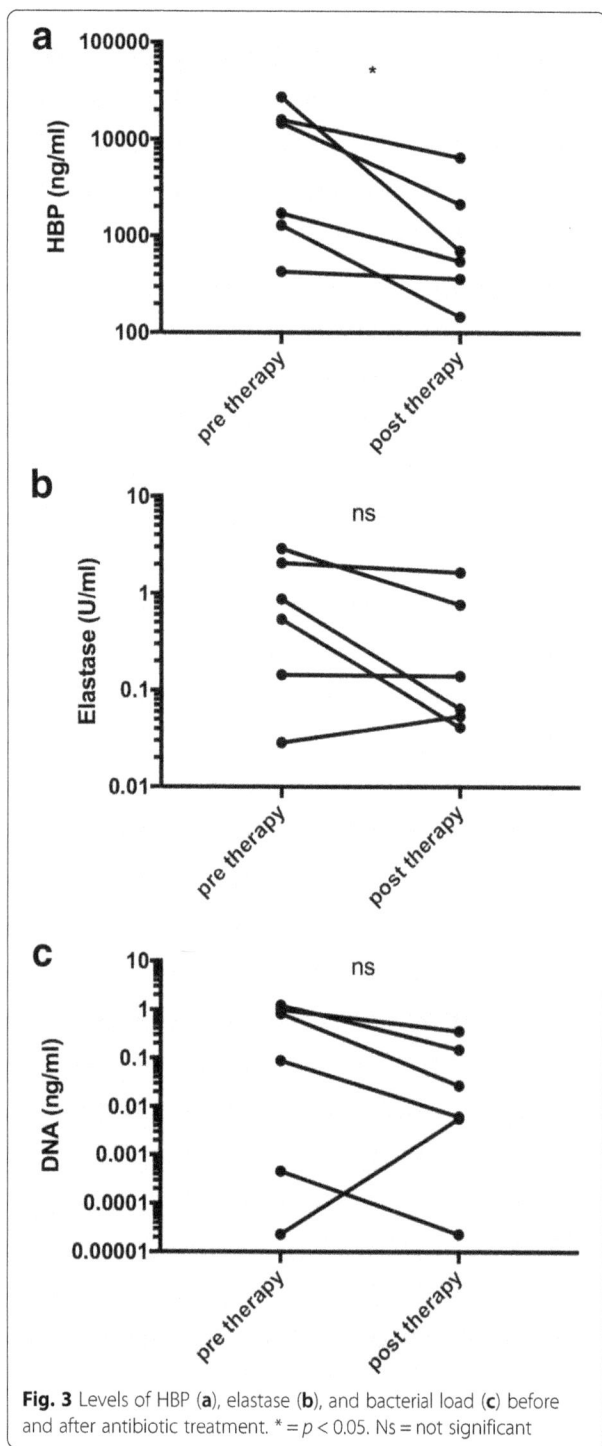

Fig. 3 Levels of HBP (**a**), elastase (**b**), and bacterial load (**c**) before and after antibiotic treatment. * = $p < 0.05$. Ns = not significant

0.80 (95% CI 0.65–0.94) for HBP and 0.78 (95% CI 0.62–0.93) for elastase. Bacterial DNA presented a lower AUC of 0.54 (95% CI 0.34–0.73) for the detection of a decrease in ΔFEV_1. Based on ROC data, cut-off values for the calculation of sensitivity, specificity and predictive values were identified for HBP, elastase and bacterial DNA. At a cut-off value of 650 ng/ml for HBP, the sensitivity was 81% and the specificity 70% for the detection of > 10% decline in ΔFEV_1. The positive and negative predictive values were 74 and 78%, respectively. Elastase performed similar to HBP, whereas bacterial DNA showed poor sensitivity and specificity (Table 2).

HBP levels in plasma

Eight patients donated a total of 9 plasma samples at the start of *iv* antibiotic treatment during the study period. The median HBP concentration in plasma was 7.0 ng/ml (range 5.1–20.5 ng/ml), which was significantly lower than the HBP concentrations in the corresponding sputum samples (median 1716 ng/ml, range 384–27,051 ng/ml, $p < 0.01$).

Discussion

HBP has received attention over the last years as a promising biomarker of infection in sepsis, urinary tract infections, meningitis, and lately also as a marker of airway infection in broncho-alveolar lavage (BAL) of lung transplant recipients [7–10]. In this prospective study on children with cystic fibrosis, HBP levels in sputum correlated to lung function and to respiratory symptoms, but not to bacterial load. HBP levels in plasma were low and in the same range as reported in healthy individuals [7]. In comparison, levels of HBP in concomitant sputum samples were at least 100-fold and up to 1000-fold higher. The high concentrations of HBP in sputum underline the heavy neutrophil-dominated airway inflammation seen in CF patients, and probably reflect that the lung is the end organ where the neutrophil becomes activated and releases its granular contents.

Expectorated and induced sputum is a non-invasive method to obtain airway samples from CF-patients, as opposed to BAL which is still the gold standard for defining airway inflammation and microbiology in infants and young children [17]. Studies have shown that sputum samples are of equal value as BAL specimens to detect *P. aeruginosa* colonization [18], indicating that sputum biomarkers for the detection of airway inflammation and infection would be a simple and useful tool in clinical practice. However, sputum collection is not as standardized as BAL, which may result in large intra- and inter-individual variations. For example, CF patients often have sputum plugs that cannot be expectorated and thus cause false low levels of inflammatory markers. Moreover, the sampling technique was not identical for all samples in the study, as 17% of samples were

Using 10% decline in ΔFEV_1 compared to baseline as cut-off, both HBP and elastase were significantly increased in the group with a decrease in ΔFEV_1 (Fig. 5). The levels of bacterial DNA were similar in both groups (data not shown). Receiver Operator Characteristics (ROC) analyses for the detection of > 10% decline in ΔFEV_1 are shown in Fig. 6. HBP and elastase performed equally well, with area under the curve (AUC) values of

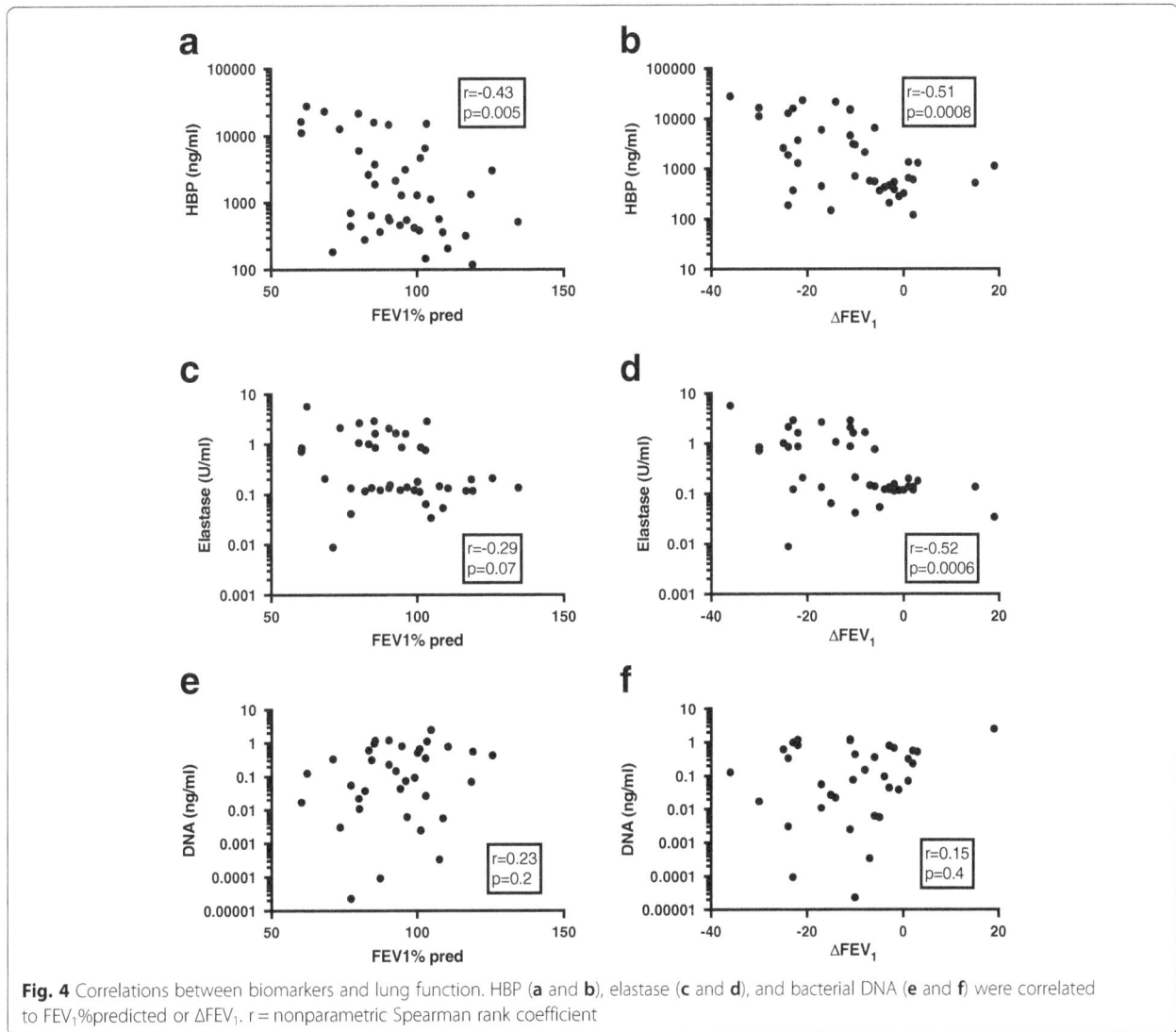

Fig. 4 Correlations between biomarkers and lung function. HBP (**a** and **b**), elastase (**c** and **d**), and bacterial DNA (**e** and **f**) were correlated to FEV_1%predicted or ΔFEV_1. r = nonparametric Spearman rank coefficient

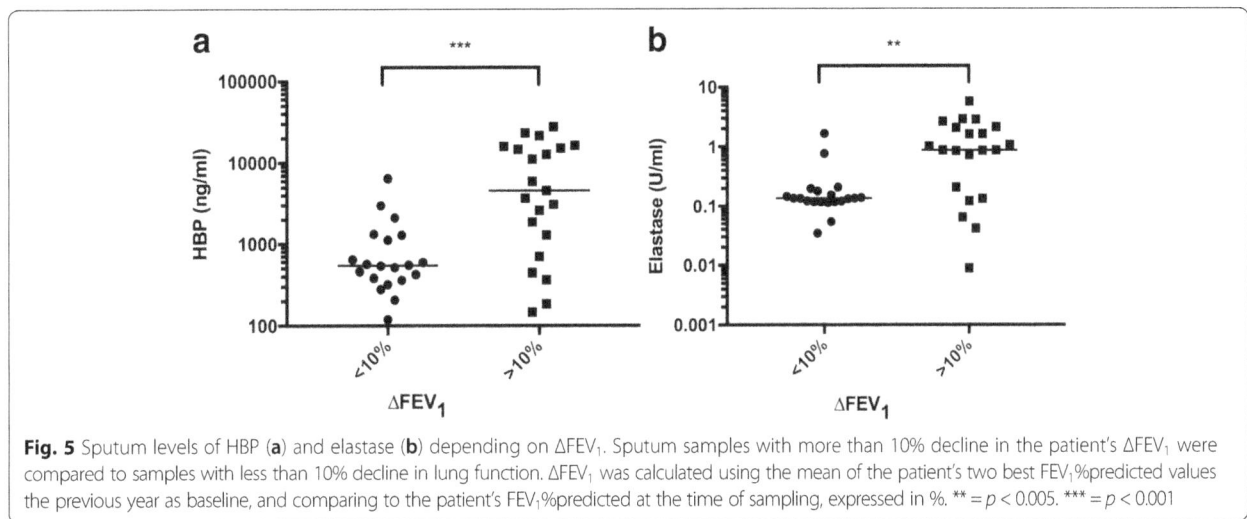

Fig. 5 Sputum levels of HBP (**a**) and elastase (**b**) depending on ΔFEV_1. Sputum samples with more than 10% decline in the patient's ΔFEV_1 were compared to samples with less than 10% decline in lung function. ΔFEV_1 was calculated using the mean of the patient's two best FEV_1%predicted values the previous year as baseline, and comparing to the patient's FEV_1%predicted at the time of sampling, expressed in %. ** $= p < 0.005$. *** $= p < 0.001$

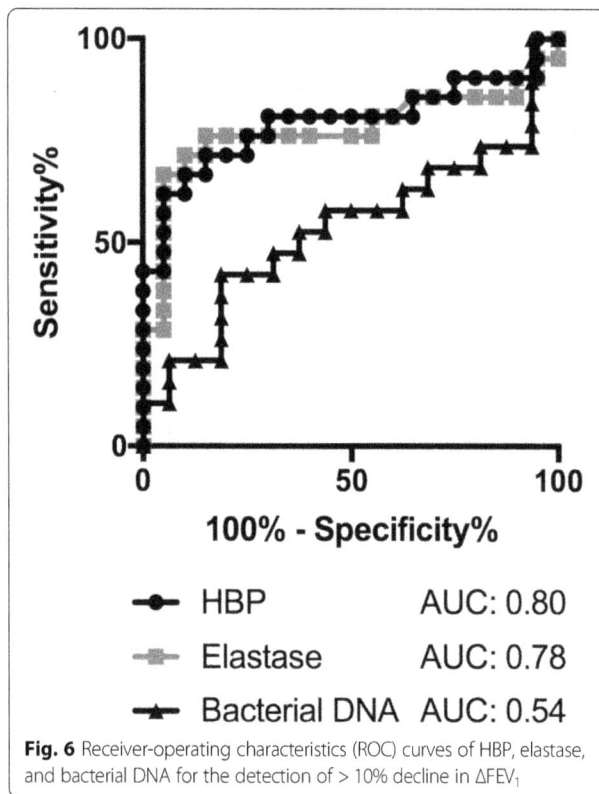

Fig. 6 Receiver-operating characteristics (ROC) curves of HBP, elastase, and bacterial DNA for the detection of > 10% decline in ΔFEV_1

colonized with pseudomonas. This PCR-method detects both viable and dead cells, which may be one reason why not more clear results were obtained.

An important shortcoming of the study is the lack of information about sputum neutrophil counts. Instead, we used neutrophil elastase as a marker of the neutrophil burden in our comparisons with HBP. Neutrophil elastase is well studied in sputum from CF patients, and has been reported to decrease after treatment of pulmonary exacerbations [21], to have a longitudinal association with lung function [23], and to be predictive of lung function decline [24]. Both elastase and HBP are neutrophil granule proteins that are released upon cellular activation. It is therefore not surprising that HBP performed equally well to elastase in most, but not all, comparisons made in this study. For example, HBP decreased significantly in sputum after antibiotic treatment, whereas elastase did not. However, only 6 patients had sputum samples taken before and after treatment, which gives the comparison poor power. Moreover, HBP was the only biomarker that remained statistically significant in all comparisons regardless of statistical analysis.

Another difficulty is the definition of airway symptoms in the study. There is no universally accepted definition of pulmonary exacerbations in CF, although Fuchs criteria are commonly used for adults. However, it has been argued that Fuchs criteria are less suited for studies on children, who have a milder lung disease and also milder symptoms of exacerbation [25]. In this study, patients were simply classified based on symptoms from the lower respiratory tract as reported by the patient or staff. Only a few patients experienced exacerbations that required *iv* antibiotic treatment during the study period. Even so, HBP increased significantly in the presence of pulmonary symptoms.

A final limitation is the small number of patients and the fact that participants donated varying numbers of samples to the study. However, even after correction for multiple measurements with mixed models and GEE, we could demonstrate that HBP correlates to ΔFEV_1 and pulmonary symptoms.

Conclusion

Sputum HBP is a promising biomarker for pulmonary inflammation and lung function in children with CF, and could thus be a simple and complementary tool in clinical practice. However, more studies are needed on larger study populations to validate the results.

expectorated and 83% were induced with sodium chloride. However, we saw no differences in biomarker levels between induced and non-induced sputum, and it has also been shown by others that there are no differences in microbiology between induced and expectorated sputum [19]. We therefore believe that the sampling technique has a minor impact on the results.

In this study, bacterial DNA tended to increase with pulmonary symptoms but did not reach statistical significance. Nor did bacterial DNA levels correlate to pulmonary function or biomarker levels. Previous work has reported conflicting results. For example, it has been shown that *P. aeruginosa* load correlate to lung function in stable patients, and also decrease after treatment of pulmonary exacerbation [20–22]. On the other hand, a large multicentre study could not attribute any important differences in FEV_1 to bacterial densities [23]. In this study, the cohort was diverse with respect to airway microbiology. We therefore chose to analyse total bacterial load with a universal 16S rDNA primer, as not all participants were

Table 2 Sensitivity, specificity and predictive values for the detection of > 10% decrease in ΔFEV_1

	Cut-off	Sensitivity (%)	Specificity (%)	PPV (%)	NPV (%)
HBP (ng/ml)	650	81	70	74	78
Elastase (U/ml)	0.15	76	70	73	74
Bacterial load (ng/ml)	0.1	47	44	50	41

PPV positive predictive value, *NPV* negative predictive value

Abbreviations
ΔFEV₁: Change in FEV₁%predicted; BAL: Broncho-alveolar lavage; CF: Cystic Fibrosis; FEV₁%predicted: Forced expiratory volume in one second, % of predicted; HBP: Heparin-binding protein; RT-PCR: Real-Time Polymerase Chain Reaction

Acknowledgements
The authors whish to thank Dr. Adam Linder for helpful discussions, and Maria Mårtensson and all other staff at the Cystic Fibrosis centre, Children's Hospital in Lund, for valuable help with sputum collection.

Funding
This work was funded by the Swedish Heart and Lung foundation, the Alfred Österlund, Magnus Bergvall, and Mats Kleeberg Foundations, Lions research fund in Skåne, The Swedish Heart and Lung Association, and the Swedish Government Funds for Clinical Research (ALF).

Authors' contributions
GH analysed sputum samples and was involved in writing of the manuscript. VP contributed to the concept and design of the study. FK helped with statistical analyses. AE contributed to the concept of the study and writing of the manuscript. LP contributed to the concept and design of the study, analysis and interpretation of samples and patient data, and writing of the manuscript. All authors read and approved the final manuscript.

Consent for publication
Not applicable.

Competing interests
The authors declare that they have no competing interests.

Author details
[1]Department of Clinical Sciences Lund, Division of Infection Medicine, BMC B14, Lund University, Skåne University Hospital, Tornavägen 10, SE-22184 Lund, Sweden. [2]Skåne University Hospital, Clinic of Paediatrics, Lund, Sweden. [3]Department of Clinical Sciences Lund, Respiratory Medicine & Allergology, Lund University, Lund, Sweden.

References
1. Stoltz DA, Meyerholz DK, Welsh MJ. Origins of cystic fibrosis lung disease. N Engl J Med. 2015;372(16):1574–5.
2. Cogen J, Emerson J, Sanders DB, Ren C, Schechter MS, Gibson RL, Morgan W, Rosenfeld M, Group ES. Risk factors for lung function decline in a large cohort of young cystic fibrosis patients. Pediatr Pulmonol. 2015;50(8):763–70.
3. Nkam L, Lambert J, Latouche A, Bellis G, Burgel PR, Hocine MN. A 3-year prognostic score for adults with cystic fibrosis. J Cyst Fibros. 2017;16(6):702-8.
4. Tapper H, Karlsson A, Morgelin M, Flodgaard H, Herwald H. Secretion of heparin-binding protein from human neutrophils is determined by its localization in azurophilic granules and secretory vesicles. Blood. 2002;99(5):1785–93.
5. Linder A, Soehnlein O, Akesson P. Roles of heparin-binding protein in bacterial infections. J Innate Immun. 2010;2(5):431–8.
6. Gautam N, Olofsson AM, Herwald H, Iversen LF, Lundgren-Akerlund E, Hedqvist P, Arfors KE, Flodgaard H, Lindbom L. Heparin-binding protein (HBP/CAP37): a missing link in neutrophil-evoked alteration of vascular permeability. Nat Med. 2001;7(10):1123–7.
7. Linder A, Arnold R, Boyd JH, Zindovic M, Zindovic I, Lange A, Paulsson M, Nyberg P, Russell JA, Pritchard D, et al. Heparin-binding protein measurement improves the prediction of severe infection with organ dysfunction in the emergency department. Crit Care Med. 2015;43(11):2378–86.
8. Linder A, Akesson P, Brink M, Studahl M, Bjorck L, Christensson B. Heparin-binding protein: a diagnostic marker of acute bacterial meningitis. Crit Care Med. 2011;39(4):812–7.
9. Kjolvmark C, Pahlman LI, Akesson P, Linder A. Heparin-binding protein: a diagnostic biomarker of urinary tract infection in adults. Open Forum Infect Dis. 2014;1(1):ofu004.
10. Stjärne, Aspelund A, Hammarström H, Inghammar M, Larsson H, Hansson L, Christensson B, Påhlman LI. Heparin-binding protein, lysozyme and inflammatory cytokines in bronchoalveolar lavage fluid as diagnostic tools for pulmonary infection in lung transplanted patients. Am J Transplant. 2018;18(2):444-52.
11. Zapletal A, Paul T, Samanek M. Significance of contemporary methods of lung function testing for the detection of airway obstruction in children and adolescents (author's transl). Z Erkr Atmungsorgane. 1977;149(3):343–71.
12. Murray PR. Manual of clinical microbiology. Washington: ASM Press; 2007.
13. Wood SN, Pya N, Säfken B. Smoothing parameter and model selection for general smooth models. J Am Stat Assoc. 2016;111(516):1548–63.
14. Yan J, Fine J. Estimating equations for association structures. Statist Med Stat Med. 2004;23(6):859–74.
15. Jaeger BC, Edwards LJ, Das K, Sen PK. An R2 statistic for fixed effects in the generalized linear mixed model. J Appl Stat. 2017;44(6):1086–105.
16. Eckrich J, Zissler UM, Serve F, Leutz P, Smaczny C, Schmitt-Grohe S, Fussbroich D, Schubert R, Zielen S, Eickmeier O. Airway inflammation in mild cystic fibrosis. J Cyst Fibros. 2017;16(1):107–15.
17. Stafler P, Davies JC, Balfour-Lynn IM, Rosenthal M, Bush A. Bronchoscopy in cystic fibrosis infants diagnosed by newborn screening. Pediatr Pulmonol. 2011;46(7):696–700.
18. Jung A, Kleinau I, Schonian G, Bauernfeind A, Chen C, Griese M, Doring G, Gobel U, Wahn U, Paul K. Sequential genotyping of Pseudomonas aeruginosa from upper and lower airways of cystic fibrosis patients. Eur Respir J. 2002;20(6):1457–63.
19. Rogers GB, Skelton S, Serisier DJ, van der Gast CJ, Bruce KD. Determining cystic fibrosis-affected lung microbiology: comparison of spontaneous and serially induced sputum samples by use of terminal restriction fragment length polymorphism profiling. J Clin Microbiol. 2010;48(1):78–86.
20. Deschaght P, Schelstraete P, Van Simaey L, Vanderkercken M, Raman A, Mahieu L, Van Daele S, De Baets F, Vaneechoutte M. Is the improvement of CF patients, hospitalized for pulmonary exacerbation, correlated to a decrease in bacterial load? PLoS One. 2013;8(11):e79010.
21. Ordonez CL, Henig NR, Mayer-Hamblett N, Accurso FJ, Burns JL, Chmiel JF, Daines CL, Gibson RL, McNamara S, Retsch-Bogart GZ, et al. Inflammatory and microbiologic markers in induced sputum after intravenous antibiotics in cystic fibrosis. Am J Respir Crit Care Med. 2003;168(12):1471–5.
22. Reid DW, Latham R, Lamont IL, Camara M, Roddam LF. Molecular analysis of changes in Pseudomonas aeruginosa load during treatment of a pulmonary exacerbation in cystic fibrosis. J Cyst Fibros. 2013;12(6):688–99.
23. Mayer-Hamblett N, Aitken ML, Accurso FJ, Kronmal RA, Konstan MW, Burns JL, Sagel SD, Ramsey BW. Association between pulmonary function and sputum biomarkers in cystic fibrosis. Am J Respir Crit Care Med. 2007;175(8):822–8.
24. Sagel SD, Wagner BD, Anthony MM, Emmett P, Zemanick ET. Sputum biomarkers of inflammation and lung function decline in children with cystic fibrosis. Am J Respir Crit Care Med. 2012;186(9):857–65.
25. Waters V, Ratjen F. Pulmonary exacerbations in children with cystic fibrosis. Ann Am Thorac Soc. 2015;12(Suppl 2):S200–6.

6

The level of lipopolysaccharide-binding protein is elevated in adult patients with obstructive sleep apnea

Yinfeng Kong[†], Zhijun Li[†], Tingyu Tang, Haiyan Wu, Juan Liu, Liang Gu, Tian Zhao and Qingdong Huang[*]

Abstract

Background: lipopolysaccharide-binding protein (LBP) has been to be a surrogate marker of inflammation in OSA. This study aimed to test the hypothesis that the concentration of LBP is elevated in adult patients with obstructive sleep apnea (OSA).

Methods: A total of 90 patients were enrolled into the study, 50 subjects were divided into OSA groups and 40 in healthy control according to PSG examination. Subsequently, patients with apnea-hypopnea index (AHI) $\geqq$ 5, were divided into different subgroups according to blood pressure, gender, body mass index (BMI) and AHI. Venous blood samples were collected for detection after polysomnography. The serum levels of LBP and proinflammatory cytokines (interleukin (IL)-1β, IL-6, tumor necrosis factor (TNF)-α) were tested by ELISA.

Results: The present study demonstrated that the serum levels of both LBP and proinflammatory cytokines were elevated in OSA patients. A stratified analysis conducted to analyze differences among subgroups indicated that OSA patients with a higher AHI or BMI had an increased level of LBP and proinflammatory cytokines (all $p < 0.05$). Furthermore, a significant correlations were observed between LBP and inflammation and AHI. Multivariate regression analysis also demonstrated that AHI, LSaO2 and BMI had impact on the concentration of LBP.

Conclusion: The research showed that the serum level of LBP and proinflammatory cytokines were elevated in adult patients with OSA, and an association with severity of disease and BMI were established. Furthermore, sleep apnea and BMI had effect on the concentration of LBP.

Keywords: Obstructive sleep apnea, Lipopolysaccharide-binding protein, Inflammation, Serum

Background

Obstructive sleep apnea (OSA) is described as repeated collapse of the upper airways during sleep, leading to repeated cycle of hypoxemia-reoxygenation and sleep disruption. Risk factors for OSA, including obesity and aging, are on the rise in the public; therefore, the prevalence of OSA is increasing worldwide, and is estimated to affect up to 17% of middle-aged men and 9% of middle-aged women [1].

The putative mechanism by which OSA has been linked to numerous pathologic conditions including stroke, cardiovascular disease, hypertension, and metabolic derangements is through the systemic inflammatory cascade [2–4]. In the past several years, it has become apparent that the increasing level of inflammation are strongly associated with OSA [5]. A meta-analysis including 1985 OSA patients and conducted by Xie et al. indicated that proinflammatory factors, such as interleukin (IL)-6, IL-8, and tumor necrosis factor (TNF)-α, are increased in patients with OSA, which is partially reversed after continuous positive airway pressure intervention [6]. However, the potential molecular mechanisms how to initiate the inflammation are not fully understood in OSA patients.

Lipopolysaccharide-binding protein (LBP) is an acute-phase reactant predominantly derived from the liver, adipose and intestinal epithelial cells. LBP binds lipopolysaccharide (LPS) through recognition of lipid A and initiates its response by forming a complex with

* Correspondence: zjyyhqd@163.com
[†]Yinfeng Kong and Zhijun Li contributed equally to this work.
Department of Respiratory Medicine in Zhejiang Hospital, 12 Lingyin Road, Xihu District, Hangzhou 310013, Zhejiang Province, China

myeloid differentiation factor 2 leading to activation of both MyD88-dependent and non-MyD88-dependent downstream signaling pathways causing subsequent inflammatory responses, such as the release of various biomediators including IL-6, TNF-α, and IL-1β [7]. Therefore, LBP usually as a biomarker of system inflammation, intestinal barrier and microbe translocation in deferent study [8–11].

Metabolic endotoxemia has been shown to be the primary contributor to the pathogenesis of chronic low-grade inflammation, characterized by increased plasma LBP levels, which are believed to originate from changes in gut microbiota and increasing of intestinal permeability [10]. Altered gut microbiota composition are key factors affecting gut barrier integrity. The gut microbiota, which serves as reservoir for bacterial LPS, could be altered by OSA and subsequently trigger inflammation. At present, several studies reported that the chronic intermittent hypoxia of OSA has a significant impact on the overall microbial community structure of mice, indicating that the homeostatic relationships between host and gut microbiota could be compromised in OSA patients [12, 13]. Moreno-Indias et al. study indicated that fecal microbiota composition and diversity were altered as a result of intermittent hypoxia realistically mimicking OSA [12]. Therefore, it is rational to deduce that the concentration of LBP is elevated in OSA patients. At present, one study from Kheirandish-Gozal et al. reported that children with OSA exhibited increased LBP levels [14]. However, only children were recruited into the Kheirandish-Gozal et al. research. There is indeed a paucity of published literature on the association between LBP levels and adult patients with OSA.

Based on previous studies, we conducted the study to test the hypothesis that the serum level of LBP is elevated in adult patients with OSA, and the correlations with proinflammatory factors and AHI were also evaluated.

Methods

Study population

A total of 50 patients with OSA (mild [n = 10], moderate [n = 15], and severe OSA [n = 25]) and 40 healthy controls were consecutively recruited in the study. The patients were examined at sleep laboratory of the respiratory department of Zhejiang Hospital from January 2016 to June 2016. Body weight and height were measured, and body mass index (BMI) was calculated as weight (kg)/height^2(m), and overweight was defined as BMI $\geq$ 25 kg/m^2. Blood pressure was recorded using a mercury sphygmomanometer, and elevated blood pressure was defined as systolic blood pressure (SBP) $\geq$ 140 mmHg and/or diastolic blood pressure (DBP) $\geq$ 90 mmHg or taking antihypertensive drug.

All subjects provided their informed written consent. The study was conducted according to the World Medical Association Declaration of Helsinki in 1975, as revised in 1983, and was approved by the Ethic Committee of Zhejiang Hospital.

Polysomnography

All participants received overnight polysomnography (PSG) according to standardized criteria [15]. The results of PSG were reviewed by two sleep specialists (Juan Liu & Liang Gu). Apnea was defined as continuous cessation of airflow for > 10 s. Hypopnea was defined as a $\geq$ 30% reduction in airflow for > 10 s with oxygen desaturation of $\geq$4%. Apnea-hypopnea index (AHI) was calculated as the sum of apneas and hypopneas per hour during overnight. A respiratory event was scored as an obstructive apnea or hypopnea if chest and abdominal respiratory movement was identified and oronasal airflow ceased, or there is an associated thoracoabdominal paradox that occurs during the hypopnea with snoring. Microarousal index (MAI) was defined according to the American Academy of Sleep Medicine Scoring Manual [16]. The oxygen desaturation index (ODI) was defined as $\geq$4% oxygen desaturation per hour during sleep. Patients with OSA were divided into the mild group (AHI: 5–15 events/h), moderate group (AHI: 15–30 events/h), and severe group (AHI > 30 events/h) [17]. Subjects with sleepy and snore who accepted PSG examination, with an AHI < 5 events/h were included in the study as healthy controls. The exclusion criteria of subjects were as follows: (1) chronic hypoxia caused by asthma, chronic obstructive pulmonary disease, interstitial lung disease and other respiratory disorders. (2) Participants with a history of drug or alcohol abuse, or taking drugs to regulate intestinal flora. (3) cardiovascular, endocrine, and other disorders that could lead to hypoxemia. (4) Diseases which may lead to the release of proinflammatory factors, such as connective tissue disease, cancer, and inflammatory bowel disease. (5) required gastrointestinal surgical procedures or had received antibiotic therapy in the preceding 8 weeks were also excluded.

Blood collection and analysis

Peripheral blood, drawn from each subject on the morning after PSG, was centrifuged at 3000 rpm for 15 min, and serum was stored at – 70 °C for analysis. Concentrations of serum LBP, IL-1β, IL-6, TNF-α were measured using commercially available ELISA kits (R&D Systems, Minneapolis, MN, USA) in duplicate according to the manufacturer's instruction. An automatic biochemical analyzer (UniCel DxC 800 Synchron, Beckman Coulter, Inc., Brea, CA, USA) was used to test the serum level of lipids.

Statistical analysis

Continuous variables are expressed as the mean ± standard deviation. Comparisons were performed using t test or χ^2 tests depending on data differences among groups. Spearman's correlation analysis were conducted to examine potential associations between LBP and proinflammatory factors. A multivariate regression analysis was also performed to evaluate the role of confounding factors on LBP. Statistical significance was determined by a level of 0.05 on two-sided tests. All statistical analysis was performed using the SPSS Statistics 19.0.0 (IBM Corporation, Somers, NY, USA).

Results

General clinical characteristics of the study participants

The basic clinical characteristics of the subjects are detailed in Table 1. The mean age of patients with OSA was 54.34 ± 14.38 years, compared with 50.42 ± 8.35 years in the control group. There are significant differences were observed between cases and controls group in terms of BMI, blood pressure (SBP and DBP), the serum concentration of triglyceride (TG), and PSG parameters (all $p < 0.05$).

The comparison of LBP and proinflammatory factors between patients and controls

There were significant differences in the serum level of LBP (36.05 ± 7.35 vs 32.11 ± 5.94, $p = 0.01$) and inflammatory factors (IL-1β, 27.15 ± 5.91 vs 21.17 ± 1.70, $p = 0.000$; IL-6, 61.59 ± 9.76 vs 54.46 ± 9.43, $p = 0.005$; TNF-α 327.34 ± 46.81 vs 307.95 ± 27.15, $p = 0.020$) between cases and control group.

To further analyze differences among subgroups, a stratified analysis was performed according to blood pressure, gender, BMI and severity of disease (AHI). The results demonstrated that a significant differences were found between normal weight and overweight patients with OSA, which suggested that OSA patients with a higher BMI had a higher serum level of LBP and proinflammatory factors (all $p < 0.05$). However, no differences were identified in other subgroups based on blood pressure and gender ($p > 0.05$) (Table 2). Alternatively, a marked differences were determined in the mild vs moderate, mild vs severe, moderate vs severe groups (all $p < 0.05$), except for IL-1β in the mild vs moderate group ($t = - 1.837$, $p = 0.091$) (Table 3).

The correlations between LBP and proinflammatory factors and severity of disease

Based on aforementioned findings, The correlations between LBP and proinflammatory cytokines and severity of diseases were also evaluated. As evident in Fig. 1, significant correlations were found between LBP and IL-1β ($r = 0.464$, $p = 0.003$), IL-6 ($r = 0.586$, $p = 0.000$), TNF-α

Table 1 Clinical characteristics of the OSA and control group

Variables	Patients	Controls	p value
Gender			0.317
Male	34	31	
Female	16	9	
Age (years)	54.34 ± 14.38	50.42 ± 8.35	0.112
BMI(kg/m^2)	26.86 ± 3.12	22.26 ± 3.54	0.000
Normal weight	11(22.00%)	27(67.50%)	
Overweight	39(78.00%)	13(32.50%)	
SBP(mmHg)	133.60 ± 16.37	120.19 ± 17.11	0.000
DBP(mmHg)	81.16 ± 14.45	74.05 ± 10.72	0.005
Respiratory events			
Obstructive	241.76 ± 106.12	17.49 ± 7.18	< 0.001
Central	1.32 ± 0.59	0.94 ± 0.37	0.551
AHI	37.34 ± 19.02	3.31 ± 1.09	< 0.001
LSaO2	75.29 ± 11.83	95.95 ± 4.65	< 0.001
mSaO2	93.01 ± 4.18	96.35 ± 3.87	< 0.001
ODI	41.83 ± 25.9	3.56 ± 1.12	< 0.001
MAI	22.61 ± 15.12	4.27 ± 2.16	< 0.001
NREM1(%)	23.21 ± 12.79	15.9 ± 13.04	0.031
NREM21(%)	52.73 ± 12.31	48.1 ± 16.21	0.335
NREM31(%)	14.51 ± 9.95	20.23 ± 8.72	0.045
REM(%)	10.23 ± 5.31	16.74 ± 7.36	0.012
TG	2.96 ± 2.53	1.71 ± 1.07	0.004
TC	4.98 ± 1.10	4.71 ± 0.91	0.189
HDL	1.04 ± 0.23	1.23 ± 0.26	0.000
LDL	2.98 ± 1.10	3.02 ± 0.89	0.847
LBP	36.05 ± 7.35	32.11 ± 5.94	0.010
IL-1β	27.15 ± 5.91	21.17 ± 1.70	0.000
IL-6	61.59 ± 9.76	54.46 ± 9.43	0.001
TNF-α	327.34 ± 46.81	307.95 ± 27.15	0.027

AHI Apnea-hypopnea index, *BMI* Body mass index, *SBP* Systolic blood pressure, *DBP* Diastolic blood pressure, *LSaO2* Lowest saturation oxygen, *mSaO2* Mean saturation oxygen, *ODI* Oxygen desaturation index, *MAI* Microarousal index, *TG* triglyceride, *TC* Total cholesterol, *LDL* Low-density lipoprotein, *HDL* High-density lipoprotein

($r = 0.490$, $p = 0.001$), and AHI ($r = 0.371$, $p = 0.001$). In addition, a multivariate regression analysis were performed to determine the role of possible confounding factor to the concentration of LBP. The result of analysis showed that AHI, LSaO2 and BMI had a significant impact on the LBP (all $p < 0.05$), which suggested that sleep apnea and obesity have effect on the levels of serum LBP. However, other variables were not identified ($p > 0.05$) (Table 4).

Discussion

This is the first study to investigate OSA has an impact on the concentration of LBP in adults. The results

Table 2 Comparison of various index in OSA subgroups according to blood pressure, gender and BMI

Variables	HBP vs Normal BP		p value	Male vs Female		p value	Normal weight vs Overweight		p value
	HBP(21)	Normal BP(29)		Male(34)	Female(16)		Normal weight(14)	Overweight(36)	
Age(years)	49.76 ± 13.28	56.46 ± 14.55	0.083	55.76 ± 12.76	52.13 ± 9.41	0.912	58.36 ± 18.68	52.78 ± 12.29	0.315
BMI(kg/m^2)	28.30 ± 3.32	25.09 ± 2.83	0.022	27.28 ± 2.79	25.44 ± 3.12	0.531	24.42 ± 1.17	27.56 ± 2.60	0.017
SBP(mmHg)	150.06 ± 7.61	123.61 ± 11.33	0.000	135.12 ± 15.61	131.50 ± 17.14	0.362	136.63 ± 16.38	126.15 ± 14.31	0.051
DBP(mmHg)	92.71 ± 13.12	74.14 ± 10.15	0.000	83.08 ± 14.23	78.42 ± 9.12	0.112	83.31 ± 15.02	75.85 ± 11.83	0.117
AHI	34.43 ± 17.72	40.19 ± 20.51	0.322	40.35 ± 16.63	29.61 ± 23.02	0.073	33.87 ± 16.52	38.69 ± 19.96	0.426
LSaO$_2$(%)	77.17 ± 10.71	71.83 ± 13.75	0.160	72.87 ± 12.24	75.85 ± 7.77	0.132	75.83 ± 11.09	75.12 ± 12.22	0.859
mSaO$_2$(%)	92.96 ± 5.37	93.67 ± 2.30	0.684	92.73 ± 4.78	94.11 ± 1.54	0.315	93.74 ± 2.67	92.89 ± 4.59	0.546
ODI	36.58 ± 23.77	48.89 ± 27.72	0.126	47.75 ± 24.49	25.91 ± 23.50	0.008	36.71 ± 22.46	43.54 ± 27.03	0.435
MAI	20.13 ± 13.27	26.33 ± 17.25	0.180	24.49 ± 16.22	17.44 ± 10.45	0.170	20.25 ± 13.07	23.56 ± 15.97	0.512
LBP	36.25 ± 8.71	35.72 ± 4.52	0.805	35.78 ± 7.73	37.14 ± 5.93	0.645	26.75 ± 3.50	37.38 ± 6.79	0.002
IL-1β	26.89 ± 6.27	27.58 ± 5.44	0.728	27.81 ± 5.93	24.52 ± 5.36	0.161	20.90 ± 2.03	28.04 ± 5.75	0.010
IL-6	61.69 ± 10.62	61.46 ± 8.47	0.944	61.52 ± 10.22	61.90 ± 8.24	0.924	46.41 ± 5.50	63.78 ± 8.18	0.000
TNF-α	325.11 ± 49.82	331.06 ± 42.73	0.703	329.95 ± 49.06	316.88 ± 37.36	0.487	252.99 ± 18.74	337.96 ± 39.29	0.000

AHI Apnea-hypopnea index, BMI Body mass index, SBP Systolic blood pressure, DBP Diastolic blood pressure, LSaO$_2$ Lowest saturation oxygen, mSaO$_2$ Mean saturation oxygen, ODI Oxygen desaturation index, MAI Microarousal index

Table 3 Comparison of various index in subgroups according to severity of disease

Variables	OSA			Mild vs Moderate		Mild vs Severe		Moderate vs Severe	
	Mild(10)	Moderate(15)	Severe(25)	t	p value	t	p value	t	p value
Age(years)	59.60 ± 15.13	56.73 ± 15.93	52.27 ± 13.54	0.352	0.729	1.104	0.277	−0.983	0.331
BMI(kg/m²)	27.04 ± 2.58	26.81 ± 3.80	27.28 ± 3.16	0.120	0.906	−0.164	0.871	0.436	0.665
SBP(mmHg) 140.40 ± 13.05	130.31 ± 16.79	133.93 ± 16.82	1.204	0.246	0.812	0.423	0.638	0.528	
DBP(mmHg)	85.20 ± 9.61	79.85 ± 15.63	81.04 ± 14.63	0.686	0.502	0.597	0.555	0.236	0.815
AHI	10.14 ± 2.95	22.88 ± 3.93	49.11 ± 14.96	−6.066	0.000	−12.848	0.000	−8.999	0.000
LSaO2	87.20 ± 1.30	79.53 ± 9.13	70.90 ± 12.00	3.159	0.006	6.958	0.000	2.429	0.020
mSaO2	94.80 ± 1.48	93.88 ± 2.27	92.38 ± 5.10	0.840	0.412	1.040	0.307	1.077	0.288
ODI	11.94 ± 5.37	26.41 ± 18.78	55.44 ± 22.17	−1.672	0.112	−9.008	0.000	−4.305	0.000
MAI	14.56 ± 2.87	16.45 ± 8.12	27.06 ± 17.40	−0.501	0.623	−3.484	0.002	−2.627	0.012
LBP	25.81 ± 7.16	33.55 ± 3.50	38.29 ± 7.40	−2.743	0.018	−2.771	0.010	−2.642	0.012
IL-1β	20.10 ± 1.47	24.35 ± 3.83	29.15 ± 5.91	−1.837	0.091	−2.604	0.015	−2.475	0.018
IL-6	46.20 ± 6.09	58.34 ± 7.09	64.76 ± 9.05	−2.686	0.020	−3.434	0.002	−2090	0.044
TNF-α	274.64 ± 4.91	308.75 ± 42.48	341.28 ± 44.80	−2.601	0.025	−2.534	0.017	−2.048	0.048

AHI Apnea-hypopnea index, *BMI* Body mass index, *SBP* Systolic blood pressure, *DBP* Diastolic blood pressure, *LSaO₂* Lowest saturation oxygen, *mSaO₂* Mean saturation oxygen, *ODI* Oxygen desaturation index, *MAI* Microarousal index

demonstrated that the serum level of LBP and inflammation were higher in OSA patients, compared with healthy subjects, and subgroups analysis indicated that OSA patients with a higher BMI and AHI had a higher serum level of LBP and proinflammatory factors. Additionally, the correlational analysis showed that serum LBP levels were positively correlated with inflammation and AHI. A multivariate regression analysis indicated that sleep apnea and BMI had a significant impact on the concentration of LBP.

To the best of our knowledge, OSA has an impact on the intestinal barrier function and gut microflora. A study conducted by Moreno-Indias et al. suggested that composition and diversity of intestinal microflora are altered caused by intermittent hypoxia [12]. The translocation or change of commensal microbiota across the intestinal barrier can result in a persistent state of low grade immune activation or inflammation. LBP is located upstream of IL-1β, IL-6, and TNF-α expression, and initiates the recognition of bacterial LPS exposure and amplifies the host immune response which, if continued long-term, results in adverse sequelae to the host. Therefore, LBP has been suggested to serve as a surrogate marker of chronic inflammatory status in several disorders, such as obesity, diabetes, hypertension and other chronic inflammation diseases [18, 19]. Kim et al. study indicated that LBP levels were positively associated with BMI, SDP, total cholesterol, low density lipoprotein-cholesterol, fasting glucose and insulin, and insulin resistance [18].

The present study showed that the levels of LBP and inflammation are increased in adult OSA patients and are positively associated with the severity of disease.

Significant correlations were also determined between LBP and AHI and proinflammatory factors, which was is in line with the previous study. Another study of Moreno-Indias et al. demonstrated that the LPS concentration was elevated at the end of intermittent hypoxia in mouse model, and a significant association was found between gut bacterial dysbiosis and the increases in plasma LPS levels [20]. In a recent study conducted by

Table 4 The effect of confounding factor on concentation of LBP in OSA patients

Variables	β	95% CI	p value
AHI	14.430	(5.152, 29.078)	0.026
ODI	−0.139	(−0.397, 0.119)	0.276
MAI	0.074	(−0.135, 0.282)	0.472
LSaO2	10.125	(3.917, 25.071)	0.035
mSaO2	−0.256	(−0.929, 0.416)	0.438
Age	0.115	(−0.150, 0.379)	0.379
BMI	8.245	(1.154, 18.386)	0.041
SBP	−0.214	(−0.470, 0.042)	0.097
DBP	0.345	(−0.008, 0.698)	0.055
TG	1.378	(−0.964, 3.719)	0.236
TC	−5.532	(−12.988, 1.924)	0.138
HDL	−4.509	(−20.564, 11.546)	0.567
LDL	5.397	(−2.166, 12.960)	0.153
IL-1β	0.373	(−0.730, 1.476)	0.492
IL-6	−0.079	(−0.363, 0.204)	0.569
TNF-α	−0.006	(−0.076, 0.064)	0.859

AHI Apnea-hypopnea index, *BMI* Body mass index, *SBP* Systolic blood pressure, *DBP* Diastolic blood pressure, *LSaO₂* Lowest saturation oxygen, *mSaO₂* Mean saturation oxygen, *ODI* Oxygen desaturation index, *MAI* Microarousal index

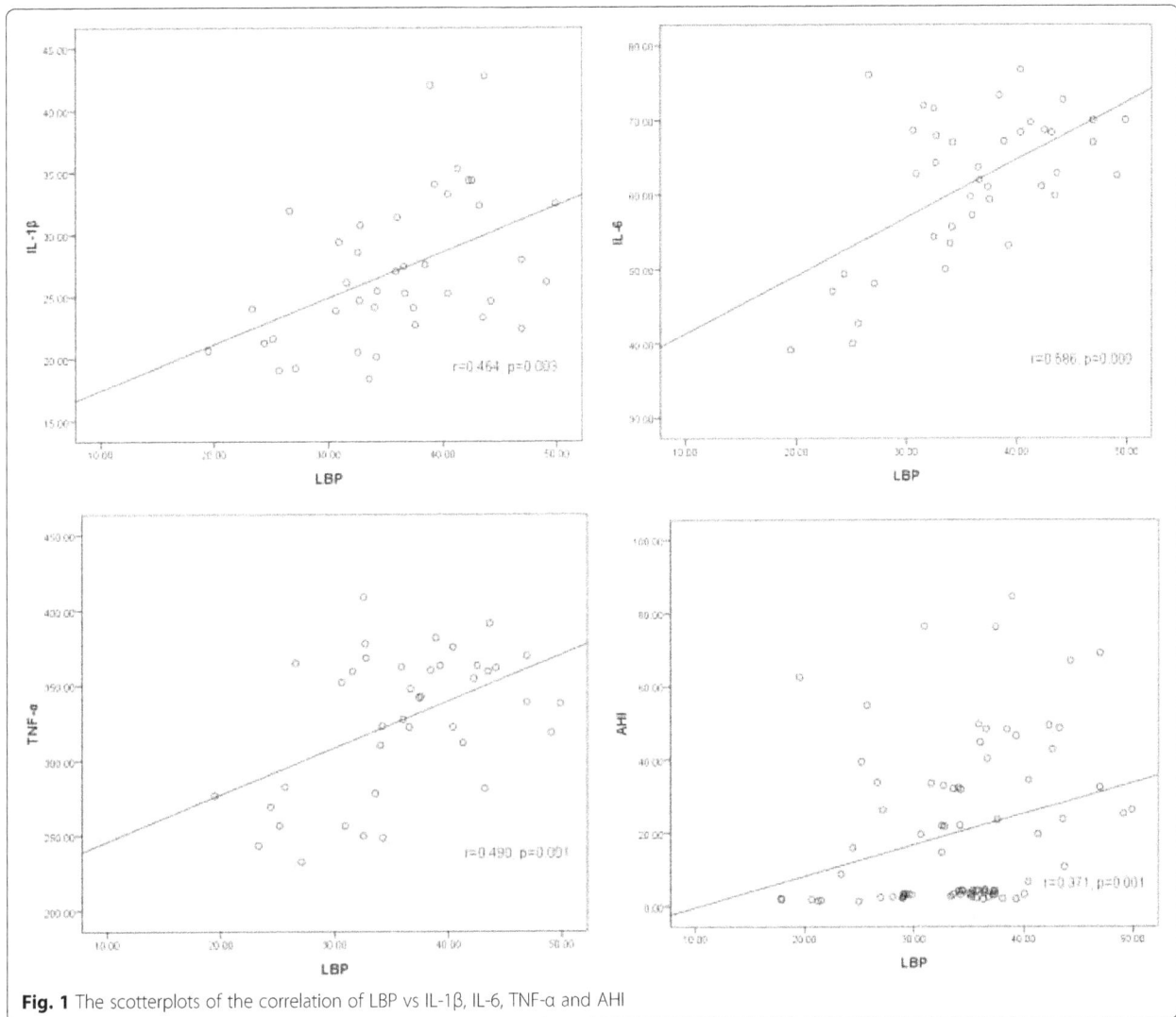

Fig. 1 The scotterplots of the correlation of LBP vs IL-1β, IL-6, TNF-α and AHI

Kheirandish-Gozal et al. [14], they assessed the LBP plasma levels of 219 child patients with OSA, and found that systemic low-level endotoxemia and elevation of LBP was established in children with OSA, associated with measures of OSA severity. However, only children with OSA were included to analyze in the study. Another research conducted by Sakura et al. also domenstrated that serum LBP levels were positively correlated with inflammation [19]. Taken together, we can deduce that chronic intermittent hypoxia of OSA may lead to elevation of systemic LBP levels with resultant inflammation by causing disorder of intestinal microflora.

As previously described, several researches reported that LBP levels and proinflammation factors had positively associated with BMI and hypertension [18]. Although a remarkable differences were obeserved between cases and controls in term of BMI and blood pressure. However, the result of present study demonstrated that the concentration of LBP and level of inflammation had only a positive association with BMI in OSA patients, and no relation with hypertension. As we known, obesity is one of the strongest risk factors for OSA, which imposes mechanical loads on the upper airway, resulting in flow limitation and apnea, with > 50% of OSA diagnoses attributable to being overweight [21]. Kheirandish-Gozal et al. also indicated that a significant increases was identified in LBP levels in children with obesity or OSA, and the highest LBP levels was observed when both conditions are present [14]. Additionally, a study came from Kim et al. showed that circulating plasma LBP levels were significantly increased in overweight/obese participants compared with those in normal weight participants [18]. The same results drew from another study conducted by Gonzalez-Quintela et al. [22]. Therefore, the current evidence supported that that sleep apnea and other factors such as obesity may disrupt intestinal barrier function or gut microbiota, and casue to increased the serum LPS concentration with resultant systemic inflammation.

In interpreting the results of the research, there are some methodological limitations requiring comment. First, disruption of gut microflora plays an important role in low-grade inflammation, we should therefore detect changes of gut microflora in future studies to explain the underlying mechanism of increased of LBP and inflammatory factors caused by OSA. Second, the study was not a clinical randomized controlled trial, and only the serum level of LBP and proinflammatory factors were evaluated in patients with OSA. It would be important to test if we can detect the changes in LBP and proinflammatory factors levels before and after intervention. Third, the sample size of the study was relatively small, with only 50 OSA patients included. These limitations could have affected the power of the conclusions. In the future, we intend to conduct an analysis of a larger sample size and a randomized controlled trial, which will include these risk factors.

Conclusions

The present study shown that higher LBP levels and inflammation are detected in the presence of obesity and in the presence of sleep-disordered breathing in a severity-dependent fashion. Furthermore, higher serum LBP levels were positively correlated with AHI, and sleep apnea and BMI had effect on the concention of LBP. Improved understanding the mechanism underlying these associations may offer not only opportunities for detection of OSA patients at risk of comorbidities, but may also enable delineation of therapeutic interventions, such as regulation of intestinal flora through probiotics, for example, to reduce end-organ damage caused by OSA.

Abbreviations

AHI: Apnea-hypopnea index; BMI: Body mass index; DBP: Diastolic blood pressure; HDL: High-density lipoprotein; IL: Interleukin; LBP: Lipopolysaccharide-binding protein; LDL: Low-density lipoprotein; LPS: Lipopolysaccharide; LSaO2: Lowest saturation oxygen; MAI: Microarousal index; mSaO2: Mean saturation oxygen; ODI: Oxygen desaturation index; SBP: Systolic blood pressure; TC: Total cholesterol; TG: Triglyceride; TNF: Tumor necrosis factor

Funding

The Medical and Health Science and Technology Plan of Zhejiang Province (2014KYA001) and TCM Science and Technology Plan of Zhejiang Province (2015ZB002) provided financial support in the form of researcher funding. The sponsor had no role in the design or conduct of this research.

Authors' contributions

YFK and ZJL planned the experimental design and drafted the manuscript, LG and JL helped PSG examination and analyze data, HYW and TYT collected the samples and prepared revision of manuscript, TZ contributed to perform detection and prepare tables, QDH conceived and participated in the study design. All authors read and approved the final manuscript.

Competing interests

The authors declare that they have no competing interests.

References

1. Peppard PE, Young T, Barnet JH, Palta M, Hagen EW, Hla KM. Increased prevalence of sleep-disordered breathing in adults. Am J Epidemiol. 2011; 177(9):1006–14.
2. Wu H, Yuan X, Wang L, Sun J, Liu J, Wei Y. The relationship between obstructive sleep apnea hypopnea syndrome and inflammatory markers and quality of life in subjects with acute coronary syndrome. Respir Care. 2016;61(9):1207–16.
3. Ifergane G, Ovanyan A, Toledano R, Goldbart A, Abu-Salame I, Tal A, Stavsky M, Novack V. Obstructive sleep apnea in acute sroke: a role for stroke inflammation. Stroke. 2016;47(5):1207–12.
4. Kim J, Yoon DW, Lee SK, Lee S, Choi KM, Robert TJ, Shin C. Concurrent presence of inflammation and obstructive sleep apnea exacerbates the risk of metabolic syndrome: A KoGES 6-year follow-up study. Medicine (Baltimore). 2017;96(7):e4488.
5. Vicente E, Marin JM, Carrizo SJ, Osuna CS, González R, Marin-Oto M, Forner M, Vicente P, Cubero P, Gil AV, et al. Upper airway and systemic inflammation in obstructive sleep apnoea. Eur Respir J. 2016;48(4):1108–17.
6. Xie X, Pan L, Ren D, Du C, Guo Y. Effects of continuous positive airway pressure therapy on systemic inflammation in obstructive sleep apnea: A meta-analysis. Sleep Med. 2013;14(11):1139–50.
7. Tobias PS, Soldau K, Ulevitch RJ. Identification of a lipid A binding site in the acute phase reactant lipopolysaccharide binding protein. J Biol Chem. 1989;264(18):10867–71.
8. Forsyth CB, Shannon KM, Kordower JH, Voigt RM, Shaikh M, Jaglin JA, Estes JD, Dodiya HB, Keshavarzian A. Increased intestinal permeability correlates with sigmoid mucosa alpha-synuclein staining and endotoxin exposure markers in early Parkinson's disease. PLoS One. 2011;6(12):e28032.
9. Sun L, Yu Z, Ye X, Zou S, Li H, Yu D, Wu H, Chen Y, Dore J, Clément K, et al. A marker of endotoxemia is associated with obesity and related metabolic disorders in apparently healthy Chinese. Diabetes Care. 2010;33(9):1925–32.
10. Cani PD, Bibiloni R, Knauf C, Waget A, Neyrinck AM, Delzenne NM, Burcelin R. Changes in gut microbiota control metabolic endotoxemia-induced inflammation in high-fat-diet-induced obesity and diabetes in mice. Diabetes. 2008;57(6):1470–81.
11. Giloteaux L, Goodrich JK, Walters WA, Levine SM, Ley RE, Hanson MR. Reduced diversity and altered composition of the gut microbiome in individuals with myalgic encephalomyelitis/chronic fatigue syndrome. Microbiome. 2016;4(1):30.
12. Moreno-Indias I, Torres M, Montserrat JM, Sanchez-Alcoholado L, Cardona F, Tinahones FJ, Gozal D, Poroyko VA, Navajas D, Queipo-Ortuño MI, et al. Intermittent hypoxia alters gut microbiota diversity in a mouse model of sleep apnoea. Eur Respir J. 2015;45(4):1055–65.
13. Durgan DJ, Ganesh BP, Cope JL, Ajami NJ, Phillips SC, Petrosino JF, Hollister EB, Bryan RM Jr. Role of the gut microbiome in obstructive sleep apnea–induced hypertension. Hypertension. 2016;67(2):469–74.
14. Kheirandish-Gozal L, Peris E, Wang Y, Tamae Kakazu M, Khalyfa A, Carreras A, Gozal D. Lipopolysaccharide-binding protein plasma levels in children: effects of obstructive sleep apnea and obesity. J Clin Endocrinol Metab. 2014;99(2):656–63.
15. Berry RB, Budhiraja R, Gottlieb DJ, Gozal D, Iber C, Kapur VK, Marcus CL, Mehra R, Parthasarathy S, Quan SF, et al. Rule for scoring respiratory events in sleep: update of the 2007 AASM Manual for the scoring of sleep and sssociated events. Deliberations of the sleep apnea definitions task force of the American academy of sleep medicine. J Clin Sleep Med. 2012;8(5):597–619.
16. EEG arousals. Scoring rules and examples: a preliminary report from the sleep disorders atlas task force of the American Sleep Disorders Association. Sleep. 1992;15(2):173–84.
17. Sleep-related breathing disorders in adults: recommendations for syndrome definition and measurement techniques in clinical research. The Report of an American Academy of Sleep Medicine Task Force. Sleep. 1999;22(5):667–89.
18. Kim KE, Cho YS, Baek KS, Li L, Baek KH, Kim JH, Kim HS, Sheen YH. Lipopolysaccharide-binding protein plasma levels as a biomarker of obesity-related insulin resistance in adolescents. Korean J Pediatr. 2016;59(5):231–8.

7

Effects of vitamin D supplementation on the outcomes of patients with pulmonary tuberculosis

Hong-xia Wu[1], Xiao-feng Xiong[1], Min Zhu[1], Jia Wei[2], Kai-quan Zhuo[3] and De-yun Cheng[1*]

Abstract

Background: Vitamin D is involved in the host immune response toward *Mycobacterium tuberculosis*. However, the efficacy of vitamin D supplementation on sputum conversion, clinical response to treatment, adverse events, and mortality in patients with pulmonary tuberculosis (PTB) remains controversial. We aimed to clarify the efficacy and safety of vitamin D supplementation in PTB treatment.

Methods: We searched Medline, Embase, Cochrane Central Register of Controlled Trials, Web of Science for double-blind, randomized controlled trials of vitamin D supplementation in patients with PTB that reported sputum conversion, clinical response to treatment, adverse events, or mortality, published from database inception to November 26, 2017. This study was registered with PROSPERO, number CRD42018081236.

Results: A total of 1787 patients with active PTB receiving vitamin D supplementation along with standard anti-tuberculosis regimen were included in the eight trials with different doses of vitamin D ranging from 1000 IU/day to 600,000 IU/month at different intervals. Primary analysis revealed that vitamin D supplementation increased the proportion of sputum smear and culture conversions (OR 1.21, 95%CI 1.05~ 1.39, $z = 2.69$, $P = 0.007$; OR 1.22, 95%CI 1.04~ 1.43, $z = 2.41$, $P = 0.02$), but did not improve the time to sputum smear and culture conversions (HR 1.07, 95%CI 0.83~ 1.37, $z = 0.50$, $P = 0.62$; HR 0.97, 95%CI 0.76~ 1.23, $z = 0.29$, $P = 0.77$). In the secondary analysis, vitamin D improved serum 25(OH)D, plasma calcium concentration, lymphocyte count, and chest radiograph (MD 103.36, 95%CI 84.20~ 122.53, $z = 10.57$, $P < 0.00001$; SMD 0.26, 95%CI 0.15~ 0.37, $z = 4.61$, $P < 0.00001$; MD 0.09, 95%CI 0.03~ 0.14, $z = 2.94$, $P = 0.003$; MD -0.33, 95% CI -0.57~ − 0.08 $z = 2.57$, $P = 0.01$), but had no impact on adverse events, mortality and other indicators(TB score, BMI, mean mid-upper arm circumference, weight gain, CRP, ESR, and other blood cells) ($P > 0.05$).

Conclusions: Vitamin D supplementation can be considered as a combination therapy in patients with PTB.

Keywords: Vitamin D, Tuberculosis, Meta-analysis, Therapy

Background

Tuberculosis (TB) is a major health problem; the World Health Organization estimates that there were 10.4 million incident cases and 1.7 million deaths due to TB worldwide in 2016. Although TB is a preventable and curable disease, the high prevalence of multidrug-resistant and extensively drug-resistant TB with the pandemics of human immunodeficiency virus infection and diabetes generates further problems [1]. The duration of anti-tuberculosis treatment is long and requires multiple drugs that often have mild to severe side effects. Thus, there is an urgent need for developing novel drugs that can shorten treatment duration and combat infection with both susceptible and resistant TB strains.

Two epidemiological studies demonstrated that seasonal variations in serum vitamin D concentration were strongly related to the incidence of TB [2, 3]. A

* Correspondence: chengdeyunscu@163.com
[1]Department of Respiratory and Critical Care Medicine, West China Hospital, Sichuan University, NO.37 Guoxue Alley, Chengdu 610041, Sichuan, China
Full list of author information is available at the end of the article

meta-analysis found that low serum vitamin D status was associated with increased risk of TB [4]. These results suggested that vitamin D supplementation is likely to have a primary preventive effect on the incidence risk as well as a beneficial effect on the anti-tuberculosis treatment.

The use of vitamin D for TB treatment started in 1849, with the observation that oil from fish liver improved appetite and strength [5]. The major circulating metabolite of vitamin D, 1,25-hydroxyvitamin D (1,25[OH]D), supports innate antimicrobial immune responses, suggesting a potential mechanism by which adjunctive vitamin D might enhance response to anti-tuberculosis therapy [6]. In recent years, vitamin D was used to treat PTB in the pre-antibiotic era. Thus far, two meta-analyses incorporating the data from trials of vitamin D supplementation as treatment in patients with PTB have been performed. A meta-analysis that included four trials did not show any improvement in the clinical parameters (mortality, sputum smear positivity, and sputum culture positivity) of vitamin D administration compared with placebo ($P = 0.05$) [7]. Another meta-analysis that included five studies (one study aimed at children) showed that vitamin D supplementation does not have any beneficial effects on improving sputum smear and culture conversion, adverse effects, and body weight [8]. Both meta-analyses had limited number of studies, sample sizes, and parameters analyzed, influencing the results. Currently, several new RCTs have been published. We conducted a meta-analysis of all published RCTs to update and further clarify the efficacy and safety of vitamin D as adjunctive therapy in patients with PTB.

Methods

Each enrolled trial was approved by the corresponding Institutional Ethical Committee. Ethics approval and consent to participate are not relevant for systematic reviews and meta-analysis. This study was registered with PROSPERO. Findings are reported according to the PRISMA guidelines.

Search strategies

In this systematic review and meta-analysis, we searched Medline, Embase, Cochrane Central Register of Controlled Trials, Web of Science for trials in process using the keywords "tuberculosis or tuberculoses" and "vitamin D or cholecalciferol," with limitations in the publication type of RCTs but not in the publication language or period. We regularly updated our searches from database inception up to and including Nov 26, 2017. We reviewed the references listed in each identified article and manually searched the related articles to identify all eligible studies and minimize potential publication bias.

Inclusion and exclusion criteria

Clinical trials were considered eligible based on the following criteria: 1) RCTs, 2) trials conducted in patients newly diagnosed with PTB who were on initial anti-tuberculosis treatment, 3) those conducted in patients aged > 16 years, and 4) those conducted in patients receiving vitamin D3 or vitamin D2 as an interventional treatment, with reported data on efficiency or safety of vitamin D supplementation. Patients had taken oral corticosteroid or other immunosuppressant therapy, or drugs known to interfere with vitamin D levels, or antituberculous therapy were excluded. Trials conducted in pregnant women; retrospective, observational, cohort, and case control studies; and congress articles were excluded.

Outcome measures

Outcome measures consisted of efficacy assessment and safety evaluation, which were divided into primary and the secondary results. Primary outcomes included proportion of sputum smear or culture conversion and time to sputum smear or culture conversion. Secondary outcomes included serum 25-hydroxy vitamin D(25(OH)D) concentration, serum calcium concentration, TB score, chest imaging, body mass index (BMI), weight gain, mean mid-upper arm circumference, C-reactive protein (CRP), erythrocyte sedimentation rate (ESR), blood indexes (total white cell, neutrophil, monocyte, lymphocyte, and hemoglobin), adverse effects, and mortality.

Study selection

The study selection was performed by two investigators in two phases to determine which studies are suitable. Duplicated and non-randomized controlled studies were discarded by screening titles and abstracts firstly. Secondly, accordance with the previously designed study inclusion criteria, eligible studies were extracted by reviewing full texts.

Data extraction

Two data collectors extracted and recorded authors, publication year, registration series, study design, participants and population, demographic characteristics, baseline characteristics, details of intervention treatment (dose, frequency, routine, and duration), follow-up period, outcome measures and study results of each enrolled study in a standard form as recommended by Cochrane [9], independently. For any missing information, corresponding authors were contacted by email.

Quality assessment

Five GRADE considerations [10] was used to assess the quality of evidence contributing to the analyses of efficacy assessment and safety evaluation. For the assessment of risk of bias in estimating the study outcomes, the Cochrane risk of bias tool [9] was used.

A third investigator was consulted to solve any disagreement on study selection, data extraction, or quality assessment.

Statistical analysis

The statistical analysis was accomplished by Cochrane systematic review software Review Manager (RevMan; Version 5.3, The Nordic Cochrane Centre, The Cochrane Collaboration, Copenhagen, 2014). The Mann-Whitney U-test was applied to verify the hypothesis and rendered statistical significance as z-value and P-value< 0.05; the results were displayed in forest plots.

The effects of the intervention on continuous outcomes, dichotomous outcomes, and time to event were expressed as mean differences or standard mean differences, odds ratios, and hazard ratios, respectively. The χ2 test with $P < 0.1$ and $I2 > 50\%$ indicated significant heterogeneity. The sensitivity analysis was performed to substitute unclear alternative decisions and ranges of values for decisions. In the presence of statistical heterogeneity, random-effects model was applied; otherwise, fixed-effects model was used.

Results
Study description

Our search identified 333 unique studies that we assessed for eligibility, of which eight studies [11–18] with 1787 randomly assigned participants who fulfilled the eligibility criteria were enrolled in our final quantitative synthesis (Fig. 1). The eight analyzed RCTs were performed in eight different countries in three continents. Among all people, 898 patients were assigned to receive vitamin D, while 889 were administered placebo. A total of 1044 patients enrolled in the studies were male, and the male/female ratios were 535:363 and 539:360 in vitamin D and placebo groups, respectively. The mean age of patients ranged from 27.8~41.6 years and 26.7~43.7 years in the intervention and control

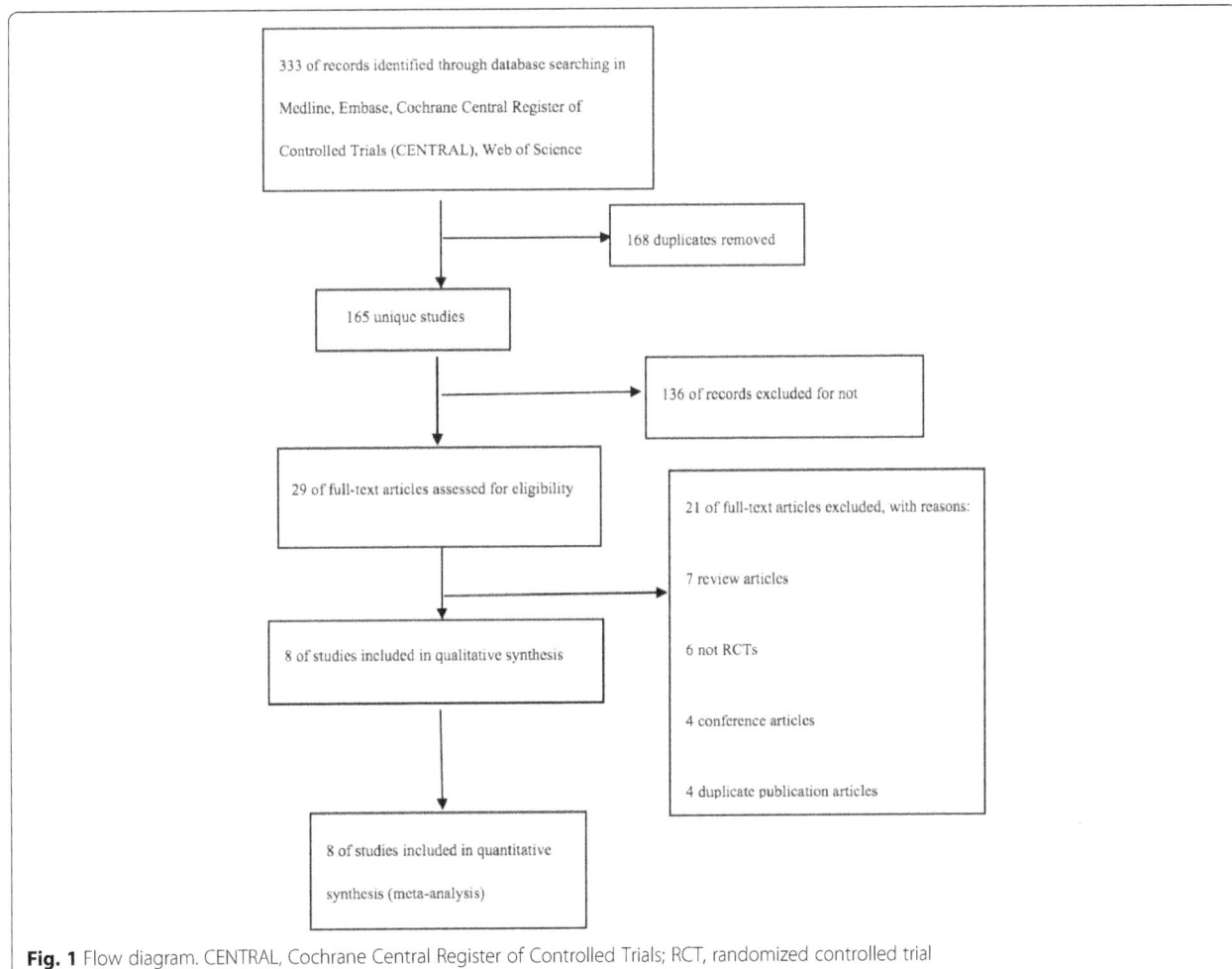

Fig. 1 Flow diagram. CENTRAL, Cochrane Central Register of Controlled Trials; RCT, randomized controlled trial

arms, respectively. Baseline serum 25(OH)D concentrations were determined in six RCTs, ranging from 7.8~ 77.5 nmol/L and 6.0~ 79.1 nmol/L in the intervention and control arms, respectively. All studies involved the administration of vitamin D to participants in the intervention arm: this was an oral bolus dose given within a 4-month period (2.5 mg per bolus × 3 doses) in one study [18], an intramuscular bolus dose administered monthly (15 mg per bolus × 2 doses) in one study [16], an oral bolus dose administered biweekly (2.5~ 3.5 mg per bolus × 4 dose) in three studies [11–13], a combination of oral bolus does administered triweekly (1.25 mg per bolus × 3 doses) and weekly (1.25 mg per bolus × 3 doses) in one study [17], an oral bolus dose administered weekly (0.875 mg per bolus × 8 doses) in one study [14], and an oral dose administered daily (0.25 mg per day for 6 weeks) in one study [15]. Study durations ranged from 6 weeks to 8 months.

Regarding the outcome measures, six studies [11–13, 15, 16, 18] reported the proportion of sputum smear conversion, five [11–14, 17] reported the proportion of sputum culture conversion and changes of plasma calcium concentrations, four [11–14] provided the time to sputum smear conversion, four [11–13, 17] provided the time to sputum culture conversion, six [12–14, 16, 17] provided the changes in serum vitamin D concentrations, three [14, 16, 18] presented the data on TB score change, four [12, 13, 15, 16] exhibited the BMI change, four [12, 13, 16, 17] showed the changes in mean mid-upper arm circumference, five [12–16, 18] showed the changes in weight gain, three [12, 13, 16] presented the data on chest radiograph change, six [12–14, 17, 18] showed the incidence of serious adverse events, three [11, 13, 18] exhibited the incidence of non-serious adverse events, seven [11–14, 16–18] provided the incidence of all-cause deaths, three [12–14] showed the changes in blood indexes, CRP and ESR. Details on patients' characteristics, intervention strategies, and outcomes are summarized in Tables 1 and 2.

Three RCTs [12–14] were at low risk of bias for all aspects analyzed. The trials conducted by Daley, Tukvadze, and Wejse as well as their colleagues had an unclear risk of attrition bias due to the missing data [11, 17, 18], which could have affected the outcome, but we found no evidence to confirm the doubt. The study conducted by Nursyam and colleagues had an unclear risk of selection, performance, and detection bias as it did not describe the definite methods used in random sequence generation, blinding of participants, and personnel and outcome assessments [15]. The study conducted by Salahuddin and colleagues had an unclear risk of performance and detection bias as it did not show the details of the blinding method [16]. Details on the risk of bias assessment are provided in Additional file 1: Figure

S1 and Additional file 2: Figure S2. No studies excluding for low quality (GRADE) or dubious decisions were found in the sensitivity analysis.

Heterogeneity

A statistical heterogeneity was not observed in the proportion of sputum smear and culture conversion, time to sputum smear and culture conversion, changes in chest radiograph, CRP, ESR, blood indexes, and number of non-serious and serious adverse events and all-cause deaths (Fig. 25; Additional file 3: Figure S3, Additional file 4: Figure S4, Additional file 5: Figure S5, Additional file 6: Figure S6, Additional file 7: Figure S7, Additional file 8: Figure S8, Additional file 9: Figure S9, Additional file 10: Figure S10, Additional file 11: Figure S11, Additional file 12: Figure S12). By contrast, a significant statistical heterogeneity was found in the changes in serum 25(OH)D, plasma calcium concentration, TB score, BMI, weight gain, mean mid-upper arm circumference, and neutrophil count ($I^2 = 99\%$, MD 103.36, 95%CI 84.2~ 122.53; $I^2 = 57\%$, MD 0.26, 95%CI 0.15~ 0.37; $I^2 = 97\%$, MD 0.33, 95%CI -1.58~ 2.24; $I^2 = 62\%$, MD 0.04, 95%CI -0.15~ 0.24; $I^2 = 60\%$, MD -0.21, 95%CI -0.44~ 0.01; $I^2 = 73\%$, MD 0.07, 95%CI -0.78~ 0.92; $I^2 = 66\%$, MD -0.13, 95%CI -0.42~ 0.16) (Additional file 13: Figure S13, Additional file 14: Figure S14, Additional file 15: Figure S15, Additional file 16: Figure S16, Additional file 17: Figure S17, Additional file 18: Figure S18, Additional file 19: Figure S19). To ensure that if any single study skewed the overall results, a sensitivity analysis was performed to evaluate the stability of the results. One study was removed at a time and the overall effect and summary MD recalculated. This analysis confirmed the stability of the results: the overall effects (P value) did not show statistically significant reversal, and summary MDs were consistent and without apparent fluctuation (range of recalculated summary MDs: 80.39~ 122.62; 0.13~ 0.33; − 0.43~ 0.72;0.02~ 0.10; − 0.23~ − 0.10; − 0.40~ 0.47;-0.18~ − 0.06).

Outcomes
Primary outcomes

Proportion of sputum conversion There were significant differences in the proportion of sputum smear conversion in the overall effects (OR 1.21, 95%CI 1.05~ 1.39, $P = 0.007$), but null was found in 2, 4, 6, 8, and 12 weeks (OR 1.26, 0.93~ 1.72, $P = 0.14$; OR 1.25, 0.97~ 1.62, $P = 0.08$; OR 1.41, 1.04~ 1.92, $P = 0.03$; OR 1.02, 0.77~ 1.35, $P = 0.90$; OR 1.05, 0.56~ 1.96, $P = 0.88$) (Fig. 2).

We found significant differences in proportion of sputum culture conversion in the overall effects (OR 1.22, 1.04~ 1.43, $P = 0.02$), but null was found in 2, 4, 6, 8, and 16 weeks (OR 1.44, 0.95~ 2.17, P = 0.08; OR 1.09, 0.84~

Table 1 Details of each enrolled study

Author (Year)	Setting	Clinical trials register No.	Pre-protocol participants (I/C)	Participants completed study (I/C)	Intervention drug	Single dose	Frequency	Total dose	Routine	Control	Study duration	Outcomes[a]
Daley 2015 [11]	India	NCT00366470	247(121/126)	211(101/110)	Vitamin D3	2.5 mg	Biweekly*4 doses	10 mg	Oral	Placebo	6 weeks	①②④⑥⑤⑯
Ganmaa 2016 [12]	Mongolia	NCT01657656	390(190/200)	352(174/178)	Vitamin D3	3.5 mg	Biweekly*4 doses	13.5 mg	Oral	Placebo	8 weeks	①②④⑥⑦⑧⑨⑩⑪⑫⑬⑭⑮⑯
Martineau 2011 [13]	UK	NCT00419068	146(73/73)	126(62/64)	Vitamin D3	2.5 mg	Biweekly*4 doses	10 mg	Oral	Placebo	8 weeks	①②③④⑥⑦⑧⑨⑩⑪⑫⑬⑭⑯
Mily 2015 [14]	Bangladesh	NCT01580007	144(72/72)	128(63/65)	Vitamin D3	0.875 mg	Weekly*8 doses	7 mg	Oral	Placebo	8 weeks	②③⑤⑦⑩⑫⑬④⑥⑯
Nursyam 2006 [15]	Indonesia	NM	67(34/33)	67(34/33)	Vitamin D3	0.25 mg	Per day*42 doses	10.5 mg	Oral	Placebo	6 weeks	①⑨⑩
Salahuddin 2013 [16]	Pakistan	NCT01130311	259(132/127)	238(119/119)	Vitamin D3	15 mg	Per month*2 doses	30 mg	Intramuscular	Placebo	8 weeks	①⑦⑧⑩⑪⑯
Tukvadze 2015 [17]	Georgia	NCT00918086	199(100/99)	192(97/95)	Vitamin D3	1.25 mg	Triweekly*3 doses and weekly*3 doses	7.5 mg	Oral	Placebo	16 weeks	②④⑤⑥⑦⑤⑧⑨⑩⑪⑯
Wejse 2009 [18]	Guinea	ISRCTN35212132	355(187/178)	281(136/145)	Cholecalciferol	2.5 mg	Four-monthly*3 doses	7.5 mg	Oral	Placebo	8 months	①②⑩⑤⑯

[a]Outcome measures include: ①proportion of sputum smear conversion;②proportion of sputum culture conversion;③proportion of sputum smear conversion;④proportion of sputum culture conversion;⑤serum 25-hydroxyvitamin D concentration;⑥serum calcium concentration;⑦TB score;⑧chest imaging;⑨Body Mass Index;⑩weight gain;⑪mean mid-upper arm circumference;⑫CRP;⑬ESR;⑭blood cell;⑮adverse effects;⑯mortality. I/C intervention/control, NM not mentioned, No. numbers, * multiply

Table 2 Baseline characteristics of patients in each enrolled trial

Author (Year)	Sex(male/ female)	Age (Years) (mean,SD) (I/C)	Baseline chest radiograph Zones affected number(%)(I/C)	Baseline BMI (mean,SD) (I/C)	Baseline body weight (mean,SD) (I/C)	Baseline TB score (mean,SD) (I/C)	Baseline 25(OH)D (mean,SD) (nmol/L) (I/C)	Baseline calcium concentrations (mean,SD) (I/C)	Baseline CRP(mean,SD) (mg/L)(I/C)	Baseline ESR (mean,SD)(mm/h) (I/C)
Daley 2015 [11]	88/33(I) 101/25(C)	41.6 (15.1)/ 43.7(14.3)	NM	18.0(2.9)/ 17.8(3.0)	NM	NM	63.1(46.6)/ 62.2(51.0)	2.27(0.15)/ 2.28(0.17)	NM	NM
Gannmaa 2016 [12]	123/ 190(I) 133/ 200(C)	31.0 (15.6)/ 35.0(16.3)	7.4(4.4)/7.3(4.4)	19.7(2.8)/ 20.1(3.1)	NM	NM	7.8(11.8)/6.0(7.2)	2.28(0.16)/ 2.26(0.18)	62.7(46.1)/63.0(46.7)	17.2(10.7)/ 15.8(11.3)
Martineau 2011 [13]	14/48(I) 14/50(C)	30.7 (12.6)/ 30.5(10.1)	2.8(1.3)/2.8(1.3)	20.1(3.1)/ 20.2(2.7)	NM	NM	21.1(20.0)/ 21.3(19.0)	2.45(0.08)/ 2.45(0.09)	71.4(49.5)/60.5(45.0)	62.1(23.1)/ 60.9(17.4)
Mily 2015 [14]	36/36(I) 36/36(C)	28.1 (9.9)/26.7(8.1)	NM	NM	44.2(9.4)/ 43.7(7.4)	7.9(5.6)/ 8.0(5.0)	28.0(17.5)/ 28.1(16.2)	8.82(0.55)/ 8.65(0.59)	26.2(0.4)/32.1(0.4)	54.0(31.1)/ 60.2(34.9)
Nursyam 2006 [15]	20/14(I) 19/14(C)	29.9 (11.1)/ 32.6(11.6)	NM	16.9(2.1)/ 17.7(2.5)	NM	NM	NM	9.73(1.28)/ 9.4(0.92)	NM	31.4(5.9)/36.7(6.1)
Salahuddin 2013 [16]	71/61(I) 70/57(C)	27.8 (13.2)/ 28.3(14.1)	3.6(1.4)/3.6(1.5)	17.2(3.5)/ 17.3(4.0)	45.2(7.6)/ 45.6(9.0)	6.7(2.0)/ 6.9(2.5)	20.6(8.5)/ 22.9(10.3)	NM	NM	NM
Tukvadze 2015 [17]	67/33(I) 60/39(C)	34.1 (12.4)/ 32.4(10.6)	NM	NM	NM	NM	NM	2.11(0.3)/ 2.17(0.29)	NM	NM
Wejse 2009 [18]	116/71(I) 106/72(C)	37.0 (13.0)/ 38.0(14.0)	NM	18.8(5.3)/ 18.5(3.8)	51.9(9.4)/ 51.1(8.7)	6.7(2.1)/ 6.8(2.0)	77.5(23.8)/ 79.1(21.8)	2.03(0.26)/ 2.03(0.24)	NM	NM

Data reported in all patients receiving vitamin D supplementation. *BMI* body mass index, *NM* not mentioned, *No.* numbers, *SD* standard derivation, *I/C* intervention/control, *ESR* Erythrocyte sedimentation rate, *CRP* C reactive protein

1.41, $P = 0.51$; OR 1.28, 0.93~ 1.76, $P = 0.13$; OR 1.30, 0.89~ 1.90, $P = 0.17$; and OR 0.93, 0.39~ 2.22, $P = 0.87$) (Fig. 3).

Time to sputum conversion Neither time to sputum smear conversion (HR 1.07, 0.83~ 1.37, $P = 0.62$) nor time to culture conversion (HR 0.97, 0.76~ 1.23, $P = 0.77$) was found with a statistical significance in vitamin D arm compared with the placebo arm (Figs. 4 and 5).

Secondary outcomes

Hematology indexes We found significant differences in increase in serum 25(OH)D concentrations from baseline in 2, 4, 6, 8, 12, 16, and 24 weeks and in the overall effects (MD 103.52, 41.34~ 165.70, $P = 0.001$; MD 116.85, 60.55~ 173.16, $P < 0.0001$; MD 128.90, 124.09~ 133.71, $P < 0.00001$;MD 125.66, 76.61~ 174.72, $P < 0.00001$;MD 83.42, 26.26~ 140.58, $P = 0.004$;MD 82.51, 69.47~ 95.55, $P < 0.00001$;MD 26.50, 12.81~ 40.19,

$P = 0.0001$;MD 103.36, 84.20~ 122.53, $P < 0.00001$) (Additional file 13: Figure S13).

Meanwhile, significant improvements in plasma calcium concentrations were found in the overall effects and between 4 and 6 weeks (SMD 0.26, 0.15~ 0.37, $P < 0.00001$;SMD 0.23, 0.04~ 0.43, $P = 0.02$;SMD 0.47, 0.30~ 0.65, $P < 0.00001$), but null in 2, 8, and 12 weeks (SMD 0.26, – 0.20~ 0.72, $P = 0.27$;SMD 0.24, – 0.01~ 0.48, $P = 0.06$;SMD 0.11, – 0.25~ 0.46, $P = 0.56$) (Additional file 14: Figure S14).

Significant differences were found in CRP in 2 and 6 weeks (MD 9.50, 1.94~ 17.06, $P = 0.01$;MD -7.20, – 12.79~ – 1.61,P = 0.01), but none in 4, 8, and 12 weeks and in the overall effects (MD -9.55, – 30.51~ 11.42, $P = 0.37$;MD -1.70, – 4.20~ 0.80, $P = 0.18$;MD -0.60, – 2.61~ 1.41, P = 0.56;MD -2.92, – 10.43~ 4.59, $P = 0.45$) (Additional file 4: Figure S4).

A non-significant difference was found in ESR in 2, 4, 6, 8, and 24 weeks and in the overall effects (MD 0.30, – 2.01~ 2.61, $P = 0.80$;MD 1.21, – 0.86~ 3.27, $P = 0.25$;MD -0.60, – 2.78~ 1.58, $P = 0.59$;MD 0.62, – 1.28~

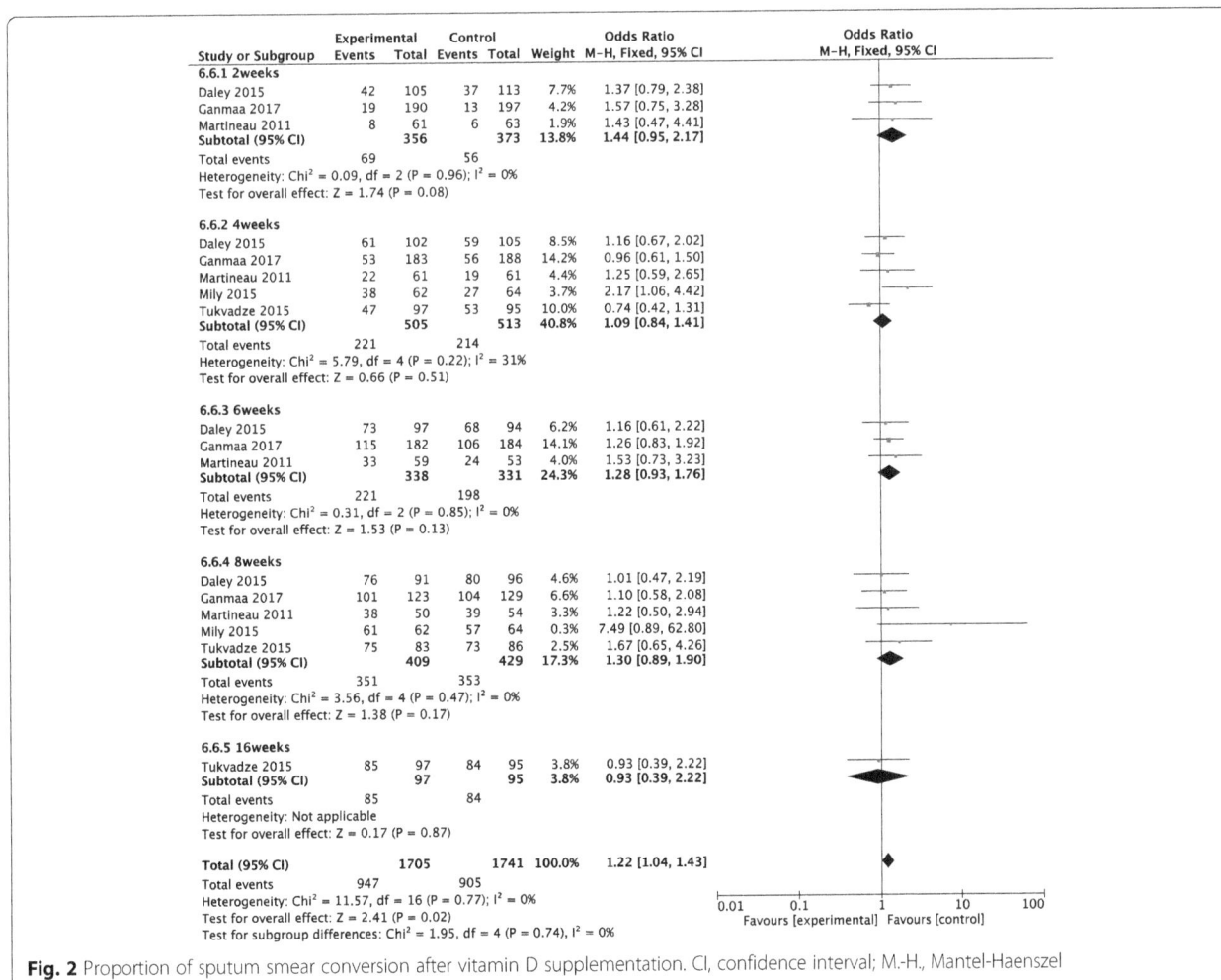

Fig. 2 Proportion of sputum smear conversion after vitamin D supplementation. CI, confidence interval; M.-H., Mantel-Haenszel

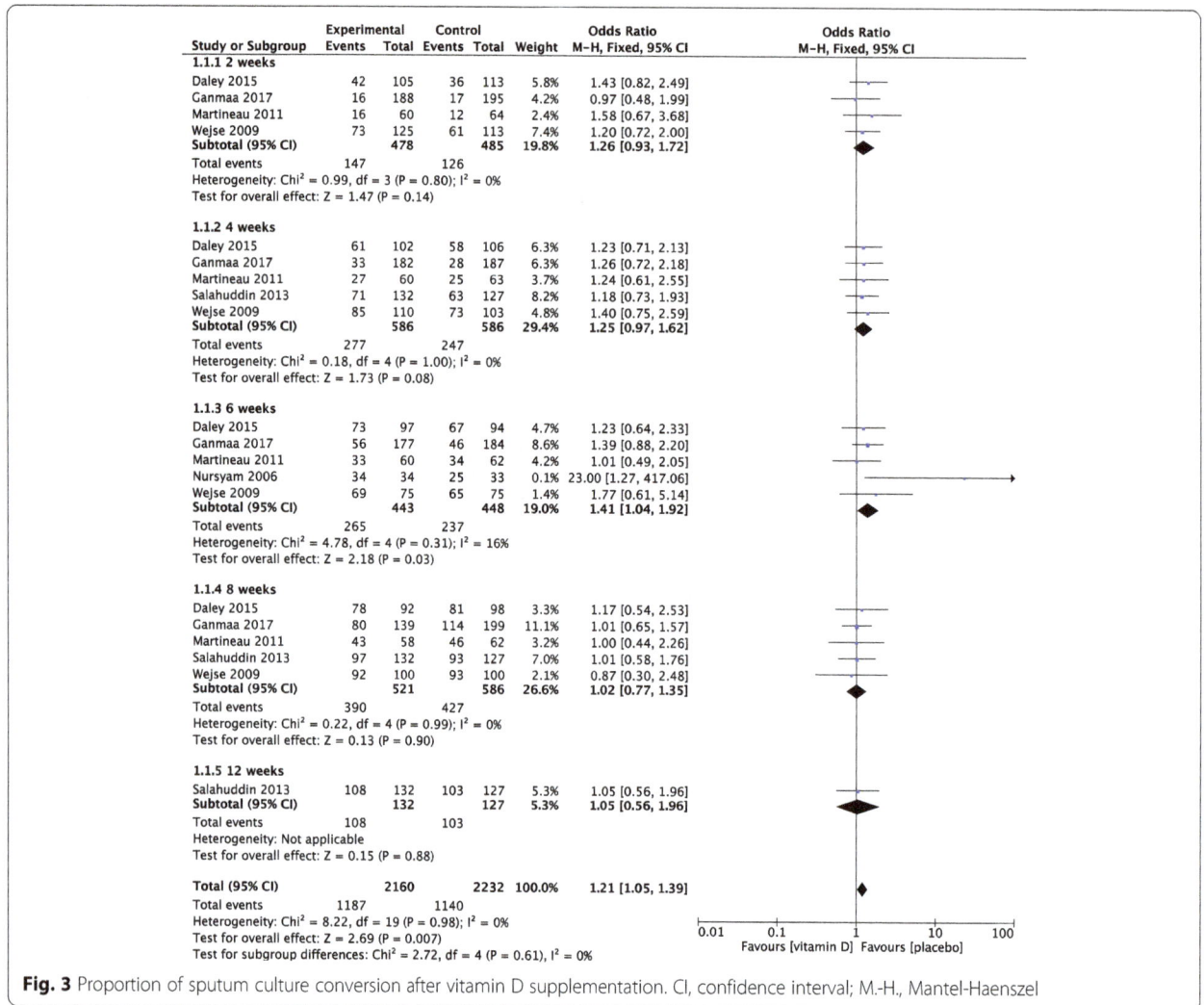

Fig. 3 Proportion of sputum culture conversion after vitamin D supplementation. CI, confidence interval; M.-H., Mantel-Haenszel

2.53, $P = 0.52$;MD -1.90, − 8.68~ 4.88, $P = 0.58$;MD 0.37, − 0.67~ 1.41, $P = 0.48$) (Additional file 5: Figure S5).

No significant difference was found in mutation in total white blood cells in 2, 4, 6, 8, and 24 weeks and in the overall effects (MD 0.40, − 0.24~ 1.04, $P = 0.22$;MD 0.20, − 0.37~ 0.77, $P = 0.49$;MD -0.20, − 0.80~ 0.40, $P = 0.51$;MD -0.29, − 0.97~ 0.40, $P = 0.41$;MD 0.32, − 0.52~ 1.16, $P = 0.46$;MD -0.02, − 0.36~ 0.32, $P = 0.91$) (Additional file 6: Figure S6).

Additionally, there was no significant difference in the changes in neutrophil count in 2, 4, 6, 8, and 24 weeks and in the overall effects (MD 0.30, − 0.31~ 0.91, $P = 0.33$;MD -0.02, − 0.33~ 0.28, $P = 0.88$;MD -0.30, − 0.87~ 0.27, $P = 0.30$;MD -0.41, − 0.92~ 0.11, $P = 0.12$;MD 0.21, − 0.19~ 0.61, $P = 0.31$;MD -0.13, − 0.42~ 0.16, $P = 0.38$) (Additional file 19: Figure S19).

No significant difference was found in alteration in monocyte count in 2, 4, 6, 8, and 24 weeks and in the

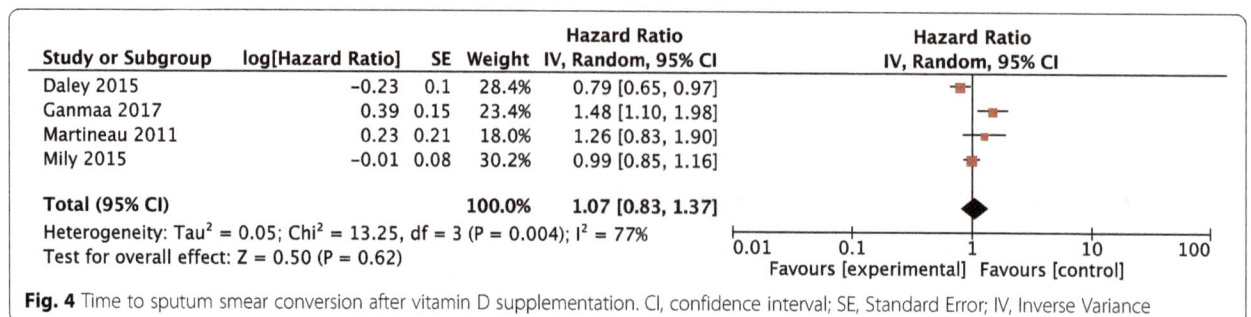

Fig. 4 Time to sputum smear conversion after vitamin D supplementation. CI, confidence interval; SE, Standard Error; IV, Inverse Variance

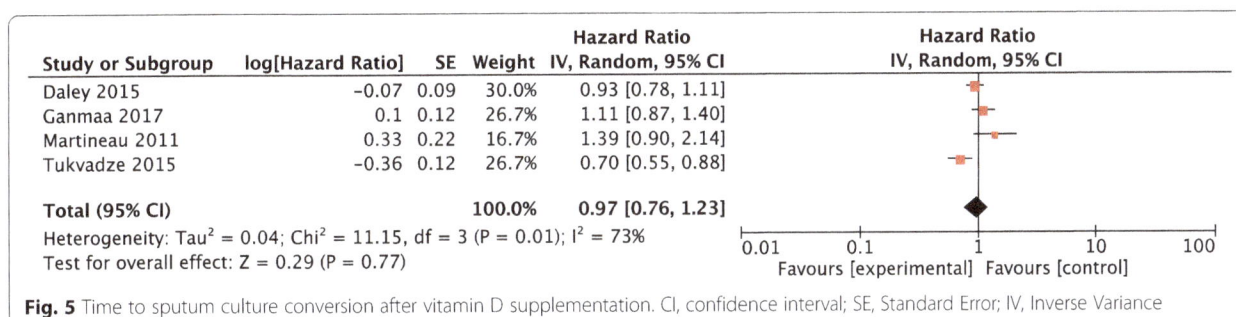

Study or Subgroup	log[Hazard Ratio]	SE	Weight	Hazard Ratio IV, Random, 95% CI	Hazard Ratio IV, Random, 95% CI
Daley 2015	-0.07	0.09	30.0%	0.93 [0.78, 1.11]	
Ganmaa 2017	0.1	0.12	26.7%	1.11 [0.87, 1.40]	
Martineau 2011	0.33	0.22	16.7%	1.39 [0.90, 2.14]	
Tukvadze 2015	-0.36	0.12	26.7%	0.70 [0.55, 0.88]	
Total (95% CI)			**100.0%**	**0.97 [0.76, 1.23]**	

Heterogeneity: Tau^2 = 0.04; Chi^2 = 11.15, df = 3 (P = 0.01); I^2 = 73%
Test for overall effect: Z = 0.29 (P = 0.77)

Fig. 5 Time to sputum culture conversion after vitamin D supplementation. CI, confidence interval; SE, Standard Error; IV, Inverse Variance

overall effects (MD 0.05, – 0.01~ 0.11, P = 0.13;MD -0.01, – 0.06~ 0.04, P = 0.78;MD -0.04, – 0.01~ 0.02, P = 0.20;MD -0.04, – 0.12~ 0.04, P = 0.36;MD -0.04, – 0.15~ 0.07, P = 0.47;MD -0.02, – 0.05~ 0.02, P = 0.34) (Additional file 7: Figure S7).

A significant difference was found in the change in lymphocyte count in 4 weeks and in the overall effects (MD 0.22, 0.10~ 0.34, P = 0.0003;MD 0.09, 0.03~ 0.14, P = 0.003), while the results in 2, 6, 8, and 24 weeks (MD 0.00, – 0.12~ 0.12, P = 1.00;MD 0.10, – 0.03~ 0.23, P = 0.13;MD 0.05, – 0.06~ 0.15, P = 0.36;MD 0.02, – 0.37~ 0.41, P = 0.92) were on the contrary (Additional file 8: Figure S8).

Imaging index A significant improvement in the chest radiograph (mean no. of zones involved) was detected in vitamin D arm compared with the placebo arm (MD -0.33, – 0.57~ – 0.08, P = 0.01) (Additional file 3: Figure S3).

Clinical indexes No significant improvement was found in TB score in 8 weeks and 5, 6, and 8 months (MD -0.01, – 0.23~ 0.22, P = 0.98; MD -0.09, – 0.26~ 0.08, P = 0.29; MD 0.01, – 1.69~ 1.71, P = 0.99; MD -0.18, – 0.36~ 0.00, P = 0.05; MD -0.21, – 0.44~ 0.01, P = 0.07), except 12 weeks (MD -1.18, – 1.78~ 0.59, P < 0.0001) (Additional file 15: Figure S15). No significant difference was found in the change in hemoglobin levels in 4, 8, and 24 weeks and in the overall effects (MD -0.13, – 0.77~ 0.51, P = 0.69; MD -0.10, – 0.51~ 0.31, P = 0.64; MD -0.25, – 0.96~ 0.46, P = 0.49; MD -0.13, – 0.45~ 0.18, P = 0.40) (Additional file 9: Figure S9). An insignificant improvement was found in the anthropometric outcomes: BMI, weight gain and mean mid-upper arm circumference (MD 0.33, – 1.58~ 2.24, P = 0.74; SMD 0.04, – 0.15~ 0.24, P = 0.68; MD 0.07, – 0.78~ 0.92, P = 0.88) (Additional file 16: Figure S16, Additional file 17: Figure S17, Additional file 18: Figure S18).

Safety and mortality Pooled analysis showed that no significant difference was found in the number of non-serious adverse events, serious adverse events, and all-cause deaths (OR 1.06, 0.65~ 1.74, P = 0.80; OR 1.02, 0.48~ 2.20, P = 0.95; OR 1.22, 0.74~ 2.04, P = 0.43)

(Additional file 10: Figure S10, Additional file 11: Figure S11, Additional file 12: Figure S12).

Discussion

This is the largest and the most comprehensive meta-analysis to investigate the effects of adjunctive vitamin D on patients with PTB currently. In this meta-analysis, we found that vitamin D could increase the proportion of sputum smear and culture conversion, but was unable to shorten the time to sputum smear and culture conversion. An increase in lymphocyte count, serum 25(OH)D, and plasma calcium concentrations and improvement in chest radiograph were observed after vitamin D supplementation. There was no evidence of improvement of other parameters (TB score, BMI, mean mid-upper arm circumference, weight gain, CRP, ESR, and blood indexes) in the vitamin D arm. No significant difference was found in the safety (non-serious and serious adverse events) and mortality (all-cause deaths) between two groups.

The results of this meta-analysis are inconsistent with those of previous meta-analyses, showing that vitamin D supplementation safely and effectively increases the proportion of sputum smear and culture conversion. A meta-analysis that included four trials did not show any improvement in the clinical parameters of the participants in the vitamin D arm compared with those in the placebo arm (P = 0.05) [7]. Unfortunately, no further information was obtained from this congress literature after contacting the corresponding author. Another meta-analysis, which included five studies (one study aimed at children) with 841 participants, showed that vitamin D supplementation does not have any beneficial effects on improving sputum smear and culture conversion, adverse effects, and body weight [8]. These two meta-analyses had limited number of studies, sample sizes, and parameters analyzed, influencing the results.

Vitamin D supplementation as adjunctive therapy had no impact on the time to sputum smear or culture conversion, the latter is recognized as a surrogate endpoint for treatment failure and relapse in patients with TB [19], despite the increase in the proportion of sputum smear and culture conversion. Thus, more rigorous and larger scale RCTs should be conducted to further verify this problem.

Besides, we detected whether adjunctive vitamin D exhibited anti-inflammatory actions on influencing the peripheral blood parameters. A significant increase in lymphocyte count was observed in the vitamin D arm, but null was found in total white blood cell count, neutrophil count, monocyte count, CRP, and ESR. The lymphocyte: monocyte ratio was verified as a biomarker of pulmonary inflammation resolution in an animal model of TB [20]. Coussens et al. [21] found that adjunctive vitamin D therapy accelerated sputum smear conversion as well as enhanced resolution of lymphopaenia and monocytosis in PTB patients. In our meta-analysis, improvements of sputum conversion and lymphocyte: monocyte ratio were compliance with previous studies. These findings propose a potential effect of vitamin D supplementation on accelerating resolution of inflammatory responses during tuberculosis therapy. Thus, we speculated that the modest immune modulatory effect of vitamin D might have a preventing role on TB [22]; this hypothesis is being solved by two ongoing clinical trials [23, 24].

Statistical differences in the improvement of chest imaging were observed between groups, but studies included in the analysis are less. However, this result needs to be verified further. A non-statistical difference in BMI, weight gain, mean mid-upper arm circumference, hemoglobin, and TB scores was observed among patients receiving vitamin D supplements compared with those in the placebo group. The indicator for weight gain used in this study was consistent with that in the previous meta-analyses.

Based on the presently available studies, serum 25(OH)D and plasma calcium concentrations returned to normal after vitamin D administration. The mostly reported non-serious adverse event is hypocalcemia. Adverse events and all-cause deaths were evenly distributed between the vitamin D and placebo groups. Results confirmed that vitamin D supplementation is safe and effective. These findings are accord with previous meta-analyses.

This study has several strengths. Our meta-analysis has the largest number of studies and participants currently, and the studies included were of high quality. This study is the first meta-analysis to examine the effects of vitamin D supplementation on the time to sputum smear or culture conversion; the latter was considered a surrogate endpoint for treatment failure and relapse [19]. Besides, 25(OH)D concentration was measured using validated assays in laboratories. The proportion of missing outcome data was small and similar in both groups. Therefore, our findings have a high degree of validity.

This study has some limitations. The administration doses of vitamin D, duration of treatment, and follow-up time were different. Heterogeneity was found in some analyses (serum 25(OH)D, plasma calcium concentration, BMI, weight gain, TB score, mean mid-upper arm circumference, and neutrophil count). For small number of published RCTs, power of some analyses was limited. These may affect the accuracy of analysis results.

Genetic variation in the gene encoding the vitamin D receptor (vitamin D receptor polymorphisms) may modify the effects of adjunctive vitamin D in PTB. Jolliffe et al. [25] suggested that single nucleotide polymorphisms(SNPs) in special gene in the vitamin D pathway have an influence on disease outcomes. Ganmaa et al. [12] showed that vitamin D_3 did not improve time to sputum culture conversion overall, but significant difference was found in patients with one or more minor alleles for SNPs. So, we speculate that vitamin D receptor polymorphisms may affect the effects of vitamin D adjunctive treatment. But unfortunately, we cannot do subgroup analysis in our meta-analysis with insufficient data of relevant studies.

For low cost of this intervention and major economic burden of PTB, vitamin D is regarded as a cost-effective adjunctive therapy.

Conclusions

In conclusion, vitamin D supplementation can safely and effectively increase the proportion of sputum smear and culture conversion, but it may not have enough beneficial effects on time to sputum conversion. As this intervention is safe and low cost, it is considered a cost-effective strategy in treating patients with PTB. Thus, future rigorous RCTs are needed, particularly with different vitamin D dose, treatment duration, and follow-up based on vitamin D receptor polymorphisms and severities of diseases, to further determine the role of vitamin D in patients with PTB.

Additional files

Additional file 1: Figure S1. Risk of bias graph. (PDF 80 kb)

Additional file 2: Figure S2. Risk of bias summary. (PDF 96 kb)

Additional file 3: Figure S3. Change of chest radiograph after vitamin D supplementation. CI, confidence interval; SD, standard derivation; IV, Inverse Variance. (PDF 101 kb)

Additional file 4: Figure S4. Change of CRP after vitamin D supplementation. CI, confidence interval; SD, standard derivation; IV, Inverse Variance. (PDF 311 kb)

Additional file 5: Figure S5. Change of ESR after vitamin D supplementation. CI, confidence interval; SD, standard derivation; IV, Inverse Variance. (PDF 102 kb)

Additional file 6: Figure S6. Change of white blood cell count after vitamin D supplementation. CI, confidence interval; SD, standard derivation; IV, Inverse Variance. (PDF 302 kb)

Additional file 7: Figure S7. Change of monocyte count after vitamin D supplementation. CI, confidence interval; SD, standard derivation; IV, Inverse Variance. (PDF 301 kb)

Additional file 8: Figure S8. Change of lymphocyte count after vitamin D supplementation. CI, confidence interval; SD, standard derivation; IV, Inverse Variance. (PDF 293 kb)

Additional file 9: Figure S9. Change of hemoglobin count after vitamin D supplementation. CI, confidence interval; SD, standard derivation; IV, Inverse Variance. (PDF 195 kb)

Additional file 10: Figure S10. Non-serious adverse events after vitamin D supplementation. CI, confidence interval; M.-H., Mantel-Haenszel. (PDF 91 kb)

Additional file 11: Figure S11. Serious adverse events after vitamin D supplementation. CI, confidence interval; M.-H., Mantel-Haenszel. (PDF 110 kb)

Additional file 12: Figure S12. All-cause deaths after vitamin D supplementation. CI, confidence interval; M.-H., Mantel-Haenszel. (PDF 124 kb)

Additional file 13: Figure S13 Serum 25(OH)D concentration after vitamin D supplementation. CI, confidence interval; SD, standard derivation; IV, Inverse Variance. (PDF 502 kb)

Additional file 14: Figure S14. Plasma calcium concentration after vitamin D supplementation. CI, confidence interval; SD, standard derivation; IV, Inverse Variance. (PDF 399 kb)

Additional file 15: Figure S15. TB score after vitamin D supplementation. CI, confidence interval; SD, standard derivation; IV, Inverse Variance. (PDF 291 kb)

Additional file 16: Figure S16. Change of Body-Mass Index after vitamin D supplementation. CI, confidence interval; SD, standard derivation; IV, Inverse Variance. (PDF 116 kb)

Additional file 17: Figure S17. Weight gain after vitamin D supplementation. CI, confidence interval; SD, standard derivation; IV, Inverse Variance. (PDF 141 kb)

Additional file 18: Figure S18. Change of Mean Mid-Upper Arm Circumference after vitamin D supplementation. CI, confidence interval; SD, standard derivation; IV, Inverse Variance. (PDF 92 kb)

Additional file 19: Figure S19. Change of neutrophil count after vitamin D supplementation. CI, confidence interval; SD, standard derivation; IV, Inverse Variance. (PDF 297 kb)

Acknowledgements
We thank all the people who participated in the primary randomized controlled trials and the teams who did them.

Funding
The authors declare that no funding was received for this work.

Authors' contributions
H-XW and D-YC initiated and coordinated the study. X-FX, MZ, JW and K-QZ were responsible for the data collection and data analysis. Studies were reviewed by D-YC. H-XW wrote the first draft of the manuscript. All authors read and approved the final manuscript.

Competing interests
The authors declare that they have no competing interests.

Author details
[1]Department of Respiratory and Critical Care Medicine, West China Hospital, Sichuan University, NO.37 Guoxue Alley, Chengdu 610041, Sichuan, China. [2]Department of Respiratory Medicine, Chengdu Second People's Hospital, Chengdu, China. [3]Department of Neurosurgery, Suining Municipal Hospital of TCM, Suining, China.

References
1. World Health Organization. Global tuberculosis report 2017. www.who.int/tb/publications/global_report/en/. Accessed 9 Nov 2017.
2. Martineau AR, Nhamoyebonde S, Oni T. Reciprocal seasonal variation in vitamin D status and tuberculosis notifications in cape town, South Africa. Proc Natl Acad Sci U S A. 2011;108:19013–7.
3. Maclachlan JH, Lavender CJ, Cowie BC. Effect of latitude on seasonality of tuberculosis, Australia, 2002-2011. Emerg Infect Dis. 2012;18:1879–81.
4. Nnoaham KE, Clarke A. Low serum vitamin D levels and tuberculosis: a systematic review and meta-analysis. Int J Epidemiol. 2008;37:113–9.
5. Williams C. Cod liver oil in phthisis. Lond J Med. 1849;1:1–18.
6. Martineau AR. Old wine in new bottles: vitamin D in the treatment and prevention of tuberculosis. Proc Nutr Soc. 2012;71:84–9.
7. Haris R, Irbaz R, Tanvir A, Maaz B, Abul M. Vitamin D as a supplementary agent in the treatment of pulmonary tuberculosis: a systematic review and meta-analysis of randomized controlled trials. European Respiratory Society annual congress 2013. Eur Respir J. 2013;42:4623.
8. Xia J, Shi L, Zhao L, Xu F. Impact of vitamin D supplementation on the outcome of tuberculosis treatment: a systematic review and meta-analysis of randomized controlled trials. Chin Med J. 2014;127:3127–34.
9. Higgins JP, Green S. Cochrane Handbook for Systematic Reviews of Interventions Version 5.3.0. Oxford: The Cochrane Collaboration, 2014. Updated March 2014. www.cochrane-handbook.org. Accessed 9 Nov 2017.
10. Guyatt GH, Oxman AD, Vist GE, Kunz R, Falck-Ytter Y, Alonso-Coello P, et al. GRADE: an emerging consensus on rating quality of evidence and strength of recommendations. BMJ. 2008;336:924–6.
11. Daley P, Jagannathan V, John KR, Sarojini J, Latha A, Vieth R, et al. Adjunctive vitamin D for treatment of active tuberculosis in India: a randomised, double-blind, placebo-controlled trial. Lancet Infect Dis. 2015;15:528–34.
12. Ganmaa D, Munkhzul B, Fawzi W, Spiegelman D, Willett WC, Bayasgalan P, et al. High-dose vitamin D3 during tuberculosis treatment in Mongolia: a randomised controlled trial. Am J Respir Crit Care Med. 2017;196:628–37.
13. Martineau AR, Hanifa Y, Islam K. High-dose vitamin D3 during intensive phase treatment of pulmonary tuberculosis: a double-blind randomised controlled trial. Lancet. 2011;377:242–50.
14. Mily A, Rekha RS, Kamal SM, Arifuzzaman AS, Rahim Z, Khan L, et al. Significant effects of oral Phenylbutyrate and vitamin D3 adjunctive therapy in pulmonary tuberculosis: a randomized controlled trial. PLoS One. 2015;10:e0138340.
15. Nursyam EW, Amin Z, Rumende CM. The effect of vitamin D as supplementary treatment in patients with moderately advanced pulmonary tuberculous lesion. Acta Med Indones. 2006;38:3–5.
16. Salahuddin N, Ali F, Hasan Z, Rao N, Aqeel M, Mahmood F. Vitamin D accelerates clinical recovery from tuberculosis: results of the SUCCINCT study [supplementary cholecalciferol in recovery from tuberculosis]. A randomized, placebo-controlled, clinical trial of vitamin D supplementation in patients with pulmonary tuberculosis. BMC Infect Dis. 2013;13:22.
17. Tukvadze N, Sanikidze E, Kipiani M, Hebbar G, Easley KA, Shenvi N, et al. High-dose vitamin D3 in adults with pulmonary tuberculosis: a double-blind randomized controlled trial. Am J Clin Nutr. 2015;102:1059–69.
18. Wejse C, Gomes VF, Rabna P, Gustafson P, Aaby P, Lisse IM, et al. Vitamin D as supplementary treatment for tuberculosis: a double-blind, randomized, placebo-controlled trial. Am J Respir Crit Care Med. 2009;179:843–50.
19. Phillips PP, Fielding K, Nunn AJ. An evaluation of culture results during treatment for tuberculosis as surrogate endpoints for treatment failure and relapse. PLoS One. 2013;8:e638r40.
20. Sabin FR, Doan CA, Cunningham RS. Studies of the blood in experimental tuberculosis: the monocyte-lymphocyte ratio; the anemia-leucopenia phase. Trans Ann Meet Natl Tuberc Assoc. 1926;22:252–6.
21. Coussens AK, Wilkinson RJ, Hanifa Y, Nikolayevskyy V, Elkington PT, Islam K, et al. Vitamin D accelerates resolution of inflammatory responses during tuberculosis treatment. PNAS. 2012;109:15449–54.
22. Davies PD, Martineau AR. Vitamin D and tuberculosis: more effective in prevention than treatment? Int J Tuberc Lung Dis. 2015;19:876–7.
23. Ganmaa D, Martineau AR. Trial of vitamin D supplementation to prevent acquisition of latent M. tuberculosis infection in Mongolian primary schoolchildren. 2015. Available from: https://clinicaltrials.gov/ct2/show/NCT02276755
24. Martineau AR, Middelkoop K. Trial of vitamin D supplementation in Cape Town primary schoolchildren. 2016. Available from: https://clinicaltrials.gov/ct2/show/NCT02880982

8

Activation and polarization of circulating monocytes in severe chronic obstructive pulmonary disease

William D. Cornwell[1,2]*, Victor Kim[2], Xiaoxuan Fan[3], Marie Elena Vega[2], Frederick V. Ramsey[4], Gerard J. Criner[1,2] and Thomas J. Rogers[1,2] (iD)

Abstract

Background: The ability of circulating monocytes to develop into lung macrophages and promote lung tissue damage depends upon their phenotypic pattern of differentiation and activation. Whether this phenotypic pattern varies with COPD severity is unknown. Here we characterize the activation and differentiation status of circulating monocytes in patients with moderate vs. severe COPD.

Methods: Blood monocytes were isolated from normal non-smokers (14), current smokers (13), patients with moderate (9), and severe COPD (11). These cells were subjected to analysis by flow cytometry to characterize the expression of activation markers, chemoattractant receptors, and surface markers characteristic of either M1- or M2-type macrophages.

Results: Patients with severe COPD had increased numbers of total circulating monocytes and non-classical patrolling monocytes, compared to normal subjects and patients with moderate COPD. In addition, while the percentage of circulating monocytes that expressed an M2-like phenotype was reduced in patients with either moderate or severe disease, the levels of expression of M2 markers on this subpopulation of monocytes in severe COPD was significantly elevated. This was particularly evident for the expression of the chemoattractant receptor CCR5.

Conclusions: Blood monocytes in severe COPD patients undergo unexpected pre-differentiation that is largely characteristic of M2-macrophage polarization, leading to the emergence of an unusual M2-like monocyte population with very high levels of CCR5. These results show that circulating monocytes in patients with severe COPD possess a cellular phenotype which may permit greater mobilization to the lung, with a pre-existing bias toward a potentially destructive inflammatory phenotype.

Keywords: COPD, Systemic inflammation, Polarization, Monocyte activation

Background

Several studies have shown that the numbers of lung macrophages are increased in patients with Chronic Obstructive Pulmonary Disease (COPD), and lung macrophage numbers increase in proportion to disease severity [1–5]. It is believed that many resident macrophages in the lungs, including those macrophages in the alveolar compartment, are derived from fetal progenitors, and

are self-renewing in the lung tissue [6–9]. However, more recent evidence shows that the extravasation of monocytes into the lungs initiates differentiation of these cells into new macrophages, and these differentiated cells can persist in the lung tissue for the life span of the animal [10]. These recent immigrant macrophages can mature (or polarize) into distinct macrophage sub-populations with divergent functional activities. The M1 (classically activated) phenotype produces high levels of several pro-inflammatory cytokines [11, 12], while the M2 (alternatively activated) phenotype express high levels of mannose receptors (CD206), scavenger receptors (including CD163), IL-10, and fibronectin. The M2 cells can promote

* Correspondence: cornwell@temple.edu
[1]Center for Inflammation, Translational and Clinical Lung Research, Lewis Katz School of Medicine, Temple University, Philadelphia, PA 19140, USA
[2]Department of Thoracic Medicine and Surgery, Lewis Katz School of Medicine, Temple University, Philadelphia, PA 19140, USA
Full list of author information is available at the end of the article

tissue fibrosis, in part, due to the expression of pro-fibrotic proteins such as fibronectin [13]. It should be pointed out that these phenotypes may actually represent two maturation stages on opposite sides of a continuum of functional capabilities.

Distinct sub-populations of monocytes can be distinguished by the expression of the surface markers CD14 and CD16. The CD14 + CD16- "classical" monocytes are considered pro-inflammatory, while the CD14 + CD16+ intermediate and CD14^{DIM} CD16+ "non-classical" cells play a role in tissue repair [14, 15]. Non-classical monocytes (5–8% of blood monocytes) expand substantially in individuals following infection or other inflammatory stimuli [16–18]. The classical monocytes are selectively recruited to inflamed tissues and lymph nodes and produce high levels of the pro-inflammatory cytokines [19]. In contrast, the non-classical monocytes, interact strongly with the luminal surface of vascular endothelial cells, and patrol the endothelial cell surface to scavenge dead cells, and certain infectious agents [14].

The non-classical monocytes remain in blood vessels until they encounter inflamed tissue, where they may extravasate [14, 20], while classical monocytes transition into and out of tissues in the absence of apparent inflammation. These monocytes continuously patrol blood vessels and most tissues, until the appropriate tissue signals are present, the cells immigrate to the lungs, and the monocyte-to-macrophage program may be initiated. Previous evidence has suggested that macrophage polarization occurs only after maturation following tissue extravasation [11, 12].

The M2 macrophage phenotype is particularly significant in the setting of COPD, since these cells can promote inappropriate tissue remodeling and fibrosis, and are believed to contribute to tissue damage in COPD [21–24]. We examined the monocytes in patients with moderate and severe COPD to determine whether these cells express markers indicative of either the M1 or M2 phenotype, and whether COPD severity varies with the pattern of phenotypic expression. We show that patients with severe COPD have unusually elevated levels of the activation marker CCR5 and M2-like markers. We propose that these populations of monocytes likely give rise to disease-promoting lung macrophages in severe COPD.

Methods
Subject selection
Subjects with moderate to severe COPD, current smokers without airflow obstruction (healthy smokers), and healthy nonsmokers were recruited. This study was conducted in accordance with the amended Declaration of Helsinki. Institutional Review Board approval was obtained from the Temple University Institutional Review Board, protocol 20,567, and all subjects signed written informed consent. COPD subjects were selected with an FEV$_1$ between 30 and 60% predicted. Healthy smokers were currently smoking, had no airflow obstruction, and had a smoking history ≥ 10 pack-years. Subjects with allergic rhinitis, acute or chronic sinusitis, upper respiratory tract infection, or COPD exacerbation ≤ 6 weeks of the screening visit were excluded. To reduce the effects of steroids, subjects receiving inhaled or oral steroids discontinued use > 4 weeks prior to enrollment. A summary of the subject demographics is presented in Table 1.

Isolation of PBMCs
Venous blood was collected into vacutainers containing EDTA. The blood was layered onto Ficoll Hypaque (GE Healthcare) and centrifuged to separate the PBMCs and plasma. PBMCs were collected, washed with HBSS, and stained for flow cytometric analysis.

Analysis of PBMCs by flow cytometry
PBMC's (1 million) were resuspended in FACS staining buffer (BD Biosciences) and blocked with human IgG (Sigma; 20μg) for 30 min on ice. Cells were washed and resuspended in FACS buffer containing a combination of antibodies including CD3-V500 (BD Biosciences; clone UCHT1), CD14-QDot605 (Life Technologies; clone Tü K4), CD16-V450 (BD Biosciences; clone 3G8), CD163-PE (Trillium; clone MAC2–158), CD206-APC-Cy7 (Biolegend; clone 15–2), CD25-Alexa700 (Biolegend; clone BC 96), CCR2-Alexa647 (BD Biosciences; clone 48,607), CCR5-PE-Cy7 (BD Biosciences; clone 2D7/CCR5), IL13 Rα1-PerCP-Cy5.5 (R&D Systems; clone 419,718), and CX3CR1-FITC (MBL International; clone 2A9–1) and incubated on ice for 30 min. Cells were washed with FACS buffer followed by centrifugation. Cells were resuspended in 2% paraformaldehyde and incubated on ice for 10 min. Cells were centrifuged and resuspended in FACS buffer for acquisition of events using and LSRII cytometer (BD Biosciences).

Cytometer Setup & Tracking, as well as mid-range ("rainbow") beads (BD Biosciences) were used daily to calibrate the instrument. In addition, compensation adjustment for each channel was performed using single stained compensation beads (BD Biosciences). At least, 250,000 events were acquired per sample using BD FACSDIVA v6.1.3 software. Debris and dead cells were gated out using forward and side light scatter. The gating strategy for the flow cytometry is presented (Additional file 1: Fig. S1).

Statistical analysis
Monocyte means (expressed as concentrations, percentages, or fluorescence intensity) for the normal, smoker, and moderate and severe COPD groups were

Table 1 Demographic data for the study subjects

	Age (years)	Gender (M/F)	Race (AA/C/H/As)	Pack-Years	FEV$_1$ (% Pred)	FEV1/FVC	Current Smoke (Y/N)
Normal	50 (2.0)	9/5	1/10/1/2	N/A	88.1 (2.9)	81.4 (4.1)	0/14
Smoker	49.6 (1.5)	4/9	11/2/0/0	26.4 (3.1)	101.9 (4.6)	96.4 (1.8)	13/0
COPD – M	59.9 (3.9)	5/4	8/1/0/0	29.6 (7.9)	55.1 (1.6)	56.6 (3.7)	6/3
COPD – S	62.3 (2.3)	10/1	10/1/0/0	39.9 (5.6)	36.6 (1.7)	38.6 (3.1)	2/11

FEV$_1$ = Forced Expiratory Volume in 1 s
FVC = Forced Vital Capacity

compared using one-way ANOVA. To adjust for multiple comparisons, post-hoc comparisons were pre-planned and limited to three pair-wise comparisons of normal (as the control group) to smoker, to moderate COPD, and to severe COPD. Adjusted p-values were calculated using Dunnett's method. For patients with COPD, relationships of patient data (i.e., spirometry or pack-years) and monocyte fluorescence intensity were assessed using univariate linear regression, where data for the moderate and severe COPD groups were aggregated and analyzed as a combined COPD group. All analyses were performed using SAS 9.4. Statistical significance was defined as $p < 0.05$.

Results

The numbers of classical and non-classical blood monocytes are altered in severe COPD

We used flow cytometry to evaluate the numbers of monocytes in the peripheral blood of normal subjects, current smokers without COPD, and both moderate and severe COPD. Flow cytometric analysis of the monocytes, based on CD14 and CD16 staining, demonstrates the typical pattern of classical (CD14 + 16-), intermediate (CD14 + 16+) and non-classical (CD14^{DIM}16+) populations (Fig. 1). Analysis of the data (Fig. 2) show that there was a statistically significant increase in the number of total monocytes in patients with severe COPD, but no

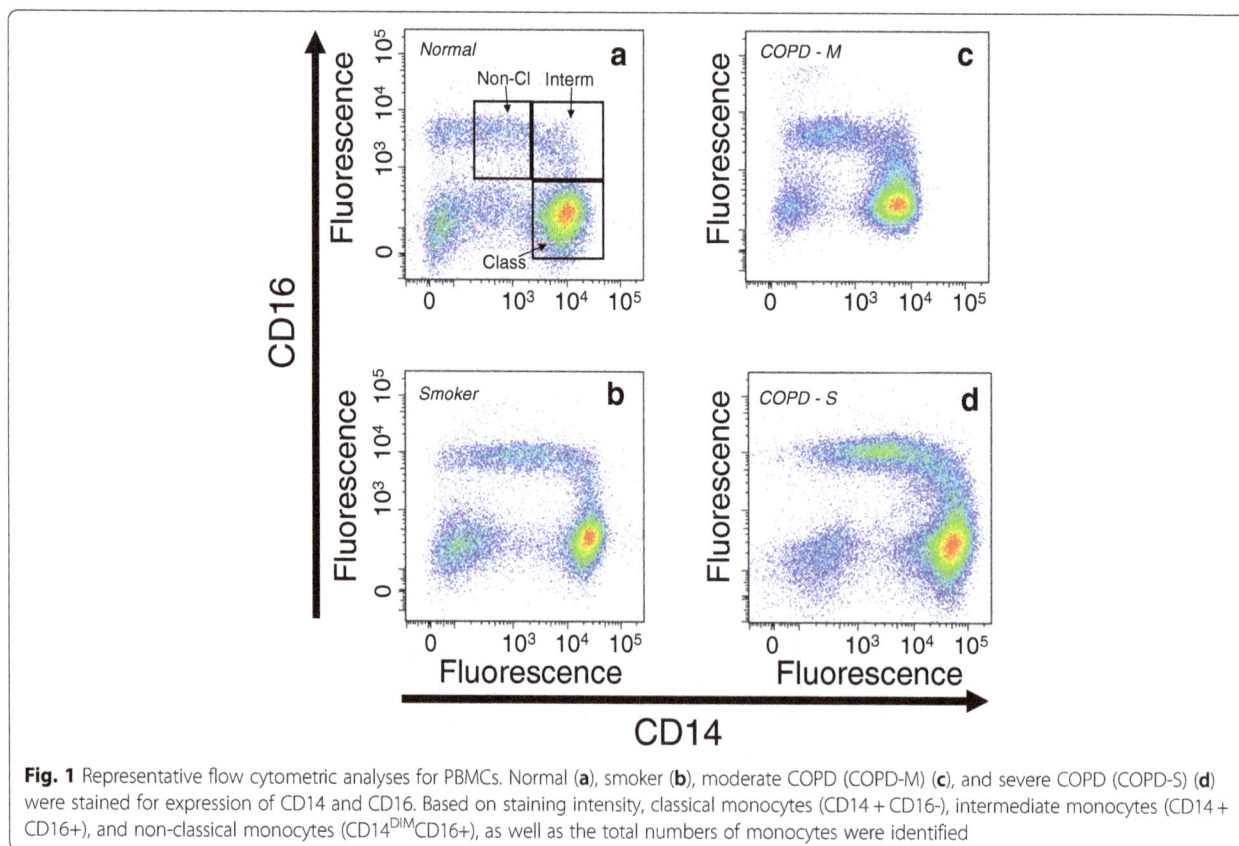

Fig. 1 Representative flow cytometric analyses for PBMCs. Normal (**a**), smoker (**b**), moderate COPD (COPD-M) (**c**), and severe COPD (COPD-S) (**d**) were stained for expression of CD14 and CD16. Based on staining intensity, classical monocytes (CD14 + CD16-), intermediate monocytes (CD14 + CD16+), and non-classical monocytes (CD14^{DIM}CD16+), as well as the total numbers of monocytes were identified

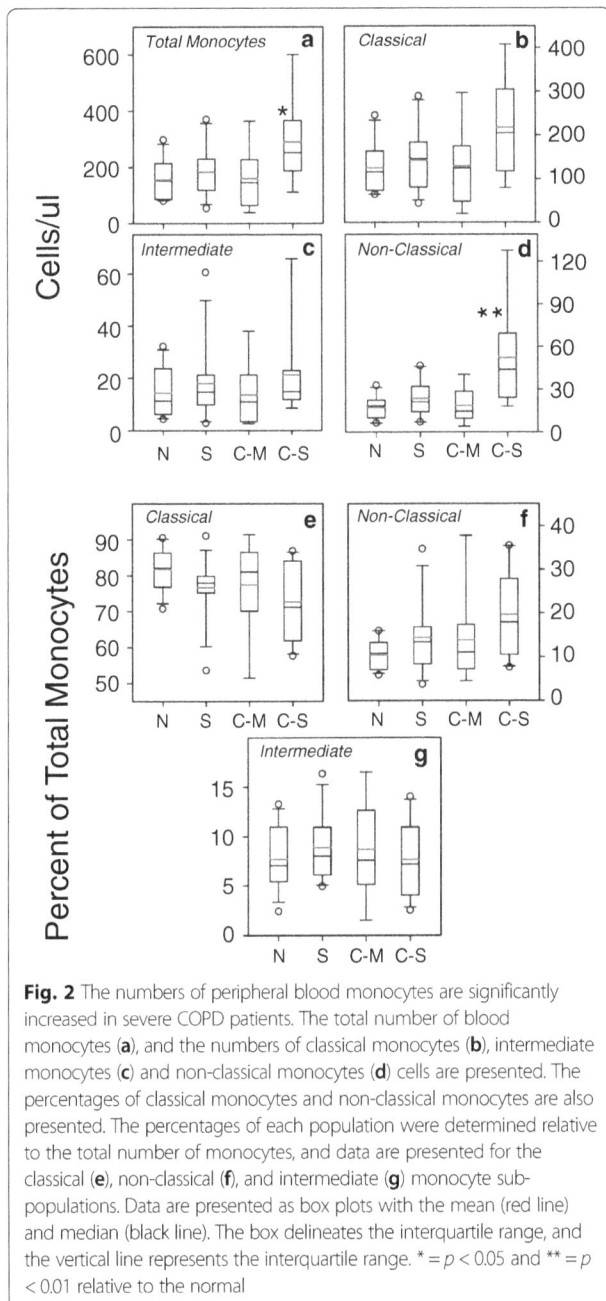

Fig. 2 The numbers of peripheral blood monocytes are significantly increased in severe COPD patients. The total number of blood monocytes (**a**), and the numbers of classical monocytes (**b**), intermediate monocytes (**c**) and non-classical monocytes (**d**) cells are presented. The percentages of classical monocytes and non-classical monocytes are also presented. The percentages of each population were determined relative to the total number of monocytes, and data are presented for the classical (**e**), non-classical (**f**), and intermediate (**g**) monocyte sub-populations. Data are presented as box plots with the mean (red line) and median (black line). The box delineates the interquartile range, and the vertical line represents the interquartile range. * = $p < 0.05$ and ** = $p < 0.01$ relative to the normal

differences in the numbers of total monocytes in any other subject groups. We also determined the numbers of circulating classical, intermediate, and non-classical monocytes in each of the subject groups (Fig. 2b-d). Our results show that the numbers of each of the classical and intermediate monocyte sub-populations was modestly increased in patients with severe COPD. However, in severe COPD, a more substantial increase in non-classical monocytes was observed.

In contrast, when judged as a proportion of the total monocytes, the data show (Fig. 2e) that classical monocytes represent a modestly reduced proportion of the

total monocytes in patients with severe COPD. At the same time, the proportion of non-classical monocytes (Fig. 2f) was also only modestly increased in severe COPD patients. Finally, the proportion of intermediate monocytes in these subject groups is not significantly different (Fig. 2g), and we chose to focus our further analysis on the classical and non-classical monocyte sub-populations.

The expression of activation markers in sub-populations of monocytes in severe COPD

We evaluated the level of expression of the activation and homing proinflammatory chemokine receptors CCR2 and CCR5 in each of our subject groups. The results from the analysis (Additional File 2: Fig. S2a-d) shows modest, but statistically insignificant, changes in the expression of both of these receptors by both classical and non-classical monocytes. We also assessed the percentage of monocytes which co-express these important chemoattractant receptors, and the results show that the level of co-expression was not significantly altered in any of the subject groups, for either classical or non-classical monocytes (Additional file 2: Fig. S2e & f).

The expression of M2 macrophage-associated markers is altered in normal smokers and patients with COPD

We assessed the numbers of monocytes expressing the M2-associated markers CD163, CD206 and IL-13Rα1. We found that the percentage of both classical and non-classical monocytes expressing CD163 (Fig. 3a & b) was significantly increased in both the moderate and severe COPD groups. There was also a significant increase in CD163 expression on classical monocytes from smokers. At the same time, the percentage of cells expressing the M1-marker CD25 was not different when comparing each of the subject groups (Fig. 3c & d) with the normal controls. In contrast, the percentage of monocytes expressing either CD206 or IL-13Rα1 were reduced in both the classical and non-classical monocytes (Fig. 3e-h) in both of the COPD subject groups, as well as the smokers. Overall these results demonstrate differential expression of the M1 and M2 markers in both smokers and COPD subjects.

The level of expression of activation markers and M2-associated markers is elevated in subjects with severe COPD

We used flow cytometry to quantitatively analyze the level of expression of each of the activation and M2 markers on monocytes. Our results show that expression (on a per cell basis) of CCR2, but not CCR5 (Additional file 3: Fig. S3a, b, d, & e), was significantly reduced on non-classical monocytes from subjects with moderate or severe COPD, or smokers. Finally, we also evaluated the level of CD14

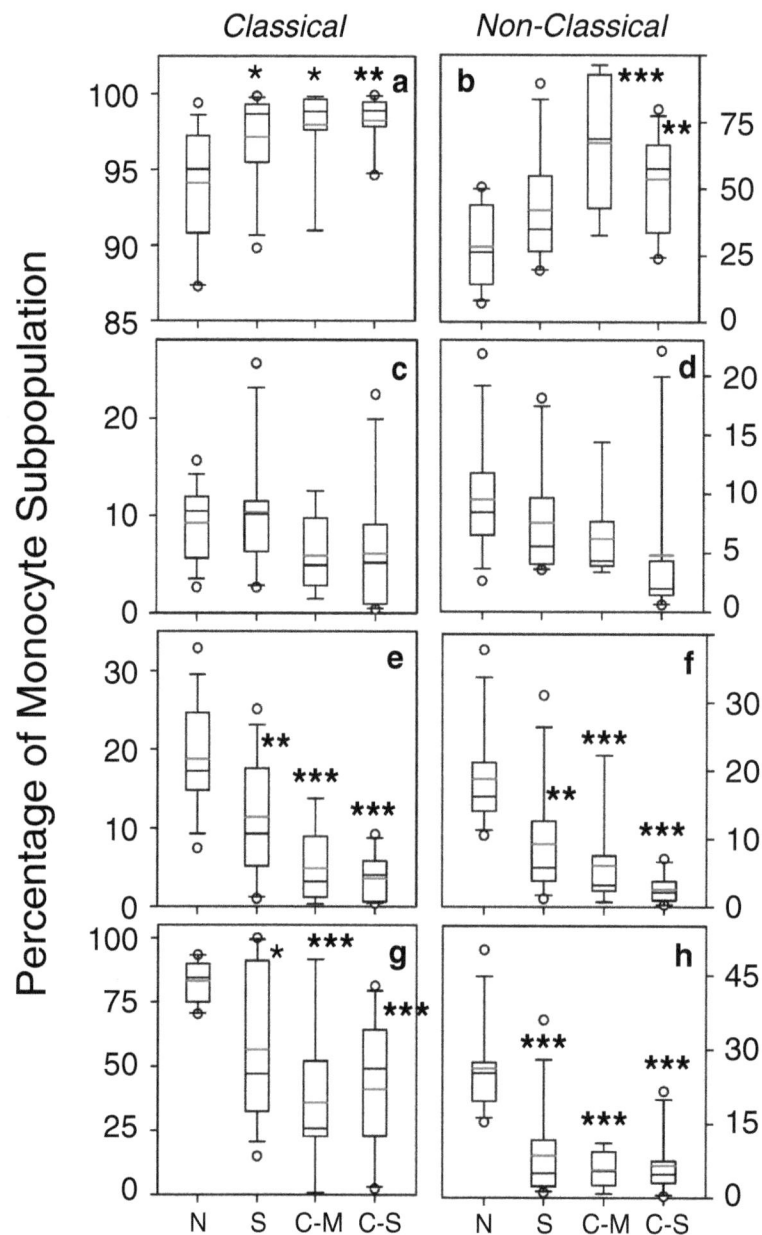

Fig. 3 Altered composition of monocyte sub-populations in smokers and COPD patients. Classical (**a**, **c**, **e**, and **g**) and non-classical (**b**, **d**, **f**, **h**) monocytes were stained for CD163 (**a**, **b**), CD25 (**c**, **d**), CD206 (**e**, **f**), and IL-13Rα1 (**g**, **h**) expression. The data are presented as the percentage of total classical or non-classical monocytes for each group. *** = $p < 0.001$ are relative to the normal

expression, a member of the bacterial endotoxin (TLR4) receptor complex, and we find that CD14 is modestly elevated on monocytes from moderate or severe COPD subjects, but not smokers (Additional file 3: Fig. S3c & f). Interestingly, the level of expression of CX3CR1, a chemokine receptor which promotes adhesion to inflamed vascular endothelia, was also significantly elevated on non-classical monocytes in severe COPD, but not the other subject groups (Additional file 4: Fig. S4).

We also analyzed the level of expression of M1 and M2-associated markers, and our results show that the level of expression of the M2-markers CD163 and CD206 are significantly elevated on both the classical and non-classical severe COPD monocytes (Fig. 4a-d). In contrast, the level of expression of the M1-associated marker CD25 in severe COPD monocytes was not significantly different from control (Fig. 4e-f). These results show that while the proportions of cells that express

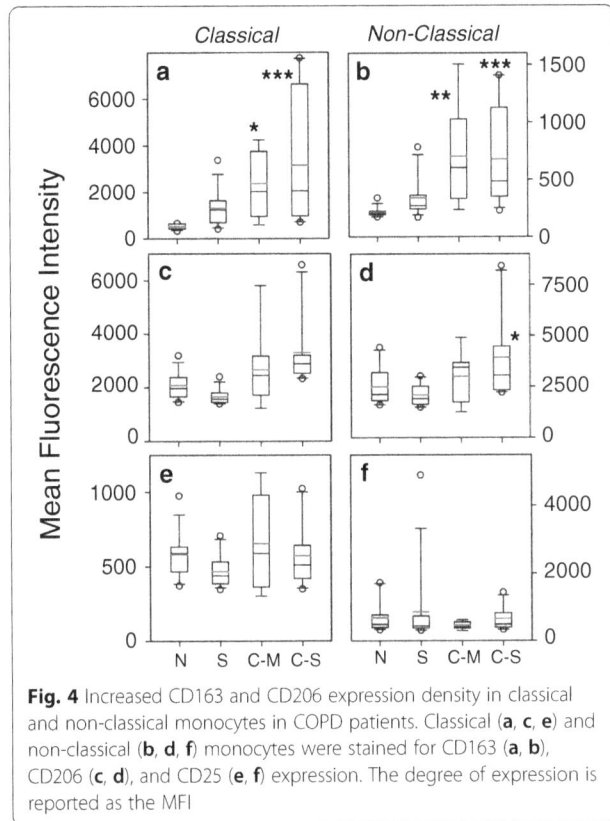

Fig. 4 Increased CD163 and CD206 expression density in classical and non-classical monocytes in COPD patients. Classical (**a**, **c**, **e**) and non-classical (**b**, **d**, **f**) monocytes were stained for CD163 (**a**, **b**), CD206 (**c**, **d**), and CD25 (**e**, **f**) expression. The degree of expression is reported as the MFI

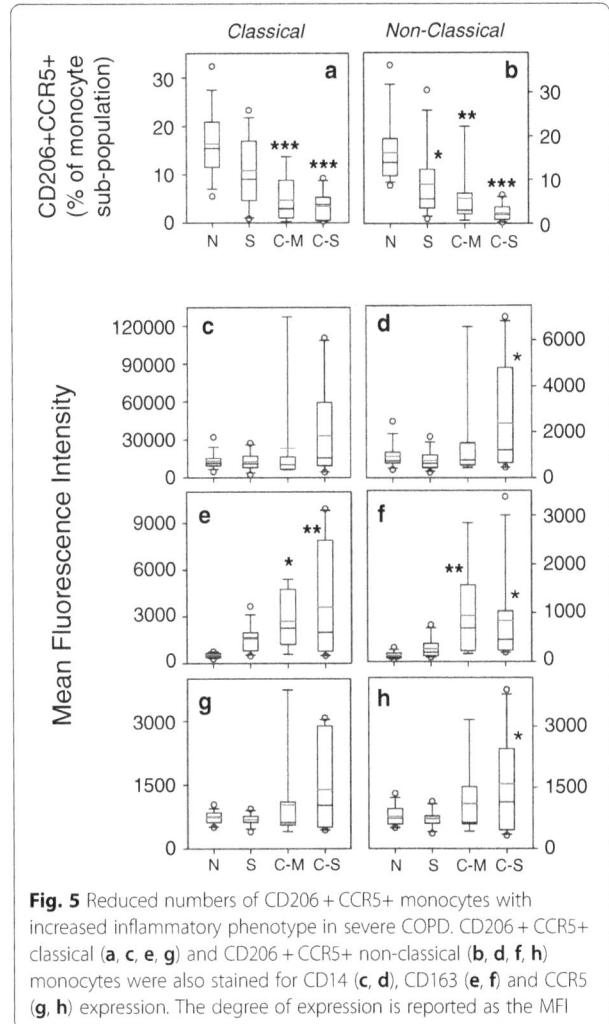

Fig. 5 Reduced numbers of CD206 + CCR5+ monocytes with increased inflammatory phenotype in severe COPD. CD206 + CCR5+ classical (**a**, **c**, **e**, **g**) and CD206 + CCR5+ non-classical (**b**, **d**, **f**, **h**) monocytes were also stained for CD14 (**c**, **d**), CD163 (**e**, **f**) and CCR5 (**g**, **h**) expression. The degree of expression is reported as the MFI

CD206 are reduced in severe COPD (Fig. 3), the level of expression of both CD163 and CD206 on the cells which are positive for these markers, was substantially increased.

Identification of a novel M2-like monocyte subset which emerges in severe COPD

We attempted to determine whether the elevated level of M2-associated marker expression in monocytes from the severe COPD subjects might reflect the presence of a specific sub-population monocytes in the subjects with severe COPD. We first assessed the presence of monocytes which co-express both CD206 and CCR5 within both the classical and non-classical monocyte populations in each group. Our results (Fig. 5a, b) show that the proportion of monocytes with the CD206 + CCR5+ phenotype was reduced in severe COPD, smokers and moderate COPD patients. Moreover, when the data are expressed on the basis of cell number, the same pattern was observed (Additional file 5: Fig. S5). However, further analysis of these CD206 + CCR5+ cells shows that the level of expression of CD14 (Fig. 5c & d), the M2-marker CD163 (Fig. 5e & f), and CCR5 (Fig. 5g & h) were substantially and significantly increased in severe COPD. The levels of expression of CD163 were also significantly elevated in moderate COPD patients, but otherwise, these markers were not elevated on monocytes from smokers or moderate COPD patients. More

detailed analysis of the expression of CCR5 on these CD206 + CCR5+ cells shows that the very high level of expression of CCR5 (Fig. 6) was unique and novel on the monocytes in severe COPD. These results show the emergence of monocytes with a unique high level of both CD206 and CCR5 expression, in both the classical and non-classical monocyte sub-populations.

Discussion

The results reported here demonstrate that the number of circulating monocytes was significantly increased in patients with severe COPD, and this increase was most prominent for the non-classical monocyte population. The elevated number of circulating monocytes was not observed for smokers without COPD, or patients with moderate COPD. These results are consistent with previous studies showing that the numbers of lung macrophages are significantly elevated in patients with COPD [25–28]. A previous report has shown that the numbers of lung macrophages increases approximately 12-fold in

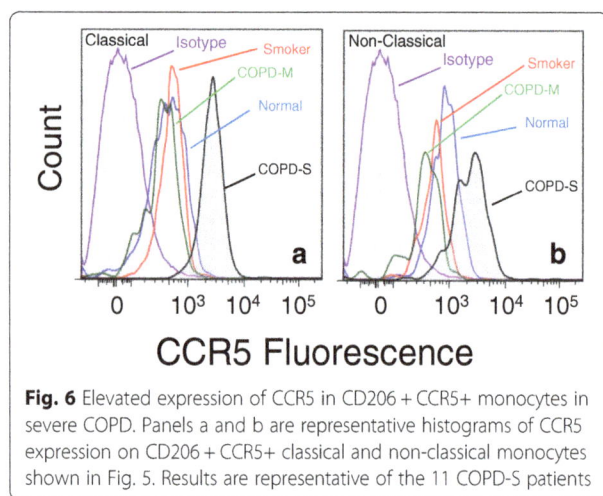

Fig. 6 Elevated expression of CCR5 in CD206 + CCR5+ monocytes in severe COPD. Panels a and b are representative histograms of CCR5 expression on CD206 + CCR5+ classical and non-classical monocytes shown in Fig. 5. Results are representative of the 11 COPD-S patients

severe COPD, and this elevation is not observed in patients with moderate COPD [28]. However, we believe the present report is the first to show that the increase in circulating monocytes in severe COPD is most significant in the non-classical population.

The non-classical sub-population functions to patrol the vasculature, in part by taking advantage of the expression of CX3CR1 [29, 30], and appears to play a significant role in clearing "damaged" endothelial cells, particularly at sites of inflammation [20, 31]. In contrast, the classical monocytes circulate in and out of normal tissues, and patrol for antigens which can be transported to lymph nodes. In inflamed tissues, these cells may also differentiate into macrophages and remain in the inflamed organ [32]. Monocytes which are recruited to the lung first reside in the parenchyma, and then under the appropriate inflammatory conditions, migrate to the alveoli [30, 33]. Indeed, the phenotype of the macrophages in the interstitium have a greater similarity to blood monocytes than to alveolar macrophages. Finally, the phenotype of monocytes which migrate into the lung is important. The non-classical monocytes when recruited to inflamed lung tissue is preferentially differentiated into the M2-type of macrophage, while the classical monocyte sub-population is a more typical source of M1-type macrophages [20]. Of course, it is important to appreciate that macrophage phenotypes are highly plastic, and environmental factors can have an effect on the functional activity of macrophages in any tissue. The M1 vs M2 paradigm should be evaluated with caution given the spectrum of phenotypes that can be derived from these cells in a given disease process [34], and the plasticity of these cells are particularly apparent in the alveolar compartment [35].

We report results here which show that the frequency of cells which express of the M2 marker CD163 (haptoglobin/hemoglobin scavenging receptor) is significantly increased for both classical and non-classical monocytes. Previous studies have shown that the expression of CD163 is significantly elevated on alveolar macrophages in patients with severe COPD [24], and recent reports show that this receptor is bound by both gram positive and negative bacteria [36, 37]. These studies suggest that bacterial binding to CD163 promotes the production of a number of cytokines and promotes lung inflammation.

In contrast with CD163, the overall percentage of cells which express the M2 marker CCR5 is not significantly altered, and the frequency of cells which express the M2 marker CD206 is actually significantly reduced among smokers and both COPD patient populations. However, we characterized the monocytes which co-express CD163, CD206 and CCR5 in an effort to assess the presence of cells with a pre-M2 phenotype. While we find that the percentage of circulating classical or non-classical monocytes which express these M2 markers is reduced in both moderate and severe COPD, we have detected the emergence of populations of classical and non-classical M2-like monocytes with an unusually high level of CCR5 expression in patients with severe, but not moderate, COPD. We hypothesize that the reduction in the percentage of these cells in the blood is due to their preferential recruitment to the inflamed lungs in these patients. The development of this population of monocytes with a pre-M2 phenotype is significant because it suggests that these cells are more likely to develop into M2 macrophages once they emigrate from the bloodstream. This would be consistent with the observation that macrophages in the lungs of COPD patients are enriched for the M2-type, and the M2 functional activity is likely to contribute to the disease process [21, 22, 24, 38]. Analysis of alveolar macrophages from COPD patients shows that expression of several M1 genes is down-regulated, while a large number of M2 genes is up-regulated [39]. Moreover, COPD alveolar macrophages have been found to exhibit impaired phagocytic activity, and in particular a reduced capacity to ingest both live and dead bacteria [40, 41], which is consistent with the reduced phagocytic activity reported for the M2-type macrophage [42].

The M2-like monocytes that we have identified in severe, but not moderate, COPD possesses unusually high levels of the chemokine receptor CCR5 and is a part of both the classical and non-classical monocyte subtype. We suggest that these cells would possess a much greater capacity to traffic to sites of inflammation, since the chemokine ligands for this receptor are typically produced at higher levels in these inflamed tissues. Experimental animal studies have shown that the severity of cigarette smoke-induced emphysema is greatly attenuated in CCR5-deficient mice [43, 44], and monocytes from patients with COPD exhibit enhanced migration in response to CCL5 [45]. Moreover, levels of CCL5 (a

CCR5 agonist) are significantly increased in the lungs of patients with COPD [46].

It should be pointed out that we were unable to match the various subject groups for race or gender, and this is a limitation in our study. In addition, the subjects in our "normal" cohort exhibited lung function which was somewhat lower than might be predicted. We recruited individuals who did not exhibit apparent cardiovascular disease, diabetes, rheumatic disease, or confounding illnesses.

Finally, we were unable to assess the capacity of the novel M2-like monocytes to traffic to the lungs of patients with severe COPD. This limitation is difficult to overcome given the limits of the technology that is currently available for studying cellular traffic in humans. Nevertheless, our data show that in severe COPD, populations of M2-like monocytes develop, and these cells may preferentially migrate to the inflamed lungs of the COPD patient. This would occur because these cells possess a much greater density of CCR5, and the lung produces an elevated level of a chemokine ligand for CCR5. We suggest that once these cells are recruited to the COPD lung, they are pre-programed to further differentiate into M2-type tissue macrophages. The emergence of these pathogenic monocytes is likely to accelerate the disease progression in the lung, and thus limit the sensitivity to therapeutic intervention.

Conclusions

Our studies reveal the emergence in severe COPD of a novel population of circulating monocytes with characteristics of the M2 lung macrophage phenotype. This monocyte phenotype was not observed in either normal subjects, smokers, or patients with moderate COPD. We suggest that cells which may be precursors of the lung M2-type of macrophage develop in the circulation, and these cells may serve as a source of these lung macrophages in severe disease.

Additional files

Additional file 1: Figure S1. Flow cytometry gating strategy to identify and characterize monocyte subpopulations. PMBCs were stained as described in the Methods section and at least 250,000 events per sample were collected. Singlets (red rectangle, panel a) were gated using the forward side-scatter area (FSC-A) vs height (FSC-H). From the singlets gate, monocytes (red oval, panel b) were gated using the FSC-A vs side-scatter area (SSC-A). The monocytes were further gated using CD14 vs CD16 and are indicated by the red boxes (panel c). The classical monocytes are CD14 + CD16-; the intermediate monocytes are CD14 + CD16+; and the non-classical monocytes are CD14^{DIM}CD16+. From the classical gate, cells stained for CCR2, CCR5, CD163, CD206, and IL-13Ra1 are shown (panels i-m), and from the non-classical gate, the staining for CCR2, CCR5, CD163, CD206, and IL-13Ra1 are shown in panels d-h. The red histograms indicate the isotype control for each marker. The black histograms indicated the expression of each marker. (PDF 311 kb)

Additional file 2: Figure S2. Analysis of CCR2 and CCR5 expression by classical and non-classical monocytes. Classical (a, c, e) and non-classical

(b, d, f) monocytes were stained for CCR2 and CCR5 expression. The data are presented for the percentage of CCR2-positive (a, b), CCR5-positive (c, d), and CCR2- and CCR5-double positive (e, f) monocytes. The data are presented as the percentage of total classical or non-classical monocytes for each group. (PDF 13 kb)

Additional file 3: Figure S3. Altered surface expression density of monocytes in COPD patients. Classical (a-c) and non-classical monocytes (panels d-f) were stained for CCR2 (a, d), CCR5 (b, e), and CD14 (c, f) expression. The degree of expression is reported as the mean fluorescence intensity (MFI). * = p < 0.05 and ** = p < 0.01 relative to the normal. (PDF 13 kb)

Additional file 4: Figure S4. Increased CX3CR1 expression density in CD206 + CCR5+ non-classical monocytes in severe COPD patients. CD206 + CCR5+ co-expressing cells were stained for CX3CR1, and the mean fluorescence intensity (MFI) for each patient population was determined. Results represent the mean MFI ± SEM of all subjects in each subject group. * = p < 0.05. (PDF 4 kb)

Additional file 5: Figure S5. Reduced numbers of CD206 + CCR5+ monocytes in severe COPD. CD206 + CCR5+ classical (a) and CD206 + CCR5+ non-classical (b) monocytes data were expressed as the number of cells per μl. * = p < 0.05; ** = p < 0.01; and *** = p < 0.001 relative to the normal. (PDF 11 kb)

Funding

Supported by grants from the National Institutes of Health (DA14230, DA25532, P30DA13429, DA040619, and S10 RR27910).

Authors' contributions

Concept and design: WDC, XF, VK, GJC, and TJR. Acquisition of data: WDC, XF, TJR. Analysis and interpretation: WDC, VK, XF, MEVS, GJC, FVR and TJR. Preparation of manuscript and important intellectual content: WDC, VK, XF, MEVS, GJC and TJR. All authors have read and approved the manuscript.

Competing interests

The authors declare that they have no competing interests.

¹
Author details

Center for Inflammation, Translational and Clinical Lung Research, Lewis Katz School of Medicine, Temple University, Philadelphia, PA 19140, USA. ²Department of Thoracic Medicine and Surgery, Lewis Katz School of Medicine, Temple University, Philadelphia, PA 19140, USA. ³Temple University Flow Cytometry Facility, Lewis Katz School of Medicine, Temple University, Philadelphia, PA 19140, USA. ⁴Department of Clinical Sciences, Lewis Katz School of Medicine, Temple University, Philadelphia, PA 19140, USA.

References

1. Grashoff WF, Sont JK, Sterk PJ, Hiemstra PS, de Boer WI, Stolk J, Han J, van Krieken JM. Chronic obstructive pulmonary disease: role of bronchiolar mast cells and macrophages. AmJPathol 1997; 151:1785–1790.
2. Finkelstein R, Fraser RS, Ghezzo H, Cosio MG, Finkelstein R, Fraser RS, Ghezzo H, Cosio MG. Alveolar inflammation and its relation to emphysema in smokers. American Journal of Respiratory & Critical Care Medicine. 1995;152: 1666–72.
3. Hogg JC, Chu F, Utokaparch S, Woods R, Elliott WM, Buzatu L, Cherniack RM, Rogers RM, Sciurba FC, Coxson HO, et al. The nature of small-airway obstruction in chronic obstructive pulmonary disease. NEnglJMed. 2004;350: 2645–53.
4. Hiemstra PS. Altered macrophage function in chronic obstructive pulmonary disease. Ann Am Thorac Soc. 2013;10(Suppl):S180–5.
5. Barnes PJ. Alveolar macrophages as orchestrators of COPD. COPD: J Chron Obstruct Pulmon Dis. 2004;1:59–70.

6. van de Laar L, Saelens W, De Prijck S, Martens L, Scott CL, Van Isterdael G, Hoffmann E, Beyaert R, Saeys Y, Lambrecht BN, et al. Yolk sac macrophages, fetal liver, and adult monocytes can colonize an empty niche and develop into functional tissue-resident macrophages. Immunity. 2016;44:755–68.

7. Yona S, Kim KW, Wolf Y, Mildner A, Varol D, Breker M, Strauss-Ayali D, Viukov S, Guilliams M, Misharin A, et al. Fate mapping reveals origins and dynamics of monocytes and tissue macrophages under homeostasis. Immunity. 2013; 38:79–91.

8. Kopf M, Schneider C, Nobs SP. The development and function of lung-resident macrophages and dendritic cells. Nat Immunol. 2015;16:36–44.

9. Guilliams M, De Kleer I, Henri S, Post S, Vanhoutte L, De Prijck S, Deswarte K, Malissen B, Hammad H, Lambrecht BN. Alveolar macrophages develop from fetal monocytes that differentiate into long-lived cells in the first week of life via GM-CSF. J Exp Med. 2013;210:1977–92.

10. Misharin AV, Morales-Nebreda L, Reyfman PA, Cuda CM, Walter JM, McQuattie-Pimentel AC, Chen CI, Anekalla KR, Joshi N, Williams KJN, et al. Monocyte-derived alveolar macrophages drive lung fibrosis and persist in the lung over the life span. J Exp Med. 2017;214:2387–404.

11. Martinez FO, Gordon S, Locati M, Mantovani A. Transcriptional profiling of the human monocyte-to-macrophage differentiation and polarization: new molecules and patterns of gene expression. J Immunol. 2006;177:7303–11.

12. Martinez FO, Helming L, Gordon S. Alternative activation of macrophages: an immunologic functional perspective. Annu Rev Immunol. 2009;27:451–83.

13. Rees AJ. Monocyte and macrophage biology: an overview. Semin Nephrol. 2010;30:216–33.

14. Auffray C, Sieweke MH, Geissmann F. Blood monocytes: development, heterogeneity, and relationship with dendritic cells. Annu Rev Immunol. 2009;27:669–92.

15. Ziegler-Heitbrock L, Ancuta P, Crowe S, Dalod M, Grau V, Hart DN, Leenen PJ, Liu YJ, MacPherson G, Randolph GJ, et al. Nomenclature of monocytes and dendritic cells in blood. Blood. 2010;116:e74-e80.

16. Nockher WA, Scherberich JE. Expanded CD14+ CD16+ monocyte subpopulation in patients with acute and chronic infections undergoing hemodialysis. Infect Immun. 1998;66:2782–90.

17. Fingerle G, Pforte A, Passlick B, Blumenstein M, Strobel M, Ziegler-Heitbrock HW. The novel subset of CD14+/CD16+ blood monocytes is expanded in sepsis patients. Blood. 1993;82:3170–6.

18. Skinner NA, MacIsaac CM, Hamilton JA, Visvanathan K. Regulation of toll-like receptor (TLR)2 and TLR4 on CD14dimCD16+ monocytes in response to sepsis-related antigens. Clin Exp Immunol. 2005;141:270–8.

19. Geissmann F, Jung S, Littman DR. Blood monocytes consist of two principal subsets with distinct migratory properties. Immunity. 2003;19:71–82.

20. Auffray C, Fogg D, Garfa M, Elain G, Join-Lambert O, Kayal S, Sarnacki S, Cumano A, Lauvau G, Geissmann F, et al. Monitoring of blood vessels and tissues by a population of monocytes with patrolling behavior. Science. 2007;317:666–70.

21. Barnes PJ. Immunology of asthma and chronic obstructive pulmonary disease. Nature Reviews. Immunology. 2008;8:183–92.

22. Vlahos R, Bozinovski S. Role of alveolar macrophages in chronic obstructive pulmonary disease. Front Immunol. 2014;5:435.

23. Bozinovski S, Cross M, Vlahos R, Jones JE, Hsuu K, Tessier PA, Reynolds EC, Hume DA, Hamilton JA, Geczy CL, et al. S100A8 chemotactic protein is abundantly increased, but only a minor contributor to LPS-induced, steroid resistant neutrophilic lung inflammation in vivo. J Proteome Res. 2005;4: 136–45.

24. Kaku Y, Imaoka H, Morimatsu Y, Komohara Y, Ohnishi K, Oda H, Takenaka S, Matsuoka M, Kawayama T, Takeya M, et al. Overexpression of CD163, CD204 and CD206 on alveolar macrophages in the lungs of patients with severe chronic obstructive pulmonary disease. PLoS One. 2014;9:e87400.

25. Shapiro SD. The macrophage in chronic obstructive pulmonary disease. AmJRespirCrit Care Med. 1999;160:S29–32.

26. Pesci A, Balbi B, Majori M, Cacciani G, Bertacco S, Alciato P, Donner CF. Inflammatory cells and mediators in bronchial lavage of patients with chronic obstructive pulmonary disease. EurRespirJ. 1998;12:380–6.

27. Keatings VM, Collins PD, Scott DM, Barnes PJ. Differences in interleukin-8 and tumor necrosis factor-alpha in induced sputum from patients with chronic obstructive pulmonary disease or asthma. Am J Respir Crit Care Med. 1996;153:530 4.

28. Retamales I, Elliott WM, Meshi B, Coxson HO, Pare PD, Sciurba FC, Rogers RM, Hayashi S, Hogg JC, Retamales I, et al. Amplification of inflammation in

29. Xiong Z, Leme AS, Ray P, Shapiro SD, Lee JS. CX3CR1+ lung mononuclear phagocytes spatially confined to the interstitium produce TNF-alpha and IL-6 and promote cigarette smoke-induced emphysema. J Immunol. 2011;186: 3206–14.

30. Landsman L, Varol C, Jung S. Distinct differentiation potential of blood monocyte subsets in the lung. J Immunol 2007; 178:2000–2007.

31. Carlin LM, Stamatiades EG, Auffray C, Hanna RN, Glover L, Vizcay-Barrena G, Hedrick CC, Cook HT, Diebold S, Geissmann F. Nr4a1-dependent Ly6C(low) monocytes monitor endothelial cells and orchestrate their disposal. Cell. 2013;153:362–75.

32. Jakubzick C, Gautier EL, Gibbings SL, Sojka DK, Schlitzer A, Johnson TE, Ivanov S, Duan Q, Bala S, Condon T, et al. Minimal differentiation of classical monocytes as they survey steady-state tissues and transport antigen to lymph nodes. Immunity. 2013;39:599–610.

33. Landsman L, Jung S. Lung macrophages serve as obligatory intermediate between blood monocytes and alveolar macrophages. J Immunol. 2007;179: 3488–94.

34. Murray PJ, Allen JE, Biswas SK, Fisher EA, Gilroy DW, Goerdt S, Gordon S, Hamilton JA, Ivashkiv LB, Lawrence T, et al. Macrophage activation and polarization: nomenclature and experimental guidelines. Immunity. 2014;41: 14–20.

35. Hussell T, Bell TJ. Alveolar macrophages: plasticity in a tissue-specific context. Nat Rev Immunol. 2014;14:81–93.

36. Abdullah M, Kahler D, Vock C, Reiling N, Kugler C, Dromann D, Rupp J, Hauber HP, Fehrenbach H, Zabel P, et al. Pulmonary haptoglobin and CD163 are functional immunoregulatory elements in the human lung. Respiration. 2012;83:61–73.

37. Fabriek BO, van Bruggen R, Deng DM, Ligtenberg AJ, Nazmi K, Schornagel K, Vloet RP, Dijkstra CD, van den Berg TK. The macrophage scavenger receptor CD163 functions as an innate immune sensor for bacteria. Blood. 2009;113:887–92.

38. Baraldo S, Bazzan E, Zanin ME, Turato G, Garbisa S, Maestrelli P, Papi A, Miniati M, Fabbri LM, Zuin R, et al. Matrix metalloproteinase-2 protein in lung periphery is related to COPD progression. Chest. 2007;132:1733–40.

39. Shaykhiev R, Krause A, Salit J, Strulovici-Barel Y, Harvey BG, O'Connor TP, Crystal RG. Smoking-dependent reprogramming of alveolar macrophage polarization: implication for pathogenesis of chronic obstructive pulmonary disease. J Immunol. 2009;183:2867–83.

40. Taylor AE, Finney-Hayward TK, Quint JK, Thomas CM, Tudhope SJ, Wedzicha JA, Barnes PJ, Donnelly LE. Defective macrophage phagocytosis of bacteria in COPD. European Respiratory J. 2010;35:1039–47.

41. Berenson CS, Garlipp MA, Grove LJ, Maloney J, Sethi S. Impaired phagocytosis of nontypeable Haemophilus influenzae by human alveolar macrophages in chronic obstructive pulmonary disease. J Infect Dis. 2006; 194:1375–84.

42. Price JV, Vance RE. The macrophage paradox. Immunity. 2014;41:685–93.

43. Ma B, Kang MJ, Lee CG, Chapoval S, Liu W, Chen Q, Coyle AJ, Lora JM, Picarella D, Homer RJ, et al. Role of CCR5 in IFN-gamma-induced and cigarette smoke-induced emphysema. J Clin Invest. 2005;115:3460–72.

44. Bracke KR, D'Hulst AI, Maes T, Demedts IK, Moerloose KB, Kuziel WA, Joos GF, Brusselle GG. Cigarette smoke-induced pulmonary inflammation, but not airway remodelling, is attenuated in chemokine receptor 5-deficient mice. Clin Exp Allergy. 2007;37:1467–79.

45. Costa C, Traves SL, Tudhope SJ, Fenwick PS, Belchamber KB, Russell RE, Barnes PJ, Donnelly LE. Enhanced monocyte migration to CXCR3 and CCR5 chemokines in COPD. Eur Respir J. 2016;47:1093–102.

46. Costa C, Rufino R, Traves SL, Lapa ESJR, Barnes PJ, Donnelly LE. CXCR3 and CCR5 chemokines in induced sputum from patients with COPD. Chest. 2008;133:26–33.

emphysema and its association with latent adenoviral infection. American Journal of Respiratory & Critical Care Medicine. 2001;164:469–73.

9

Fatal interstitial lung disease associated with Crizotinib pathologically confirmed by percutaneous lung biopsy in a patient with ROS1-rearranged advanced non-small-cell lung cancer

Shibo Wu[1†] (iD), Kaitai Liu[2†], Feng Ren[3], Dawei Zheng[4] and Deng Pan[5*]

Abstract

Background: Crizotinib is a multi-target inhibitor approved for the treatment of advanced non-small-cell lung cancer patients with a ROS1 rearrangement. However, interstitial lung disease is a rare but severe and fatal side effect of crizotinib that should lead to immediate discontinuation of the drug. Unfortunately, the pathophysiology, molecular mechanism and risk factors for crizotinib-induced interstitial lung disease remain poorly understood.

Case presentation: We first identified and reported interstitial lung disease induced de novo by crizotinib in a 47-year-old female patient who was diagnosed with advanced lung adenocarcinoma with a ROS1 rearrangement in a malignant pleural effusion. Subsequent next-generation sequencing analysis revealed both ROS1 rearrangement and an EGFR exon 19 deletion mutation in lung biopsy specimens, which were histologically confirmed to be interstitial lung disease. Although crizotinib treatment was ceased immediately and a shock treatment with high-dose methylprednisolone as well as other necessary treatment procedures was applied to reverse the interstitial lung disease process, the patient died.

Conclusions: The present case indicates that while treating non-small-cell lung cancer patients with crizotinib, it is important to constantly monitor any newly emerging respiratory symptoms and unexplained imaging changes, which may suggest an adverse effect related to drug-induced interstitial lung disease or even lethality. Histopathology and molecular pathological examination of lung biopsy specimens may help clinicians understand the development mechanism and exclude other causes.

Keywords: Interstitial lung disease, Crizotinib, ROS1 rearrangement, EGFR mutation

Background

Crizotinib is a multi-target inhibitor, which was granted a full approval by the Food and Drug Administration (FDA) for the treatment of advanced non-small-cell lung cancer (NSCLC) patients with a ROS1 rearrangement in March 2016. However, interstitial lung disease (ILD) is a rare but severe and fatal side effect of crizotinib that should lead to immediate discontinuation of the drug.

Unfortunately, the pathophysiology, molecular mechanism and risk factors for crizotinib-induced ILD remain poorly understood. Here, we describe a case of SDC4-ROS1 rearrangement-positive advanced lung adenocarcinoma with de novo crizotinib-induced ILD.

Case presentation

A 47-year-old female Chinese patient was admitted to our hospital in January 2018 due to complaints of continuous cough and a feeling of breathlessness for more than a week. The patient did not have a history of alcohol consumption or smoking. She refused to reveal a

* Correspondence: pand2008@yeah.net; 178042519@qq.com
†Shibo Wu and Kaitai Liu contributed equally to this work.
5Department of Diagnosis, Ningbo Diagnostic Pathology Center, No. 79, Huan'cheng Road, Ningbo 315021, China
Full list of author information is available at the end of the article

special occupational history and the medical history of her family.

A chest computed tomography (CT) scan revealed a large, irregularly shaped mass on the upper right lobe, accompanied by multiple nodules, plaques and consolidated masses of different sizes, randomly distributed in both lung fields. Nodular thickening of the interlobular septa and fissures, which suggested lymphangitis carcinomatosa, hilar and mediastinal lymphadenopathy and bilateral pleural effusions, was identified by the CT scan as well (Fig. 1a).

An immediate drainage was conducted for the right pleural effusion, followed by a series of tests. Methylprednisolone (MP) at 80 mg/day was administered to alleviate dyspnoea associated with lymphangitis carcinomatosa. With oxygen therapy via a nasal catheter at a flow rate of 6 L/min, her arterial blood gas was measured to have values of a PaO_2 of 55.0 mmHg, a $PaCO_2$ of 32.0 mmHg, and a pH of 7.49. The carcinoembryonic antigen (CEA) level in hydrothorax was 7.5 µg/L (normal 0–5 µg/L), whereas the serum CEA level was 12.4 µg/L. The rest of the important blood and sputum test indicators are described in Table 1.

With a poor performance status (PS = 4), the patient was unable to withstand tissue biopsy acquisition. A great number of tumour cells positive for thyroid transcription factor-1 (TTF-1) and cytokeratin 7 (CK 7)

were confirmed by pathological haematoxylin-eosin (HE) staining examination of hydrothorax, combined with immunohistochemical staining. These observations led to a diagnosis of advanced lung adenocarcinoma with extensive dissemination in the chest (Fig. 2a-c).

Next-generation sequencing was then conducted on tumour cells of hydrothorax. The SDC4-ROS1 fusion gene was detected at an abundance of 19.8% in the malignant pleural effusion (MPE). Other mutations, such as those in the EGFR, ALK, KRAS, BFAF, HER2, PIK3CA, MET, and RET genes, were not detected (Fig. 3 Z17L06517, Fig. 4b). The patient was thus orally administered crizotinib at a dose of 250 mg twice per day. After three days of crizotinib treatment, the orthopnoea was greatly relieved, and MP medication was withdrawn. However, oxygen therapy was still required within a one-week time frame of administration. On the tenth day of medication, the patient had a low-grade fever and slight aggravation of dyspnoea. A chest CT re-scan revealed a significant shrinkage of intrapulmonary neoplastic lesions, lymphadenitis and lymphadenectasis. However, multiple new-onset ground-glass opacities and consolidations were detected throughout both lungs (Fig. 1b). The patient was then additionally treated with cefoperazone/sulbactam to exclude the possibility of infection.

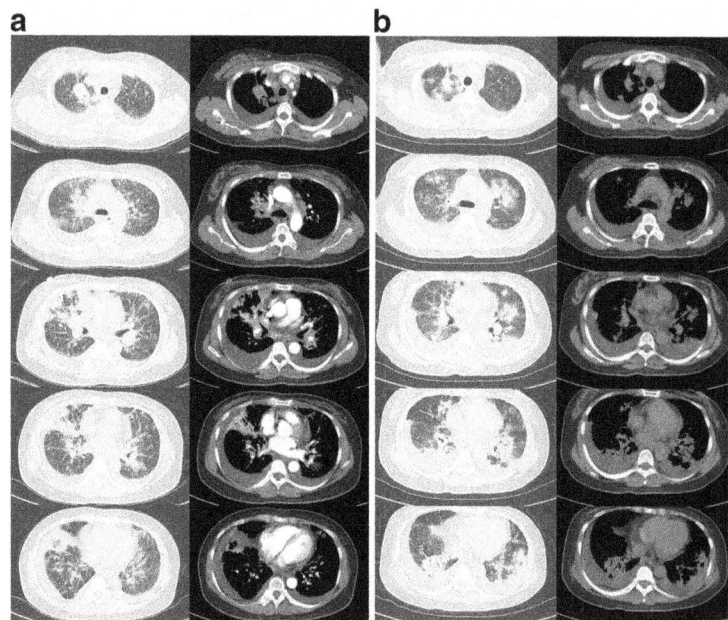

Fig. 1 a. Prior to treatment with crizotinib, a chest CT scan revealed a large irregularly shaped mass on the upper right lobe, accompanied by multiple nodules, plaques and consolidated masses of diverse sizes randomly distributed in both lung fields. Nodular thickening of the interlobular septa and fissures, which suggested lymphangitis carcinomatosa, hilar and mediastinal lymphadenopathy, and bilateral pleural effusions, were identified as well. **b** Ten days after the initiation of crizotinib, chest CT revealed a significant shrinkage of intrapulmonary neoplastic lesions, lymphadenitis and lymphadenectasis but not of multiple new-onset ground-glass opacities and consolidation lesions throughout both lungs

Table 1 The rest important blood and sputum testing indicators of pre- and post-treatment with Crizotinib

	Blood testing indicators							Sputum indicators
	Carbohydrate antigen 199 (IU/ml)	Cytokeratin fragment (ug/L)	Neuron-specific enolase (ug/L)	Squamous cell carcinoma antigen (ug/L)	White blood cell count ($\times 10^9$/L)	Erythrocyte sedimentation rate (mm/h)	C-reactive protein (mg/L)	Sputum culture
Normal range	0.0~37.0	0.00~7.00	0.00~10.00	0.00~2.50	3.5~9.5	0~20	0~8	NA
Pre-treatment	100.8	14.31	4.85	22.94	11.3	32	95.1	negative
Post-treatment	57.3	15.14	5.84	7.89	16.7	10	4.1	negative

In addition, a re-examination of blood tumour markers, infection-related indicators, and characteristics of hydrothorax, combined with percutaneous lung biopsy, was undertaken to clarify the cause. CEA in the pleural fluid and serum increased to 13.6 μg/L and 52.7 μg/L, respectively, after crizotinib medication. Other important indicators are described in Table 1. Consistent with the CT scan, the pathology of hydrothorax suggested a significantly reduced number of tumour cells. Three columnar specimens of percutaneous biopsy from the new-onset consolidation area on the lower left pulmonary were collected promptly, all of which were 1 cm in length and 18 gauge in diameter. Histological observation of these biopsies revealed a diffuse alveolar oedema, thickening of the septa (Fig. 2d), macrophages or foamy macrophages prominently present in differently sized alveolar spaces (Fig. 2e), mild infiltration of inflammatory lymphocytes, monocytes, fibroblasts, and myofibroblasts in the interstitium (Fig. 2f), rare and atypical hyaline membrane formations in alveolar spaces (Fig. 2g), multiple hyaline thrombi (microthrombi) in pulmonary arterioles of partial areas (Fig. 2h), and atypical hyperplasia of type II alveolar epithelial cells in localized areas (Fig. 2i). There was no evidence of infections and

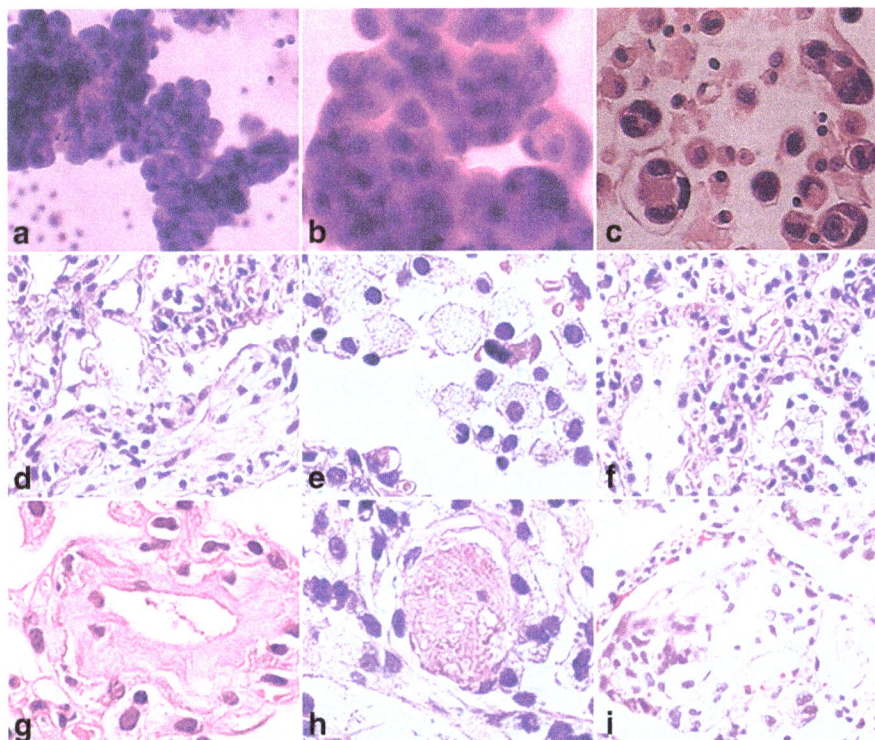

Fig. 2 a-c HE staining (×200), (×400), (×200), liquid-based cell smear and a cell wax block revealed that tumour cells with gigantic nucleoli were distributed in clusters and presented with a round-edge, strongly encapsulated, obviously three-dimensional structure. Fig. 2**d-l** HE staining showed histological characteristics of acute interstitial pneumonia. Fig. 2**d** (×200) Diffuse alveolar oedema, thickening of the septa. Fig. 2**e** (×400) Macrophages or foamy macrophages prominently present in differently sized alveolar spaces. Fig. 2**f** (×200) Mild infiltration of inflammatory cells in the interstitium. Fig. 2**g** (×400) Rare and atypical hyaline membrane formations in alveolar spaces. Fig. 2**h** (×400) Multiple hyaline thrombi (microthrombi) in pulmonary arterioles of partial areas. Fig. 2**i** (×400) Atypical hyperplasia of type II alveolar epithelial cells in localized areas

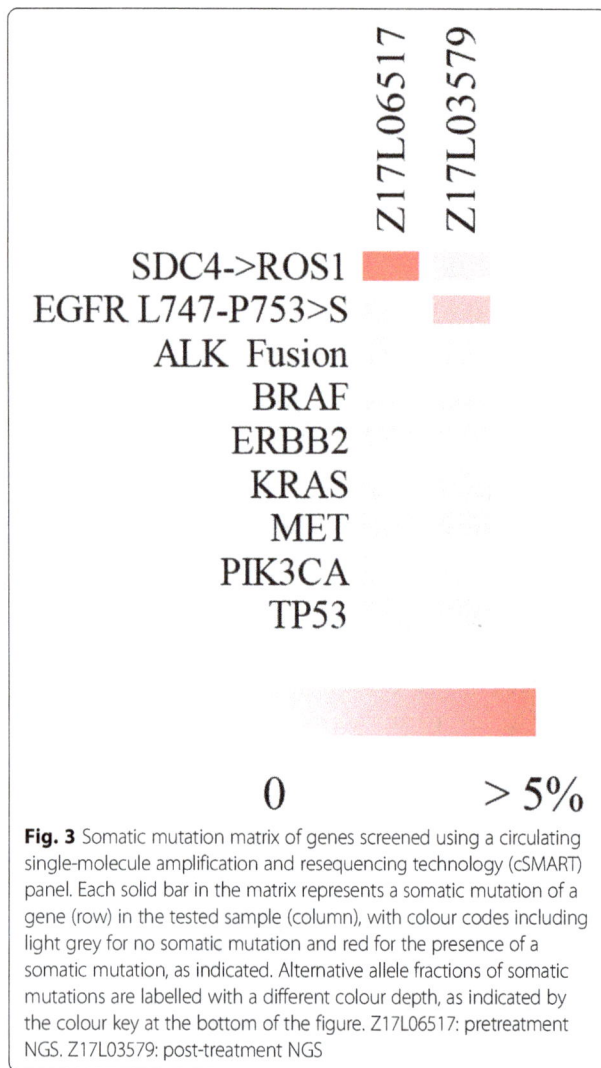

Fig. 3 Somatic mutation matrix of genes screened using a circulating single-molecule amplification and resequencing technology (cSMART) panel. Each solid bar in the matrix represents a somatic mutation of a gene (row) in the tested sample (column), with colour codes including light grey for no somatic mutation and red for the presence of a somatic mutation, as indicated. Alternative allele fractions of somatic mutations are labelled with a different colour depth, as indicated by the colour key at the bottom of the figure. Z17L06517: pretreatment NGS. Z17L03579: post-treatment NGS

invasion of tumour cells. All these pathological changes were consistent with acute lung injury. The pathological stage was assumed to be a transition from exudation to organization. The patient denied having previous pulmonary-related diseases, and there were no other drugs that might potentially cause lung toxicity during crizotinib treatment. Therefore, we made a diagnosis of crizotinib-induced ILD.

MP pulse therapy (0.5 g once per day) was immediately substituted for the original crizotinib treatment and applied for three days. Tracheal intubation and mechanical ventilation were also undertaken because of progressive deterioration leading to respiratory failure. All necessary and additional treatment procedures were conducted to prevent ILD, but the patient died 20 days after the first administration of crizotinib. Upon approval of her family, next-generation sequencing analysis of a lung biopsy sample was performed, which revealed a de novo exon 19 deletion mutation in EGFR, not detected in MPE before treatment with crizotinib (Fig. 3 Z17L03579, Fig. 4a). On the other hand, the frequency of ROS1 rearrangement decreased after crizotinib treatment (Fig. 3). The occurrence of this phenomenon deserves special consideration and investigation of current crizotinib treatment in NSCLC patients.

Ethics, consent and permissions

Written informed consent has been obtained from the patient's family for the publication of this case report and accompanying images.

Discussion

In this study, we report the first case of fatal crizotinib-induced ILD in a ROS1-positive NSCLC patient. ROS1 rearrangements are identified in 1 to 2% of patients with NSCLC [1]. Up to now, crizotinib is still the only targeted agent approved for NSCLC patients

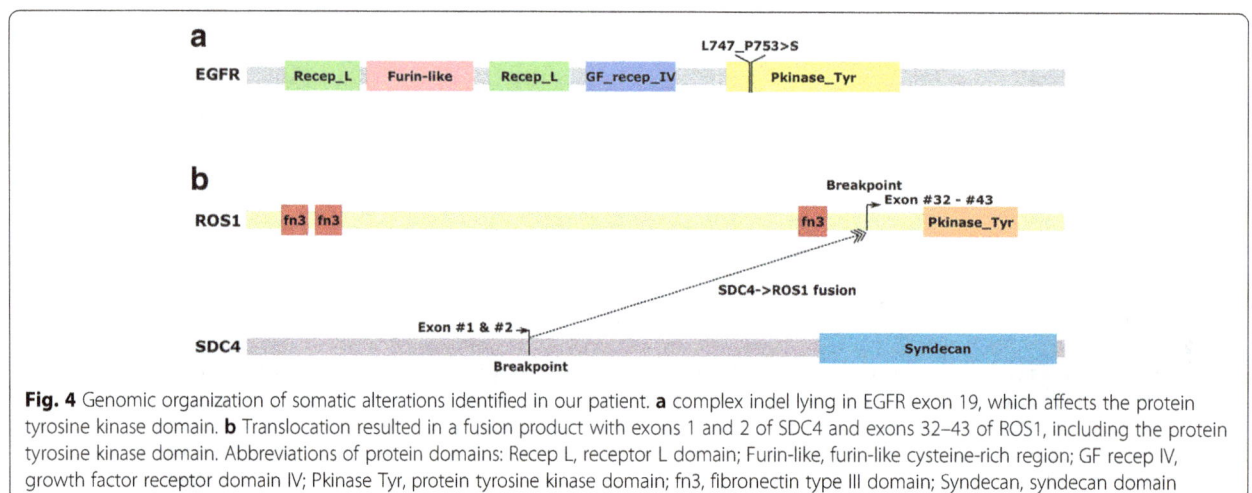

Fig. 4 Genomic organization of somatic alterations identified in our patient. **a** complex indel lying in EGFR exon 19, which affects the protein tyrosine kinase domain. **b** Translocation resulted in a fusion product with exons 1 and 2 of SDC4 and exons 32–43 of ROS1, including the protein tyrosine kinase domain. Abbreviations of protein domains: Recep L, receptor L domain; Furin-like, furin-like cysteine-rich region; GF recep IV, growth factor receptor domain IV; Pkinase Tyr, protein tyrosine kinase domain; fn3, fibronectin type III domain; Syndecan, syndecan domain

with ROS1 rearrangements. A retrospective review of 4 PROFILE clinical trials indicated that the overall incidence of crizotinib-induced ILD was 1.2%, but its mortality rate was up to 50% [2]. It is a rare but serious adverse event in patients on crizotinib therapy.

Although crizotinib-induced ILD in ROS1-positive NSCLC patients has not been systematically characterized before, patients with ROS1 rearrangements had a similar incidence (1.9%, 1 of 53) of ILD as those containing ALK rearrangements (1.7%, 2 of 119) in a phase I PROFILE 1001 study of crizotinib [3]. In addition, the safety profiles of crizotinib are similar for ALK-positive and ROS1-positive NSCLC patients [4]. The factors contributing to crizotinib-induced ILD in ROS1-positive patients remain unclear, whereas risk factors significantly correlated with the development of ILD in ALK-positive NSCLC patients have been described and include age, poor performance status, smoking status, past/concomitant ILD and concomitant pleural effusion [5]. In this case report, a compromised performance status, lymphangitis carcinomatosa and bilateral pleural effusions were observed in the chest and, hence, could be the key factors contributing to the development of ILD.

The median duration from the initiation of crizotinib therapy to the onset of ILD was found to be 23 days (range: 3–763 days) [2]. Créquit et al. described that a severe, usually fatal ILD developed within the 1st month of treatment, and its chest CT manifestation included an early onset of ground-glass opacity, which diffused and spread rapidly in both lungs [6]. In our case, in addition to multiple ground-glass opacity lesions, multiple consolidation lesions were found simultaneously, which coincided with our pathological staging features of the transition from exudation to the organizing period. Moreover, it was reasonable to assume that the clinical symptoms and imaging changes of interstitial pneumonia would be observed earlier than the tenth day without MP administration at the time of admission.

Possible pathological causation of crizotinib-induced ILD has been discussed in several studies [6–8]. In these studies, specimens were obtained either from bronchoscopic lung biopsy, alveolar lavage fluid or corpse biopsy. Limited by the quality and phase of biopsy specimen collection, these pathological findings could only reveal incomplete characteristics of interstitial pneumonia. To explore the pathology of the case reported in this study, we applied an HE staining technique to three freshly coloured, cylindrical percutaneous biopsy samples, which fully met the requirements for diagnosis of ILD. We first excluded the possibility of infection, and no invasion of tumour cells could be observed either. Histological characteristics, such as a thickened alveolar septa, infiltration of inflammatory cells in the interstitium, foamy macrophages and hyalinosis in alveolar cavities,

hyaline thrombi (microthrombi) in pulmonary arterioles, and atypical hyperplasia of type II alveolar epithelial cells, corresponded to typical diffuse alveolar damage. The pathological stage of transition from exudation to the organizing period was also proposed. As far as we are aware, all these detailed pathological features have not been reported in the literature so far.

It is worth noting that a de novo EGFR mutation was detected in the ILD biopsy, which was not found at the time of admission. One possible reason could be a low abundance of EGFR-mutated subclones that already existed in tumour tissue at the time of admission. These cells survived the crizotinib treatment, and their abundance increased. Recently, several studies have suggested that ROS1 rearrangements co-occur with mutations in EGFR at clinically relevant frequencies [9–11]. Another reason might be that crizotinib treatment induces acquired mutations in EGFR. Activation of EGFR, which enables cancer cells to bypass crizotinib-mediated inhibition of ROS1 signalling, has been described as a mechanism of resistance to crizotinib in ROS1-rearranged NSCLC [12]. Interestingly, in ROS1-rearranged and other fusion kinase-driven cell line models, EGFR activation and signalling appear to serve as an important early adaptive survival response to TKI exposure [13]. In this case, a decrease in original tumour lesions was observed before the time of lung biopsy, suggesting that the detectable EGFR mutations had not triggered crizotinib resistance in this period. ILD can be frequently caused by targeted therapy in EGFR-positive patients; however, the link between EGFR mutations, targeted therapy and ILD requires further investigation. It is also notable that there were no tumour cells detected in the second round of pathological diagnosis in the patient. Therefore, the detection of the EGFR mutation could be due to DNA fragments of ruptured tumour cells merging with interstices. In summary, there is not sufficient evidence to demonstrate that the EGFR mutation resulted in crizotinib resistance in this case because of radiological shrinkage of original tumour lesions and pathological features of new-onset lesion biopsy. Nevertheless, it is worth investigating the relationship between EGFR mutations and ILD in the future.

The limitations of this case report are that we did not detect hydrothorax after the treatment, and other gene mutation-detecting methods were not used to further examine all the specimens to exclude detection error.

Conclusions

In conclusion, advanced non-small-cell lung cancer in patients with ROS1 rearrangements, treated with crizotinib, may be accompanied by fatal ILD in the initial period. Histopathology and molecular pathological examination of lung biopsy specimens is crucial for differential diagnosis and treatment guidance.

Authors' contributions

SBW and KTL conceived and designed the study. FR, DP and FR performed the analyses. SBW and DP prepared all tables. KTL and DWZ wrote the main manuscript. All authors reviewed the manuscript. All authors read and approved the final manuscript.

Competing interests

The authors declare that they have no competing interests.

Author details

[1]Department of Respiratory Medicine, Lihuili Hospital, Ningbo Medical Center, No. 57, Xin'ning Road, Ningbo 315041, China. [2]Department of Radiation Oncology, Lihuili Hospital, Ningbo Medical Center, Ningbo 315041, China. [3]Department of Radiology, Lihuili Hospital, Ningbo Medical Center, Ningbo 315041, China. [4]Department of Thoracic Surgery, Lihuili Hospital, Ningbo Medical Center, Ningbo 315041, China. [5]Department of Diagnosis, Ningbo Diagnostic Pathology Center, No. 79, Huan'cheng Road, Ningbo 315021, China.

References

1. Bergethon K, Shaw AT, Ou SH, et al. ROS1 rearrangements define a unique molecular class of lung cancers. J Clin Oncol. 2012;30:863–70.
2. Yoneda KY, Scranton JR, Michael A, et al. Interstitial lung disease associated with Crizotinib in patients with advanced none small cell lung Cancer: independent review of four PROFILE trials. Clin Lung Cancer. 2015;18(5):472–9.
3. Data on file (62a). Pfizer.
4. Shaw AT, Ou S-HI, Bang Y-J, et al. Crizotinib in ROS1-rearranged non–small-cell lung Cancer. N Engl J Med. 2014;371:1963–71.
5. Gemma A, Kusumoto M, Kurihara Y, et al. Analysis of Data on Interstitial Lung Disease Onset and Its Risk Following Treatment of ALK-positive NSCLC with Xalkori [poster]. Presented at WCLC 2017, October 15–18; Yokohama, Japan. Abstract no. 9146.
6. Créquit P, Wislez M, Fleury Feith J, et al. Crizotinib associated with ground-glass opacity predominant pattern interstitial lung disease. J Thorac Oncol. 2015;10:1148–55.
7. Tamiya A, Okamoto S, Miyazaki M, Shimizu S, Kitaichi M, Nakagawa K. Severe acute interstitial lung disease after Crizotinib therapy in a patient with EML4-ALKepositive none-small-cell lung cancer. J Clin Oncol. 2013;31:149–51.
8. Tachihara M, Kobayashi K, Ishikawa Y, et al. Successful Crizotinib Rechallenge after Crizotinib-induced interstitial lung disease. Jpn J Clin Oncol. 2014;44(8):762–4.
9. Rimkunas VM, Crosby KE, Li D, et al. Analysis of receptor tyrosine kinase ROS1-positive tumors in non-small cell lung cancer: identification of a FIG-ROS1 fusion. Clin Cancer Res. 2012;18:4449–57.
10. Wiesweg M, Eberhardt WE, Reis H, et al. High prevalence of concomitant oncogene mutations in prospectively identified patients with ROS1-positive metastatic lung cancer. J Thorac Oncol. 2017;12:54–64.
11. Lin JJ, Ritterhouse LL, Ali SM, et al. ROS1 fusions rarely overlap with other oncogenic drivers in non-small cell lung cancer. J Thorac Oncol. 2017;12:872–7.
12. Davies KD, Mahale S, Astling DP, et al. Resistance to ROS1 inhibition mediated by EGFR pathway activation in non-small cell lung cancer. PLoS One. 2013;8(12):e82236.
13. Vaishnavi A, Schubert L, Rix U, et al. EGFR mediates responses to small-molecule drugs targeting oncogenic fusion kinases. Cancer Res. 2017;77:3351–63.

10

Physical activity and sedentary time are related to clinically relevant health outcomes among adults with obstructive lung disease

Shilpa Dogra[1*], Joshua Good[1], Matthew P. Buman[2], Paul A. Gardiner[3], Jennifer L. Copeland[4] and Michael K. Stickland[5]

Abstract

Background: The purpose of the current study was to determine the association between sedentary time and physical activity with clinically relevant health outcomes among adults with impaired spirometry and those with or without self-reported obstructive lung disease (asthma or COPD).

Methods: Data from participants of the Canadian Longitudinal Study on Aging were used for analysis ($n = 4156$). Lung function was assessed using spirometry. Adults were said to have impaired spirometry if their Forced Expiratory Volume in 1 s was <5th percentile lower limit of normal (LLN). A modified version of the Physical Activity Scale for the Elderly was used to assess sitting time and physical activity levels. Healthcare use and quality of life outcomes were assessed using self report.

Results: Among those with asthma, participating in strengthening activities was associated with lower odds of reporting poor perceived health (OR = 0.65, CI: 0.53, 0.79), poor perceived mental-health (OR = 0.73, CI: 0.60, 0.88), unhealthy aging (OR = 0.68, CI: 0.56, 0.83), and reporting an emergency department visit in the past 12 months (OR = 0.76, CI: 0.60, 0.95). Among those with COPD, those who reported highest weekly sedentary time had higher odds of reporting poor perceived health (OR = 2.70, CI: 1.72, 4.24), poor perceived mental-health (OR = 1.99, CI: 1.29, 3.06), and unhealthy aging (OR = 3.04, CI: 1.96, 4.72). Among those below the LLN, sitting time (OR = 2.57, CI: 1.40, 4.72) and moderate intensity physical activity (OR = 0.23, CI: 0.09, 0.63) were associated with overnight hospital stays.

Conclusions: Higher physical activity levels and lower sedentary time may be associated with lower healthcare use and better quality of life. This research may have implications related to the use of physical activity for improving health outcomes and quality of life among adults with obstructive lung disease or impaired spirometry.

Keywords: Asthma, COPD, Physical activity, Hospitalization

Background

Chronic obstructive lung diseases such as asthma and chronic obstructive pulmonary disease (COPD) are estimated to affect 4.3 and 4.7% of the global population, respectively [1, 2], with the prevalence as high as 20–25% in some countries [1, 3]. Obstructive lung diseases are typically associated with suboptimal quality of life, and an increased burden on the healthcare system [4, 5]. Importantly, adults with chronic lung diseases who are physically active have better health outcomes, and lower health care use than their inactive peers [6–8]. Among those with COPD, systematic reviews of the literature have shown that physical inactivity is associated with worse lung function [9], lower health-related quality of life, and greater dyspnea [10]. Similarly, while regular exercise is not associated with improved lung function among adults with asthma, it leads to significant improvements in health related quality of life [11].

* Correspondence: Shilpa.Dogra@uoit.ca
[1]Faculty of Health Sciences (Kinesiology), University of Ontario Institute of Technology, 2000 Simcoe St N, Oshawa, ON L1H-7K4, Canada
Full list of author information is available at the end of the article

Evidence suggests that individuals with obstructive lung disease are often misdiagnosed using previously established fixed ratio lung function cut-points [12]. It has been suggested that clinicians use the lower limit of normal (LLN), that is, spirometry values below the 5th percentile, instead [12]. Not surprisingly, the risk of hospitalization is higher among those with COPD who are below the LLN compared to those above the LLN [13]. However, no evidence is available on the association between physical activity and health outcomes among those below the LLN, regardless of whether they have a diagnosed lung disease.

There is also a dearth of research on the association between sedentary time and health outcomes among those with obstructive lung disease. Sedentary behavior is any activity performed in a seated or reclined position requiring low energy expenditure while awake [14], and a growing body of literature suggests an association between time spent in sedentary activities and health [15], particularly among older adults [16]. Among those with COPD and asthma, sedentary time may be associated with dyspnea, higher health care use, worse disease management, and all-cause mortality [17–20]. Recent evidence suggests that both physical activity and sedentary time are associated with lung function among healthy adults (Dogra S, Good J, Buman MP, Gardiner P, Stickland MK, Copeland J. Movement behaviours are associated with lung function in middle-aged and older adults: a cross-sectional analysis of the Canadian longitudinal study on aging, unpublished). However, the association between sedentary time and clinically relevant health outcomes among those with existing obstructive lung diseases or among those with impaired spirometry is not known.

Physical activity levels among those with obstructive lung disease remain suboptimal [21], and sedentary time is likely high due to dyspnea and deconditioning. Both sedentary time and physical activity may be modifiable determinants of clinically relevant health outcomes among those with obstructive lung disease or those with impaired spirometry, and could be used clinically to understand symptom management. However, large database analysis is needed to establish correlations before clinical investigation can be undertaken. Thus, the purpose of the present analysis was to determine the association between sedentary time as well as different modes and intensities of physical activity with clinically relevant outcomes of lung function, healthcare use, and quality of life, among middle-aged and older adults with self-reported obstructive lung disease (i.e. COPD, asthma). We also examined these associations separately among those who had impaired spirometry as per the LLN, regardless of whether they had a diagnosed lung disease.

Methods

Data source and participants

The Canadian Longitudinal Study on Aging (CLSA) is a nationally representative, stratified, random sample of 51,338 Canadian women and men aged 45 to 85 years (at baseline). The purpose of this survey is to collect data on the health and quality of life of Canadians to better understand the processes and dimensions of aging. The study contains two samples: the CLSA Comprehensive, and the CLSA Tracking. Data from participants in the first sample were collected through questionnaires, physical examinations and biological samples. These participants live within a 25-50 km radius of one of the 11 data collection sites across Canada (Vancouver/Surrey (two sites), Victoria, Calgary, Winnipeg, Hamilton, Ottawa, Montreal, Sherbrooke, Halifax, and St. John's). This sample contains approximately 30,000 participants, recruited between 2012 and 2015, and was used for the current study.

Inclusion in the CLSA was limited to those who were able to read and speak either French or English. Residents in the three territories and some remote regions, persons living on federal First Nations reserves and other First Nations settlements in the provinces, and full-time members of the Canadian Armed Forces were excluded. Individuals living in long-term care institutions (i.e., those providing 24-h nursing care) were excluded at baseline; however, those living in households and transitional housing arrangements (e.g., seniors' residences, in which only minimal care is provided) were included. Finally, those with a cognitive impairment at the time of recruitment were excluded.

The protocol of the CLSA has been reviewed and approved by 13 research ethics boards across Canada. Changes to the CLSA protocol are reviewed annually. Written consent is obtained from all participants. The University of Ontario Institute of Technology Research Ethics Board approved secondary analysis of the CLSA dataset (REB #1367).

Measures

Outcome variables

Forced expiratory volume in 1 s (FEV$_1$) Spirometry was conducted using the TruFlow Easy-On Spirometer. Only those with major contraindications did not perform the test [22]. Maximal inspiratory and expiratory maneuvers were performed to obtain FEV$_1$ and forced vital capacity (FVC). Only participants who performed at least three acceptable efforts, with their best two FVC and FEV$_1$ within 150 ml, were included. The best FEV$_1$ and FVC were used for analysis.

Healthcare use Participants were asked "Have you been seen in an Emergency Department during the past 12 months?" and "Were you a patient in a hospital over-night during the past 12 months?". Response options were yes or no.

Quality of life Participants were asked "In general, would you say your health is excellent, very good, good, fair, or poor?", "In general, would you say your mental health is excellent, very good, good, fair, or poor?", and "In terms of your own healthy aging, would you say it is excellent, very good, good, fair, or poor?". Each variable was re-categorized in to "Good" (excellent, or very good,) and "Poor" (good, fair, or poor) based on the distribution of the sample.

Lung disease categories

Participants were asked whether a doctor had ever told them that they have asthma, and whether a doctor had ever told them that they have emphysema, chronic bronchitis, chronic obstructive pulmonary disease (COPD), or chronic changes to their lungs due to smoking. Participants who responded "yes" to either question were considered to have an obstructive lung disease, regardless of spirometry data. Thus, asthma and COPD were self-reported.

Participants with a $FEV_1 > 10$ Litres were excluded. Predicted FEV_1 ($FEV_{1\%pred}$) and LLN were calculated based on age, height, and sex using formulas developed on the Canadian population [23]. The LLN for each participant was calculated using the formula:

$$LLN = \text{predicted value} - (1.645 \times \text{Standard Error of the Estimate})$$

Individuals with an $FEV_1 <$ 5th percentile LLN were considered to have impaired spirometry, regardless of whether they reported a diagnosed obstructive lung disease.

Exposure variables

Physical activity and sitting time A modified version of the Physical Activity Scale for Elderly (PASE) was used to collect information on sitting time and physical activity. The PASE is a valid and reliable tool for assessing physical activity and sitting time among older adults. It has been shown to have good test-retest reliability over a 3 to 7-week interval (0.75, 95% CI = 0.69–0.80). Construct validity has also been established [24].

With regard to sitting time, participants were asked "Over the past 7 days, how often did you participate in sitting activities such as reading, watching TV, computer activities or doing handicrafts?" and "On average, how many hours per day did you engage in these sitting activities?". The frequency of individual sitting activities

was recorded in categories of never, seldom (1 to 2 days), sometimes (3 to 4 days), or often (5 to 7 days) for frequency, and the duration of individual sitting activities was recorded in categories of < 30 min, 30 min to < 1 h, 1 h to < 2 h, 2 h to < 4 h, or 4 h or more. The midpoint of each frequency and duration category (except for the 4 h or more hours category, which was coded as 4 h), was used to estimate weekly total sitting time in hours per week.

The PASE also asks a series of questions pertaining to physical activity over the past 7 days. Specifically, participants were asked how often they took a walk outside, engaged in light sports or recreational activities, engaged in moderate sports or recreational activities, engaged in strenuous sports or recreational activities, and engaged in exercises specifically to increase muscle strength and endurance. The frequency and duration for each activity was recorded in the same way as for sitting time; the same midpoints were used to calculate hours per week spent in each type/intensity of activity.

Weekly physical activity and sitting time variables were categorized for logistic regressions. For sitting time (0 to 14 h, 14.1 to 18 h, and 18.1 to 24 h) and walking (0 to 2.25 h, 2.26 to 4.5 h, 4.6 to 24 h), there was enough variability to categorize the variables based on tertiles. For light intensity PA (0 h, > 0 h), moderate intensity physical activity (0 h, > 0 h), strenuous intensity PA (0 h, > 0 h), and muscle strengthening activity (0 h, > 0 h), variables were dichotomized due to lack of variability.

Covariates

Smoking status Pack years were calculated using eight variables from the CLSA. Participants who responded negatively to "Have you smoked at least 100 cigarettes in your life? (about 4 - 5 packs)" were categorized as "Never Smoked". Participants who were current smokers were asked "For how many total years have you smoked daily?" and "During the total years that you have smoked daily, about how many cigarettes per day have you usually smoked? (If your smoking pattern has changed over the years, make your best guess of the average number of cigarettes you have smoked per day.)" The number of cigarettes smoked per day was recorded in categories of 1–5, 6–10, 11–15, 16–20, 21–25, and 26+ cigarettes. The midpoint of each of category was used to determine the number of cigarettes smoked per day with the exception of 26+ cigarettes in which case an exact number was recorded. Similar questions were asked to former daily smokers.

Pack years was calculated as: [(number of cigarettes smoked per day/20 cigarettes per pack) x number of years smoked]. Pack years was then categorized into

Never Smoked, < 10 pack years, and 10 or more pack years. Participants who were never daily smokers but had smoked more than 100 lifetime cigarettes were included in the < 10 pack years category.

Others Participants were asked to report their age and sex, and provided information on several additional relevant covariates. For *sleep*, participants were asked "During the past month, on average, how many hours of actual sleep did you get at night?". This was categorized into < 6 h, 6–8 h, and > 8 h according to previous research on the association between sleep and health [25]. For *retirement status*, participants were asked "At this time, do you consider yourself to be completely retired, partly retired or not retired". Those who responded partly retired were merged with the not retired group due to sample size. For *education levels*, participants were asked four questions pertaining to their highest level of education. These responses were combined to categorize the sample as: Less than secondary school graduation, secondary school graduation, no post-secondary education, some post-secondary education, or post-secondary degree/diploma. Height and weight were measured by trained professionals, and used to calculate *body mass index* (kg/m^2).

For the present analysis, only those who reported an obstructive lung disease (defined above, $n = 5094$) or those with impaired spirometry ($n = 1747$) were included for analysis. Of note, participants may have been in multiple groups, that is, those with asthma may also have reported COPD, or had an FEV_1 below the LLN. Those who reported a history of lung cancer ($n = 103$) were not included, and only those with complete data for spirometry ($n = 4493$), physical activity and sitting time, quality of life, healthcare use ($n = 4212$), and all covariates ($n = 4156$) were included. In this select sample, 1939 had asthma only, 432 had COPD only, and 1021 were below LLN; 764 were in multiple groups. Of those with COPD, only 224 were below the LLN. Individuals who responded positively to "Have you taken any long acting inhalers in the last 12 hours?" and/or "Have you taken any short acting inhalers in the last 6 hours?" were excluded ($n = 713$) from analyses where spirometry was the main outcome.

Statistical analysis

Means and frequencies were used to describe the sample. Crude beta coefficients for the associations of $FEV_{1\%pred}$ and FEV_1/FVC with sitting time, walking, light physical activity, moderate physical activity, strenuous physical activity, and muscle strengthening activity were assessed using linear regression models. Hierarchical models were used to generate adjusted associations

for $FEV_{1\%pred}$. Specifically, block 1 contained all of the covariates (age, sex, sleep, retirement status, education level, and body mass index) while block 2 included each of the sedentary and physical activity variables. Models (containing both blocks) were run separately for those with asthma, COPD, and those who demonstrated impaired spirometry (FEV_1 below LLN).

Crude and adjusted odds ratios were calculated for quality of life (perceived general health, perceived mental health, and healthy aging) and healthcare use outcomes (emergency department visit and overnight hospitalization) for sitting time, walking, light physical activity, moderate physical activity, strenuous physical activity, and muscle strengthening activity using logistic regression models. Adjusted models included age, sex, sleep, retirement status, education level, body mass index, and $FEV_{1\%pred}$. Models were run separately for those with asthma, COPD, and those with impaired spirometry (FEV_1 below LLN).

All analyses were performed using SPSS v.24. To ensure national representation and to compensate for under-represented groups, sampling weights were applied to regression models. Significance was set at $p < 0.05$. Additional details on sampling, methods and weighting on the CLSA can be found in the protocol document [26, 27].

Results

The overall sample was 61.6 ± 9.9 years of age, with 45.5% being male. Per week, participants were averaging 18.3 ± 6.1 h of sitting time, 4.2 ± 4.6 h of walking, 0.8 ± 2.5 h of light intensity physical activity, 0.7 ± 2.4 h of moderate intensity physical activity, 1.3 ± 2.9 h of strenuous intensity physical activity, and 0.7 ± 1.7 h of strengthening activity. The sample had an average $FEV_{1\%pred}$ of $84.4 \pm 19.2\%$. Additional sample characteristics can be found by lung condition in Table 1.

In crude models assessing the association with $FEV_{1\%pred}$, participating in strenuous intensity physical activity was associated with better $FEV_{1\%pred}$ among those with asthma (β: 0.31, CI: 1.00–0.52), COPD (β: 0.78, CI: 0.21–1.35), and those below the LLN (β: 0.27, CI: 0.11–0.42) (Additional file 1: Figure S1). There were no significant associations once models were adjusted for covariates (age, sex, sleep, retirement status, education level, and body mass index, Fig. 1). The association between sitting time and FEV_1/FVC was significant among those with COPD (β: -0.18, CI:-0.28, – 0.08) such that a higher FEV_1/FVC was associated with lower sitting time. A significant association was also noted between FEV_1/FVC with strenuous intensity physical activity, such that those with COPD participating in strenuous intensity physical activity had a higher FEV_1/FVC. Finally, there was an inverse association with light intensity physical activity such that those below the LLN

Table 1 Sample Characteristics of Adults with Asthma, COPD, and those below the LLN

Characteristics		Asthma (n = 2569)	COPD (n = 877)	Below LLN for FEV$_1$ (n = 1545)
Age (years)		60.9 ± 9.7	65.0 ± 9.9	61.7 ± 9.9
BMI (kg/m^2)		29.0 ± 6.1	29.2 ± 6.3	29.6 ± 6.6
Height (cm)		167.0 ± 9.6	166.3 ± 9.5	170.8 ± 9.7
FEV$_1$ (L)		2.5 ± 0.7	2.2 ± 0.8	2.0 ± 0.6
FEV$_1$% predicted		91.2 ± 17.3	85.1 ± 20.4	65.4 ± 9.7
FVC (L)		3.4 ± 0.9	3.1 ± 0.9	2.9 ± 0.8
FVC % predicted		90.6 ± 14.6	85.9 ± 16.1	70.6 ± 10.8
FEV$_1$/FVC		0.75 ± 0.07	0.72 ± 0.09	0.69 ± 0.09
FEV$_1$/FVC % predicted		99.9 ± 9.4	97.3 ± 12.0	92.9 ± 12.0
Education (% of sample)	Less than secondary school graduation	4.0%	9.2%	6.2%
	Secondary school graduation, no post-secondary education	7.3%	10.3%	9.6%
	Some post-secondary education	6.8%	9.9%	8.3%
	Post-secondary degree/diploma	81.9%	70.6%	75.9%
Retirement Status (% of sample)	Retired	38.1%	54.0%	41.1%
	Not or partly retired	61.9%	46.0%	58.9%
Activity Levels (hours/week)	In sitting activities	18.2 ± 6.1	19.1 ± 5.9	18.5 ± 6.1
	Walking	4.3 ± 4.7	3.9 ± 4.3	4.1 ± 4.7
	Light activities	0.8 ± 2.5	0.9 ± 2.6	0.8 ± 2.6
	Moderate sports or recreational activities	0.7 ± 2.4	0.7 ± 2.6	0.6 ± 2.3
	Strenuous sports or recreational activities	1.5 ± 3.0	0.8 ± 2.2	1.1 ± 2.7
	Increase muscle strength and endurance	0.7 ± 1.7	0.7 ± 1.9	0.6 ± 1.5
Sleep (% of sample)	Less than 6 h	14.4%	19.8%	14.4%
	6 to 8 h	80.1%	71.2%	80.8%
	More than 8 h	5.4%	9.0%	4.8%
Perceived health (% of sample)	Good (excellent and very good	56.3%	42.9%	48.3%
	Poor (good, fair, and poor)	43.7%	57.1%	51.7%
Self-rated healthy aging (% of sample)	Good (excellent and very good	59.0%	46.2%	49.6%
	Poor (good, fair, and poor)	41.0%	53.8%	50.4%
Self-rated mental health (% of sample)	Good (excellent and very good	66.6%	57.8%	66.0%
	Poor (good, fair, and poor)	33.4%	42.2%	34.0%
Emergency visit in last 12 months (% Yes)		21.1%	26.7%	20.5%
Overnight hospitalization in last 12 months (% Yes)		8.8%	12.5%	9.9%

participating in light intensity physical activity had lower FEV$_1$/FVC. No other associations were significant in crude models (Additional file 2: Figure S2).

The associations for healthcare use outcomes are presented in Table 2. In crude models, sedentary time, walking, moderate intensity, and strenuous intensity physical activity were associated with overnight hospital stays in both adults with asthma and those below the LLN. In models adjusted for covariates (age, sex, sleep, retirement status, education level, body mass index, and FEV$_{1\%pred}$), participating in light intensity activity (OR:

0.61, CI: 0.40–0.92) was associated with lower odds of reporting an overnight hospital stay among those with asthma compared to those who were not physically active at light intensities. Among those below the LLN, sedentary time appeared to be important for overnight hospital stays such that those who reported 14.1–18 h/week (OR: 2.03, CI: 1.09–3.78) and those who reported 18.1–24 h per week (OR: 2.57, CI: 1.40–4.72) were approximately 2 times more likely to report an overnight hospital stay than those who reported < 14 h per week of sedentary time.

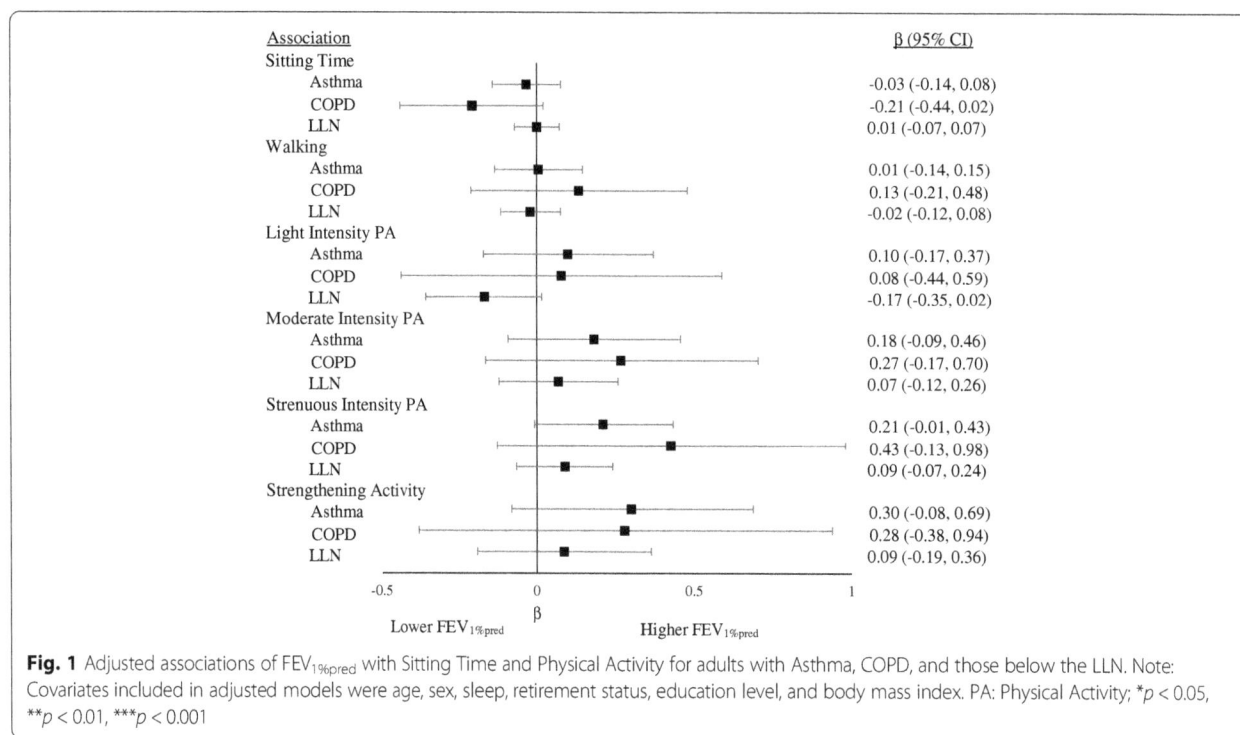

Fig. 1 Adjusted associations of $FEV_{1\%pred}$ with Sitting Time and Physical Activity for adults with Asthma, COPD, and those below the LLN. Note: Covariates included in adjusted models were age, sex, sleep, retirement status, education level, and body mass index. PA: Physical Activity; *$p < 0.05$, **$p < 0.01$, ***$p < 0.001$

Associations for poor perceived health, poor perceived mental health, and unhealthy aging are presented in Figs. 2, 3 and 4 (crude associations are presented in Additional file 3: Figure S3, Additional file 4: Figure S4, Additional file 5: Figure S5). Among those with asthma, participating in strengthening activities was associated with lower odds of reporting poor perceived health (OR: 0.65, CI: 0.53–0.79), poor perceived mental-health (OR: 0.73, CI: 0.60–0.88), and unhealthy aging (OR: 0.68, CI: 0.56–0.83) compared to those who did not participate in strengthening activity in fully adjusted models. Among those with COPD, those who reported higher weekly sedentary time had higher odds of reporting poor perceived health, poor perceived mental-health, and unhealthy aging in fully adjusted models. Finally, among those below the LLN, participating in strenuous intensity physical activity was associated with lower odds of reporting poor perceived health (OR: 0.59, CI: 0.46–0.76), perceived mental-health (OR: 0.62, CI: 0.48–0.81), and unhealthy aging (OR: 0.54, CI: 0.42–0.69) compared to those who did not participate in strenuous physical activity in fully adjusted models.

Discussion

These data are the first, to our knowledge, to assess the associations of sitting time, strenuous intensity physical activity, and strengthening activity among adults with obstructive lung disease, and the first to conduct such analyses among those who fall below the LLN for FEV_1. Our primary finding is that physical activity and sedentary time *may be* important risk factors for hospitalization. Specifically, light intensity physical activity was associated with lower odds of reporting an overnight hospital stay, and strengthening activity was associated with lower odds of an emergency department visit among adults with asthma. Further, among those with a FEV_1 below the LLN, engaging in less than 14 h of sedentary time or participating in moderate intensity physical activity were associated with lower odds of reporting an overnight hospital stay. In addition to hospitalization, physical activity and sedentary time were consistently associated with quality of life measures amongst the three groups. These findings provide insight into the importance of physical activity and sedentary time for disease management among individuals with obstructive lung disease or among those with impaired spirometry.

Asthma

The association between physical activity and clinically relevant health outcomes among adults with asthma is not surprising [6, 19], however, associations with sedentary time and strengthening activity are poorly studied. To date, most of the available literature in the area of asthma and sedentary time is from young samples [28]. In a Canadian study of Indigenous adults, it was found that healthcare use was higher among those who watched more than 10 h of television per week after adjustment for physical activity [19]. Little additional data are available in adults. Similarly, for the association between strengthening activity and asthma outcomes,

Table 2 Associations of Healthcare Use with Sitting Time and Physical Activity among adults with Asthma, COPD, and those below the LLN

Activity (referent category)	Category	Asthma		COPD		Below LLN for FEV$_1$	
		Overnight hospital visit	Emergency department visit	Overnight hospital visit	Emergency department visit	Overnight hospital visit	Emergency department visit
		OR (95% CI)	OR (95% CI)	OR (95% CI)	OR (95% CI)	OR (95% CI)	OR (95% CI)
a) Crude associations							
Sitting Time (14 h/ week or less)	14.1 to 18 h/ week	1.10 (0.74–1.63)	1.16 (0.90–1.49)	1.10 (0.55–2.20)	1.42 (0.89–2.26)	2.40** (1.30–4.43)	1.45* (1.02–2.05)
	18.1 to 24 h/ week	1.63* (1.12–2.38)	1.32* (1.03–1.70)	1.70 (0.89–3.25)	1.44 (0.91–2.27)	3.48*** (1.92–6.29)	1.39 (0.99–1.97)
Walking (2.25 h/week or less)	2.26 to 4.5 h/ week	0.62** (0.45–0.86)	0.78* (0.62–0.96)	0.67 (0.38–1.18)	0.93 (0.64–1.37)	0.65* (0.43–0.99)	0.81 (0.60–1.10)
	4.6 to 24 h/ week	0.58** (0.40–0.83)	0.86 (0.68–1.08)	1.04 (0.61–1.75)	1.15 (0.78–1.69)	0.55* (0.35–0.87)	0.76 (0.56–1.04)
Light Intensity PA (No time reported)	Greater than 0 h/ week	0.58** (0.39–0.86)	0.90 (0.71–1.14)	1.07 (0.63–1.83)	1.75** (1.21–2.52)	0.77 (0.47–1.25)	1.15 (0.84–1.58)
Moderate Intensity PA (No time reported)	Greater than 0 h/ week	0.49** (0.29–0.83)	0.76 (0.57–1.03)	0.61 (0.27–1.36)	0.76 (0.46–1.26)	0.22** (0.08–0.59)	0.82 (0.55–1.24)
Strenuous PA (No time reported)	Greater than 0 h/ week	0.57*** (0.41–0.78)	0.78* (0.64–0.95)	0.50* (0.27–0.92)	1.01 (0.70–1.45)	0.53** (0.34–0.81)	0.79 (0.60–1.04)
Strengthening Activity (No time reported)	Greater than 0 h/ week	0.87 (0.63–1.19)	0.70** (0.56–0.87)	0.94 (0.56–1.59)	1.22 (0.85–1.75)	0.83 (0.55–1.25)	1.15 (0.87–1.52)
b) Adjusted associations							
Sitting Time (14 h/ week or less)	14.1 to 18 h/ week	0.92 (0.61–1.38)	1.07 (0.82–1.38)	1.08 (0.52–2.22)	1.41 (0.87–2.29)	2.03* (1.09–3.78)	1.38 (0.97–1.97)
	18.1 to 24 h/ week	1.04 (0.69–1.55)	1.11 (0.85–1.44)	1.25 (0.63–2.51)	1.39 (0.86–2.26)	2.57** (1.40–4.72)	1.30 (0.91–1.87)
Walking (2.25 h/week or less)	2.26 to 4.5 h/ week	0.75 (0.53–1.05)	0.86 (0.68–1.08)	0.80 (0.43–1.47)	0.97 (0.65–1.46)	0.74 (0.47–1.14)	0.84 (0.62–1.14)
	4.6 to 24 h/ week	0.69 (0.47–1.00)	0.93 (0.74–1.18)	1.31 (0.75–2.30)	1.20 (0.80–1.81)	0.70 (0.43–1.12)	0.82 (0.59–1.12)
Light Intensity PA (No time reported)	Greater than 0 h/ week	0.61* (0.40–0.92)	0.95 (0.75–1.20)	1.28 (0.73–2.27)	1.99* (1.35–2.93)	0.95 (0.57–1.56)	1.25 (0.90–1.73)
Moderate Intensity PA (No time reported)	Greater than 0 h/ week	0.58 (0.34–1.00)	0.85 (0.63–1.14)	0.74 (0.32–1.73)	0.75 (0.43–1.29)	0.23** (0.09–0.63)	0.85 (0.56–1.29)
Strenuous PA (No time reported)	Greater than 0 h/ week	0.80 (0.56–1.13)	1.01 (0.81–1.25)	0.61 (0.32–1.16)	0.99 (0.67–1.48)	0.69 (0.44–1.11)	0.86 (0.63–1.17)
Strengthening Activity (No time reported)	Greater than 0 h/ week	1.13 (0.80–1.58)	0.76* (0.60–0.95)	1.20 (0.68–2.11)	1.37 (0.93–2.01)	1.08 (0.70–1.69)	1.35* (1.00–1.82)

A higher OR indicates a higher odds of having an overnight hospitalization or emergency room visit in the last 12 months relative to the referent category (as indicated in title). Covariates included in adjusted models were age, sex, sleep, retirement status, education level, body mass index, and FEV$_{1\%pred}$. PA: Physical Activity; *p < 0.05, **p < 0.01, ***p < 0.001

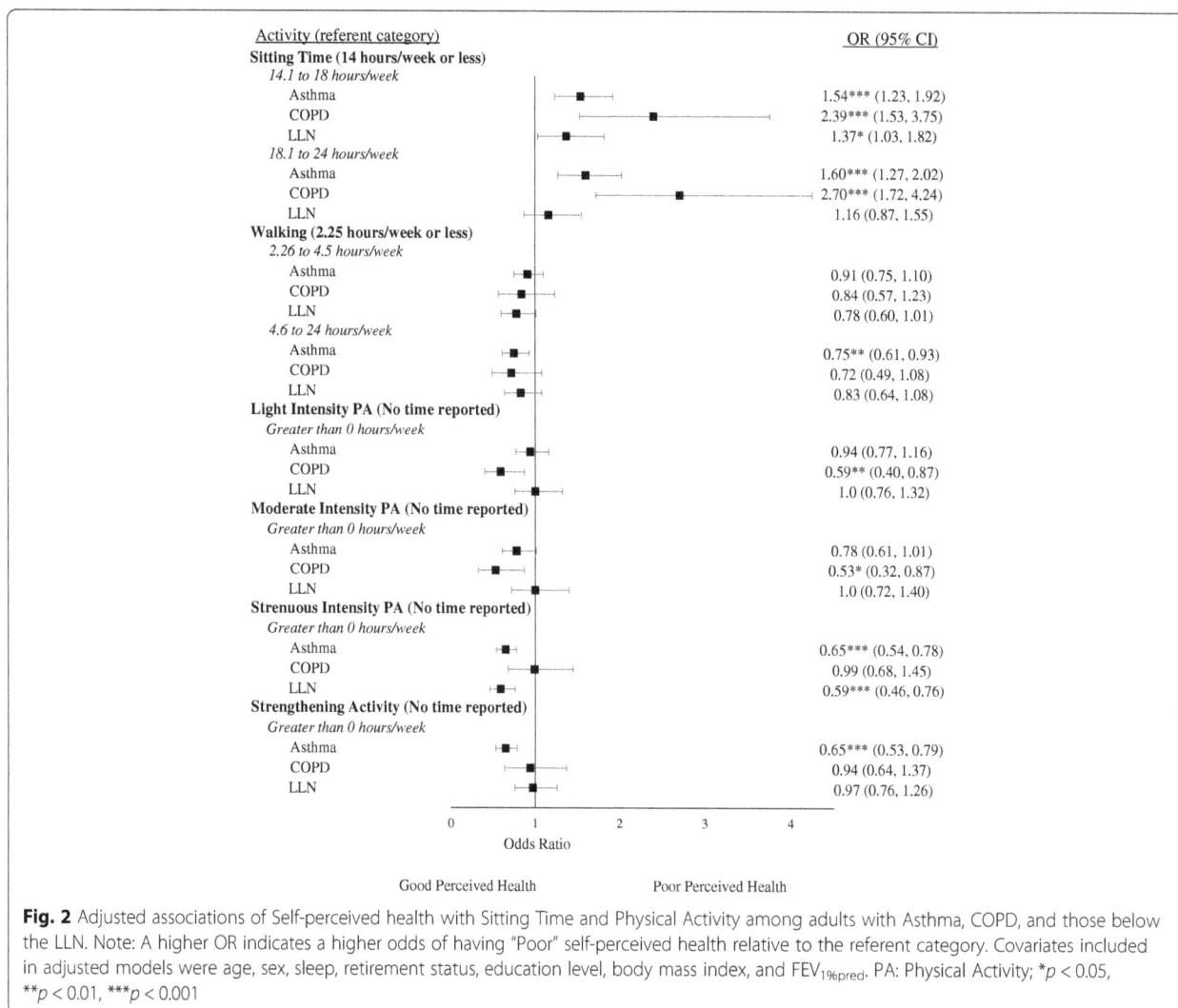

Fig. 2 Adjusted associations of Self-perceived health with Sitting Time and Physical Activity among adults with Asthma, COPD, and those below the LLN. Note: A higher OR indicates a higher odds of having "Poor" self-perceived health relative to the referent category. Covariates included in adjusted models were age, sex, sleep, retirement status, education level, body mass index, and FEV$_{1\%pred}$. PA: Physical Activity; *$p < 0.05$, **$p < 0.01$, ***$p < 0.001$

evidence from RCTs in obese adults with asthma indicate that concurrent strengthening and endurance training improve a variety of asthma specific outcomes [29], however the independent effect of strength training is not clear. Strength training may be a particularly important activity to assess among adults with asthma as it has a low ventilatory requirement and thus less likely to induce bronchoconstriction. Given that adults with asthma tend to be less active than their peers, reducing sedentary time or engaging in strengthening activities may be an effective method for initiating an active lifestyle. The present study highlights several opportunities for future research among adults with asthma.

Chronic obstructive pulmonary disease

Associations between physical activity and a variety of quality of life and healthcare use measures have been previously reported among adults with COPD [30–33]. The novelty of the present study is the assessment of different intensities of physical activity, as well the inclusion of strengthening activity and sedentary time. Previous work has found that light intensity physical activity, but not high intensity physical activity, is important for hospitalization avoidance among those with COPD [33]. Surprisingly, the current study found that engaging in light intensity physical activity was associated with *increased* risk of emergency department visits in COPD patients, whereas no association was found between moderate or strenuous physical activity and emergency department visits. Previous work that found that light intensity physical activity was associated with hospitalization avoidance used an activity monitor (Sensewear Armband) to record physical activity, whereas the CLSA uses a self-reported tool. Self-reported physical activity may lack precision, and additional follow-up studies using physical activity monitors are needed to better understand how different intensities of physical activity relate to healthcare utilization in COPD. Furthermore, it is possible that those with severe COPD experienced exacerbations or severe

Physical activity and sedentary time are related to clinically relevant health outcomes among adults...

77

Activity (referent category)	OR (95% CI)
Sitting Time (14 hours/week or less)	
14.1 to 18 hours/week	
Asthma	1.15 (0.93, 1.44)
COPD	2.21*** (1.43, 3.40)
LLN	0.82 (0.61, 1.09)
18.1 to 24 hours/week	
Asthma	1.15 (0.91, 1.44)
COPD	1.99** (1.29, 3.06)
LLN	0.92 (0.69, 1.23)
Walking (2.25 hours/week or less)	
2.26 to 4.5 hours/week	
Asthma	0.93 (0.76, 1.13)
COPD	1.05 (0.73, 1.50)
LLN	0.71* (0.54, 0.92)
4.6 to 24 hours/week	
Asthma	1.00 (0.82, 1.23)
COPD	1.02 (0.70, 1.49)
LLN	0.87 (0.66, 1.13)
Light Intensity PA (No time reported)	
Greater than 0 hours/week	
Asthma	0.89 (0.73, 1.10)
COPD	0.58** (0.39, 0.85)
LLN	0.88 (0.65, 1.17)
Moderate Intensity PA (No time reported)	
Greater than 0 hours/week	
Asthma	0.74* (0.57, 0.96)
COPD	0.62 (0.38, 1.00)
LLN	1.07 (0.76, 1.52)
Strenuous Intensity PA (No time reported)	
Greater than 0 hours/week	
Asthma	0.93 (0.77, 1.12)
COPD	1.04 (0.72, 1.49)
LLN	0.62*** (0.48, 0.81)
Strengthening Activity (No time reported)	
Greater than 0 hours/week	
Asthma	0.73** (0.60, 0.88)
COPD	0.67* (0.47, 0.97)
LLN	1.20 (0.93, 1.56)

Odds Ratio

Good Perceived Mental Health   Poor Perceived Mental Health

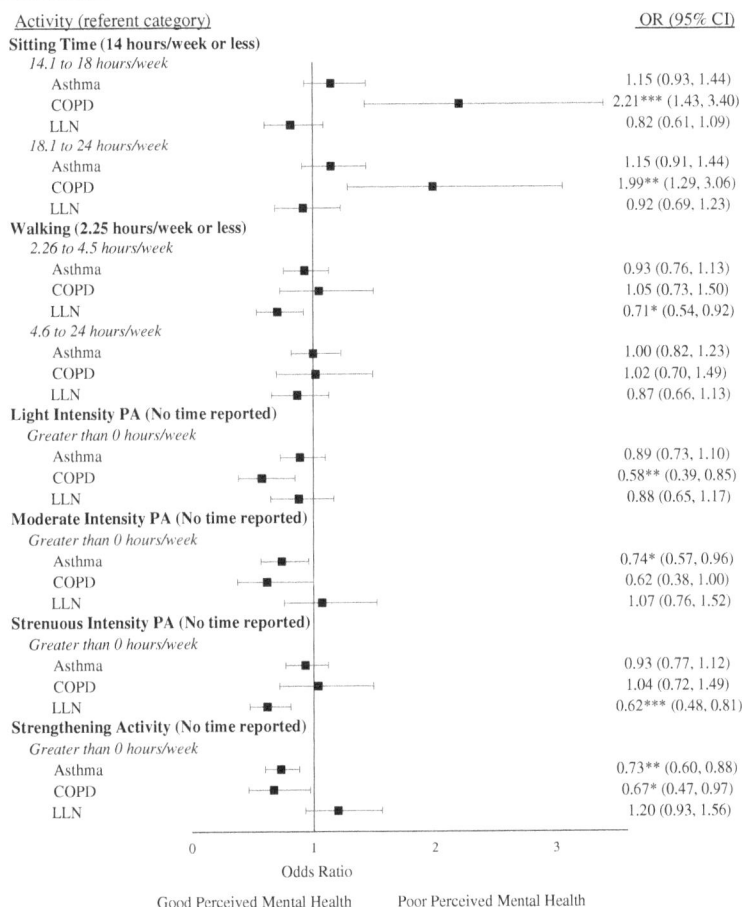

Fig. 3 Adjusted associations of Self-perceived mental health with Sitting Time and Physical Activity among adults with Asthma, COPD, and those below the LLN. Note: A higher OR indicates a higher odds of having "Poor" self-perceived mental health relative to the referent category. Covariates included in adjusted models were age, sex, sleep, retirement status, education level, body mass index, and $FEV_{1\%pred}$. PA: Physical Activity; *$p < 0.05$, **$p < 0.01$, ***$p < 0.001$

dyspnea due to engagement in light intensity physical activity, thus increasing their odds of emergency medical needs. Of note, the examples provided for light intensity physical activity in the questionnaire (eg: bowling, golf with a cart) may be of higher relative intensity for individuals with severe COPD. Future research is needed to better understand the effects of disease severity and comorbidity on healthcare use outcomes.

While we did not observe an association between strenuous activity and hospitalizations, it should be noted that strenuous intensity physical activity is beneficial for dyspnea and ventilatory parameters [34], and leads to significant improvements in exercise capacity [35]. Higher exercise capacity is also associated with better health outcomes in COPD [36]. Therefore, future research should further investigate the potential role of strenuous intensity physical activity for COPD management.

The relationship between exercise capacity and health outcomes may further explain why strength training was important among those with COPD. Some research has shown that when compared to endurance training, strength training has the same effect on exercise capacity in COPD [37]; this may be explained by the marked skeletal muscle dysfunction in COPD [38]. Skeletal muscle dysfunction contributes to dyspnea, which may explain why sitting time was associated with quality of life measures and healthcare use measures in our sample. Specifically, poor lung function or disease management may lead to an increase in sedentary behaviours to avoid dyspnea. Although it has been documented that those with COPD have lower physical activity levels and higher sedentary time [39], no research to date has assessed the association of sedentary time with clinically relevant health outcomes in COPD.

Impaired spirometry

Only one other study, to our knowledge, has looked at the association between sedentary time and health outcomes in those with spirometry values below the

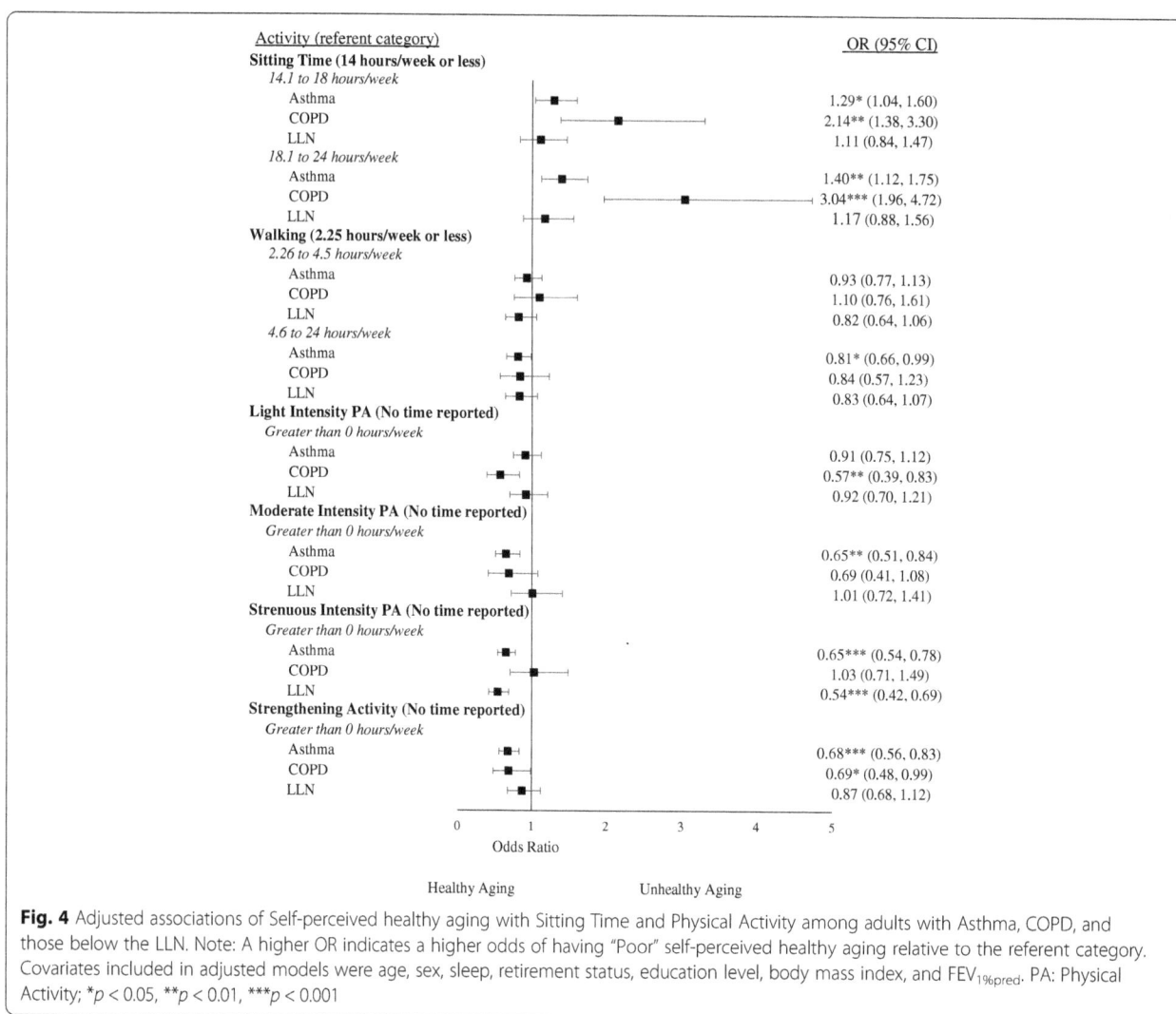

Activity (referent category)	OR (95% CI)
Sitting Time (14 hours/week or less)	
14.1 to 18 hours/week	
Asthma	1.29* (1.04, 1.60)
COPD	2.14** (1.38, 3.30)
LLN	1.11 (0.84, 1.47)
18.1 to 24 hours/week	
Asthma	1.40** (1.12, 1.75)
COPD	3.04*** (1.96, 4.72)
LLN	1.17 (0.88, 1.56)
Walking (2.25 hours/week or less)	
2.26 to 4.5 hours/week	
Asthma	0.93 (0.77, 1.13)
COPD	1.10 (0.76, 1.61)
LLN	0.82 (0.64, 1.06)
4.6 to 24 hours/week	
Asthma	0.81* (0.66, 0.99)
COPD	0.84 (0.57, 1.23)
LLN	0.83 (0.64, 1.07)
Light Intensity PA (No time reported)	
Greater than 0 hours/week	
Asthma	0.91 (0.75, 1.12)
COPD	0.57** (0.39, 0.83)
LLN	0.92 (0.70, 1.21)
Moderate Intensity PA (No time reported)	
Greater than 0 hours/week	
Asthma	0.65** (0.51, 0.84)
COPD	0.69 (0.41, 1.08)
LLN	1.01 (0.72, 1.41)
Strenuous Intensity PA (No time reported)	
Greater than 0 hours/week	
Asthma	0.65*** (0.54, 0.78)
COPD	1.03 (0.71, 1.49)
LLN	0.54*** (0.42, 0.69)
Strengthening Activity (No time reported)	
Greater than 0 hours/week	
Asthma	0.68*** (0.56, 0.83)
COPD	0.69* (0.48, 0.99)
LLN	0.87 (0.68, 1.12)

0   1   2   3   4   5
Odds Ratio

Healthy Aging   Unhealthy Aging

Fig. 4 Adjusted associations of Self-perceived healthy aging with Sitting Time and Physical Activity among adults with Asthma, COPD, and those below the LLN. Note: A higher OR indicates a higher odds of having "Poor" self-perceived healthy aging relative to the referent category. Covariates included in adjusted models were age, sex, sleep, retirement status, education level, body mass index, and $FEV_{1\%pred}$. PA: Physical Activity; *$p < 0.05$, **$p < 0.01$, ***$p < 0.001$

LLN. Vas Fragoso and colleagues [40] found that among community dwelling older adults, respiratory impairment (defined using $FEV_1 < LLN$) was associated with sedentary time and mobility impairment. Although we did not assess mobility impairment, our finding that strenuous intensity physical activity was important for perceived health and healthy aging suggests that perhaps exercise capacity or mobility are critical indicators of the impact that declining lung function has on functional ability and quality of life. In addition, perceived health has been associated with chronic conditions such as depression, anxiety, and mortality [41–44]. Therefore strenuous physical activity may be important for potential comorbidities among individuals with poor lung function. This study is the first to our knowledge to report on sedentary time and physical activity among adults below the LLN, and indicates that both sitting time and

strenuous intensity physical activity may be indicative of symptom management, and could be a valuable clinical tool.

Strengths of this study include the large sample of adults with asthma and COPD, the separate analysis of those with impaired spirometry (i.e. FEV_1 below the LLN), and use of a validated questionnaire for sitting time and physical activity. Nevertheless, device- measured physical activity and sitting time would provide more valid data, as well as the opportunity to analyze differences between prolonged and interrupted sitting time. Similarly, data on cardiorespiratory and musculo-skeletal fitness would have allowed for better understanding of the impact that physical activity and sedentary time have on health outcomes, as both physical activity and sedentary time are known to impact fitness levels, and fitness is likely a stronger predictor than the behaviours assessed.

Another limitation is the self-reported asthma, COPD, and healthcare use variables. It is possible that participants did not accurately recall hospital stays or emergency department visits; however, given that these are prominent events, and that response options were yes or no, the risk of misclassification is low. Furthermore, we did not have data on walk-in clinic use, which may be important among those with poorly controlled disease. It should also be noted that healthcare use could have been related to other comorbidities. While we did remove those with lung cancer, we did not adjust for additional chronic conditions. Thus, care should be taken when interpreting the findings, as individuals with COPD tend to have more comorbidities than individuals with asthma. Another limitation is that the FVC appears to be underestimated as the mean $FVC_{\%predicted}$ in the overall CLSA cohort was 93% (85.0 ± 16.3 in the selected sample for this study). Although the FVC data were reproducible, the reduced FVC suggests that participants may not have exhaled for the maximal possible duration, thereby overestimating the FEV_1/FVC and under reporting the degree of airflow obstruction.

Finally, it is important to note that data from the CLSA are cross-sectional, thus, reverse-causality cannot be ruled out at this time. In the next 5 years, the CLSA will provide its first round of longitudinal data where these associations can be further analyzed. Currently, it is not clear whether physical activity and sitting time change as a result of declining lung function, or whether low levels of physical activity and high levels of sitting time accelerate the decline in lung function. Given the previously described cyclical association between deconditioning and dyspnea, this association may be bi-directional. However, mechanistic studies are needed to understand how physical activity and sedentary time may affect outcomes such as lung function. For example, inflammation is associated with chronic lung disease, and is attenuated with participation in regular physical activity [45, 46], thus, it is possible that increasing physical activity and reducing sedentary time can directly affect respiratory disease physiology. With regard to healthcare use and quality of life, the role of functional autonomy, chronic comorbidities, medications, and disease control need to be assessed to better understand why physical activity and sitting time impact these outcomes.

Conclusion

In conclusion, data from a nationally representative sample of adults with asthma, COPD, and lung function below LLN indicate that physical activity and sedentary time may be predictors of healthcare use and quality of life. This research may have implications related to the use of physical activity for improving health outcomes and quality of life among adults with obstructive lung disease.

Additional files

Additional file 1: Figure S1. Crude associations of $FEV1_{\%pred}$ with Sitting Time and Physical Activity for adults with Asthma, COPD, and those below the LLN. Note: PA: Physical Activity; *$p < 0.05$, **$p < 0.01$, ***$p < 0.001$. (DOCX 23 kb)

Additional file 2: Figure S2. Crude associations of FEV_1/FVC with Sitting Time and Physical Activity for adults with Asthma, COPD, and those below the LLN. Note: β values for the change in FEV_1/FVC rather than the ratio (e.g. 70 to 70.2 rather than 0.70 to 0.702). PA: Physical Activity; *$p < 0.05$, **$p < 0.01$, ***$p < 0.001$. (DOCX 22 kb)

Additional file 3: Figure S3. Crude associations of Self-perceived health with Sitting Time and Physical Activity among adults with Asthma, COPD, and those below the LLN. Note: A higher OR indicates a higher odds of having "Poor" self-perceived health relative to the referent category. PA: Physical Activity; *$p < 0.05$, **$p < 0.01$, ***$p < 0.001$. (DOCX 23 kb)

Additional file 4: Figure S4. Crude associations of Self-perceived mental health with Sitting Time and Physical Activity among adults with Asthma, COPD, and those below the LLN. Note: A higher OR indicates a higher odds of having "Poor" self-perceived mental health relative to the referent category. PA: Physical Activity; *$p < 0.05$, **$p < 0.01$, ***$p < 0.001$. (DOCX 24 kb)

Additional file 5: Figure S5. Crude associations of Self-reported healthy aging with Sitting Time and Physical Activity among adults with Asthma, COPD, and those below the LLN. Note: A higher OR indicates a higher odds of having "Poor" self-reported healthy aging relative to the referent category. PA: Physical Activity; *$p < 0.05$, **$p < 0.01$, ***$p < 0.001$. (DOCX 23 kb)

Abbreviations

CI: Confidence interval; CLSA: Canadian Longitudinal Study on Aging; COPD: Chronic obstructive pulmonary disease; FEV_1: Forced expiratory volume in 1 seconds; FVC: Forced vital capacity; LLN: Lower limit of normal; PA: Physical activity; PASE: Physical Activity Scale for Elderly

Acknowledgements

This research was made possible using the data/biospecimens collected by the Canadian Longitudinal Study on Aging (CLSA).

Funding

This work was supported by the Canadian Institutes of Health Research [funding reference number 372547]. The funding body was not involved in the design of the study, collection, analysis, interpretation of data, and in writing the manuscript. Funding for the Canadian Longitudinal Study on Aging (CLSA) is provided by the Government of Canada through the Canadian Institutes of Health Research (CIHR) under grant reference: LSA 9447 and the Canada Foundation for Innovation. This research has been conducted using the CLSA dataset Baseline Comprehensive version 3.1 and Maintaining Contact version MCQ v2.0, under Application Number 170315. The CLSA is led by Drs. Parminder Raina, Christina Wolfson and Susan Kirkland.

Authors' contributions

SD contributed to the study design, data analysis, and writing of the manuscript. JG analyzed the data and contributed to the writing of the manuscript. MPB, PG, JLC, and MS contributed to the development of data analysis procedures and editing of the manuscript. All authors read and approved the final manuscript.

Competing interests
The authors declare that they have no competing interests.

Author details
[1]Faculty of Health Sciences (Kinesiology), University of Ontario Institute of Technology, 2000 Simcoe St N, Oshawa, ON L1H-7K4, Canada. [2]College of Health Solutions, Arizona State University, 550 N 3rd Street, Phoenix, AZ 85004, USA. [3]Faculty of Medicine, The University of Queensland, Level 2, Building 33, Princess Alexandra Hospital, Woolloongabba, QLD 4102, Australia. [4]Department of Kinesiology and Physical Education, University of Lethbridge, 4401 University Drive, Lethbridge, AB T1K 3M4, Canada. [5]Faculty of Medicine and Dentistry, University of Alberta, and G.F. Macdonald Centre for Lung Health, 3-135 Clinical Sciences Building, 11304 - 83 Avenue, Edmonton, Alberta T6G 2J3, Canada.

References

1. To T, Stanojevic S, Moores G, Gershon AS, Bateman ED, Cruz AA, et al. Global asthma prevalence in adults: findings from the cross-sectional world health survey. BMC Public Health. 2012;12(1):204.
2. Terzikhan N, Verhamme KM, Hofman A, Stricker BH, Brusselle GG, Lahousse L. Prevalence and incidence of COPD in smokers and non-smokers: the Rotterdam study. Eur J Epidemiol. 2016;31(8):785–92.
3. Buist AS, McBurnie MA, Vollmer WM, Gillespie S, Burney P, Mannino DM, et al. International variation in the prevalence of COPD (the BOLD study): a population-based prevalence study. Lancet. 2007;370(9589):741–50.
4. Crighton EJ, Ragetlie R, Luo J, To T, Gershon A. A spatial analysis of COPD prevalence, incidence, mortality and health service use in Ontario. Health Rep. 2015;26(3):10.
5. Bahadori K, Doyle-Waters MM, Marra C, Lynd L, Alasaly K, Swiston J, et al. Economic burden of asthma: a systematic review. BMC Pulm Med. 2009;9(1):24.
6. Dogra S, Baker J, Ardern CI. The role of physical activity and body mass index in the health care use of adults with asthma. Ann Allergy Asthma Immunol. 2009;102(6):462–8.
7. Garcia-Aymerich J, Lange P, Benet M, Schnohr P, Antó JM. Regular physical activity reduces hospital admission and mortality in chronic obstructive pulmonary disease: a population based cohort study. Thorax. 2006;61(9):772–8.
8. Seidel D, Cheung A, Suh E, Raste Y, Atakhorrami M, Spruit M. Physical inactivity and risk of hospitalisation for chronic obstructive pulmonary disease. Int J Tuberc Lung Dis. 2012;16(8):1015–9.
9. Hartman JE, Boezen HM, De Greef MH, Bossenbroek L, ten Hacken NH. Consequences of physical inactivity in chronic obstructive pulmonary disease. Expert Rev Respir Med. 2010;4(6):735–45.
10. Gimeno-Santos E, Frei A, Steurer-Stey C, De Batlle J, Rabinovich RA, Raste Y, et al. Determinants and outcomes of physical activity in patients with COPD: a systematic review. Thorax. 2014;69(8):731–9.
11. Carson KV, Chandratilleke MG, Picot J, Brinn MP, Esterman AJ, Smith BJ. Physical training for asthma. Cochrane Database Syst Rev. 2013;(9): CD001116. https://doi.org/10.1002/14651858.CD001116.pub4.
12. Miller MR, Quanjer PH, Swanney MP, Ruppel G, Enright PL. Interpreting lung function data using 80% predicted and fixed thresholds misclassifies more than 20% of patients. Chest J. 2011;139(1):52–9.
13. Zaigham S, Wollmer P, Engström G. Lung function, forced expiratory volume in 1 s decline and COPD hospitalisations over 44 years of follow-up. Eur Respir J. 2016;47(3):742–50.
14. Tremblay MS, Aubert S, Barnes JD, Saunders TJ, Carson V, Latimer-Cheung AE, et al. Sedentary behavior research network (SBRN)–terminology consensus project process and outcome. Int J Behav Nutr Phys Act. 2017; 14(1):75.
15. de Rezende LF, Rey-Lopez JP, Matsudo VK, do Carmo Luiz O. Sedentary behavior and health outcomes among older adults: a systematic review. BMC Public Health. 2014;14:333.
16. Copeland JL, Ashe MC, Biddle SJ, Brown WJ, Buman MP, Chastin S, et al. Sedentary time in older adults: a critical review of measurement, associations with health, and interventions. Br J Sports Med. 2017;51(21):1539.
17. Fragoso CA, Beavers DP, Hankinson JL, Flynn G, Berra K, Kritchevsky SB, et al. Respiratory impairment and dyspnea and their associations with physical inactivity and mobility in sedentary community-dwelling older persons. J Am Geriatr Soc. 2014;62(4):622 8.
18. Furlanetto KC, Donária L, Schneider LP, Lopes JR, Ribeiro M, Fernandes KB, et al. Sedentary behavior is an independent predictor of mortality in subjects with COPD. Respir Care. 2017;62(5):579–87.
19. Doggett N, Dogra S. Physical inactivity and television-viewing time among aboriginal adults with asthma: a cross-sectional analysis of the aboriginal peoples survey. Health promotion and chronic disease prevention in Canada: research, policy and. Practice. 2015;35(3):54.
20. Vlaski E, Stavric K, Seckova L, Kimovska M, Isjanovska R. Influence of physical activity and television-watching time on asthma and allergic rhinitis among young adolescents: preventive or aggravating? Allergol Immunopathol (Madr). 2008;36(5):247–53.
21. Vorrink SN, Kort HS, Troosters T, Lammers JW. Level of daily physical activity in individuals with COPD compared with healthy controls. Respir Res. 2011;12:33.
22. Canadian Longitudinal Study on Aging Spirometry Standard Operating Procedures. 2014. https://clsa-elcv.ca/researchers/physical-assessments.
23. Tan WC, Bourbeau J, Hernandez P, Chapman K, Cowie R, FitzGerald M, et al. Canadian prediction equations of spirometric lung function for Caucasian adults 20 to 90 years of age: results from the Canadian obstructive lung disease (COLD) study and the lung health Canadian environment (LHCE) study. Can Respir J. 2011;18(6):321–6.
24. Washburn RA, Smith KW, Jette AM, Janney CA. The physical activity scale for the elderly (PASE): development and evaluation. J Clin Epidemiol. 1993; 46(2):153–62.
25. Hirshkowitz M, Whiton K, Albert SM, Alessi C, Bruni O, DonCarlos L, et al. National Sleep Foundation's sleep time duration recommendations: methodology and results summary. Sleep Health. 2015;1(1):40–3.
26. Canadian Longitudinal Study on Aging. Sampling and Computation of Response Rates and Sample Weights for the Tracking (Telephone Interview) Participants and Comprehensive Participants. 2011. https://clsa-elcv.ca/researchers/data-collection.
27. Raina PS, Wolfson C, Kirkland SA, Griffith LE, Oremus M, Patterson C, et al. The Canadian longitudinal study on aging (CLSA). Can J Aging/La Revue canadienne du vieillissement. 2009;28(3):221–9.
28. Konstantaki E, Priftis K, Antonogeorgos G, Papoutsakis C, Drakouli M, Matziou V. The association of sedentary lifestyle with childhood asthma. The role of nurse as educator. Allergol Immunopathol (Madr). 2014;42(6):609–15.
29. Freitas PD, Ferreira PG, Silva AG, Stelmach R, Carvalho-Pinto RM, Fernandes FL, et al. The role of exercise in a weight-loss program on clinical control in obese adults with asthma. A randomized controlled trial. Am J Respir Crit Care Med. 2017;195(1):32–42.
30. Esteban C, Quintana J, Aburto M, Moraza J, Egurrola M, Pérez-Izquierdo J, et al. Impact of changes in physical activity on health-related quality of life among patients with COPD. Eur Respir J. 2010;36(2):292–300.
31. Dürr S, Zogg S, Miedinger D, Steveling EH, Maier S, Leuppi JD. Daily physical activity, functional capacity and quality of life in patients with COPD. COPD: J Chron Obstruct Pulmon Dis. 2014;11(6):689–96.
32. Durheim MT, Smith PJ, Babyak MA, Mabe SK, Martinu T, Welty-Wolf KE, et al. Six-minute-walk distance and accelerometry predict outcomes in chronic obstructive pulmonary disease independent of global initiative for chronic obstructive lung disease 2011 group. Ann Am Thorac Soc. 2015;12(3):349–56.
33. Donaire-Gonzalez D, Gimeno-Santos E, Balcells E, de Batlle J, Ramon MA, Rodriguez E, et al. Benefits of physical activity on COPD hospitalisation depend on intensity. Eur Respir J. 2015;46(5):1281–9.
34. Osterling K, MacFadyen K, Gilbert R, Dechman G. The effects of high intensity exercise during pulmonary rehabilitation on ventilatory parameters in people with moderate to severe stable COPD: a systematic review. Int J Chron Obstruct Pulmon Dis. 2014;9:1069.
35. Morris NR, Walsh J, Adams L, Alision J. Exercise training in COPD: what is it about intensity? Respirology. 2016;21(7):1185–92.
36. Oga T, Nishimura K, Tsukino M, Sato S, Hajiro T. Analysis of the factors related to mortality in chronic obstructive pulmonary disease: role of exercise capacity and health status. Am J Respir Crit Care Med. 2003;167(4):544–9.
37. Zambom-Ferraresi F, Cebollero P, Gorostiaga EM, Hernández M, Hueto J, Cascante J, et al. Effects of combined resistance and endurance training versus resistance training alone on strength, exercise capacity, and quality of life in patients with COPD. J Cardiopulm Rehabil Prev. 2015; 35(6):446–53.
38. Maltais F, Jobin J, Sullivan MJ, Bernard S, Whittom F, Killian KJ, et al. Metabolic and hemodynamic responses of lower limb during exercise in patients with COPD. J Appl Physiol. 1998;84(5):1573–80.

39. Park SK, Richardson CR, Holleman RG, Larson JL. Physical activity in people with COPD, using the National Health and nutrition evaluation survey dataset (2003–2006). Heart Lung. 2013;42(4):235–40.

40. Vaz Fragoso CA, Beavers DP, Hankinson JL, Flynn G, Berra K, Kritchevsky SB, et al. Respiratory impairment and dyspnea and their associations with physical inactivity and mobility in sedentary community-dwelling older persons. J Am Geriatr Soc. 2014;62(4):622–8.

41. Wittchen H-U, Carter R, Pfister H, Montgomery S, Kessler R. Disabilities and quality of life in pure and comorbid generalized anxiety disorder and major depression in a national survey. Int Clin Psychopharmacol. 2000;15(6):319–28.

42. Harlow SD, Goldberg EL, Comstock GW. A longitudinal study of risk factors for depressive symptomatology in elderly widowed and married women. Am J Epidemiol. 1991;134(5):526–38.

43. Kennedy GJ, Kelman HR, Thomas C. The emergence of depressive symptoms in late life: the importance of declining health and increasing disability. J Community Health. 1990;15(2):93–104.

44. Idler EL, Benyamini Y. Self-rated health and mortality: a review of twenty-seven community studies. J Health Soc Behav. 1997:21–37.

45. Edwards MK, Loprinzi PD. Systemic inflammation as a function of the individual and combined associations of sedentary behaviour, physical activity and cardiorespiratory fitness. Clin Physiol Funct Imaging. 2018;38(1):93–9.

46. Willoughby TN, Doan J, Currie CL, Copeland JL. Short-term changes in daily movement behaviour influence salivary C-reactive protein in healthy women. Appl Physiol Nutr Metab. 2018; In Press

11

Viruses in bronchiectasis: a pilot study to explore the presence of community acquired respiratory viruses in stable patients and during acute exacerbations

Alicia B. Mitchell[1,2,4]* (iD), Bassel Mourad[1,4], Lachlan Buddle[2], Matthew J. Peters[2,3], Brian G. G. Oliver[1,4,5,6] and Lucy C. Morgan[2,3]

Abstract

Background: Bronchiectasis is a chronic respiratory condition. Persistent bacterial colonisation in the stable state with increased and sometimes altered bacterial burden during exacerbations are accepted as key features in the pathophysiology. The extent to which respiratory viruses are present during stable periods and in exacerbations is less well understood.

Methods: This study aimed to determine the incidence of respiratory viruses within a cohort of bronchiectasis patients with acute exacerbations at a teaching hospital and, separately, in a group of patients with stable bronchiectasis. In the group of stable patients, a panel of respiratory viruses were assayed for using real time quantitative PCR in respiratory secretions and exhaled breath. The impact of virus detection on exacerbation rates and development of symptomatic infection was evaluated.

Results: Routine hospital-based viral PCR testing was only requested in 28% of admissions for an exacerbation. In our cohort of stable bronchiectasis patients, viruses were detected in 92% of patients during the winter season, and 33% of patients during the summer season. In the 2-month follow up period, 2 of 27 patients presented with an exacerbation.

Conclusions: This pilot study demonstrated that respiratory viruses are commonly detected in patients with stable bronchiectasis. They are frequently detected during asymptomatic viral periods, and multiple viruses are often present concurrently.

Keywords: Bronchiectasis, Respiratory viruses, Viral infection, Influenza

Background

Bronchiectasis is a progressive disease characterised by permanent dilatation of bronchi, impairment of muco-ciliary clearance, and retention of secretions. Recurrent respiratory infections are a key feature of bronchiectasis, with the majority of research focusing on the role of bacteria in stable patients, during acute exacerbations and particularly in disease progression [1, 2]. Despite

* Correspondence: amit9422@uni.sydney.edu.au
[1]Respiratory Cellular and Molecular Biology, Woolcock Institute of Medical Research, The University of Sydney, Sydney, NSW 2006, Australia
[2]Department of Respiratory Medicine, Concord Repatriation General Hospital, Concord, NSW 2139, Australia
Full list of author information is available at the end of the article

significant advances in diagnostic immunology and radiology, and a growing global awareness of bronchiectasis as a significant twenty-first century clinical problem, the underlying cause of bronchiectasis in a given patient is not always clear. Approximately 40% of cases remain idiopathic [3], after the most common causes (immunodeficiencies, cystic fibrosis (CF), primary ciliary dysfunction (PCD), allergic bronchopulmonary aspergillosis (ABPA), connective tissue disorders, chronic obstructive pulmonary disease (COPD)-related, or asthma-related) have been excluded [4, 5].

Respiratory infections in early childhood are an important cause of airway damage with the potential to initiate the vicious cycle of epithelial damage, airway dilatation, mucostasis, and bacterial colonisation [6]. Prior to widespread vaccination in the mid twentieth century, measles and pertussis played a major role in post-infectious damage leading to bronchiectasis [7]. The incidence and mortality of pneumonia associated with influenza and pneumococcal infection has also been reduced in both paediatric [8–10] and adult populations with access to vaccination programs [11, 12]. Pneumonia in childhood caused by common respiratory viruses has been associated with significant early airway damage and these viruses are emerging as major factors in the subsequent development of bronchiectasis [4, 13]. While research has focused on defining the aetiology of bronchiectasis due to its implications in individualised treatment and management of the disease, little work has been done to define the role of respiratory viruses in stable and acute bronchiectasis.

As there is considerable phenotypic overlap between bronchiectasis, CF and COPD, the basic understanding gained from investigating the role of viruses in exacerbations and asymptomatic viral detection during stable phases in these diseases may guide our knowledge regarding bronchiectasis.

The association between viral infection and bacterial superinfection is well described in the literature, and more recently, with changes in the microbiome. In COPD and CF, respiratory viruses precipate exacerbations, which in turn, are associated with accelerated disease progression [14]. Mallia et al. [15] demonstrated that experimental rhinovirus infection in patients with COPD could induce symptoms associated with exacerbations, and induce changes in the microbiota. These findings in COPD have been further confirmed by a serial analysis of the lung microbiome following rhinovirus infection [16]. In patients with CF, significantly higher levels of respiratory viruses were detected during exacerbations (46%) compared to stable phases (17%) [17]. The detection of viruses during exacerbation has also been associated with an increase in colony counts of Pseudomonas aeruginosa, suggesting that viruses may also affect the stability of the microbiome in cystic fibrosis [18]. In these diseases, increased viral presence was often observed during exacerbations which also lead to changes in the resident microbial communities. Bacterial colonisation is a common and key feature of the pathophysiology of bronchiectasis. Less is known about the role of viruses in stable state bronchiectasis, or the effect of viruses on the equilibrium between symbiotic and pathogenic bacterial species.

Therefore, this pilot study aimed to determine the incidence of respiratory virus testing ordered by physicians within a cohort of bronchiectasis patients with acute exacerbations at a teaching hospital and separately, to determine the incidence of viral detection within a group of patients with stable bronchiectasis to establish baseline viral prevalence. The incidence of symptomatic viral infections and rates of exacerbations in this cohort was also evaluated.

Methods
Part 1
A retrospective clinical audit was undertaken to determine the rate of testing for respiratory viruses for patients admitted to Concord Repatriation General Hospital July 2011 to June 2016 with an acute exacerbation of bronchiectasis. Patient data regarding exacerbation frequency, previous lung function and hospital admissions were collected from the Australian Bronchiectasis Registry.

Part 2
Clinical measures
Two cohorts of patients were recruited from an outpatient clinic whilst clinically stable. All patients attending the specialised bronchiectasis clinic during the recruitment months were asked to participate. Bronchiectasis was deemed to be clinically stable from the point of view by the consultant physician in clinic based on the patient's history, and no deterioration in clinical symptoms in the month prior to their clinic visit. A history of viral-related symptoms was not an exclusion criteria. One cohort was recruited during the winter months in Australia (May – September), while the other was recruited during the summer months (January – March). Samples were collected from each patient during their clinic visit, to determine if viruses were present within the lungs of bronchiectasis patients when clinically stable, similar to resident bacterial species. This is a tertiary referral centre for PCD, where the diagnosis of PCD was made based on ciliary motility studies and electron microscopy. Patients provided a basic medical history and filled out a common cold questionnaire at the time of recruitment [19]. The common cold questionnaire (CCQ) assesses viral symptoms on an 11-point scale. Based on the presence or absence of these symptoms, the questionnaire predicts the likelihood of a viral infection. Results are classified into three categories; 'no virus', 'possible virus' or 'probable virus' depending on how many symptoms are reported [19]. The results of the questionnaires were considered at the time of analysis in conjunction with the viral PCR results, and were not used as inclusion or exclusion criteria.

Spirometry was performed at the time of sample collection (according to ATS/ERS guidelines) [20] and compared to previous results to ensure that patients were at baseline. FEV_1 was used as a surrogate measure of severity in this cohort of patients. The filters from the spirometer mouthpieces were frozen during storage, then processed for RNA extraction from exhaled breath using a methodology described previously [21], and spontaneously expectorated sputum samples were also collected. All patients were reviewed by the physiotherapist in clinic if sputum was not easily spontaneously expectorated.

To investigate if asymptomatic infections could develop into acute exacerbations, information regarding exacerbations and hospitalisations in the following 2 months were collected for all patients. Other patient outcomes, including lung function, acute viral or bacterial infections, were also collected.

Sample molecular processing

Filters and sputum samples were analysed for a panel of respiratory viruses using PCR. Virus RNA was extracted from the exhaled breath captured in spirometry filters using a methodology published previously [21]. Filters were first removed from the spirometry mouthpieces and 1 ml of Bioline Lysis Buffer RLY (Bioline, Alexandria, Australia) was then added. This was centrifuged for 2 min at 10 000 rpm. The eluate was collected after the final spin and stored at − 20 °C until RNA extraction. Sputum samples were homogenised by mixing the secretion with 1 ml of 1% B-ME Lysis Buffer RLY to achieve a final volume of 1.5 ml, which was then stored at − 20 °C. Following this, RNA was purified using the Isolate II RNA Mini Kit (Bioline, Alexandria, Australia) before conversion to cDNA using the Bioline SensiFAST cDNA Synthesis Kit (Bioline, Alexandria, Australia).

cDNA was assayed by uniplex real time reverse transcription polymerase chain reactions for human rhinovirus (HRV), respiratory syncytial virus (RSV), influenza virus type A and influenza virus type B, parainfluenza virus (PIV) 1, 2 and 3, and human metapneumovirus (HMPV). Real Time quantitative PCR (qPCR) assays utilised the StepOnePlus Real-Time PCR System (Applied Biosystems, ThermoFisher, Massachusetts, USA). All samples were run in triplicate, with 2 μl of cDNA template added to Bioline SensiFAST Probe Hi-ROX Master Mix. PCR primers were sourced from the literature [21–25], and have been previously optimised using clinical samples. Forward and reverse primers were added along with virus specific probe. The qPCR was run for 40 cycles, and the cycle threshold (CT) value was defined for each reaction.

Statistical analysis

T-tests were used to compare parametric data sets, Mann-Whitney tests for non-parametric data, and Fisher's exact test was completed for contingency table analyses using GraphPad Prism version 6.

Results

Part 1

During the study period 47 patients were identified from the Bronchiectasis Registry as having been admitted to Concord Repatriation General Hospital for an exacerbation of bronchiectasis with a total of 83 admissions. The average age for this cohort was 72 ± 14 years, mean ± SD (range 24–88) (male = 19).

Of the 83 total admissions, viral PCR was requested in only 23. In comparison, bacterial and fungal cultures were requested in 73 admissions.

Viral PCR was positive in 9 of 23 cases (39%), with 3 cases of influenza A and 6 cases of HRV.

Bacterial and fungal cultures were positive in 22/73 admissions (30%). The most commonly detected pathogen by culture was *Pseudomonas aeruginosa* in 9 admissions, followed by *Haemophilus influenzae* in 7 cases, *Burkholderia cepacia* in 1, and *Achromobacter xylosoxidans* in 1 case. Fungal species were less common, with *Aspergillus* spp. detected during 3 exacerbations, and *Candida albicans* in 1 case.

Part 2

Winter cohort

Twelve patients with stable bronchiectasis were recruited in the winter cohort. The clinical characteristics of these patients are summarised in Table 1. Four patients were on maintenance therapy with an inhaled corticosteroid (ICS) /long acting beta agonist (LABA) combination inhaler, while the majority had been prescribed a short acting beta agonist (SABA) as needed. Only one patient reported being a past smoker, all other patients had never smoked.

Of the 12 patients with bronchiectasis recruited during the winter period, 9 of these also had a concurrent diagnosis of PCD. The majority of these patients (11/12) had relatively preserved lung function with an FEV_1 greater than the lower limit of normal. One patient had severely reduced lung function, with an FEV_1 of only 21% predicted (0.56 L), and an FEV_1/FVC ratio of 50% based on ATS/ERS guidelines [26].

All patients completed the CCQ on the day of secretion sampling. None reported enough symptoms on the 11-point scale to be categorised as "probable virus". All patients remained stable, with no reported exacerbations or hospital admissions within a month prior to or 2 months after sample collection.

Filters and sputum samples were processed for a panel of respiratory viruses. Nine of 12 patients had respiratory virus RNA identified in filter samples. In the filters, influenza was the most commonly detected respiratory virus (9/12), with 3 patients having influenza A, 3 with influenza B, 2 with concurrent influenza A and B detection and one patient who demonstrated co-detection of

Table 1 Summary of patient characteristics and respiratory virus detection and exacerbation rates in both the winter and summer cohorts

Season	Mean age ± SD	Gender (F/M)	Mean FEV$_1$ ± SD	Comorbid PCD	Overall viral detection rate	Number of patients with Influenza	Multiple virus detection rate	Exacerbation rate during follow up period
Winter (n = 12)	36 ± 12	10/2	77% ± 22%	9/12 (75%)	11/12 (92%)	10/12 (83%)	10/12 (83%)	0/12 (0%)
Summer (n = 15)	60 ± 17	12/3	60% ± 33%	3/15 (20%)	5/15 (33%)	5/15 (33%)	0/15 (0%)	1/15 (7%)
Overall (n = 27)	49 ± 19	22/5	67% ± 29%	12/27 (44%)	16/27 (59%)	15/27 (56%)	10/27 (37%)	1/27 (4%)

human rhinovirus and influenza A (Table 2). Using qPCR, in the samples where the same virus was detected in the filter as the sputum sample, the CT value was lower (approximately 33 cycles) compared with those viruses found in the sputum alone (approximately 37 cycles).

Table 2 Specific viruses detected in the filter and sputum samples of patients in Summer and Winter cohorts

Patient	Winter	
	Filter positive	Sputum positive
1	Flu A	RV, RSV, Flu A + B
2	Flu B	RV, RSV, Flu A + B
3	Flu B	RV, RSV, Flu A + B
4	Flu B	RV, RSV, Flu A + B
5	Flu A	RV, RSV + Flu A
6		RV + RSV
7		Flu A
8	RV + Flu A	RV + Flu A
9	Flu A + B	RV, RSV, Flu A + B
10	Flu A + B	RV, RSV, Flu A + B
11	Flu A	RV, RSV, Flu A + B
12		
Patient	Summer	
	Filter positive	Sputum positive
13		
14	FluA	FluA
15		
16		
17		
18	FluA	FluA
19		FluA
20		FluA
21		
22		
23		
24		
25		
26	FluA	FluA
27		

In sputum samples, 11 of 12 patients had a respiratory virus identified. A single patient had only influenza A identified. Co-infection was more common with 7 patients showing concurrent detection of HRV, RSV, influenza A and B; 1 patient with HRV, RSV and influenza A; 1 with HRV and RSV; 1 with HRV and influenza A. All 9 subjects with virus detected in exhaled breath also had virus detected in the matched sputum sample. As 11 of 12 patients in the winter cohort were viral positive, it was not possible to correlate virus detection with disease severity based on FEV1. Similarly, a correlation between viral detection and use of SABA, or ICS/LABA combination treatment could not be deduced.

Summer cohort

Fifteen patients were recruited in the summer cohort. Their clinical characteristics are summarised in Table 1. Ten patients were on maintenance therapy with an ICS/LABA combination inhaler, two had additional tiotropium therapy; 12/15 had been prescribed a SABA PRN. All patients reported never smoking.

In this cohort, 3 of 15 patients had a concomitant PCD diagnosis, while 2 of 15 also had a diagnosis of asthma. This was a slightly more severe cohort of bronchiectasis patients based on spirometry when compared with the group recruited during the winter season. The mean FEV$_1$ in this group was 59% of predicted, however this was not significantly different to the winter group. Only one patient reported symptoms of viral infection at the time of sample collection, the rest of the patients reported feeling well at the time of their clinic visit which was confirmed by responses to the common cold questionnaire. Two patients with severe bronchiectasis (one with comorbid asthma) were subsequently admitted to hospital for an exacerbation within 2 months of sample collection.

During the summer season, respiratory viruses were less commonly detected, with 3 of 15 patients demonstrating influenza A detection in the filters and 5 of 15 samples detecting Influenza A in the sputum sample (Table 2). No other respiratory viruses on our panel were detected in these samples. Furthermore, none of the patients in the summer cohort had a "probable virus" based on the CCQ. In the patients who were viral positive in the summer cohort, the average FEV1 was lower

($p > 0.05$), compared with the viral negative group. However, no associations between medication usage and viral detection were observed.

One patient was admitted to hospital within 2 weeks of the clinic visit with an exacerbation of bronchiectasis, and influenza A was again detected in both exhaled breath and sputum samples. Another patient who experienced an exacerbation 6 weeks after their clinic visit, did not have any viruses detected in either sample.

Comparison of cohorts

There was a significant difference in viral detection between Summer and Winter cohorts ($p < 0.01$), with a greater rate of viral detection observed during the winter months (Fig. 1). These cohorts were not age or severity matched, and there was a significantly higher rate of underlying PCD in the winter cohort ($p < 0.05$).

Discussion

Our small retrospective audit of admissions for exacerbation of bronchiectasis revealed how infrequently viral PCR testing was requested in a large teaching hospital with ready access to on site rapid respiratory viral PCR. Reflecting the current state of the literature, bacterial and fungal species were more frequently assumed to be the etiological agents and therefore, tested for in the majority of patients presenting with an exacerbation. Viral PCR testing was only requested in 28% of the bronchiectasis exacerbations included in the audit, compared with 88% of admissions where bacterial and fungal culture were requested.

However, despite the greater frequency of request for bacterial and fungal culture, viruses were still detected in 39% of the samples when viral PCR was requested, compared with bacterial or fungal pathogen detection in 30% of samples sent for testing. It is important that sampling rates increase, and prospective, longitudinal studies of both bacterial and viral pathogens in stable and exacerbating bronchiectasis are undertaken, if we are to understand with more precision, the role of viruses in exacerbations and their seasonality.

Due to the low rate of viral testing in acute exacerbations of bronchiectasis at our centre, we designed a study to determine the incidence of respiratory virus detection during stable periods and whether this was associated with an increased risk of exacerbation or developing a symptomatic viral infection. Studying stable patients with bronchiectasis provides information regarding the background level of viruses to inform future analysis of results obtained during acute exacerbations. Our pilot study demonstrated that respiratory viruses are commonly detected in respiratory secretions and the exhaled breath of patients with stable bronchiectasis. They are frequently detected during asymptomatic periods, and multiple viruses are often present concurrently.

In this study, there was a 92% detection rate in the winter cohort, and a 33% detection rate in the summer cohort. Other studies have detection rates of around 20% in stable bronchiectasis rising to around 40–50% in exacerbations in non-CF bronchiectasis in adults [27, 28]. One potential reason for obtaining such high virus detection by PCR is contamination within the PCR reaction. We are confident that high viral detection rates in the winter cohort this is not caused by poor PCR technique or experimental contamination as out negative controls were always negative. Furthermore, whilst the samples were collected during different periods of the year, the PCRs were carried out simultaneously. However, we used a highly sensitive PCR which can detect as few as 5 virions. In our study, even low CT values were classified as viral positive whereas in other studies these might be classified as negative. Whist not a part of this study, we have compared our research lab virus PCR results to virus positivity by PCR obtained from a diagnostic lab. We found almost 100% agreement for all viruses, apart from rhinovirus, where we found our PCR was more sensitive (twice the detection frequency). We think that the most plausible explanation for the high sample detection in our winter cohort happened to be sampled during a year that was recognised to have a heavy burden of influenza infections. Other possible reasons might be the increased severity of bronchiectasis based on FEV_1 values in our cohort, and

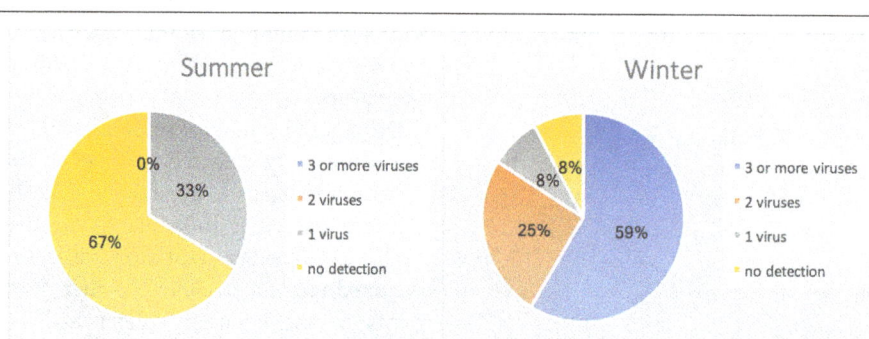

Fig. 1 Rates of single or multiple respiratory virus detection during stable state in the summer and winter cohorts

also, the high incidence of PCD as our clinic is a state-wide referral centre for PCD. However, it is unusual to have found such high rates of multiple virus detection, and further studies are needed in PCD to confirm these findings. There is currently little literature regarding the detection and persistence of respiratory viruses in the respiratory tract of individuals with PCD.

Respiratory viruses were more common during winter season, compared with the summer season. This study confirms previously reported seasonality of respiratory viruses [29] for RSV, however rhinovirus has been shown to occur all year round in respiratory specimens which was not observed in this cross-sectional study of bronchiectasis patients. Influenza has also demonstrated peak detection during the winter months in temperate zones, and year-round distribution in tropical areas [30]. In this study, we observed a heavy burden of influenza during the winter season, however influenza A virus was still detected in multiple asymptomatic individuals during the summer months.

Detection of respiratory viruses in the exhaled breath and sputum samples of this bronchiectasis cohort, was not significantly associated with disease severity or risk of exacerbation within the 2 month follow up period. In the one patient who was admitted to hospital with a bronchiectasis exacerbation within 2 weeks of their clinic visit, influenza A was present within both the exhaled breath and sputum sample. However, this was the only case where an exacerbation was associated with virus detection in our study. The short duration of this follow up time may not be adequate, however, to make a clear determination of exacerbation risk in this cohort. A longitudinal study design with regular viral sampling during periods of both stable disease and exacerbation, and more in depth analysis of patient outcomes may be needed to elucidate this risk.

No association was observed between viral detection and treatment with ICS/LABA or SABA alone. In the summer cohort, viruses were more commonly detected in patients with more severe disease as indicated by spirometry, with 80% patients who had influenza A detection demonstrating an FEV_1 below 30% predicted based on the GLI-2012 reference set [31]. In the winter cohort, viral detection had no significant association with spirometry values.

Real time PCR allowed quantification of viral load, with higher viral load detection in the sputum sample predicting detection in the exhaled breath sample collected using the spirometry filters. Huang et al. [32] showed that presence of influenza virus within the respiratory tract is necessary but not sufficient to cause a symptomatic influenza infection. Host immune responses play an important role, and activation of multiple simultaneous pattern recognition receptors to cause antiviral and inflammatory responses are associated with symptomatic infection. Individuals who retain tight control over these responses usually remain asymptomatic, and may explain why asymptomatic infection was so prevalent in our cohort. These patients with bronchiectasis all have chronic bacterial lung colonisation, which may play a role in downregulating immune responses [33].

A surprising finding was that of influenza A detection only during the summer months. Traditionally, influenza A activity peaks during the winter months and viruses such as rhinovirus are more commonly seen in summer and early autumn. The Australian influenza surveillance network showed that there was a higher than normal level of influenza A detected during January to March of 2017, the sampling period of our summer cohort. Likely due to the fact that this group of bronchiectasis patients have an underlying respiratory disease, and impaired muco-ciliary clearance, it is possible that these individuals were more susceptible to acquiring these circulating viruses.

A large proportion of those recruited during the winter months had PCD as the underlying cause of bronchiectasis, as this study was undertaken at a tertiary referral centre for PCD. Ciliary dysmotility impairs mucociliary clearance and it seems plausible that this might result in persistence of viral nucleic acids within sputum, even if the virus is not actively replicating. Whilst the number of subjects in this pilot is small, it raises the possibility that differences in underlying pathophysiology of bronchiectasis extend to heterogeneity in the pathogenesis of viruses.

Since the introduction of culture-independent techniques, a substantial increase in bacterial detection has been observed [34]. Molecular methods that identify bacterial species based on nucleic acid presence has greatly improved diagnostic accuracy [35, 36], and has allowed discovery of a whole range of bacterial species that are present within the lower respiratory tract. The introduction of these molecular based methods such as PCR, have also allowed the detection of respiratory viral species to become faster and easier [37]. This greatly increased the rate of respiratory infections that were found to be attributable to viruses, as this is a much more sensitive and specific tool. This was an important step in realising the high frequency of respiratory viral infections, and thus their importance in clinical disease. It also allowed a more guided approach to treatment, with a decrease in the use of antibacterial agents in some cases. Characterising the role of viruses in both stable bronchiectasis and during exacerbations may allow a greater understanding of disease pathogenesis.

Conclusions

Our pilot study provides preliminary data supporting the notion that respiratory viruses are an important part of the lung microbiome in patients with bronchiectasis. The high rates of respiratory virus detection in patients with stable bronchiectasis encourages further studies in this area to determine how viruses may impact both chronic and transient bacterial species within the lung, and the role that viruses may have in exacerbations. This is the first study to investigate the potential impact of viruses in bronchiectasis. Many fundamental questions have been raised regarding the role of respiratory viruses in this disease process, and as outlined, recent advances in metagenomic techniques have provided the tools to investigate this area. We are just beginning to understand the role of viruses in many chronic respiratory diseases and it is now timely to apply this work in patients with bronchiectasis.

Abbreviations

ABPA: Allergic bronchopulmonary aspergillosis; ATS: American thoracic society; CCQ: Common cold questionnaire; CF: Cystic fibrosis; COPD: Chronic obstructive pulmonary disease; CT: Cycle threshold; ERS: European respiratory society; HMPV: Human metapneumovirus; HRV: Human rhinovirus; PCD: Primary ciliary dyskinesia; PCR: Polymerase chain reaction; PIV: Parainfluenza virus; qPCR: Quantitative polymerase chain reaction; RSV: Respiratory syncytial virus

Acknowledgements

The authors would like to thank the lab and physiotherapy staff at Concord Repatriation General Hospital for their aid in patient recruitment and sample collection.

Funding

This research is supported by an Australian Government Research Training Program Scholarship.

Authors' contributions

ABM, BGGO, LCM were involved in the design of this study; ABM, LB were involved in participant recruitment and sample collection; ABM, BM were involved in sample processing and experimentation; ABM, BM, LB, MJP, BGGO, LCM were all involved in manuscript preparation and editing. All authors approved the final manuscript.

Competing interests

The authors declare that they have no competing interests.

Author details

[1]Respiratory Cellular and Molecular Biology, Woolcock Institute of Medical Research, The University of Sydney, Sydney, NSW 2006, Australia. [2]Department of Respiratory Medicine, Concord Repatriation General Hospital, Concord, NSW 2139, Australia. [3]Concord Clinical School, University of Sydney, Sydney, NSW 2006, Australia. [4]Molecular Biosciences, School of Life Sciences, University of Technology Sydney, Building 4, 15 Broadway, Ultimo, NSW 2007, Australia. [5]Centre for Health Technologies, University of Technology Sydney, Sydney, NSW 2007, Australia. [6]Emphysema Centre, Woolcock Institute of Medical Research, The University of Sydney, Sydney, NSW 2006, Australia.

References

1. Rogers GB, van der Gast CJ, Cuthbertson L, Thomson SK, Bruce KD, Martin ML, Serisier DJ. Clinical measures of disease in adult non-CF bronchiectasis correlate with airway microbiota composition. Thorax. 2013;68(8):731–7.
2. Tunney MM, Einarsson GG, Wei L, Drain M, Klem ER, Cardwell C, Ennis M, Boucher RC, Wolfgang MC, Elborn JS. Lung microbiota and bacterial abundance in patients with bronchiectasis when clinically stable and during exacerbation. Am J Respir Crit Care Med. 2013;187(10):1118–26.
3. Suarez-Cuartin G, Chalmers JD, Sibila O. Diagnostic challenges of bronchiectasis. Respir Med. 2016;116:70–7.
4. Chalmers JD, Aliberti S, Blasi F. Management of bronchiectasis in adults. Eur Respir J. 2015;45(5):1446–62.
5. Shoemark A, Ozerovitch L, Wilson R. Aetiology in adult patients with bronchiectasis. Respir Med. 2007;101(6):1163–70.
6. Cole PJ. Inflammation: a two-edged sword–the model of bronchiectasis. Eur J Respir Dis Suppl. 1986;147:6–15.
7. Pasteur MC, Helliwell SM, Houghton SJ, Webb SC, Foweraker JE, Coulden RA, Flower CD, Bilton D, Keogan MT. An investigation into causative factors in patients with bronchiectasis. Am J Respir Crit Care Med. 2000;162(4 Pt 1):1277–84.
8. Dagan R, Sikuler-Cohen M, Zamir O, Janco J, Givon-Lavi N, Fraser D. Effect of a conjugate pneumococcal vaccine on the occurrence of respiratory infections and antibiotic use in day-care center attendees. Pediatr Infect Dis J. 2001;20(10):951–8.
9. Huang SS, Hinrichsen VL, Stevenson AE, Rifas-Shiman SL, Kleinman K, Pelton SI, Lipsitch M, Hanage WP, Lee GM, Finkelstein JA. Continued impact of pneumococcal conjugate vaccine on carriage in young children. Pediatrics. 2009;124(1):e1–11.
10. Luksic I, Clay S, Falconer R, Pulanic D, Rudan I, Campbell H, Nair H. Effectiveness of seasonal influenza vaccines in children – a systematic review and meta-analysis. Croat Med J. 2013;54(2):135–45.
11. Suzuki M, Dhoubhadel BG, Ishifuji T, Yasunami M, Yaegashi M, Asoh N, Ishida M, Hamaguchi S, Aoshima M, Ariyoshi K, et al. Serotype-specific effectiveness of 23-valent pneumococcal polysaccharide vaccine against pneumococcal pneumonia in adults aged 65 years or older: a multicentre, prospective, test-negative design study. Lancet Infect Dis. 2017;17(3):313–21.
12. Stohr K. Preventing and treating influenza. BMJ. 2003;326(7401):1223–4.
13. Lonni S, Chalmers JD, Goeminne PC, McDonnell MJ, Dimakou K, De Soyza A, Polverino E, Van de Kerkhove C, Rutherford R, Davison J, et al. Etiology of non-cystic fibrosis bronchiectasis in adults and its correlation to disease severity. Ann Am Thorac Soc. 2015;12(12):1764–70.
14. Anzueto A, Sethi S, Martinez FJ. Exacerbations of chronic obstructive pulmonary disease. Proc Am Thorac Soc. 2007;4(7):554–64.
15. Mallia P, Message SD, Gielen V, Contoli M, Gray K, Kebadze T, Aniscenko J, Laza-Stanca V, Edwards MR, Slater L, et al. Experimental rhinovirus infection as a human model of chronic obstructive pulmonary disease exacerbation. Am J Respir Crit Care Med. 2011;183(6):734–42.
16. Molyneaux PL, Mallia P, Cox MJ, Footitt J, Willis-Owen SA, Homola D, Trujillo-Torralbo MB, Elkin S, Kon OM, Cookson WO, et al. Outgrowth of the bacterial airway microbiome after rhinovirus exacerbation of chronic obstructive pulmonary disease. Am J Respir Crit Care Med. 2013;188(10):1224–31.
17. Wat D, Gelder C, Hibbitts S, Cafferty F, Bowler I, Pierrepoint M, Evans R, Doull I. The role of respiratory viruses in cystic fibrosis. J Cyst Fibros. 2008;7(4):320–8.
18. Wark PA, Tooze M, Cheese L, Whitehead B, Gibson PG, Wark KF, McDonald VM. Viral infections trigger exacerbations of cystic fibrosis in adults and children. Eur Respir J. 2012;40(2):510–2.
19. Powell H, Smart J, Wood LG, Grissell T, Shafren DR, Hensley MJ, Gibson PG. Validity of the common cold questionnaire (CCQ) in asthma exacerbations. PLoS One. 2008;3(3):e1802.
20. Miller MR, Hankinson J, Brusasco V, Burgos F, Casaburi R, Coates A, Crapo R, Enright P, van der Grinten CP, Gustafsson P, et al. Standardisation of spirometry. Eur Respir J. 2005;26(2):319–38.
21. Mitchell AB, Mourad B, Tovey E, Buddle L, Peters M, Morgan L, Oliver BG. Spirometry filters can be used to detect exhaled respiratory viruses. J Breath Res. 2016;10(4):046002.
22. Kuypers J, Wright N, Morrow R. Evaluation of quantitative and type-specific real-time RT-PCR assays for detection of respiratory syncytial virus in respiratory specimens from children. J Clin Virol. 2004;31(2):123–9.

23. Selvaraju SB, Selvarangan R. Evaluation of three influenza a and B real-time reverse transcription-PCR assays and a new 2009 H1N1 assay for detection of influenza viruses. J Clin Microbiol. 2010;48(11):3870–5.

24. Terlizzi ME, Massimiliano B, Francesca S, Sinesi F, Rosangela V, Stefano G, Costa C, Rossana C. Quantitative RT real time PCR and indirect immunofluorescence for the detection of human parainfluenza virus 1, 2, 3. J Virol Methods. 2009;160(1–2):172–7.

25. Pabbaraju K, Wong S, McMillan T, Lee BE, Fox JD. Diagnosis and epidemiological studies of human metapneumovirus using real-time PCR. J Clin Virol. 2007;40(3):186–92.

26. Pellegrino R, Viegi G, Brusasco V, Crapo RO, Burgos F, Casaburi R, Coates A, van der Grinten CP, Gustafsson P, Hankinson J, et al. Interpretative strategies for lung function tests. Eur Respir J. 2005;26(5):948–68.

27. Gao YH, Guan WJ, Xu G, Lin ZY, Tang Y, Lin ZM, Gao Y, Li HM, Zhong NS, Zhang GJ, et al. The role of viral infection in pulmonary exacerbations of bronchiectasis in adults: a prospective study. Chest. 2015;147(6):1635–43.

28. Kapur N, Mackay IM, Sloots TP, Masters IB, Chang AB. Respiratory viruses in exacerbations of non-cystic fibrosis bronchiectasis in children. Arch Dis Child. 2014;99(8):749–53.

29. Brittain-Long R, Andersson LM, Olofsson S, Lindh M, Westin J. Seasonal variations of 15 respiratory agents illustrated by the application of a multiplex polymerase chain reaction assay. Scand J Infect Dis. 2012;44(1):9–17.

30. Tamerius JD, Shaman J, Alonso WJ, Bloom-Feshbach K, Uejio CK, Comrie A, Viboud C. Environmental predictors of seasonal influenza epidemics across temperate and tropical climates. PLoS Pathog. 2013;9(3):e1003194.

31. Quanjer PH, Stanojevic S, Cole TJ, Baur X, Hall GL, Culver BH, Enright PL, Hankinson JL, Ip MS, Zheng J, et al. Multi-ethnic reference values for spirometry for the 3-95-yr age range: the global lung function 2012 equations. Eur Respir J. 2012;40(6):1324–43.

32. Huang Y, Zaas AK, Rao A, Dobigeon N, Woolf PJ, Veldman T, Oien NC, McClain MT, Varkey JB, Nicholson B, et al. Temporal dynamics of host molecular responses differentiate symptomatic and asymptomatic influenza a infection. PLoS Genet. 2011;7(8):e1002234.

33. Finlay BB, McFadden G. Anti-immunology: evasion of the host immune system by bacterial and viral pathogens. Cell. 2006;124(4):767–82.

34. Proctor LM. The human microbiome project in 2011 and beyond. Cell Host Microbe. 2011;10(4):287–91.

35. Jarvinen AK, Laakso S, Piiparinen P, Aittakorpi A, Lindfors M, Huopaniemi L, Piiparinen H, Maki M. Rapid identification of bacterial pathogens using a PCR- and microarray-based assay. BMC Microbiol. 2009;9:161.

36. Tissari P, Zumla A, Tarkka E, Mero S, Savolainen L, Vaara M, Aittakorpi A, Laakso S, Lindfors M, Piiparinen H, et al. Accurate and rapid identification of bacterial species from positive blood cultures with a DNA-based microarray platform: an observational study. Lancet. 2010;375(9710):224–30.

37. Xiang X, Qiu D, Chan KP, Chan SH, Hegele RG, Tan WC. Comparison of three methods for respiratory virus detection between induced sputum and nasopharyngeal aspirate specimens in acute asthma. J Virol Methods. 2002;101(1–2):127–33.

Relative lymphocyte count as an indicator of 3-year mortality in elderly people with severe COPD

Domenico Acanfora[1], Pietro Scicchitano[2]* (iD), Mauro Carone[1], Chiara Acanfora[1], Giuseppe Piscosquito[1], Roberto Maestri[3], Annapaola Zito[2], Ilaria Dentamaro[2], Marialaura Longobardi[1], Gerardo Casucci[4], Raffaele Antonelli-Incalzi[5] and Marco Matteo Ciccone[2]

Abstract

Background: Prognostic stratification of elderly patients with chronic obstructive pulmonary disease (COPD) is difficult due to the wide inter-individual variability in the course of the disease. No marker can exactly stratify the evolution and natural history of COPD patients. Studies have shown that leukocyte count is associated with increased risk of mortality in COPD patients. The aim of this study was to evaluate the possible role of relative lymphocyte count as a risk marker for mortality in elderly patients with COPD.

Methods and results: This is a3-year prospective study. A total of 218patients, mean age 75.2±7 years, with moderate to severe COPD and free from conditions affecting lymphocyte count were enrolled. The population was divided into two groups according to the relative lymphocyte count, with a cut-off of 20%. Eighty-five patients (39%) had a relative lymphocyte count ≤20%. Three-year mortality rates from any cause in patients with relative lymphocyte count ≤ or > 20% were 68 and 51%, respectively ($p = 0.0012$). Survival curve analysis showed higher mortality in patients with relative lymphocyte count ≤20% ($p = 0.0005$). After adjustment for age and sex, the hazard ratio for mortality risk according to lymphocyte count was 1.79 (95% confidence interval [CI]: 1.26–2.57, $p = 0.0013$), even in the analysis limited to the 171 patients without congestive heart failure (1.63; 95% CI: 1.03–2.58, $p = 0.038$).

Conclusions: Low relative lymphocyte count was associated with higher mortality in elderly patients with severe COPD.

Keywords: Lymphocyte, Mortality, Elderly, COPD

Background

Chronic obstructive pulmonary disease (COPD) is a frequent cause of death in elderly patients.

Older age, reduced gas exchange and airflow obstruction, right atrial overload and ventricular overload and hypertrophy and selected comorbidities are the main negative prognostic indicators as they could account for early death in these patients [1–3].

The prognostic stratification of elderly patients with COPD is difficult due to wide inter-individual variability the course of the disease. No marker can exactly stratify

the evolution and natural history of COPD patients. Therefore, efforts are made in order to detect new prognostic markers and to verify whether they substantially add further prognostic value to well-recognized indicators [2, 4, 5]. Incalzi et al. [2] identified electrocardiographic signs (S1S2S3 pattern or right atrial overload (RAO)) as able to predict survival rates in patients with COPD.

The common plasmatic measures and biomarkers such as (procalctionin (PCT), C-reactive protein (CRP), white blood cell count (WBC)) are not able to reproducibly predict mortality in COPD patients [4].

Variables reflecting either inflammation or immune depression emerged as possible prognostic markers in patients with COPD. The increase in leukocyte count in peripheral blood shows a statistical trend towards the

* Correspondence: piero.sc@hotmail.it; pietrosc.83@libero.it
[2]Section of Cardiovascular Diseases, Department of Emergency and Organ Transplantation, School of Medicine, University of Bari, Bari, Italy
Full list of author information is available at the end of the article

prediction of long-term all-cause mortality risk in COPD patients but it did not reach a statistical significance in previous studies [4, 6].

More insights come from the analysis of reduced WBCs and, in particular, lymphocyte count. A low relative lymphocyte count is already known to exert a detrimental prognostic role in the setting of acute myocardial infarction, stable coronary heart disease and congestive heart failure [7–11]. It also has a negative prognostic role in the elderly population [12], and, to some extent, it could be considered as a marker of the stress response [13, 14]. Although a low relative lymphocyte count is a physiological adaptation of the immune system to increasing age, it may account for the frailty of elderly people compared with younger individuals [15–17]. As patients with COPD may show a further decrease in lymphocyte count [18, 19], elderly individuals with COPD may have a combined reduction in lymphocytes due to both age and characteristics of the pulmonary disease.

Despite the established role of low relative lymphocyte count in many diseases, its prognostic value remains to be specifically evaluated in elderly patients with COPD.

The aim of the present study was to investigate the prognostic value of relative lymphocyte count in elderly patients with COPD.

Methods

Patients

The study was conducted on elderly patients with COPD who were consecutively admitted to our Institute for Research and Care related to Cardiac and Pulmonary Rehabilitation. The diagnosis of COPD was made according to American Thoracic Society (ATS) criteria [20]. A total of 218 patients (114 men and 104 women), mean age 75.2±7 years, were recruited from October 1, 2011 to March 30, 2012.

Inclusion criteria were: age ≥65 years and presence of severe and very severe COPD, as identified by ATS criteria [20]. Severe COPD was defined in agreement with forced expiratory volume in the 1st second (FEV1) ≤50% of predicted value. Patients were excluded if they were lacking complete blood count within 1 week of study entry, or on the basis of conditions known to affect lymphocyte count [12, 13]: recent coronary revascularization or recent myocardial infarction (within 6 months of entry), long-term disorders of the hemopoietic system, history of malignancy, chemotherapy, or radiation therapy, trauma, surgery, infection and glucocorticoid therapy within 6 weeks of study entry. Patients were also excluded if dyspnoea, phlegm or weakness had worsened in the two weeks prior to admission. This precautionary measure was utilized to limit the risk of enrolling patients with exacerbated COPD.

Study design

Extensive baseline data were collected for all eligible patients within one week of hospital admission. Patients underwent physical examination, spirometry, chest X-ray, arterial blood gas analysis, electrocardiogram and laboratory tests (including complete blood count); their clinical history was accurately recorded. Spirometry was performed with a VMAX 2200 spirometer (Sensor Medics Co., Yorba Linda, USA), meeting the American College of Physicians, American College of Chest Physicians, American Thoracic Society, and European Respiratory Society 2011 recommendations for diagnostic spirometry [20, 21]. Arterial blood gas analysis was performed (during room air breathing) with an ABL 520 Radiometer analyzer (Copenhagen, Denmark).

Patients' characteristics were reported: age, gender, body mass index, history of smoking (defined as subjects who had regularly smoked at least 5 cigarettes/day during the previous 3 months or who had stopped smoking less than 1 year before admittance into our study), alcohol use, lung function [FEV_1, forced vital capacity (FVC), both in milliliters and as percent of predicted], arterial blood gases [partial arterial oxygen tension (PaO_2), partial arterial carbon dioxide tension ($PaCO_2$), pH], presence of ischemic heart disease, history of myocardial infarction, congestive heart failure, diabetes, systemic hypertension, cerebro-vascular disease, peripheral vascular disease, use of bronchodilators, mucolytics and aminophylline, heart rate, systolic and diastolic blood pressure. None of the enrolled patients were in long-term oxygen therapy. Furthermore, their $PaO2$ (mmHg) at rest was 70.4 ± 8 mmHg (range 60–91 mmHg).

Individual clinical history was diagnosed according to the International Classification of Diseases, Ninth Revision, Clinical Modification [22]. Patients were classified as affected by congestive heart failure only on the basis of a concordant diagnosis according to the physician's clinical judgment, Boston criteria [23] and a clinical diagnostic score which was previously validated on hospitalized patients [24]. We used this conservative diagnostic approach due to the great difficulty in distinguishing chronic cor pulmonare from congestive heart failure.

Baseline clinical evaluation, complete blood count, electrocardiography, lung function, blood gas analysis, and data on patient's clinical history were collected by a trained and experienced physician.

Follow-up

The follow-up covered a period of 36 months after hospital discharge. Physicians phoned all the patients at 6, 12, 24 and 36 months after hospital discharge in order to assess the data regarding their health condition. In particular, the primary end-point of the study was "death from any cause".

Death certificates and hospital records were considered and checked when patients and/or relatives were not available for phone recall. All available data were reviewed by two investigators (DA, MMC) to determine and define the cause of death. If a consensus of opinion could not be reached, the opinion of the senior investigator (RAI) prevailed.

Laboratory methods

All patients underwent complete blood count evaluation and a leukocyte differential count analysis at baseline. The percentage of lymphocytes was defined as: (total lymphocytes/total leukocytes)× 100. In our laboratories, the normal range of the percentage of lymphocytes is 20 to 50%, as defined by the central 95% range in a separate population of 52 healthy adults [11].

We evaluated the short- and long-term reproducibility of relative lymphocyte count by considering three blood samples from 24 healthy volunteers over a period of 360 days, spaced at 6 ± 1 and 136 ± 67 days.

Study approval

All procedures were in accordance with the ethical standards of the institutional research committee and with the 1964 Declaration of Helsinki. Informed written consent was obtained from all individual participants included in the study.

Statistical analysis

Data analysis was performed with SPSS software (SPSS, Chicago, USA). Results were given as means (±standard deviation) for continuous variables or as percentages for dichotomous variables.

Short-term and long-term reproducibility of relative lymphocyte count was assessed by first testing for systematic changes, between baseline and second measurement, and between baseline and the final measurement, respectively. To quantify the reproducibility, we used the standard error of measurement, which was computed as the root mean square error of the 1-way random effects analysis of variance on short-term and long-term paired measurements. From the same 1-way analysis of variance, the intra-class correlation coefficient (an index of reliability of measurements) was derived and remained significantly higher at long-term follow-up (Additional file 1: Table S1).

Differences between groups were assessed by unpaired t-test or Mann-Whitney test for continuous variables with or without normal distribution and homogeneous variance, and by chi square test for dichotomous variables. Kaplan-Meier estimates of the survival functions were plotted for relative lymphocyte count [25]. Univariate and multivariate Cox regression models were used to investigate the association of selected variables with the incidence of death [26].

All hypothesis tests were tested using a significance level of 0.05. All p-values were two-sided.

Results

Relative lymphocyte count showed high short- (standard error of measurement = 2.11) and long-term (standard error of measurement = 1.15) reproducibility. The estimates of intra-class correlation coefficient for the short- (intra-class correlation coefficient = 0.95) and long-term (intra-class correlation coefficient = 0.97) indicated excellent reproducibility for the relative lymphocyte count measurement. These values indicate that obtaining a single sample from a subject is fairly representative of that individual's relative lymphocyte count over an extended period of time.

In the study sample, 85 patients (39%) had relative lymphocyte counts≤20%.

The study sample included 218 patients with mean age of 75.2 ± 7 years, 52% male. The population sample was divided into two groups according to relative lymphocyte count: group 1 with relative lymphocyte count ≤20%; group 2 with relative lymphocyte count > 20%. About 39% of patients showed a relative lymphocyte count ≤20%.

Demographic, respiratory function and clinical characteristics of the patients in the two groups are shown in Table 1. Groups did not differ according to demographic characteristics or anthropometric status, as expressed by body mass index (BMI). All of the patients were white Caucasic individuals. A lymphocyte count ≤20% was associated with a lower six-minute walking distance and higher basal heart rate (Additional file 2: Figure S1 and Additional file 3: Figure S2). The reproducibility of the white cells count can be observed in Additional file 1: Table S1.

Lung function indices were significantly lower in patients with relative lymphocyte count ≤20%; the greatest difference was evident in FVC, expressed as a percentage of the predicted value. The FEV1/FVC index did not distinguish between groups because both terms in the ratio had reduced by a comparable extent in the two groups (Table 1).

Ischemic heart disease and previous myocardial infarction were less prevalent in patients with relative lymphocyte count ≤20% (group 1), while congestive heart failure, diabetes and chronic cor pulmonare were more prevalent in group 1. Neither arterial blood gases nor pharmacologic therapy distinguished between the groups, except for a slightly higher use of mucolytics by patients with a lymphocyte count > 20% (group 2).

Only one patient was lost at the 36-months follow-up time (he was known to be alive at 25th month follow up) and was censored. Mean follow-up time was 22 months, with 118 deaths. One- and 3-year survival rates were 67 and 42.2%, respectively. Patients died from acute or chronic

Table 1 Clinical characteristics in patients with severe COPD in relation to the relative lymphocyte count at baseline

Variable[a]	Relative lymphocyte count ≤20% (N = 85)	Relative lymphocyte count > 20% (N = 133)	p-value
Sex (M/F)	46/39	68/65	0.67
Age (years)	76±7	74±7	0.06
Bodymass index (BMI)	25.7±5	25.4±4	0.66
History of smoking (n/%)	43 (51%)	72 (54%)	0.61
Alcohol use (n/%)	30 (35%)	48 (36%)	0.90
Lung Function			
FEV₁ (ml)	762±268	870±268	0.004
FEV₁ (percent of predicted)	30±9	34±8	0.005
FVC (ml)	1720±656	2038±687	0.001
FVC (percent of predicted)	53±17	62±17	< 0.0001
FEV₁/FVC (percent)	47±13	44±11	0.16
Arterial Blood Gases			
PaO₂ (mmHg)	71±9	70±8	0.79
PaCO₂ (mmHg)	38±5	37±4	0.12
pH	7.40±0.39	7.40±0.41	0.47
Disease (n/%)			
Ischemic heart disease	21 (25%)	49 (37%)	0.027
History of myocardial infarction	20 (24%)	54 (41%)	0.0091
Congestive heart failure	32 (38%)	15 (11%)	0.0001
Corpulmonale	43 (51%)	49 (37%)	0.031
Diabetes	19 (22%)	25 (19%)	0.52
Systemic hypertension	40 (47%)	65 (49%)	0.79
Cerebro-vascular disease	20 (24%)	32 (24%)	0.93
Peripheral vascular disease	11 (13%)	17 (13%)	0.97
Therapy (n/%)			
Bronchodilators	66 (78%)	100 (75%)	0.68
Mucolytics	70 (82%)	101 (76%)	0.26
Aminophylline	53 (62%)	112 (69%)	0.029
Heart rate (bpm)	95±22	82±19	< 0.0001
Systolic blood pressure (mmHg)	139±25	142±20	0.42
Diastolic blood pressure (mmHg)	78±11	81±9	0.031

Differences between groups were assessed by unpaired t-test or Mann-Whitney test for continuous variables having or not both normal distribution and homogeneous variance, and by the chi square test for dichotomous variables

COPD chronic obstructive pulmonary disease, FEV₁ forced expiratory volume at 1 s, FVC forced vital capacity, FEV₁/FVC Tiffeneau, PaO₂ partial arterial oxygen tension, PaCO₂ partial arterial carbon dioxide tension, MI myocardial infarction. Plus-minus values are means±SD

[a]Bodymass index is expressed as weight (kg)/height² (m) ratio

respiratory failure [34 (27%)], acute myocardial infarction [31 (25%)], stroke [21 (17%)], cor pulmonare [12 (10%)], respiratory infections [10 (8%)], cancer [9 (7%)], sudden death [4 (3%)], or other causes [5 (4%)].

Low relative lymphocyte count at baseline was associated with an increased incidence of death from any causes [58 (68%) vs. 68 (51%); p = 0.0012] (data not shown).

In the Additional file 4: Figure S3 the hazard ratio is shown as a function of relative lymphocyte count threshold. A clear maximum around 20% can be appreciated indicating this value as the optimal cutoff-point.

Table 2 compared causes of early (within 6 months from discharge) and late (after 6 months from discharge) mortality. Worsening of cardiopulmonary failure prevailed as a cause of early mortality, while acute myocardial infarction, stroke and cancer accounted for most late mortality.

Kaplan-Meier estimates of the probability of death are shown in Fig. 1a. Patients with relative lymphocyte count ≤20% had worse prognosis, which became evident in the earliest phases of the follow up and remained unchanged for the whole observation period.

The relationship between tertiles of relative lymphocyte count at study entry and 3-year mortality is shown in Fig. 1b. Mortality decreased significantly, from 69.3% in the first tertile to 45.7% in the third.

Table 3 outlines the results of Cox proportional-hazard model comparing mortality in patients with lymphocyte count≤ 20 and > 20%. The age- and sex-adjusted hazard ratio was significantly different from 1.0, suggesting an excess of mortality in patients with lower relative lymphocyte count. The result remained statistically significant even after further adjustment for smoking, body mass index, FEV1 (percent of predicted) and also after adjusting for all variables potentially associated with death.

Table 4 shows the Cox proportional-hazard model limited to patients without a diagnosis of congestive heart failure. The hazard ratio for lymphocyte count ≤ 20% (group1) remained significant after excluding those with congestive heart failure.

Discussion

Relative lymphocyte count was significantly related to survival in elderly patients with moderate to severe COPD. The present findings are in agreement with those of Lehtonen et al. who found that a reduction in both B and T cells could predict mortality in very old

Table 2 Causes of early (0–6 months from discharge) and late (> 6 months from discharge) mortality

Cause of death	n Early death	n Late death
Progressive pulmonary failure	44	12
Acute myocardial infarction	11	20
Stroke	8	13
Cancer	0	9
Sudden death	1	3
Others	2	3

Pearson's χ² = 39.57, p < 0.001

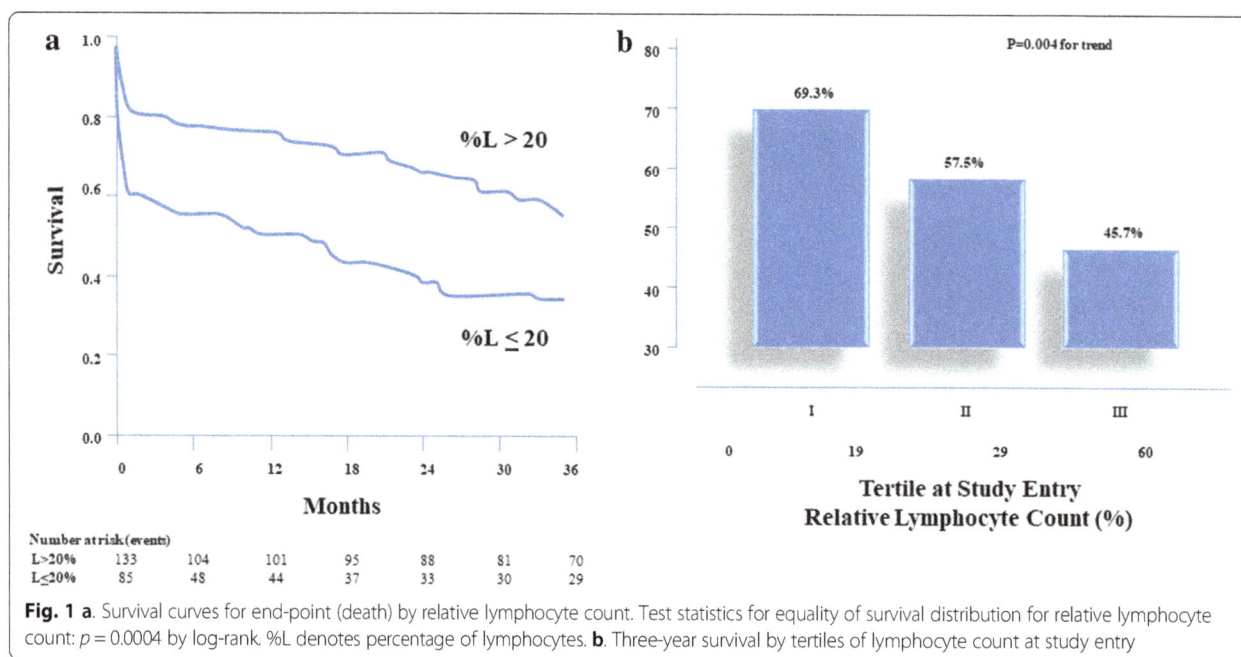

Fig. 1 a. Survival curves for end-point (death) by relative lymphocyte count. Test statistics for equality of survival distribution for relative lymphocyte count: $p = 0.0004$ by log-rank. %L denotes percentage of lymphocytes. **b.** Three-year survival by tertiles of lymphocyte count at study entry

people with severe chronic illnesses [15]. The differences in survival at 1 and 3 years between groups with and without relative lymphopenia were similar, with the excess deaths in those with low relative lymphocyte count mostly due to very early events. Figure 1 shows that the difference in survival is early on, and the slopes are the same (i.e. the same relative death rate) from about 6 months afterwards.

Analysis of the causes of death shows that worsening of cardiopulmonary failure was responsible for most of the early deaths, whereas late mortality was related mainly to cardiovascular or cerebrovascular disease and cancer (Table 2). As a sign of impaired immunity, lymphopenia should carry a higher risk of infections, which are the main cause of fatal COPD exacerbations and, thus, should be related mainly to early mortality [5]. The significant difference in both early and late mortality between patients with and without lymphopenia suggests that reduced lymphocyte count qualifies as a comprehensive indicator of health status rather than as a

pure immunologic marker. The very high mortality in the six months after discharge from a rehabilitation unit suggests that COPD should not be considered as a stable condition even if clinical judgment is consistent with such a diagnosis. Thus, careful supervision of patients with COPD seems desirable in order promptly to recognize and treat impending cardiopulmonary failure.

There are contradictory results regarding lymphocyte number and function in senescence [15, 27].

Rea et al. demonstrated a 10% decrease in both B and T cell number and percentage of absolute lymphocyte count in elderly subjects [28]. According to B cells, the relative reduction in B cells can provoke alterations in the production of specific antibodies. As B cells can switch immunoglobulins among the different types and in agreement with specific actions toward the pathogenic agents, the reduction in B cell count can negatively affect outcome in elderly patients [29, 30]. Furthermore, T cells can promote the production of cytokines able to enhance the response to pathogens from different actors in the immune

Table 3 Results of Cox proportional hazards model comparing mortality in patients with severe COPD with relative lymphocyte count ≤20%

Variable	Hazard ratio for relative lymphocytes count ≤20% (95% CI)	p-value
Adjusted for age and sex	1.81 (1.27–2.59)	0.0012
Adjusted for age, sex, smoking, body mass index, FEV₁ (percent of predicted)	1.79 (1.22–2.62)	0.003
Adjusted for age, sex, smoking, body mass index, FEV₁ (percent of predicted), FVC (percent of predicted), FEV₁/FVC (percent), PaO₂, PaCO₂, pH, ischemic heart disease, history of myocardial infarction, congestive heart failure, heart rate, systolic and diastolic blood pressure.	1.56 (1.02–2.38)	0.04

COPD chronic obstructive pulmonary disease, *CI* confidence interval, *FEV₁* forced expiratory volume in one second, *FVC* forced vital capacity, *FEV₁/FVC* Tiffeneau, *PaO₂* partial arterial oxygen tension, *PaCO₂* partial arterial carbon dioxide tension

Table 4 Results of Cox proportional hazards model comparing mortality in COPD patients free from CHF with relative lymphocyte count ≤20%

Variable	Hazard ratio for relative lymphocytes count ≤20% (95% CI)	p-value
Adjusted for age and sex	1.65 (1.04–2.61)	0.034
Adjusted for age, sex, smoking, body mass index, FEV₁ (percent of predicted), FVC (percent of predicted), FEV₁/FVC (percent), PaO₂, PaCO₂, pH, ischemic heart disease, history of myocardial infarction, heart rate, systolic and diastolic blood pressure.	1.63 (1.03–2.58)	0.038

COPD chronic obstructive pulmonary disease, *CHF* congestive heart failure, *CI* confidence interval, *FEV₁* forced expiratory volume in one second, *FVC* forced vital capacity, *FEV₁/FVC* Tiffeneau, *PaO₂* partial arterial oxygen tension, *PaCO₂* partial arterial carbon dioxide tension

system, as well as the switch of immunoglobulins and the promotion of B cell growth and reproduction [28]. All of these data demonstrate that a deficit in either the B or T cell population or both could increase the risk of infection and, thus, morbidity and mortality in elderly patients. Lehtonen et al. suggested that, in very old people, both T and B cell function are significantly reduced and that there are major changes in lymphocyte subsets [15].

The mechanisms leading to the reduction in lymphocyte count and immunological impairment are still far from clear. Aging and COPD are associated with psychological stress [27].

It has been long known that psychological and physiological stresses result in a significant increase in systemic cortisol production [31]. The physiological diurnal variation and pulsatile pattern of secretion are thought to limit the lymphocyte-depleting effect of cortisol. However, elderly people secrete large amounts of cortisol, whose levels may remain elevated for a longer time than in younger adults [32, 33]. Increased cortisol levels can result in a gradual decrease in relative lymphocyte count. Therefore, it may be supposed that a decrease in relative lymphocyte count in elderly patients with COPD, as a consequence of the combined action of age and cortisol pathway, would impair the distribution of white blood cells. Such a theory should be tested in further studies.

The hypothalamus-hypophysis-adrenal axis is a sensitive feedback system for various pathophysiological conditions leading to neurohumoral activation. Several lines of evidence demonstrate that severe COPD is associated with a generalized increase in circulating catecholamines and cytokines [34]. By increasing the production of selected cytokines, mainly of interleukin-6, cathecolamines indirectly stimulate the corticotropin-releasing hormone, which leads to increased secretion of cortisol and a consequent reduction in circulating lymphocytes [35]. Therefore, neurohumoral activation and the immune system demodulation produce a vicious circle that may worsen the prognosis in elderly patients with severe COPD and low relative lymphocyte count. The demonstration that plasma interleukin-6 levels increase with age [36–39] and in patients with COPD [40] supports this interpretation.

Furthermore, activation of the inflammatory systems could be responsible for the cachexia and hypermetabolic state found in some patients with severe COPD [34, 40]. A low relative lymphocyte count can be considered as a surrogate marker for malnutrition in patients with severe COPD, and thus as a negative prognostic factor. Fuenzalida et al. [41] demonstrated a partial recovery in immune system components, and lymphocyte count in particular, in patients with COPD who underwent a dedicated nutritional program. Therefore, the negative prognostic value of low lymphocyte count in elderly patients with COPD could be related to different conditions (cortisol and adrenergic hyperactivation, malnutrition, comorbidities, etc.), which impair the survival of such individuals. Thus, the relative lymphocyte count represents more than a simple marker of immunological deficit.

This study has some limitations, as follows: 1) lymphocyte subpopulations were not measured, and thus the respective prognostic role of deficits of the cellular and humoral immunity could not be assessed; 2) some degree of uncertainty exists in determining the cause of death in this kind of study, and, theoretically, this could affect the interpretation of the relationship between lymphopenia and mortality; 3) orthopnea and fluid retention are not uncommon in severe COPD complicated by hypoxemia and hypercapnia, and could simulate congestive heart failure. However, the stringent criteria used to diagnose congestive heart failure and the results of survival analysis for patients without congestive heart failure support the reliability of the current conclusions. Nevertheless, the proposed prognostic model should be tested in a population with only moderate COPD in order to limit further the potential confounding effect of congestive heart failure.

Conclusions

Relative lymphopenia has a homogeneous and strong effect on mortality across the whole follow-up period, but the inherent mechanisms remain to be clarified. To our knowledge, this study is the first to demonstrate that relative lymphopenia is associated with a poor prognosis in elderly patients with severe COPD. This finding seems worthy of attention because lymphocyte count is a simple, reproducible, widely available and inexpensive prognostic tool. Further research is needed to verify to which extent lymphopenia improves the prognostic definition based on well-established markers, as well as to assess the relationship linking lymphopenia with indices of neurohormonal activation and inflammation. Clarifying these issues would enable quantification of the weight of this new prognostic marker and, possibly, the design of interventions, e.g. immunological therapy, aimed at its correction.

Additional files

Additional file 1: Table S1. Evaluation of the reproducibility of measurements during the follow-up period. (DOCX 17 kb)

Additional file 2: Figure S1. Correlation between relative lymphocyte count and 6-min walking test. (TIF 100 kb)

Additional file 3: Figure S2. Correlation between relative lymphocyte count and heart rate. (TIF 126 kb)

Additional file 4: Figure S3. Hazard ratio as a function of relative lymphocyte count threshold. (TIF 151 kb)

Funding
The study did not receive any funding.

Authors' contributions
MMC, DA, RAI conceived and designed the study, analysed and interpreted the data, drafted the article and critically reviewed its intellectual content, and finally approved the version to be submitted for publication. AZ, ID, PS, MC, CA, GP, ML, GC analysed the data, reviewed the article's intellectual content, and finally approved the version to be submitted for publication. All authors read and approved the final manuscript.

Competing interests
The authors declare that they have no competing interests.

Author details
[1]Maugeri Scientific Clinical Institutes, SpA SB, Institute of Care and Scientific Research, Rehabilitation Institute of TeleseTerme, Benevento, Italy. [2]Section of Cardiovascular Diseases, Department of Emergency and Organ Transplantation, School of Medicine, University of Bari, Bari, Italy. [3]Maugeri Scientific Clinical Institutes, SpA SB, Institute of Care and Scientific Research, Rehabilitation Institute of Montescano, Pavia, Italy. [4]San Francesco Hospital-TeleseTerme, Telese, BN, Italy. [5]Institute of Internal Medicine, Chair of Geriatry, Policlinico Gemelli, School of Medicine, Rome, Italy.

References
1. Antonelli Incalzi R, Fuso L, De Rosa M, Forastiere F, Rapiti E, Nardecchia B, et al. Co-morbidity contributes to predict mortality of patients with chronic obstructive pulmonary disease. EurRespir J. 1997;10:2794–800.
2. Incalzi RA, Fuso L, De Rosa M, Di Napoli A, Basso S, Pagliari G, et al. Electrocardiographic signs of chronic corpulmonale: a negative prognostic finding in chronic obstructive pulmonary disease. Circulation. 1999;99:1600–5.
3. Song S, Yang PS, Kim TH, Uhm JS, Pak HN, Lee MH, et al. Relation of chronic obstructive pulmonary disease to cardiovascular disease in the general population. Am J Cardiol. 2017;120:1399–404.
4. Grolimund E, Kutz A, Marlowe RJ, Vögeli A, Alan M, Christ-Crain M, et al. Long-term prognosis in COPD exacerbation: role of biomarkers, clinical variables and exacerbation type. COPD. 2015;12:295–305.
5. Fuso L, Incalzi RA, Pistelli R, Muzzolon R, Valente S, Pagliari G, et al. Predicting mortality of patients hospitalized for acutely exacerbated chronic obstructive pulmonary disease. Am J Med. 1995;98:272 7.
6. Yamamoto E, Sugiyama S, Hirata Y, Tokitsu T, Tabata N, Fujisue K, et al. Prognostic significance of circulating leukocyte subtype counts in patients with coronary artery disease. Atherosclerosis. 2016;255:210–6.
7. Núñez J, Miñana G, Bodí V, Núñez E, Sanchis J, Husser O, et al. Low lymphocyte count and cardiovascular diseases. Curr Med Chem. 2011;18:3226–33.
8. Levinas T, Eshel E, Sharabi-Nov A, Marmur A, Dally N. Differentiating ischemic from non-ischemic chest pain using white blood cell-surface inflammatory and coagulation markers. J Thromb Thrombolysis. 2012;34:235–43.
9. Núñez J, Sanchis J, Bodí V, Núñez E, Mainar L, Heatta AM, et al. Relationship between low lymphocyte count and major cardiac events in patients with acute chest pain, a non-diagnostic electrocardiogram and normal troponin levels. Atherosclerosis. 2009;206:251–7.
10. Ommen SR, Hodge DO, Rodeheffer RJ, McGregor CG, Thomson SP, Gibbons RJ. Predictive power of the relative lymphocytes count in patients with advanced heart failure. Circulation. 1998;97:19–22.
11. Acanfora D, Gheorghiade M, Trojano L, Furgi G, Pasini E, Picone C, et al. Relative lymphocyte count: a prognostic indicator of mortality in elderly patients with congestive heart failure. Am Heart J. 2001;142:167–73.
12. Bender BS, Nagel JE, Adler WH, Andres R. Absolute peripheral blood lymphocyte count and subsequent mortality of elderly men: the Baltimore longitudinal study of aging. J Am Geriatr Soc. 1986;34:649–54.
13. Nelson DH, Sandberg AA, Palmer JG, Tyler FH. Blood levels of 17-hydroxycorticosteroids following the administration of adrenal steroids and their relation to levels of circulating lymphocytes. J Clin Invest. 1952;31:843–9.
14. Thomson SP, McMahon LJ, Nugent CA. Endogenous cortisol: a regulator of the number of lymphocytes in peripheral blood. Clin Immunol Immunopathol. 1980;17:506–14.
15. Lehtonen L, Eskola J, Vainio O, Lehtonen A. Changes in lymphocyte subsets and immune competence in very advanced age. J Gerontol. 1990;45:M108–12.
16. Tavares SM, Junior Wde L, Lopes E, Silva MR. Normal lymphocyte immunophenotype in an elderly population. Rev Bras Hematol Hemoter. 2014;36:180–3.
17. Morley JE, Vellas B, van Kan GA, Anker SD, Bauer JM, Bernabei R, et al. Frailty consensus: a call to action. J Am Med Dir Assoc. 2013;14:392–7.
18. Lee SJ, Lee HR, Lee TW, Ju S, Lim S, Go SI, et al. Usefulness of neutrophil to lymphocyte ratio in patients with chronic obstructive pulmonary disease: a prospective observational study. Korean J Intern Med. 2016;31:891–8.
19. Furutate R, Ishii T, Motegi T, Hattori K, Kusunoki Y, Gemma A, et al. The neutrophil to lymphocyte ratio is related to disease severity and exacerbation in patients with chronic obstructive pulmonary disease. Intern Med. 2016;55:223–9.
20. Qaseem A, Wilt TJ, Weinberger SE, Hanania NA, Criner G, van der Molen T, et al. Diagnosis and management of stable chronic obstructive pulmonary disease: a clinical practice guideline update from American College of Physicians, American College of Chest Physicians, American Thoracic Society, and European Respiratory Society. Ann Intern Med. 2011;155:179–91.
21. Bakke PS, Rönmark E, Eagan T, Pistelli F, Annesi-Maesano I, Maly M, et al. Recommendations for epidemiological studies on COPD. Eur Respir J. 2011; 38:1261–77.
22. [No authors listed]. ICD-9-CM : international classification of diseases, ninth revision, clinical modification, sixth edition. Centers for Disease Control and Prevention (US); Centers for Medicare & Medicaid Services (US). Official version. [Atlanta, Ga.] : [Baltimore, Md.] : U.S. Dept. of Health and Human Services, Centers for Disease Control and Prevention; Centers for Medicare and Medicaid Services, [2011].
23. Carlson KJ, Lee DC, Goroll AH, Leahy M, Johnson RA. An analysis of physicians' reason for prescribing long-term digitalis therapy in outpatients. J Chron Dis. 1985;38:733–9.
24. Acanfora D, Trojano L, Maggi S, Furgi G, Rengo C, Iannuzzi GL, et al. Development and validation of a clinical history form for the diagnosis of congestive heart failure. Aging Clin Exp Res. 1998;10:39–47.
25. Benedetti J, Yuen K, Young L. Life tables and survivor functions. In: Dixon WJ, editor. BMDP standard software manual. Berkley, CA: University of California Press; 1988. p. 689–718.
26. Snedecor GW, Cochran WG. Statistical methods. 8th ed. Ames: Iowa State University Press; 1989. p. 333–73.
27. Guidi L, Tricerri A, Frasca D, Vangeli M, Errani AR, Bartoloni C. Psychoneuroimmunology and aging. Gerontology. 1998;44:247–61.
28. Rea IM, Stewart M, Campbell P, Alexander HD, Crockard AD, Morris TC. Changes in lymphocyte subsets, interleukin 2, and soluble interleukin 2

receptor in old and very old age. Gerontology. 1996;42:69–78.

29. Kishimoto T, Ishikaza K. Regulation of antibody response in vitro: V1 carrier specific helper cells of IgG and IgE antibody response. J Immunol. 1993;111: 720–31.

30. Vitetta ES, Berton MT, Burger C, Kepron M, Lee WT, Yin XM. Memory B and T cells. Ann Rev Immunol. 1991;9:193–217.

31. Taylor AL, Fishman LM. Corticotropin-releasing hormone. N Egl J Med. 1988; 319:213–22.

32. Simpkins JW, Millard WJ. Influence of age on neurotrasmitter function. Endocrinol Metab Clin North Am. 1987;16:893.

33. Martin JB, Reichlin S. Clinical neuroendocrinology. 2nd ed. Philadelphia: F. A. Davis; 1987.

34. Hofford JM, Milakofsky L, Vogel WH, Sacher RS, Savage GJ, Pell S. The nutritional status in advanced emphysema associated with chronic bronchitis. A study of aminoacid and catecholamine levels. Am Rev Respir Dis. 1990;141:902–8.

35. Papanicolaou DA, Wilder RL, Manolagas SC, Chrousos GP. The pathophysiologic roles of interleukin-6 in human disease. Ann Intern Med. 1998;128:127–37.

36. Hager K, Machein U, Krieger S, Platt D, Seefried G, Bauer J. Interleukin-6 and selected plasma proteins in healthy persons of different ages. Neurobiol Aging. 1994;15:771–2.

37. Ershler WB, Sun WH, Binkley N, Gravenstein S, Volk MJ, Kamoske G, et al. Interleukin-6 and aging: blood levels and mononuclear cell production increase with advancing age and in vitro production is modifiable by dietary restriction. Lymphokine Cytokine Res. 1993;12:225–30.

38. Chiappelli M, Tampieri C, Tumini E, Porcellini E, Caldarera CM, Nanni S, et al. Interleukin-6 gene polymorphism is an age-dependent risk factor for myocardial infarction in men. Int J Immunogenet. 2005;32:349–53.

39. Ershler WB, Keller ET. Age-associated increased interleukin-6 gene expression, late-life diseases, and frailty. Annu Rev Med. 2000;51:245–70.

40. Schols AM, Buurman WA, Staal van den Brekel AJ, Dentener MA, Wouters EF. Evidence for a relation between metabolic derangements and increased levels of inflammatory mediators in a subgroup of patients with chronic obstructive pulmonary disease. Thorax. 1996;51:819–24.

41. Fuenzalida CE, Petty TL, Jones ML, Jarrett S, Harbeck RJ, Terry RW, et al. The immune response to short-term nutritional intervention in advanced chronic obstructive pulmonary disease. Am Rev Respir Dis. 1990;142:49–56.

13

Risk factors for interstitial lung disease: a 9-year Nationwide population-based study

Won-Il Choi[1]*† , Sonila Dauti[1,2†], Hyun Jung Kim[1], Sun Hyo Park[1], Jae Seok Park[1] and Choong Won Lee[3]

Abstract

Background: Understanding the risk factors that are associated with the development of interstitial lung disease might have an important role in understanding the pathogenetic mechanism of interstitial lung disease as well as prevention. We aimed to determine independent risk factors of interstitial lung disease development.

Methods: This was a retrospective cohort study with nationwide population-based 9-year longitudinal data. We selected subjects who were aged > 40 years at cohort entry and with a self-reported history of cigarette smoking. Cases were selected based on International Classification of Diseases codes. A cohort of 312,519 subjects were followed until December 2013. We used Cox regression analysis to calculate the hazard ratios (HRs) for interstitial lung disease development.

Results: Interstitial lung disease developed in 1972 of the 312,519 subjects during the 9-year period. Smoking (HR: 1.2; 95% confidence interval [CI]: 1.1–1.4), hepatitis C (HR: 1.6; 95% CI: 1.1–2.3), history of tuberculosis (HR: 1.5; 95% CI: 1.1–1.9), history of pneumonia (HR: 1.6; 95% CI: 1.3–2.0), and chronic obstructive pulmonary disease (HR: 1.8; 95% CI: 1.6–2.1), men (HR: 1.9; 95% CI: 1.7–2.1) were significantly associated with the development of interstitial lung disease. The risk of interstitial lung disease development increases with age, and the risk was 6.9 times higher (95% CI: 5.9–8.0) in those aged over 70 than in their forties.

Conclusions: Smoking, hepatitis C, history of tuberculosis, history of pneumonia, chronic obstructive pulmonary disease, male sex, and older age were significantly associated with interstitial lung disease development.

Keywords: Interstitial lung disease, Epidemiology, Risk factor

Background

If bilateral reticular or reticulonodular opacities are found on chest radiography, interstitial lung disease (ILD) is suspected. ILD is not an uncommon disease [1]. In 2012, prevalence estimates of ILD with fibrosis ranged from 42.7–63 per 100.000 population in USA, and 1.25–23.4 per 100.000 population in Europe [2].

Patients with ILD are often asymptomatic until the lesion progresses significantly. Interstitial pulmonary abnormality (ILA), which is considered to be an early lesion of interstitial lung disease, has a higher mortality rate than patients without ILA [3] as well as ILD [4]. Furthermore, in patients with ILD, a study using health insurance claim data found that lung cancer incidence is higher than

chronic obstructive pulmonary disease (COPD) [5]. ILD could have significant impact on health.

Three different population-based studies determined that cigarette smoking is a risk factor for lung parenchymal as well as interstitial abnormalities in addition to airway abnormalities [6–8]. However, previous studies examined risk factors from a limited sample size, and most of them used case-control methodology and did not consider many of the potential confounding variables as risk factors for ILD.

Determining the risk factors that are associated with the development of ILD might have an important role in understanding the pathogenetic mechanism of ILD, early diagnosis, adequate treatment and prevention.

The purpose of this study was to identify the independent risk factors for the development of ILD in a 9-year follow-up longitudinal population-based study.

* Correspondence: wichoi@dsmc.or.kr
†Won-Il Choi and Sonila Dauti contributed equally to this work.
[1]Department of Internal Medicine, Keimyung University Dongsan Hospital, Daegu 41931, Republic of Korea
Full list of author information is available at the end of the article

Methods

Database

The National Health Insurance Service (NHI) covers more than 99% of all Korean residents and includes all health claim data, including diagnostic codes, procedures, prescription drugs, patient personal information, and hospital information. There is one health insurance system with a unique resident registration number for each citizen; therefore, duplication of subjects can be avoided. This study used data from the National Health Insurance Service-National Sample Cohort(NHIS-NSC) 2002–2013 [9], which was released by the KNHIS in 2015. It includes all medical claims filed from January 2002 to December 2013 for 1,099,094 nationally representative randomly selected subjects, accounting for approximately 2.2% of the entire population in the KNHIS in 2002. The data were produced by the KNHIS using a systematic sampling method to generate a representative sample of all 46,605,433 Korean residents in 2002. The cohort population underwent biennial medical evaluations through the NHI Corporation between January 1, 2002, and December 31, 2013.

Study population

This was a nationwide population-based 9-year longitudinal study. We included subjects with a self-reported smoking history, who were ≥ 40 years old, and with co-morbidities diagnosed before the index date. Health examination data confirmed self-reported cigarette smoking history. The health examination data every 2 years was linked with the cohort data.

We did not include patients with ILD from 2002 to 2004 to exclude preexisting cases of ILD during the two medical evaluations and 1 year of follow-up. We also excluded patients with ILD who did not visit the clinic 30 days after the index date. The final sample included 312,519 subjects. Then, we identified patients with newly diagnosed ILD between January 2005 and December 2013. Among the 312,519 subjects, the control group was selected by excluding those who had ILD between 2005 and 2013.

Definition of interstitial lung disease

Cases of ILD were selected based on International Classification of Disease-10 (ICD-10) code J84 for other interstitial lung diseases, excluding drug-induced interstitial lung disorders, interstitial emphysema, and lung diseases caused by external agents. Connective tissue disease-associated ILD, hypersensitivity pneumonitis, and sarcoidosis were excluded.

Comorbidities

Comorbidities diagnosed before the index date that could be associated with an increased risk of lung fibrosis were identified using ICD-10, including COPD, hepatitis C, gastroesophageal reflux disorder (GERD), and diabetes [10–13].

Statistical analysis

Baseline characteristics (including age, sex, and comorbidities) for cases and controls are summarized using descriptive statistics such as proportion. A chi-squared test was used to compare frequencies of risk factors between ILD and the control group. Cox proportional hazards regression models were used to evaluate the risk factors for ILD and analyze the associations between ILD and different variables and comorbidities. The final multivariate models included age, sex, smoking status (former or current smoker vs. never smoker), household income, and comorbidities such as hepatitis C, herpes, tuberculosis, pneumonia, GERD, COPD, diabetes, and hepatitis B. Risk factor models for ILD were selected according to sex and smoking as sensitivity analysis. Model selection method was forward stepwise procedure using likelihood ratio test with p-value < 0.05 as entry criterion, and p-value ≥0.10 as removal criterion.

A P value < 0.05 considered to be statistically significant. All statistical analyses were performed using SAS V.9.2 (SAS Institute, Cary, North Carolina, USA).

Results

Incidence and baseline characteristics

The final sample included 312,519 subjects, of which 1972 developed ILD during the 9-year study period (Fig. 1). ILD incidence was 70.1 cases per 100,000 person-year.

All subjects were tracked by December 31, 2013, Follow up duration was median 65.6 months (interquartile range: 35.5, 89.0) in the ILD group and median 107.5 months (interquartile range; 100.2, 109.5) in the non-ILD group.

The ILD group had a higher percentage of men than the control. Compared with the control, subjects with ILD were older, and more likely to be smokers. The ILD group was more likely to have comorbidities such as respiratory diseases (tuberculosis and pneumonia), diabetes, chronic renal failure, malignancy, GERD, hepatitis C, and COPD than the control (Table 1).

Risk factors for developing ILD

Based on a multivariate Cox regression analysis of all variables (Table 2), smoking was significantly associated with the development of ILD (HR: 1.2; 95% CI: 1.1–1.4).

Co-morbidities such as hepatitis C (HR: 1.6; 95% CI: 1.1–2.3), history of tuberculosis (HR: 1.5; 95% CI: 1.1–1.9), history of pneumonia (HR: 1.6; 95% CI: 1.3–2.0), and COPD (HR: 1.8; 95% CI: 1.6–2.1) were significantly associated with the development of ILD. Men were almost twice

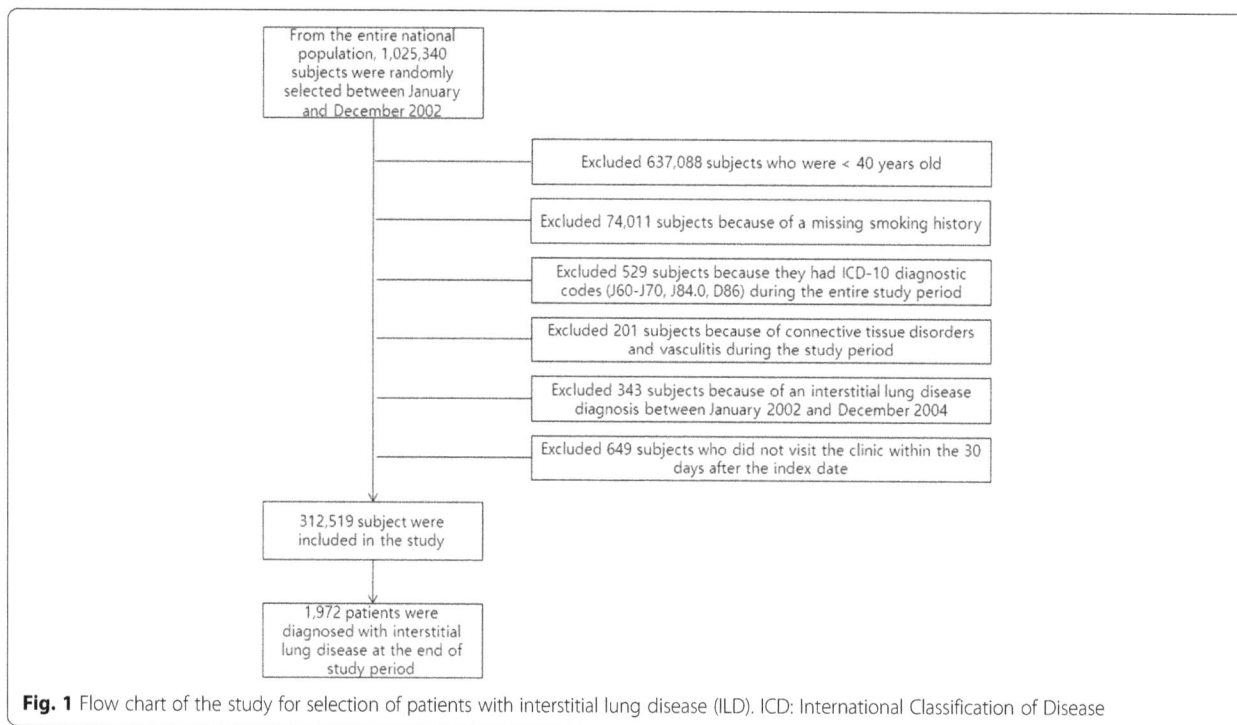

Fig. 1 Flow chart of the study for selection of patients with interstitial lung disease (ILD). ICD: International Classification of Disease

as likely to associated with the development of ILD as women.

The risk of ILD development was 1.9 times in the 50s, 4.1 times in the 60s, and 6.9 times in the 70s, which increased sharply with age. In multivariate analysis, age was found to be most associated to ILD development showing dose response. All the risk factors included in the model showed relatively narrow confidence intervals.

There were no variables that changed the direction of the hazard ratio in the univariate and multivariate analyses except hepatitis B, which was statistically not significant. The hazard ratios of COPD and history of tuberculosis were reduced by almost half after multivariate analysis. History of pneumonia, hepatitis C and diabetes showed also reduced hazard ratios in multivariate analysis. Smoking was associated with the occurrence of ILD, but its magnitude was relatively small compared to other variables.

Multivariate analysis stratified by smoking showed same direction and similar magnitude of hazard ratios in all variables. However, hazard ratios stratified by sex were somewhat different in several variables. As a result of stratified analysis on the basis of gender, the hazard ratios of COPD according to man and woman were similar 1.8 and 1.9, respectively. In the case of GERD, multivariate analysis of male subjects showed that GERD was not a significant risk factor, but the hazard ratio for women was 1.3, which was consistent with the 1.3 observed in the univariate analysis (Table 3). GERD, Hepatitis C are significant risk factors in females, in contrast malignancy and diabetes are significant risk factors in males.

Discussion

In the present study, the development of ILD was associated with older age, male sex, cigarette smoking, hepatitis C, history of tuberculosis, history of pneumonia, and COPD.

Smokers were at greater risk of developing ILD than non-smokers (HR: 1.2). Similarly, a previous study showed that smoking might contribute to the development of ILD by fibrosis (Odds Ratio: 1.6) [14]. The findings of three different studies also support a strong association between ILA and exposure to tobacco smoke and smoking status [6–8]. In this study, the risk of developing ILD was 1.4 in smokers compared to non-smokers in the univariate analysis, but decreased 1.2-fold in multivariate analysis. The lowest risk among the variables associated with ILD occurrence is low, indicating that smoking is less involved in ILD development.

COPD was associated with the development of ILD in the present study. A 2012 review of the pathogenesis of IPF and COPD showed similarities between the basic pathogenic mechanisms involved in the development of either emphysema or fibrosis [13]. Coexisting pulmonary fibrosis and emphysema is now a distinct entity [15], and studies show that the pathologic changes associated with these coexisting entities are mostly found in smokers [16–19]. In this study, the risk of developing ILD in COPD was 3.7 in univariate analysis but decreased 1.8-fold in multivariate analysis. This is presumably due to the control of cigarette smoking variables.

Table 1 Baseline characteristics of patients with interstitial lung disease (n = 1972) and controls (n = 310,547)

Variable	Interstitial lung disease No. (%)		Control No. (%)		P value
Sex					
Male	1265	(64.1)	151,124	(48.7)	< 0.001
Female	707	(35.9)	159,423	(51.3)	
Age group (years)					
40–49	354	(18.0)	136,576	(44.0)	< 0.001
50–59	474	(24.0)	89,952	(29.0)	
60–69	662	(33.6)	57,189	(18.4)	
≥ 70	482	(24.4)	26,830	(8.6)	
Baseline comorbidity					
Malignancy	357	(18.1)	43,007	(13.8)	< 0.001
Diabetes	479	(24.3)	48,507	(15.6)	< 0.001
Chronic renal failure	27	(1.4)	2187	(0.7)	< 0.001
COPD[a]	242	(12.3)	11,204	(3.6)	< 0.001
Past history					
Herpes (B00, B02)	65	(3.3)	9997	(3.2)	0.85
Tuberculosis (A15, A16, B90)	102	(5.2)	5467	(1.8)	< 0.001
Pneumonia (J12-J18)	98	(5.0)	6709	(2.2)	< 0.001
Hepatitis C (B18.2)	28	(1.4)	2068	(0.7)	< 0.001
Hepatitis B (B18.0, B18.1)	66	(3.3)	9859	(3.2)	0.66
GERD[b] (K21)	227	(11.5)	26,643	(8.6)	< 0.001
Smoker (ex-smoker or current smoker)	748	(37.9)	93,573	(30.1)	< 0.001
Household income (Quartiles), %					
81–100	870	(44.1)	131,363	(42.3)	0.11
41–80	635	(32.2)	107,310	(34.6)	
11–40	437	(22.2)	66,372	(21.4)	
0–10	30	(1.5)	5502	(1.8)	

[a]COPD chronic obstructive pulmonary disease, [b] GERD gastroesophageal reflux disorder

Hepatitis C was another risk factor associated with the development of ILD in the present study. There have been conflicting results regarding the prevalence of anti-hepatitis C virus (HCV) antibody in patients with IPF [10, 20, 21]. However, a 2008 study with HCV-infected patients and HBV-infected controls showed that ILD with fibrosis developed at a significantly greater rate in the HCV group than in the HBV group [22]. In 2002, Idilman et al. reported an increased bronchoalveolar lavage neutrophil count in individuals with hepatitis C, suggesting an inflammatory reaction in the lungs leading to fibrotic changes [23]. The findings of these studies suggest that systemic factors stimulating fibrosis, such as HCV infection, may affect the development of lung fibrosis.

Local factors such as history of pneumonia or tuberculosis may be associated with lung fibrosis. Nonresolving pneumonia may result in organizing pneumonia commonly in bacterial infections [24]. Pneumonia due to mycoplasma and Legionnaires' disease has been mostly implicated with development of pulmonary fibrosis [25, 26].

However, the occurrence of organization in cases of pneumonia is more common than expected. In 1952, Auerbach et al. studied the material from 307 necropsies and found organization in 38 cases [27]. In 1989, Shachor et al. found that the incidence of tuberculosis in subjects with ILD was 4.5 times higher than that of the general population [28]. Dheda et al. studied lung remodeling and fibrosis associated with lung injury from tuberculosis infection. Lung remodeling can result in extensive fibrosis and may be interstitial [29]. Therefore, ILD may develop due to tuberculosis or other lung infections.

GERD is a well-known risk factor for IPF [11, 30–32]. However, our data did not show a significant association between GERD and ILD. In patients with esophagitis, the associated odds ratio of pulmonary fibrosis was 1.3–1.6 [30, 33], but there was no significant association between reflux esophagitis and pulmonary fibrosis in this study (Table 2). However, GERD were observed only in women as a significant risk factor for the development of ILD (Table 3). In the present study, ICD-10 code defined a

Table 2 Univariate and multivariate Cox regression analyses for development of interstitial lung disease during the 9-year follow-up period

Risk factor	Univariate analysis		Multivariate analysis	
	HR (95% CI)	P value	HR (95% CI)	P value
Men (reference: women)	1.9 (1.7–2.1)	< 0.001	1.9 (1.7–2.1)	< 0.001
Age group (years) (reference: 40–49)				
50–59	1.9 (1.7–2.2)	< 0.001	1.9 (1.7–2.2)	< 0.001
60–69	4.3 (3.8–4.9)	< 0.001	4.1 (3.6–4.7)	< 0.001
≥70	7.1 (6.2–8.2)	< 0.001	6.9 (5.9–8.0)	< 0.001
Diabetes (reference: no)	1.6 (1.5–1.8)	< 0.001	1.1 (0.9–1.2)	0.06
COPD (reference: no)	3.7 (3.2–4.2)	< 0.001	1.8 (1.6–2.1)	< 0.001
GERD (reference: no)	1.3 (1.1–1.5)	< 0.001	1.0 (0.9–1.3)	0.31
History of herpes (reference: no)	0.97 (0.7–1.2)	0.85	0.9 (0.7–1.2)	0.92
History of tuberculosis (reference: no)	3.0 (2.4–3.7)	< 0.001	1.5 (1.1–1.9)	0.003
History of pneumonia (reference: no)	2.2 (1.8–2.7)	< 0.001	1.6 (1.3–2.0)	< 0.001
Hepatitis C (reference: no)	2.1 (1.4–3.0)	< 0.001	1.6 (1.1–2.3)	0.01
Hepatitis B (reference: no)	1.0 (0.8–1.3)	0.84	0.8 (0.7–1.1)	0.39
Smoker (reference: never smoker)	1.4 (1.3–1.6)	< 0.001	1.2 (1.1–1.4)	< 0.001
Household income, % (reference: 81–100)				
41–80	0.8 (0.8–0.9)	0.04	0.9 (0.8–1.0)	0.35
11–40	1.0 (0.9–1.1)	0.85	0.9 (0.8–1.1)	0.87
0–10	1.1 (0.8–1.6)	0.39	1.1 (0.7–1.5)	0.59

HR hazard ratio, *CI* confidence interval, *COPD* chronic obstructive pulmonary disease, *GERD* gastroesophageal reflux disorder

wider range of ILD. Therefore, in this study, it is estimated that mild cases of pulmonary fibrosis are more involved than previous studies, and that there was no significant association between reflux esophagitis and ILD in men.

Diabetes is also prevalent with IPF [12, 33]. Although diabetes was an important risk factor for developing ILD

in the univariate analysis, the significance reduced to borderline in the multivariate analysis (HR 1.1, $P = 0.06$).

Our study shows that men and older individuals have a higher risk of developing ILD. Two other studies conducted with subjects with interstitial abnormalities found that they were significantly older [7, 8]. Several studies have shown that the incidence of ILD with fibrosis is

Table 3 Multivariate Cox regression analyses with forward stepwise variable selection method for development of interstitial lung disease during the 9-year follow-up period

Risk factor	Males		Females	
	HR (95% CI)	P value	HR (95% CI)	P value
Age group (years) (reference: 40–49)				
50–59	2.3 (1.9–2.7)	< 0.001	1.4 (1.1–1.7)	0.004
60–69	4.6 (3.9–5.5)	< 0.001	3.3 (2.6–4.1)	< 0.001
≥70	8.1 (6.7–9.7)	< 0.001	5.4 (4.3–6.7)	< 0.001
Malignancy	1.1 (1.0–1.3)	0.045	1.0 (0.8–1.2)	0.68
Diabetes (reference: no)	1.2 (1.0–1.3)	0.006	0.9 (0.7–1.1)	0.38
COPD (reference: no)	1.8 (1.5–2.2)	< 0.001	1.9 (1.5–2.4)	< 0.001
History of tuberculosis (reference: no)	1.5 (1.2–2.0)	< 0.001	1.8 (1.2–2.6)	0.001
History of pneumonia (reference: no)	1.5 (1.1–2.0)	0.002	1.7 (1.2–2.3)	0.001
Hepatitis C (reference: no)	1.3 (0.8–2.1)	0.26	2.1 (1.1–3.8)	0.014
GERD (reference: no)	1.0 (0.9–1.3)	0.38	1.3 (1.0–1.6)	0.013
Smoker (reference: never smoker)	1.2 (1.1–1.4)	< 0.001	1.5 (1.1–2.0)	0.005

HR hazard ratio, *CI* confidence interval, *COPD* chronic obstructive pulmonary disease, *GERD* gastroesophageal reflux disorder

higher in men and increases with advanced age [34–37]. In our study, the HR for developing ILD in those aged ≥70 years was almost 7 times higher than for those aged 40–49 years. We suggest that ILD would be a result of the aging process.

We found reduction of risk estimates from the univariate to the multivariate analysis of some variables such as COPD and GERD. We did sensitivity analysis based on gender. Both males and females have similar risk estimates for ILD development in relation to COPD. However, GERD is significant risk factor in females but not in males.

ILD is known as non-homogeneous diseases. Although assessing risk factors for developing specific forms of ILD would be ideal, it might be difficult performing such kinds of study because surgical lung biopsy was rarely performed. In addition, assessing risk factors for the ILD development, the control group should be a general population. Therefore, we assess risk factors for developing ILD by population-based cohort database, though it does not provide information on specific forms of ILD.

The incidence of ILD was 70.1 cases per 100,000 per year, which is higher than previously reported [38]. However, the present incidence was calculated for individuals > 40 years old.

Limitations of the present study

The most important limitation of the present study is that the diagnoses of ILD and other comorbidities were defined based on ICD codes, which may be inaccurate compared to the diagnoses obtained from a medical chart. Underreporting of asymptomatic ILD or misclassification was also possible.

The validity of the medical insurance claims data for ILD has not been determined in Korea. This database consists of random samples of national insurance claim data without identification numbers. Therefore, it was impossible to validate individual cases through a chart review.

We may have underestimated ILD incidence because of inaccurate ILD data. However, previous studies of ILD incidence using data from the Health Insurance Review and Assessment Service of Korea [38] reported similar results to those of previous studies [35, 36, 39]. The incidence rate of ILD was reportedly 48.5 per 100,000 person-years in Korea based on all claims data from 2008 to 2012 [38]. In the present study, the incidence rate was 70.1 per 100,000 patients from 2005 to 2013, which appears reasonable because we excluded subjects aged < 40 years.

The present study did not take into consideration of relevant risk factor such as occupational and environmental exposure. However, annual income could be a weak proxy of the occupational exposure [40].

The present study may be affected by selection bias because the controls were identified based on medical claims. Thus, the controls were more likely to have co-morbidities than controls selected from the general population. Although we excluded patients with a diagnosis of ILD between January 2002 and December 2004 to exclude pre-existing ILD diagnosed before the first year of our study (2005), patients with ILD could be miscounted as new cases if the patient did not require medical care between 2002 and 2004, which may have caused inaccuracies. In addition, other risk factors, such as pulmonary function and high-resolution computed tomography findings for ILD, could not be evaluated because of the NHIS-NSC 2002–2013 primarily included medical claims.

Conclusions

The population is aging, and the incidence of ILD increases with advancing age. Aged men with the history of previous lung infection or COPD could be a clinical marker of suspect ILD. The demonstration of the association of these clinical attributes with ILD may encourage the search for these factors in health examination and stimulate the translational research on ILD development.

Abbreviation
CI: Confidence interval; COPD: Chronic obstructive pulmonary disease; GERD: Gastroesophageal reflux disorder; HR: Hazard ratio; ICD: International classification of disease; ILD: Interstitial lung disease; IPF: Idiopathic pulmonary fibrosis; NHI: National health insurance

Acknowledgements
We would like to thanks to Ms. Byeong Ju Park for the preparing data sets.

Funding
This work was supported by the National Research Foundation of Korea (NRF) grant funded by the Korean Government (MSIP) (No. 2014R1A5A2010008).

Authors' contributions
All authors have contributed either to the conception, original hypothesis, and design of the cohort. All authors have contributed to the writing and revisions of this article. Data acquisition was performed by CWL and W-IC, and analysis was performed by DS, HJK, JSP, SHP, W-IC, and CWL All authors had full access to all the data in the study. W-IC had final responsibility for the integrity of the data and the accuracy of the data analysis and the decision to submit for publication. All authors read and approved the final manuscript.

Competing interests
The authors state that they have no competing interests.

Author details
[1]Department of Internal Medicine, Keimyung University Dongsan Hospital, Daegu 41931, Republic of Korea. [2]Department of Allergology, Hospital Serive of Kavaje, Kavaje, Albania. [3]Department of Occupational & Environmental Medicine, Sungso Hospital, Andong, Republic of Korea.

References

1. Coultas DB, Zumwalt RE, Black WC, Sobonya RE. The epidemiology of interstitial lung diseases. Am J Respir Crit Care Med. 1994;150(4):967–72.
2. Nalysnyk L, Cid-Ruzafa J, Rotella P, Esser D. Incidence and prevalence of idiopathic pulmonary fibrosis: review of the literature. Eur Respir Rev. 2012;21(126):355–61.
3. Putman RK, Hatabu H, Araki T, Gudmundsson G, Gao W, Nishino M, Okajima Y, Dupuis J, Latourelle JC, Cho MH, et al. Association between interstitial lung abnormalities and all-cause mortality. Jama. 2016;315(7):672–81.
4. Choi WI, Park SH, Dauti S, Park BJ, Lee CW. Interstitial lung disease and risk of mortality: 11-year nationwide population-based study. Int J Tuberc Lung Dis. 2018;22(1):100–5.
5. Choi WI, Park SH, Park BJ, Lee CW. Interstitial lung disease and lung Cancer development: a 5-year Nationwide population-based study. Cancer Res Treat. 2017;50(2):374–81.
6. Lederer DJ, Enright PL, Kawut SM, Hoffman EA, Hunninghake G, van Beek EJ, Austin JH, Jiang R, Lovasi GS, Barr RG. Cigarette smoking is associated with subclinical parenchymal lung disease: the multi-ethnic study of atherosclerosis (MESA)-lung study. Am J Respir Crit Care Med. 2009;180(5):407–14.
7. Washko GR, Hunninghake GM, Fernandez IE, Nishino M, Okajima Y, Yamashiro T, Ross JC, Estepar RS, Lynch DA, Brehm JM, et al. Lung volumes and emphysema in smokers with interstitial lung abnormalities. N Engl J Med. 2011;364(10):897–906.
8. Hunninghake GM, Hatabu H, Okajima Y, Gao W, Dupuis J, Latourelle JC, Nishino M, Araki T, Zazueta OE, Kurugol S, et al. MUC5B promoter polymorphism and interstitial lung abnormalities. N Engl J Med. 2013;368(23):2192–200.
9. Lee J, Lee JS, Park SH, Shin SA, Kim K. Cohort profile: the National Health Insurance Service-National Sample Cohort (NHIS-NSC), South Korea. Int J Epidemiol. 2017;46(2):e15.
10. Ueda T, Ohta K, Suzuki N, Yamaguchi M, Hirai K, Horiuchi T, Watanabe J, Miyamoto T, Ito K. Idiopathic pulmonary fibrosis and high prevalence of serum antibodies to hepatitis C virus. Am Rev Respir Dis. 1992;146(1):266–8.
11. Tobin RW, Pope CE 2nd, Pellegrini CA, Emond MJ, Sillery J, Raghu G. Increased prevalence of gastroesophageal reflux in patients with idiopathic pulmonary fibrosis. Am J Respir Crit Care Med. 1998;158(6):1804–8.
12. Enomoto T, Usuki J, Azuma A, Nakagawa T, Kudoh S. Diabetes mellitus may increase risk for idiopathic pulmonary fibrosis. Chest. 2003;123(6):2007–11.
13. Chilosi M, Poletti V, Rossi A. The pathogenesis of COPD and IPF: distinct horns of the same devil? Respir Res. 2012;13:3.
14. Baumgartner KB, Samet JM, Stidley CA, Colby TV, Waldron JA. Cigarette smoking: a risk factor for idiopathic pulmonary fibrosis. Am J Respir Crit Care Med. 1997;155(1):242–8.
15. Travis WD, Costabel U, Hansell DM, King TE Jr, Lynch DA, Nicholson AG, Ryerson CJ, Ryu JH, Selman M, Wells AU, et al. An official American Thoracic Society/European Respiratory Society statement: update of the international multidisciplinary classification of the idiopathic interstitial pneumonias. Am J Respir Crit Care Med. 2013;188(6):733–48.
16. Auerbach O, Garfinkel L, Hammond EC. Relation of smoking and age to findings in lung parenchyma: a microscopic study. Chest. 1974;65(1):29–35.
17. Katzenstein AL, Mukhopadhyay S, Zanardi C, Dexter E. Clinically occult interstitial fibrosis in smokers: classification and significance of a surprisingly common finding in lobectomy specimens. Hum Pathol. 2010;41(3):316–25.
18. Cottin V, Nunes H, Brillet PY, Delaval P, Devouassoux G, Tillie-Leblond I, Israel-Biet D, Court-Fortune I, Valeyre D, Cordier JF, et al. Combined pulmonary fibrosis and emphysema: a distinct underrecognised entity. Eur Respir J. 2005;26(4):586–93.
19. Inomata M, Ikushima S, Awano N, Kondoh K, Satake K, Masuo M, Kusunoki Y, Moriya A, Kamiya H, Ando T, et al. An autopsy study of combined pulmonary fibrosis and emphysema: correlations among clinical, radiological, and pathological features. BMC Pulm Med. 2014;14:104.
20. Irving WL, Day S, Johnston ID. Idiopathic pulmonary fibrosis and hepatitis C virus infection. Am Rev Respir Dis. 1993;148(6 Pt 1):1683–4.
21. Meliconi R, Andreone P, Fasano L, Galli S, Pacilli A, Miniero R, Fabbri M, Solforosi L, Bernardi M. Incidence of hepatitis C virus infection in Italian patients with idiopathic pulmonary fibrosis. Thorax. 1996;51(3):315–7.
22. Arase Y, Suzuki F, Suzuki Y, Akuta N, Kobayashi M, Kawamura Y, Yatsuji H, Sezaki H, Hosaka T, Hirakawa M, et al. Hepatitis C virus enhances incidence of idiopathic pulmonary fibrosis. World J Gastroenterol. 2008;14(38):5880–6.
23. Idilman R, Cetinkaya H, Savas I, Aslan N, Sak SD, Bastemir M, Sarioglu M, Soykan I, Bozdayi M, Colantoni A, et al. Bronchoalveolar lavage fluid analysis in individuals with chronic hepatitis C. J Med Virol. 2002;66(1):34–9.
24. Cordier JF, Cottin V, Lazor R, Thivolet-Bejui F. Many faces of bronchiolitis and organizing pneumonia. Semin Respir Crit Care Med. 2016;37(3):421–40.
25. Kaufman JM, Cuvelier CA, Van der Straeten M. Mycoplasma pneumonia with fulminant evolution into diffuse interstitial fibrosis. Thorax. 1980;35(2):140–4.
26. Chastre J, Raghu G, Soler P, Brun P, Basset F, Gibert C. Pulmonary fibrosis following pneumonia due to acute Legionnaires' disease. Clinical, ultrastructural, and immunofluorescent study. Chest. 1987;91(1):57–62.
27. Auerbach SH, Mims OM, Goodpasture EW. Pulmonary fibrosis secondary to pneumonia. Am J Pathol. 1952;28(1):69–87.
28. Shachor Y, Schindler D, Siegal A, Lieberman D, Mikulski Y, Bruderman I. Increased incidence of pulmonary tuberculosis in chronic interstitial lung disease. Thorax. 1989;44(2):151–3.
29. Dheda K, Booth H, Huggett JF, Johnson MA, Zumla A, Rook GA. Lung remodeling in pulmonary tuberculosis. J Infect Dis. 2005;192(7):1201–9.
30. el-Serag HB, Sonnenberg A. Comorbid occurrence of laryngeal or pulmonary disease with esophagitis in United States military veterans. Gastroenterology. 1997;113(3):755–60.
31. Lee JS, Collard HR, Anstrom KJ, Martinez FJ, Noth I, Roberts RS, Yow E, Raghu G, Investigators IP. Anti-acid treatment and disease progression in idiopathic pulmonary fibrosis: an analysis of data from three randomised controlled trials. Lancet Respir Med. 2013;1(5):369–76.
32. Lee JS, Ryu JH, Elicker BM, Lydell CP, Jones KD, Wolters PJ, King TE Jr, Collard HR. Gastroesophageal reflux therapy is associated with longer survival in patients with idiopathic pulmonary fibrosis. Am J Respir Crit Care Med. 2011;184(12):1390–4.
33. Gribbin J, Hubbard R, Smith C. Role of diabetes mellitus and gastro-oesophageal reflux in the aetiology of idiopathic pulmonary fibrosis. Respir Med. 2009;103(6):927–31.
34. Navaratnam V, Fleming KM, West J, Smith CJ, Jenkins RG, Fogarty A, Hubbard RB. The rising incidence of idiopathic pulmonary fibrosis in the UK. Thorax. 2011;66(6):462–7.
35. Esposito DB, Lanes S, Donneyong M, Holick CN, Lasky JA, Lederer D, Nathan SD, O'Quinn S, Parker J, Tran TN. Idiopathic pulmonary fibrosis in United States automated claims. Incidence, prevalence, and algorithm validation. Am J Respir Crit Care Med. 2015;192(10):1200–7.
36. Raghu G, Chen SY, Yeh WS, Maroni B, Li Q, Lee YC, Collard HR. Idiopathic pulmonary fibrosis in US Medicare beneficiaries aged 65 years and older: incidence, prevalence, and survival, 2001-11. Lancet Respir Med. 2014;2(7):566–72.
37. Raghu G, Chen SY, Hou Q, Yeh WS, Collard HR. Incidence and prevalence of idiopathic pulmonary fibrosis in US adults 18-64 years old. Eur Respir J. 2016;48(1):179–86.
38. Gjonbrataj J, Choi WI, Bahn YE, Rho BH, Lee JJ, Lee CW. Incidence of idiopathic pulmonary fibrosis in Korea based on the 2011 ATS/ERS/JRS/ALAT statement. Int J Tuberc Lung Dis. 2015;19(6):742–6.
39. Hutchinson J, Fogarty A, Hubbard R, McKeever T. Global incidence and mortality of idiopathic pulmonary fibrosis: a systematic review. Eur Respir J. 2015;46(3):795–806.
40. Evans GW, Kantrowitz E. Socioeconomic status and health: the potential role of environmental risk exposure. Annu Rev Public Health. 2002;23:303–31.

14

Symptom prevalence of patients with fibrotic interstitial lung disease: a systematic literature review

Sabrina Carvajalino[1], Carla Reigada[2], Miriam J. Johnson[2], Mendwas Dzingina[3] and Sabrina Bajwah[3*] ⓘ

Abstract

Background: Those affected by advanced fibrotic interstitial lung diseases have limited treatment options and in the terminal stages, the focus of care is on symptom management. However, quantitatively, little is known about symptom prevalence. We aimed to determine the prevalence of symptoms in Progressive Idiopathic Fibrotic Interstitial Lung Disease (PIF-ILD).

Methods: Searches on eight electronic databases including MEDLINE for clinical studies between 1966 and 2015 where the target population was adults with PIF-ILD and for whom the prevalence of symptoms had been calculated.

Results: A total of 4086 titles were screened for eligibility criteria; 23 studies were included for analysis. The highest prevalence was that for breathlessness (54–98%) and cough (59–100%) followed by heartburn (25–65%) and depression (10–49%). The heterogeneity of studies limited their comparability, but many of the symptoms present in patients with other end-stage disease were also seen in PIF-ILD.

Conclusions: This is the first quantitative review of symptoms in people with Progressive Idiopathic Fibrotic Interstitial Lung Diseases. Symptoms are common, often multiple and have a comparable prevalence to those experienced in other advanced diseases. Quantification of these data provides valuable information to inform the allocation of resources.

Keywords: Pulmonary fibrosis, Symptom prevalence and interstitial lung disease

Background

Patients with Interstitial Lung Disease have a wide range of diagnoses and prognoses. Many patients can live many years with their diagnosis and some are responsive to treatments. However, a subset of patients with Progressive Idiopathic Fibrotic Interstitial Lung Diseases (PIF-ILD) such as idiopathic pulmonary fibrosis have a short disease trajectory and a similar prognosis to people with lung cancer [1]. The clinical manifestation of advanced fibrotic Non Specific Interstitial Pneumonia (NSIP) is similar to IPF [2]. It is important to differentiate NSIP from IPF in the early stages when the disease is potentially responsive to therapy [2] .However, when the disease is advanced and irreversible, this becomes less important and the focus should be on symptom control.

The United Kingdom (UK) End of life care strategy aimed to promote high quality care for all adults at the end of life [3]. In addition, the British Thoracic [4] and NICE idiopathic pulmonary fibrosis guidance [5] emphasize the importance of a proactive approach in managing symptoms.

Recent qualitative work in this group has shown uncontrolled symptoms, for example, shortness of breath, cough and insomnia, which impact on every aspect of patients and carers lives [6, 7]. However, quantitative work assessing prevalence of symptoms is limited and there has been no systematic review of this literature. Synthesising the quantitative evidence for symptom prevalence for this group will add to previous qualitative

* Correspondence: sabrina.bajwah@kcl.ac.uk
[3]Cicely Saunders Institute, Bessemer Rd, London, UK
Full list of author information is available at the end of the article

work, raise awareness of these symptoms and focus clinical intervention.

Methods

Aim

To estimate the symptom prevalence in people with PIF-ILD.

Design

Systematic review of the literature.

Search strategy

We performed comprehensive searches of databases including MEDLINE, Cochrane, EMBASE, Science Citation Index Expanded (Web of Knowledge), pre-Medline, CINAHL and PSYCINFO from 1966 to November 2013 using a combination of MESH headings and keywords (for full search strategy see online Additional file 1 APPENDIX A). In addition, key journals hand searched included THORAX, American Journal of Respiratory and Critical Care Medicine and CHEST (2000 to 2013). The search was updated to March 2015. Only studies in English or Spanish were included.

Selection

Study population

Published data of adults (≥ 18 years old), with all stages of the following ILD types: interstitial pulmonary fibrosis (IPF), nonspecific interstitial pneumonia (NSIP), cryptogenic fibrosing alveolitis and idiopathic interstitial pneumonia from any setting were included.

Studies in which patients had COPD and/or cancer in addition to PIF-ILD were excluded.

Types of studies included

A scoping search identified a paucity of data. Therefore all study types reporting quantitative data were included. Case reports of fewer than five patients were excluded. Qualitative studies were included if quantitative data were available for extraction.

Types of outcomes included

Symptoms included were based on a previous systematic review looking at interventions to improve symptoms and quality in patients with PIF-ILD [8] and encompassed both physical and psychological domains.

Data extraction

One independent reviewer (SC) selected the studies against the inclusion criteria using the title and, if the title did not offer enough information, abstracts and/or full text were read. Data were extracted using a form that included the main author, year of publication, setting, type and number of participants, disease group,

aims of the study, study design, measurement methods and prevalence of individual symptoms (See Additional file 2 APPENDIX B).

Data analysis

The Strengthening the Reporting of Observational Studies in Epidemiology (STROBE) Statement checklist for observational studies [9] was used to appraise each of the final studies. A palliative symptom grid was used and the number of patients in each study was calculated for each of the symptoms. Meta-synthesis and descriptive statistics were used for analysis and to present the findings. Where appropriate, a meta-analysis of each symptom from multiple studies was conducted using a random-effects model with inverse-variance weighting. Symptoms which were reported in only two studies or less were excluded from the meta-analysis. Heterogeneity was also quantified using the I-squared measure [10]. The confidence intervals are based on exact binomial (Clopper-Pearson) procedures [11]. Meta-analysis was conducted in Stata (StataCorp 2015) release 14 [12].

Results

Overview of included studies

Twenty-three articles describing symptoms were selected for this review (see Fig. 1) potentially relevant but excluded studies have been listed separately in Additional file 3 APPENDIX C. Included studies represented $N = 3171$ patients from European, Asian, and North and South American countries, conducted on outpatients at different disease stages; four studies included patients with end-stage disease [13–16]. The mean age across all studies varied between the fifth and sixth decade of life, and one study included patients older than 65 years [17]. Overall, studies found prognosis ranged between 12.9 to 46 months from time of diagnosis.

Study designs varied with a variety of retro and prospective designs (Table 1).

Symptom prevalence

Respiratory symptoms such as breathlessness and cough were measured in 13 studies [14, 15, 17–27]; fatigue and weight loss in five [18, 19, 21, 24, 28]; digestive tract symptoms in eight [13–16, 19, 20, 29, 30] sleep disorder in four [19, 28, 31, 32]; and other symptoms such as pain and urinary tract disorders in five [19–21, 24, 29]. The incidence of depression and/or anxiety was calculated in four studies [19, 33–35]. No studies documented delirium, constipation, halitosis, hemoptysis, hiccups, hyperphagia, polydipsia or mouth problems. A summary of findings is presented in Fig. 2.

PRISMA Flow chart

Records identified through database searching (*n*=4402)

Additional records identified through other sources (*n*=4)

Records after duplicates removed (*n*=4093)

Records excluded by title (*n*=3396)

Studies performed on animals=157
Pediatric population=245
No PIF-ILD =2994

Records screened (*n*=697)

Records excluded by abstract (*n*=450)

Review articles=72
No symptom prevalence =298
Different population =80

Records screened (*n*=247)

Articles excluded by full text (*n*=224)

Language=13
No PIF-ILD=24
Review article=12
Not available=35
Less than 5 patients=8
No symptom prevalence= 132

Studies included in quantitative synthesis (*n*=23)

Fig. 1 Pooled estimates of prevalence (proportion) of symptoms- random effects model ES = Estimated proportion

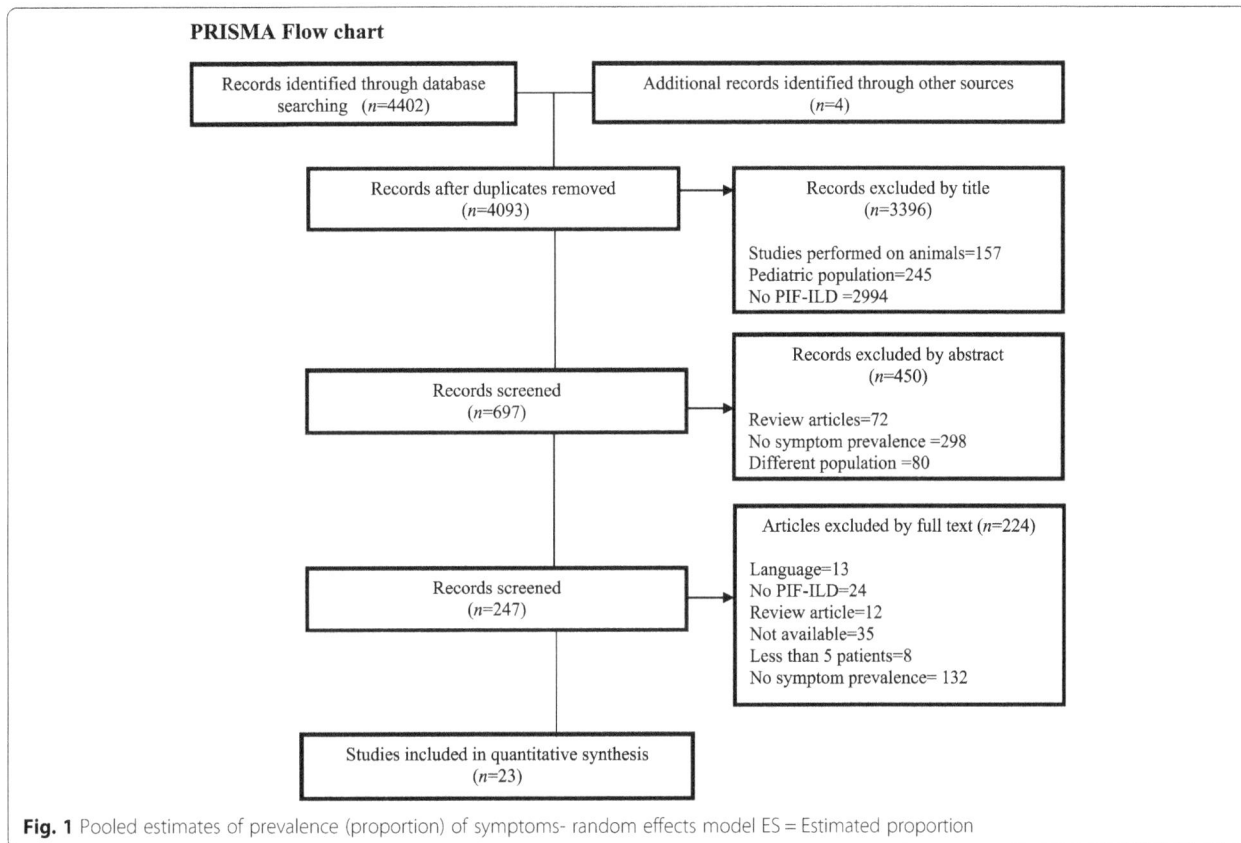

Respiratory symptoms

The overwhelming majority of patients had breathlessness (68.2–98%) and cough (59–94%) [14, 15, 17–27]. These were not only common symptoms, but preceded diagnosis by 6.8 months to 4 years [18]. Only one study documented breathlessness using the modified Medical Research Council scale (mMRC) (range 0 to 4) in 45.3% of the participants [17]. Nearly one in ten (9.3%) had mMRC grade 4. Severe breathlessness was associated with poor prognosis and those with mMRC scale score 3 and 4 had a median survival of 0.5 years [17].

Depression

A variety of depression measurement tools were used to provide prevalence estimates of depression ranking between 10% [34] and 49.2% [19, 33, 35]. A worse depression score was found to be associated with reduced Forced Expiratory Volume (FEV), Forced Vital Capacity (FVC), gas transfer factor and gas constant, increased duration of diagnosis, greater number of comorbidities [33]; worse breathlessness severity, pain severity, sleep quality, 4-m walk time, grip strength and diffusing capacity of the lung for carbon monoxide (DLco) [35].

The prevalence of anxiety was estimated to be as high as 58% in one study of health-related quality of life (HRQoL) and symptom burden [34].

Digestive tract symptoms

Upper gastro-intestinal symptoms are described in IPF and have been investigated in several studies. Gastro-oesophageal reflux prevalence was shown in 35.7 to 100% [13–16, 20, 30].

Although in some patients this appeared to be asymptomatic, symptoms were reported by a significant proportion: belching (51%) [29], regurgitation (16–40%) [13–16, 20, 29], heartburn (29–48%) [13–16, 20, 29], dysphagia (11–43%) [13, 16, 20, 29, 30], and dysphonia (11%) [20]. Typical acid reflux symptoms were found [13–15, 20] and usually related to other causes such as cough (83% in these studies). A correlation between cough and acid reflux in the oesophagus was seen in 28% of the episodes of reflux [25]. However, 33% of those without evidence of dysmotility had at least one oesophageal symptom [20].

Sleep related symptoms

A relationship between obstructive sleep apnoea and IPF was observed in a 50 patients study with stable breathlessness, which a quarter of participants had an Epworth sleepiness score higher than 10 representing significant daytime sleepiness [31]. In one study of 30 patients, the following sleep related symptoms were reported: insomnia (46.6%), snoring (40%), excessive daytime sleepiness

Table 1 Summary of studies included

Author/ Year	Aim	Study Design and symptom assessment used	Participants (n)	Diagnosis	Diagnosis method	Baseline % predicted lung function mean (SD)	Symptoms prevalence
Akhtar 2013 [33]	To assess the presence of depressive symptoms	Prospective study Wakefield Self-assessment of Depression Inventory score ≥ 15 screening tool	Outpatients (n = 118)	IPF	High resolution computed tomography, Lung biopsy	Not available	Depression 49.2%
Alhamad 2008 [18]	Describe the clinical course and prognosis of IPF among Middle Eastern patients, and to attempt to identify variables that would predict prognosis.	Retrospective study Chart reviews, telephone interviews	Hospital patients (n = 61)	IPF	ATS/ERS criteria	FVC 64.8 (21.6)[a]	Dyspnoea 93%; Cough 82%; Weight loss 12%
Araki 2003 [17]	To investigate the outcome of IPF in elderly patients whose pathological diagnosis corresponded to usual interstitial pneumonia on autopsy findings.	Retrospective study MRC dyspnoea scale, medical records	Patients older than 65y, based on histological findings on autopsy, complete medical records (n = 86)	UIP, IPF	Lung biopsy: Histological findings consistent with UIP, IPF	VC 72.6 (25.2) DLCO 62.8 (30.1)	Dyspnoea 54.7% Cough 93.2%
Bajwah 2012 [19]	To compare the palliative care needs, treatments, and end-of-life preferences of PIF-ILD patients	Retrospective study Medical records	Outpatients Hospital; Ages 37–99 (n = 45)	PIF-ILD	ATS/ERS criteria	Not available	Dyspnoea 93%; Cough 60%; Fatigue 29%; Insomnia 6%; Depress ion/anxiety 22%; Anorexia/weight loss 18%; Chest pain 29%; Generalized pain 9%; Dyspepsia 4%; Polyuria/polydipsia 4%; Diarrhea 2%; Dysphagia 2%
Bandeira 2009 [20]	To determine prevalence of GERD and to evaluate its clinical presentation	Prospective study General questionnaire, Quality of Life Scale for Gastroesophageal Reflux Disease	Outpatients (n = 28)	IPF	ATS/ERS criteria in 11 patients, lung biopsy 17 patients	FVC 66.6 (16.0) DLCO 44.5 (22.0)	Heartburn 29%; Nocturnal heartburn 14%; Regurgitation 40%; Nocturnal regurgitation 18%; Epigastric pain 18%; Dysphagia 11%; Cough 77%; Nocturnal cough 37%; Dysphonia 11%; Chest pain 25%
D'Ovidio 2005 [13]	To determine the prevalence of gastroesophageal reflux in lung transplant candidates	Interviews and Esophageal manometer.	Outpatients (n = 26)	IPF	Not specified	FVC median (range) 67 (33–96) DLCO median (range) 40 (13–77)	Heartburn Regurgitation Dysphagia 65%
Hashemi Sadraei 2013 [21]	To evaluate the clinical characteristics of IPF patients from The National Research Institute of Tuberculosis and Lung Diseases	Retrospective descriptive study Medical records and interviews	(n = 132)	IPF	Clinical presentation, radiographic and or/ pathological findings ATS criteria	Not available	Breathlessness 68.2%; Cough 60.6%; Chest pain 8.3%; Fatigue 7.6%

Table 1 Summary of studies included *(Continued)*

Author/ Year	Aim	Study Design and symptom assessment used	Participants (n)	Diagnosis	Diagnosis method	Baseline % predicted lung function mean (SD)	Symptoms prevalence
Hoppo 2012 [14]	To determine the prevalence of GERD and assess the proximity of reflux events in patients with histologically proven IPF	Retrospective study	(n = 35)	IPF	Lung biopsy	Not available	Cough 74%; Heartburn 25%; Regurgitation 25%
Jeon 2006 [22]	To investigate the prognostic factors at initial presentation and the causes of death in Korean patients with IPF	Retrospective study Medical records	Outpatients (n = 88)	IPF	Surgical lung biopsy compatible with UIP, ATS criteria	FVC 74.0 (19.2) DLCO 65.2 (21.4)	Exertional dyspnoea 89%
Lancaster 2009 [31]	To analyze obstructive sleep apnea in clinically stable patients with IPF	Epworth sleepiness scale (ESS) ≥10 consistent with daytime sleepiness	(n = 35)	IPF	ATS criteria (2000)	FVC 68.8 (13.7)[a]	Daytime sleepiness 25%
Lindell 2010 [34]	To test the ability of a complex intervention (PRISM) to decrease symptom burden, stress and improve HRQoL perceptions of patients with IPF and their carers.	Nested mixed method design (experimental, qualitative) Beck Anxiety Inventory, Beck Depression Inventory-II	Outpatients (n = 37)	IPF	Biopsy and/or High resolution computed tomography	70% FVC > 55 15% FVC 50– 55 15% FVC < 50%	Anxiety 58% Depression 4 (10%)
Mermigkis 2009 [32]	To describe sleep quality associated to daytime consequences in IPF	Cross-sectional control study Epworth Sleepiness Scale Pittsburgh Sleep Quality Index Functional Outcomes in Sleep Questionnaire Fatigue Severity Scale Polysomnography Interview	Outpatients (n = 15)	IPF	ATS/ERS criteria or lung biopsy	FVC 77.4 (21.2) DLCO 56.3 (17.8)	Daytime sleepiness 20%; Snoring 40%; Insomnia 46.6%; Witnessed apnoea's 13.3%
Mermigkis 2007 [28]	To describe the clinical and polysomnographic features of SRBD and to identify predictors of OSA in IPF patients	Retrospective study Cleveland Clinic Sleep Disorders Questionnaire, Epworth Sleepiness scale, Polysomnography	Outpatients (n = 18)	IPF	ATS/ERS criteria	FVC 65.7 (10.4) DLCO 49.9 (15.3)	Excessive daytime sleepiness 77.7%; Snoring 88%; Daytime fatigue 61%; Witnessed apnoea's 44.4%
Ohno 2007 [23]	Not specified	Retrospective Clinical personal records	(n = 1322) Patients covered by public insurance	IIP	Medical records: 12% pathological diagnosis from lung biopsy, rest clinical findings (respiratory function test, images, serology)	Not available	Cough 94%; Exertional dyspnoea 98%
Patti 2005 [15]	To determine the prevalence of GERD, the clinical presentation of GERD and reflux profiles in patients with IPF	Patients rated severity of symptoms 5 point scale (0 = no symptom to 4 = disabling symptom)	Outpatients (n = 18)	IPF	Not specified	Not available	Heartburn 55%; Regurgitation 33%; Cough 83%
Raghu 2006 [29]	To assess the prevalence and clinical symptoms of GER in patients with	Prospective study 24 h oesophageal pH probe, oesophageal	Outpatients (n = 65)	IPF	ATS criteria	FVC 59.9 (20.0)[a] DLCO	Belching 51%; Heartburn 47%; Regurgitation 16%; Abdominal pain 7%;

Table 1 Summary of studies included *(Continued)*

Author/Year	Aim	Study Design and symptom assessment used	Participants (n)	Diagnosis	Diagnosis method	Baseline % predicted lung function mean (SD)	Symptoms prevalence
	IPF and compare findings to patients with intractable asthma manifesting symptoms of GER.	manometry, symptom questionnaire form				34.8 (15.7)[a]	Bloating 27%; Chest pain 24% Choking 13%; Globus 13%; Hoarseness 31%; Liquid dysphagia 7%; Solid dysphagia 16%; Odynophagia 4%; Nausea 13%
Ryerson 2012 [35]	To investigate the prevalence of clinically meaningful depress ion at baseline, characterize the association of depression with patient and disease specific variables, and describe the natural history of depress ion over a period of 6 months	Cohort	Outpatients (n=)52	ILD (21 with IPF)	ATS/ERS criteria	FVC 74.3 (18.5) DLCO 50.8 (16.3)	Depression 24%
Schoenheit 2011 [24]	To generate in depth insights regarding the patient journey, including symptoms triggers to seeking medical care, referral patterns, initial diagnoses, follow up and current disease management.	Qualitative Interviews conducted in the participants at home	Outpatients (n = 45)	IPF	Physician confirmed diagnosis	Not available	Exertional dyspnoea 68%; Cough 59%; Fatigue 28%; Chest pain 6%; Weight loss 2%
Sweet 2007 [16]	To determine the prevalence of distal and proximal reflux, the oesophageal manometric profile and whether or not reflux symptoms could be used to screen for reflux	Retrospective Study Standardized interview with a physician or technician. Patients rated severity of symptoms 5 point scale (0 = no symptom to 4 = disabling symptom)	Outpatients (n = 30)	IPF	Pathological findings in 25 patients, ATS/ERS criteria in 5 patients	Not available	Heartburn 48%; Regurgitation 43%; Dysphagia 30%
Tobin 1998 [25]	To investigate the possible association of GER and IPF	Qualitative study Structured interview	Outpatients (n = 17)	UIP	Lung biopsy compatible with UIP	DLCO mean (range) 35.9 (9–62)	Cough 100%
Von Plessen 2003 [26]	To study the incidence and prevalence of physician diagnosed and hospitalized cryptogenic fibrosing alveolitis in a well-defined adult popula-tion in Norway	Retrospective study Registration form, hospital registers (2 physicians extracted the information)	Hospital patients 158 incident cases (1984–1998) and 61 prevalent cases (until 31.12. 1998)	CFA	Progressive dyspnoea, crackles on auscultation and bilateral shadowings on chest X-ray with no exposure to a known fibrogenic agent	83 and 80% of incident and prevalent cases TLCO < 80% predicted	Incident cases dyspnoea 87%; Prevalent cases 79%
Aksu 2014 [30]	To investigate the possibility that IPF is involved in the pathogenic of GERD	Prospective study	Outpatients (N = 21)	IPF	Pulmonary function tests (spirometry, carbon monoxide diffusion capacity,	FVC 94.9 (11.2)[a] TLCO	Reflux symptoms 52.4% Severe dysphagia 23.8% Epigastric pain 91%

Table 1 Summary of studies included *(Continued)*

Author/ Year	Aim	Study Design and symptom assessment used	Participants (n)	Diagnosis	Diagnosis method	Baseline % predicted lung function mean (SD)	Symptoms prevalence
					alveolar volume), study of BAL fluid (cell count and lymphocyte subsets, IL-1 β, TNF-α)	114.1 (16.7)	
Huang 2014 [27]	To describe the clinical features and prognosis of microscopic polyangiitis (MPA) patients whose initial respiratory presentation was pulmonary fibrosis	Retrospective study Hospital computer-assisted search	Hospital patients MPA cases (N = 67)	IPF patients (N = 19)	Radiological findings (CT), clinical manifestations consistent with UIP pattern according to the ATS/ERS/JRS/ALAT statement 2011	DLCO range 30–76	Of IPF patients: Cough 84.2% Sputum 68.4% Hemoptysis 21.1% Dyspnoea 78.9%

^a mean estimates were pooled using the inverse variance weighting method

(20%), and witnessed apnoea's (13.3%) [32]. Studies used variety of outcome measures and showed problems with daytime fatigue (The Functional Systems Scores (FSS)), daytime dysfunction (Functional Outcomes of Sleep Questionnaire (FOSQ)) and poor sleep quality (Pittsburgh Sleep Quality Index (PSQI)). Patients reported excessive daytime sleepiness (77.7%), snoring (88%), daytime fatigue (29%), witnessed apnoeas (44.4%), and insomnia (6–46%) [19, 28, 31, 32].

Anorexia, weight loss, fatigue
The prevalence of weight loss was estimated as 2–18% (out of N = 151), and the prevalence of fatigue as 7.6–29% out of N = 240 [18, 19, 21, 24, 28].

Pain
Non-specified pain was found in 9% of the population, while chest pain affected 6–29% [19–21, 24, 29]. Two studies found epigastric pain in 18 and 91% of the population [20, 30].

Other symptoms
A prevalence of polyuria/polydipsia prevalence of 4% was found in one study [19].

Discussion
This is the first systematic review to draw together the symptom profile of people with PIF-ILD and shows a wide array of symptoms; comparable with those reported in other advanced diseases [36] (see Table 2). Breathlessness is seen to be a major problem, as prevalent as for people with COPD and heart disease. Likewise, psychological problems (depression and anxiety) and insomnia are prevalent in PIF-ILD. However, given the comparable

high prevalence of both breathlessness, anxiety and sleep disturbance, the estimate for daytime fatigue was surprisingly low [28]. This may be explained, at least in part, by the different outcome measures used to assess sleep quality in the different studies and only one study accounted for comorbid conditions that might interfere with sleep quality and quality of life [28].

Two other symptoms stand out as particular problems for people with PIF-ILD. Firstly, cough is identified as not only highly prevalent, but also of major significance in terms of symptom burden, often preceding the diagnosis by some time. Secondly, although reports of nausea and vomiting are relatively low, there are significant problems associated with gastro-intestinal dysmotility leading to reflux which is likely to aggravate cough and may be associated with chest/epigastric pain.

Most people with respiratory disease have multiple co-morbidities which contribute long- term symptoms [37]. In addition, symptoms do not occur in isolation with demonstrated interactions between many symptoms, particularly in lung cancer, where a respiratory distress cluster of cough, breathlessness and fatigue has been described [38, 39]. The possibility of specific symptom clusters (clinically observed symptoms associations) for PIF-ILD which could benefit from a combined symptomatic approach is an area for further research. Knowledge of symptom clusters in PIF-ILD may help prompt clinical investigation of associated symptoms when one symptom is detected. It is clear from these data that a single symptom does not occur in isolation. Therefore is important that symptom assessment in people with PIF-ILD should focus on all commonly encountered symptoms and not just breathlessness alone. The significant prevalence of anxiety, depression and social isolation

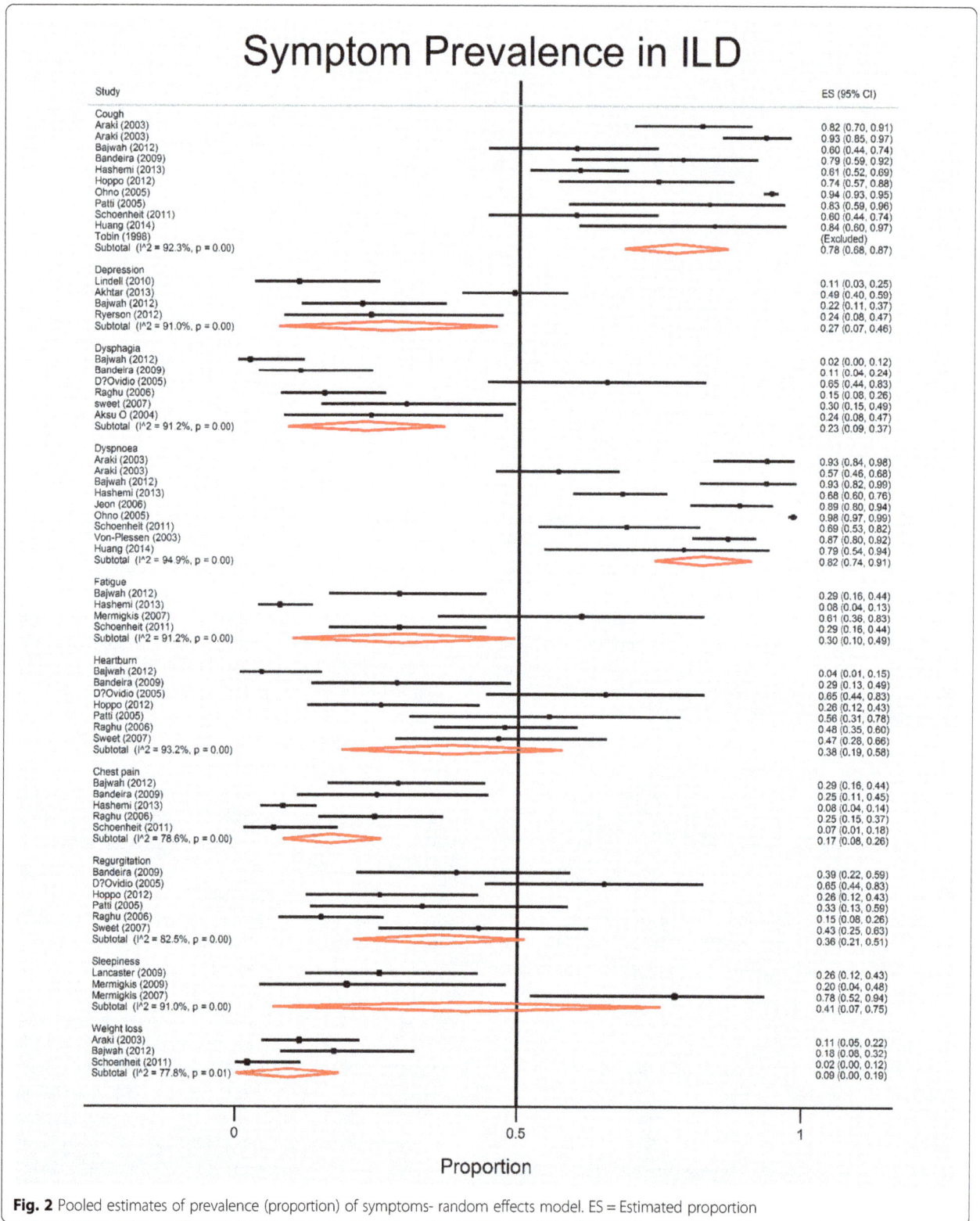

Symptom Prevalence in ILD

Study	ES (95% CI)
Cough	
Araki (2003)	0.82 (0.70, 0.91)
Araki (2003)	0.93 (0.85, 0.97)
Bajwah (2012)	0.60 (0.44, 0.74)
Bandeira (2009)	0.79 (0.59, 0.92)
Hashemi (2013)	0.61 (0.52, 0.69)
Hoppo (2012)	0.74 (0.57, 0.88)
Ohno (2005)	0.94 (0.93, 0.95)
Patti (2005)	0.83 (0.59, 0.96)
Schoenheit (2011)	0.60 (0.44, 0.74)
Huang (2014)	0.84 (0.60, 0.97)
Tobin (1998)	(Excluded)
Subtotal (I^2 = 92.3%, p = 0.00)	0.78 (0.68, 0.87)
Depression	
Lindell (2010)	0.11 (0.03, 0.25)
Akhtar (2013)	0.49 (0.40, 0.59)
Bajwah (2012)	0.22 (0.11, 0.37)
Ryerson (2012)	0.24 (0.08, 0.47)
Subtotal (I^2 = 91.0%, p = 0.00)	0.27 (0.07, 0.46)
Dysphagia	
Bajwah (2012)	0.02 (0.00, 0.12)
Bandeira (2009)	0.11 (0.04, 0.24)
D?Ovidio (2005)	0.65 (0.44, 0.83)
Raghu (2006)	0.15 (0.08, 0.26)
sweet (2007)	0.30 (0.15, 0.49)
Aksu O (2004)	0.24 (0.08, 0.47)
Subtotal (I^2 = 91.2%, p = 0.00)	0.23 (0.09, 0.37)
Dyspnoea	
Araki (2003)	0.93 (0.84, 0.98)
Araki (2003)	0.57 (0.46, 0.68)
Bajwah (2012)	0.93 (0.82, 0.99)
Hashemi (2013)	0.68 (0.60, 0.76)
Jeon (2006)	0.89 (0.80, 0.94)
Ohno (2005)	0.98 (0.97, 0.99)
Schoenheit (2011)	0.69 (0.53, 0.82)
Von-Plessen (2003)	0.87 (0.80, 0.92)
Huang (2014)	0.79 (0.54, 0.94)
Subtotal (I^2 = 94.9%, p = 0.00)	0.82 (0.74, 0.91)
Fatigue	
Bajwah (2012)	0.29 (0.16, 0.44)
Hashemi (2013)	0.08 (0.04, 0.13)
Mermigkis (2007)	0.61 (0.36, 0.83)
Schoenheit (2011)	0.29 (0.16, 0.44)
Subtotal (I^2 = 91.2%, p = 0.00)	0.30 (0.10, 0.49)
Heartburn	
Bajwah (2012)	0.04 (0.01, 0.15)
Bandeira (2009)	0.29 (0.13, 0.49)
D?Ovidio (2005)	0.65 (0.44, 0.83)
Hoppo (2012)	0.26 (0.12, 0.43)
Patti (2005)	0.56 (0.31, 0.78)
Raghu (2006)	0.48 (0.35, 0.60)
Sweet (2007)	0.47 (0.28, 0.66)
Subtotal (I^2 = 93.2%, p = 0.00)	0.38 (0.19, 0.58)
Chest pain	
Bajwah (2012)	0.29 (0.16, 0.44)
Bandeira (2009)	0.25 (0.11, 0.45)
Hashemi (2013)	0.08 (0.04, 0.14)
Raghu (2006)	0.25 (0.15, 0.37)
Schoenheit (2011)	0.07 (0.01, 0.18)
Subtotal (I^2 = 78.6%, p = 0.00)	0.17 (0.08, 0.26)
Regurgitation	
Bandeira (2009)	0.39 (0.22, 0.59)
D?Ovidio (2005)	0.65 (0.44, 0.83)
Hoppo (2012)	0.26 (0.12, 0.43)
Patti (2005)	0.33 (0.13, 0.59)
Raghu (2006)	0.15 (0.08, 0.26)
Sweet (2007)	0.43 (0.25, 0.63)
Subtotal (I^2 = 82.5%, p = 0.00)	0.36 (0.21, 0.51)
Sleepiness	
Lancaster (2009)	0.26 (0.12, 0.43)
Mermigkis (2009)	0.20 (0.04, 0.48)
Mermigkis (2007)	0.78 (0.52, 0.94)
Subtotal (I^2 = 91.0%, p = 0.00)	0.41 (0.07, 0.75)
Weight loss	
Araki (2003)	0.11 (0.05, 0.22)
Bajwah (2012)	0.18 (0.08, 0.32)
Schoenheit (2011)	0.02 (0.00, 0.12)
Subtotal (I^2 = 77.8%, p = 0.01)	0.09 (0.00, 0.18)

Proportion
0   0.5   1

Fig. 2 Pooled estimates of prevalence (proportion) of symptoms- random effects model. ES = Estimated proportion

as the disease progresses highlights the importance of a holistic approach embodied by palliative care [6].

Palliative care is the active, total care of people with advanced, progressive disease [40]. Currently, the vast majority of palliative care services are provided to patients with cancer, and access to specialist palliative care is inconsistent for people with non-malignant disease. This inequity has been highlighted in the recent NICE

Table 2 Summary of the prevalence of symptoms in Cancer, AIDS, CHF, COPD, ESRD and PIF-ILD (figures for other conditions taken from Solano et al. 2006 [36])

Symptoms	PIF-ILD	Cancer	AIDS	CHF	COPD	ESRD
Pain	9%	30–94%	30–98%	14–78%	21–77%	11–93%
Depression	10–49.2%	4–80%	17–82%	6–59%	17–77%	2–61%
Anxiety	22–58%	3–74%	13–76%	2–49%	23–53%	7–52%
Fatigue	7.6–29%	23–100%	43–95%	42–82%	32–96%	13–100%
Breathlessness	54.7–98%	16–77%	43–62%	18–88%	56–98%	11–82%
Insomnia	6–46.6%	3–67%	40–74%	36–48%	15–77%	1–83%
Nausea	13%	2–78%	41–57%	2–48%	4%	8–52%
Diarrhea	2%	1–95%	29–53%	12%		8–36%

AIDS Adult Immune Deficiency Syndrome, *CHF* Chronic Heart Failure, *COPD* Chronic Obstructive Pulmonary Disease, *ESRD* End-stage Renal Disease

guidance for IPF [5]. These stated that the ILD specialist services should have the skills to assess and manage most supportive and palliative care needs of the people under their care. In addition, robust joint working and pathways of care should also be in place to ensure access to specialist palliative care for those issues that the ILD services are unable to address. However, this policy has been largely unimplemented, and in everyday practice as currently configured, patients have unmet palliative care needs [7, 41].

Implications for clinical practice and research

People with PIF-ILD face a sombre prognosis and deterioration in their quality of life with little hope of successful disease modification. Therefore, improvement in quality of life and palliation of significant symptoms are crucially important treatment goals [5, 42]. Recognition that these are prevalent is the first step, the next is to incorporate systematic assessment of symptoms and other palliative care concerns as a routine part of clinical management by respiratory health professionals. There needs to be a recognition that other symptoms alongside breathlessness are present. This is likely to have implications for education and training needs, extended team working between respiratory, palliative and primary care, and service configuration. Validated clinical tools to aid the clinician to identify and triage symptoms and other needs are needed for everyday practice and has been highlighted in the recent NICE quality standard for IPF [42]. An example of such tool is the recently adapted and validated Needs Assessment Tool-Interstitial Lung Disease (NAT-ILD) [43].

Good quality prospective observational studies are needed to get better estimates of symptom prevalence in PIF-ILD over the duration of the disease. Such prospective evaluation would allow investigation of symptoms not found in this review such as confusion, constipation and anorexia. In particular, the natural history of symptoms as the disease progresses to advanced disease and end of life along with the impact upon the individual

and their family needs to be described in order to be able to understand the clinical care needs of this patient group, inform palliative and supportive care service planning and to inform study designs for clinical trials of symptom interventions. To facilitate this, disease severity with baseline lung function should be published for all studies.

Symptoms which seem to be of particular concern to people with PIF-ILD such as cough and gastro-intestinal dysmotility are under-researched and deserve focus. In addition, validation of questionnaires to determine the presence of conditions such as depression and fatigue in this group would be useful.

Limitations

Only one reviewer screened, selected and extracted data from the articles included. Those not published in the English or Spanish language were excluded. Grey literature was not searched. It was difficult to give an accurate estimate of symptom prevalence due to the varying quality of cohort formation, measurement tools and definition of the symptom in question. Period prevalence time ranges, varying definitions of symptoms, sample size proportions and the various different measurement methods across the studies may all have contributed to variations in the minimum and maximum prevalence ranges. Due to the heterogeneity of the study populations and poor reporting, meta-analyses and sub-analyses by disease and severity of disease was not possible. Patients included in these studies had stable disease and were not receiving oxygen therapy.

Conclusion

This study aimed to determine from existing studies, the prevalence of a group of symptoms in patients with PIF-ILD. Symptoms are common, often multiple and have a comparable prevalence to those experienced by people with other advanced diseases. Symptoms extend far beyond respiratory symptoms such as breathlessness and cough, and include fatigue, sleep disturbance as well as a broad variety of gastrointestinal symptoms. Breathlessness and anxiety are as prevalent as in COPD and heart disease, yet patients rarely have access to breathlessness management programs. Cough and gastrointestinal dysmotility appear to be particular issues for people with PIF-ILD and warrant further work which should include exploration of a possible PIF-ILD symptom clusters.

Quantification of these symptoms provide valuable information to inform the education and training needs of ILD services to allow routine assessment and management by ILD clinicians and appropriate use and allocation of specialist palliative care resources.

These findings highlight and support the need for a systematic and validated approach to assessment of symptoms in every day clinical practice by ILD services. This would ensure close attention to symptom management with appropriate and timely referral to palliative care services according to need, in order to optimise quality of life and provide good care during advanced disease and end of life.

Additional files

Additional file 1: Appendix A Full search strategy – Medicine search strategy. (DOCX 14 kb)

Additional file 2: Appendix B Data extraction form. (DOCX 13 kb)

Additional file 3: Appendix C Potentially Relevant but Excluded Studies. (DOCX 12 kb)

Abbreviations

DLco: Diffusing capacity of the lung for carbon monoxide; FEV: Forced Expiratory Volume; FOSQ : Functional Outcomes of Sleep Questionnaire; FSS: Functional Systems Scores; FVC: Forced Vital Capacity; HRQoL : Health-related quality of life; mMRC: Modified Medical Research Council scale; MPA: Microscopic polyangiitis; NAT-ILD : Needs Assessment Tool-Interstitial Lung Disease; NSIP: Non Specific Interstitial Pneumonia; PIF-ILD : Progressive Idiopathic Fibrotic Interstitial Lung Disease; PSQI : Pittsburgh Sleep Quality Index; STROBE: Strengthening the Reporting of Observational Studies in Epidemiology

Funding

This systematic review was self-funded by SC who completed it as part of a MSc in Palliative Care.

Authors' contributions

SC and SB conceived the idea for the review. SC drafted the original review. CR, MJ and SB adapted the review into a paper for publication. MD conducted analysis. All authors reviewed the final version and approved it for publication.

Competing interests

The authors declares that they have no competing interests.

Author details

[1]Fundación Santa Fé de Bogotá, Bogotá, Colombia. [2]Hull York Medical School, Hertford Building, University of Hull, Hull, UK. [3]Cicely Saunders Institute, Bessemer Rd, London, UK.

References

1. Vancheri C. Idiopathic pulmonary fibrosis and cancer: do they really look similar? BMC Med. 2015;13(1):220.
2. du Bois R, King TE Jr. Challenges in pulmonary fibrosis x 5: the NSIP/UIP debate. Thorax. 2007;62(11):1008–12.
3. Richards M. The End of Life Care Strategy: Promoting high quality care for all adults at the end of life. End of Life Care Strategy; 2008.
4. Bradley B, Branley HM, Egan JJ, Greaves MS, Hansell DM, Harrison NK, et al. Interstitial lung disease guideline: the British Thoracic Society in collaboration with the Thoracic Society of Australia and New Zealand and the Irish Thoracic Society. Thorax. 2008;63(Suppl 5):v1–58.
5. Excellence NIfHaC. Idiopathic pulmonary fibrosis: the diagnosis and management of suspected idiopathic pulmonary fibrosis. 2013.
6. Bajwah S, Higginson IJ, Ross JR, Wells AU, Birring SS, Riley J, et al. The palliative care needs for fibrotic interstitial lung disease: a qualitative study of patients, informal caregivers and health professionals. Palliat Med. 2013;27(9):869–76.
7. Sampson C, Gill BH, Harrison NK, Nelson A, Byrne A. The care needs of patients with idiopathic pulmonary fibrosis and their carers (CaNoPy): results of a qualitative study. BMC Pulm Med. 2015;15(1):1.
8. Bajwah S, Ross JR, Peacock JL, Higginson IJ, Wells AU, Patel AS, et al. Interventions to improve symptoms and quality of life of patients with fibrotic interstitial lung disease: a systematic review of the literature. Thorax. 2013;68(9):867–79.
9. Knottnerus A, Tugwell P. STROBE–a checklist to strengthen the reporting of observational studies in epidemiology. J Clin Epidemiol. 2008;61(4):323.
10. Higgins JP, Thompson SG, Deeks JJ, Altman DG. Measuring inconsistency in meta-analyses. BMJ. 2003;327(7414):557–60.
11. Newcombe RG. Two-sided confidence intervals for the single proportion: comparison of seven methods. Stat Med. 1998;17(8):857–72.
12. StataCorp. Stata Statistical Software. 14th ed. College Station: StatCorp LP; 2015.
13. D'Ovidio F, Singer LG, Hadjiliadis D, Pierre A, Waddell TK, de Perrot M, et al. Prevalence of gastroesophageal reflux in end-stage lung disease candidates for lung transplant. Ann Thorac Surg. 2005;80(4):1254–60.
14. Hoppo T, Komatsu Y, Jobe BA. Su1529 is idiopathic pulmonary fibrosis really idiopathic?: patterns of reflux analyzed by bi-positional high-resolution manometry and Hypopharyngeal multichannel intraluminal impedance. Gastroenterology. 2012;142(5):S-1056.
15. Patti MG, Tedesco P, Golden J, Hays S, Hoopes C, Meneghetti A, et al. Idiopathic pulmonary fibrosis: how often is it really idiopathic? J Gastrointest Surg. 2005;9(8):1053–6. discussion 6–8
16. Sweet MP, Patti MG, Leard LE, Golden JA, Hays SR, Hoopes C, et al. Gastroesophageal reflux in patients with idiopathic pulmonary fibrosis referred for lung transplantation. J Thorac Cardiovasc Surg. 2007;133(4):1078–84.
17. Araki T, Katsura H, Sawabe M, Kida K. A clinical study of idiopathic pulmonary fibrosis based on autopsy studies in elderly patients. Intern Med. 2003;42(6):483–9.
18. Alhamad EH, Masood M, Shaik SA, Arafah M. Clinical and functional outcomes in middle eastern patients with idiopathic pulmonary fibrosis. Clin Respir J. 2008;2(4):220–6.
19. Bajwah S, Higginson IJ, Ross JR, Wells AU, Birring SS, Patel A, et al. Specialist palliative care is more than drugs: a retrospective study of ILD patients. Lung. 2012;190(2):215–20.
20. Bandeira CD, Rubin AS, Cardoso PF, Moreira Jda S, Machado Mda M. Prevalence of gastroesophageal reflux disease in patients with idiopathic pulmonary fibrosis. J Bras Pneumol. 2009;35(12):1182–9.
21. Hashemi Sadraei N, Riahi T, Masjedi MR. Idiopathic pulmonary fibrosis in a referral center in Iran: are patients developing the disease at a younger age? Arch Iran Med. 2013;16(3):177–81.
22. Jeon K, Chung MP, Lee KS, Chung MJ, Han J, Koh WJ, et al. Prognostic factors and causes of death in Korean patients with idiopathic pulmonary fibrosis. Respir Med. 2006;100(3):451–7.
23. Ohno S, Nakaya T, Bando M, Sugiyama Y. Nationwide epidemiological survey of patients with idiopathic interstitial pneumonias using clinical personal records. Nihon Kokyuki Gakkai Zasshi. 2007;45(10):759–65.
24. Schoenheit G, Becattelli I, Cohen AH. Living with idiopathic pulmonary fibrosis: an in-depth qualitative survey of European patients. Chron Respir Dis. 2011;8(4):225–31.
25. Tobin RW, Pope CE 2nd, Pellegrini CA, Emond MJ, Sillery J, Raghu G. Increased prevalence of gastroesophageal reflux in patients with idiopathic pulmonary fibrosis. Am J Respir Crit Care Med. 1998;158(6):1804–8.

26. Von Plessen C, Grinde Ø, Gulsvik A. Incidence and prevalence of cryptogenic fibrosing alveolitis in a Norwegian community. Respir Med. 2003;97(4):428–35.

27. Huang H, Wang YX, Jiang CG, Liu J, Li J, Xu K, et al. A retrospective study of microscopic polyangiitis patients presenting with pulmonary fibrosis in China. BMC Pulm Med. 2014;14:8.

28. Mermigkis C, Chapman J, Golish J, Mermigkis D, Budur K, Kopanakis A, et al. Sleep-related breathing disorders in patients with idiopathic pulmonary fibrosis. Lung. 2007;185(3):173–8.

29. Raghu G, Freudenberger TD, Yang S, Curtis JR, Spada C, Hayes J, et al. High prevalence of abnormal acid gastro-oesophageal reflux in idiopathic pulmonary fibrosis. Eur Respir J. 2006;27(1):136–42.

30. Aksu O, Songur N, Songur Y, Ozturk O, Adiloglu AK, Kapucuoglu N, et al. Is gastroesophageal reflux contribute to the development chronic cough by triggering pulmonary fibrosis. Turk J Gastroenterol. 2014;25(Suppl 1):48–53.

31. Lancaster LH, Mason WR, Parnell JA, Rice TW, Loyd JE, Milstone AP, et al. Obstructive sleep apnea is common in idiopathic pulmonary fibrosis. Chest. 2009;136(3):772–9.

32. Mermigkis C, Stagaki E, Amfilochiou A, Polychronopoulos V, Korkonikitas P, Mermigkis D, et al. Sleep quality and associated daytime consequences in patients with idiopathic pulmonary fibrosis. Med Princ Pract. 2009;18(1):10–5.

33. Akhtar AA, Ali MA, Smith RP. Depression in patients with idiopathic pulmonary fibrosis. Chron Respir Dis. 2013;10(3):127–33.

34. Lindell KO, Olshansky E, Song M, Zullo TG, Gibson KF, Kaminski N, et al. Impact of a disease-management program on symptom burden and health-related quality of life in patients with idiopathic pulmonary fibrosis and their care partners. Heart Lung. 2010;39(4):304–14.

35. Ryerson CJ, Arean PA, Berkeley J, Carrieri-Kohlman VL, Pantilat SZ, Landefeld CS, et al. Depression is a common and chronic comorbidity in patients with interstitial lung disease. Respirology. 2012;17(3):525–32.

36. Solano JP, Gomes B, Higginson IJ. A comparison of symptom prevalence in far advanced cancer, AIDS, heart disease, chronic obstructive pulmonary disease and renal disease. J Pain Symptom Manag. 2006;31(1):58–69.

37. Currow DC, Clark K, Kamal A, Collier A, Agar MR, Lovell MR, et al. The population burden of chronic symptoms that substantially predate the diagnosis of a life-limiting illness. J Palliat Med. 2015;18(6):480–5.

38. Molassiotis A, Lowe M, Blackhall F, Lorigan P. A qualitative exploration of a respiratory distress symptom cluster in lung cancer: cough, breathlessness and fatigue. Lung Cancer. 2011;71(1):94–102.

39. Dodd MJ, Miaskowski C, Paul SM, editors. Symptom clusters and their effect on the functional status of patients with cancer. Oncol Nurs Forum; 2001.

40. WHO. Definition of palliative care: World Health Organisation. 2002 [Available from: http://www.who.int/cancer/palliative/definition/en/.

41. Bajwah S, Ross JR, Wells AU, Mohammed K, Oyebode C, Birring SS, et al. Palliative care for patients with advanced fibrotic lung disease: a randomised controlled phase II and feasibility trial of a community case conference intervention. Thorax. 2015;70(9):830–9.

42. Excellence NIfC. NICE. Idiopathic Pulmonary Fibrosis in adults Quality Standard. Quality standard for idiopathic pulmonary fibrosis DRAFT. In: NICE, editor. Manchester: NICE; 2014. https://www.nice.org.uk/guidance/qs79/resources/idiopathic-pulmonary-fibrosis-in-adults-pdf-2098856506309. Accessed May 2018.

43. Boland JW, Reigada C, Yorke J, Hart SP, Bajwah S, Ross J, et al. The adaptation, face, and content validation of a needs assessment tool: progressive disease for people with interstitial lung disease. J Palliat Med. 2016;19(5):549–55.

15

Mobile health applications in self-management of patients with chronic obstructive pulmonary disease: a systematic review and meta-analysis of their efficacy

Fen Yang[1†], Yuncui Wang[1†], Chongming Yang[2], Hui Hu[1*] and Zhenfang Xiong[1*†]

Abstract

Background: Mobile health applications are increasingly used in patients with Chronic Obstructive Pulmonary Disease (COPD) to improve their self-management, nonetheless, without firm evidence of their efficacy. This meta-analysis was aimed to assess the efficacy of mobile health applications in supporting self-management as an intervention to reduce hospital admission rates and average days of hospitalization, etc.

Methods: PubMed, Web of Science (SCI), Cochrane Library, and Embase were searched for relevant articles published before November 14th, 2017. A total of 6 reports with randomized controlled trials (RCTs) were finally included in this meta-analysis.

Results: Patients using mobile phone applications may have a lower risk for hospital admissions than those in the usual care group (risk ratio (RR) = 0.73, 95% CI [0.52, 1.04]). However, there was no significant difference in reducing the average days of hospitalization.

Conclusion: Self-management with mobile phone applications could reduce hospital admissions of patients with COPD.

Keywords: Chronic obstructive pulmonary disease, Self-management, Hospital admissions, Mobile applications

Background

Chronic Obstructive Pulmonary Disease (COPD) is a major global chronic disease which affected millions of people worldwide [1], causing considerable hospital admissions. The World Health Organization (WHO) has estimated that COPD which causes considerable hospital admission will become the third cause of global deaths by 2020 [2–5]. These patients are heavy users of healthcare and social service resources [6, 7]. As there is currently no cure for COPD, appropriate self-care and management may play an important role in the patients' lifetime. Self-management techniques, such as adherence to medication, exercises, and prompt medical care, are crucial to improve the health status and have the potential to reduce hospital admissions [8–11].

Mobile health (mHealth), is now widely used for self-management of COPD, a term used to describe medical practice and healthcare in support of mobile computing and mobile devices (such as tablets, mobile phones, etc.). However, it is unclear whether these applications are beneficial to patients [12]. The deployment of eHealth applications is conducive to the availability of health care, which in turn enhances the patient's understanding of his illness, sense of control, and willingness to manage himself [13]. However, cheaper and widely available mobile phones are not other specialized medical devices. Mobile phones with applications to monitor, prompt, and record health behaviors have become a feasible and acceptable intervention [14]. Some reviews

* Correspondence: xiong_zhenfang@126.com; xiong_zhenfang@126.com
†Fen Yang, Yuncui Wang and Zhenfang Xiong contributed equally to this work.
[1]School of Nursing, Hubei University of Chinese Medicine, Wuhan, China
Full list of author information is available at the end of the article

reported that mHealth applications were effective in promoting disease self-management and daily lifestyle changes [15–17]. Several studies showed that mobile phones could deliver effective behavior change interventions and had many positive evidences [9, 18–20]. Mobile phones were also found effective in promoting COPD patients' physical activity and exercise capacity [21]. However, another study found that COPD patients with telephone-based care had greater mortality than usual care [22]. It is not clear how effectively mobile phone interventions could improve hospital admissions and lengths of hospitalization of COPD patients. Therefore, this study was aimed to compare the efficacy of mobile phone intervention with usual care in self-management, in terms of hospital admissions and the lengths of hospitalization.

Methods

Data sources and searches

A literature search without language restriction was performed using PubMed, Web of Science, the Cochrane Library, and Embase databases to identify potentially eligible studies published prior to November 14, 2017. All titles, keywords, and abstracts were examined in accordance with our search criteria. Full reports also were reviewed in case of uncertainty. In addition, references of retrieved studies and review articles were also manually checked to identify additional relevant studies. Some authors were even contacted for further information.

Study selection

Each study had to meet four criteria to be included in this study. First, studies were RCTs reported in full text with a title and abstract. Second, it included adults with a clinical diagnosis of COPD and compare mobile phone application interventions with the control group in usual care only (namely, routine or standard care). Third, telemonitoring studies entailed a self-management by COPD patients with ≥1 month follow-up. Fourth, the trials evaluated at least one of the following primary or secondary outcomes. The primary outcome was a hospital admission. The secondary outcome was the length of hospitalization, activity level, and lung function (e.g., predicted FEV1 percentage). Inclusion of each study was evaluated and determined independently by two reviewers. Exclusion criteria included: (1) reports based on systematic reviews and meta-analyses; (2) mobile-based interventions only via phone calls or sending messages.

Data extraction and quality assessment

From the articles that met the inclusion criteria, two reviewers independently extracted descriptions of the objectives, design, participants, interventions, and follow-up time. Any disagreements in data extraction were resolved by a discussion among the reviewers, and a final decision was made by another reviewer. If it is difficult or unclear to extract data from an article, its author was directly contacted to request the original data. The Cochrane Group's predesigned table [23] was used to assess the quality of the studies, including randomization, allocation concealment, similarity of baseline, criteria of inclusion/exclusion, blinding of participants and researchers, blinding of assessors, attrition rates, reporting of lost participants, and other sources of biases. Studies were scored one point for each fulfilled criterion. The quality of the studies was divided into three levels: low (≤3 points), moderate (4–6 points), and high (7–9 points).

Data synthesis and analysis

Eight studies were selected for the systematic review [24–31] and six of that were included for the meta-analysis with a random-effects model [24–29]. The outcomes reported by similar multiple studies were combined for the analysis. Also, meta-analyzed were the RCTs that reported the number of readmissions and the average days of hospitalization of each group (usual care vs. eHealth).

Data were obtained from the original selected studies or calculated [32] from the raw data. Risk ratios (RRs) were calculated for hospital admissions and mortality rates. Statistical heterogeneity was measured with the chi-square (χ^2) and I^2 statistics whose values greater than 50% indicate a high heterogeneity for the latter [33]. Publication bias was depicted with Begg's plot. Standard Mean Differences (SMD) were estimated with random effects modeling. All analyses were performed using Stata 12.0.

Results

Basic characteristics of the studies

From the 4072 potentially relevant reports initially identified, 3350 publications were excluded. The remainder of 722 retrieved reports were selected for full-text assessments and detailed evaluations. Finally, eight articles fulfilled our inclusion criteria [24–31] and only six articles were included in our meta-analysis [24–29] because two didn't report the patients' hospital admission [30, 31]. Figure 1 shows the literature flow diagram. We also extracted some additional information, such as country, mean age, the sample size of each group, sex, FEV1, the intervention methods, the length of follow-up and BMI, as shown in Table 1. Most RCTs compared a continued care with a usual care. Six RCTs reported the primary outcome of hospital admissions [24–29]. Only one study was a multicenter RCTs, and the others were conducted in single centers. There were totally 391 participants with COPD,

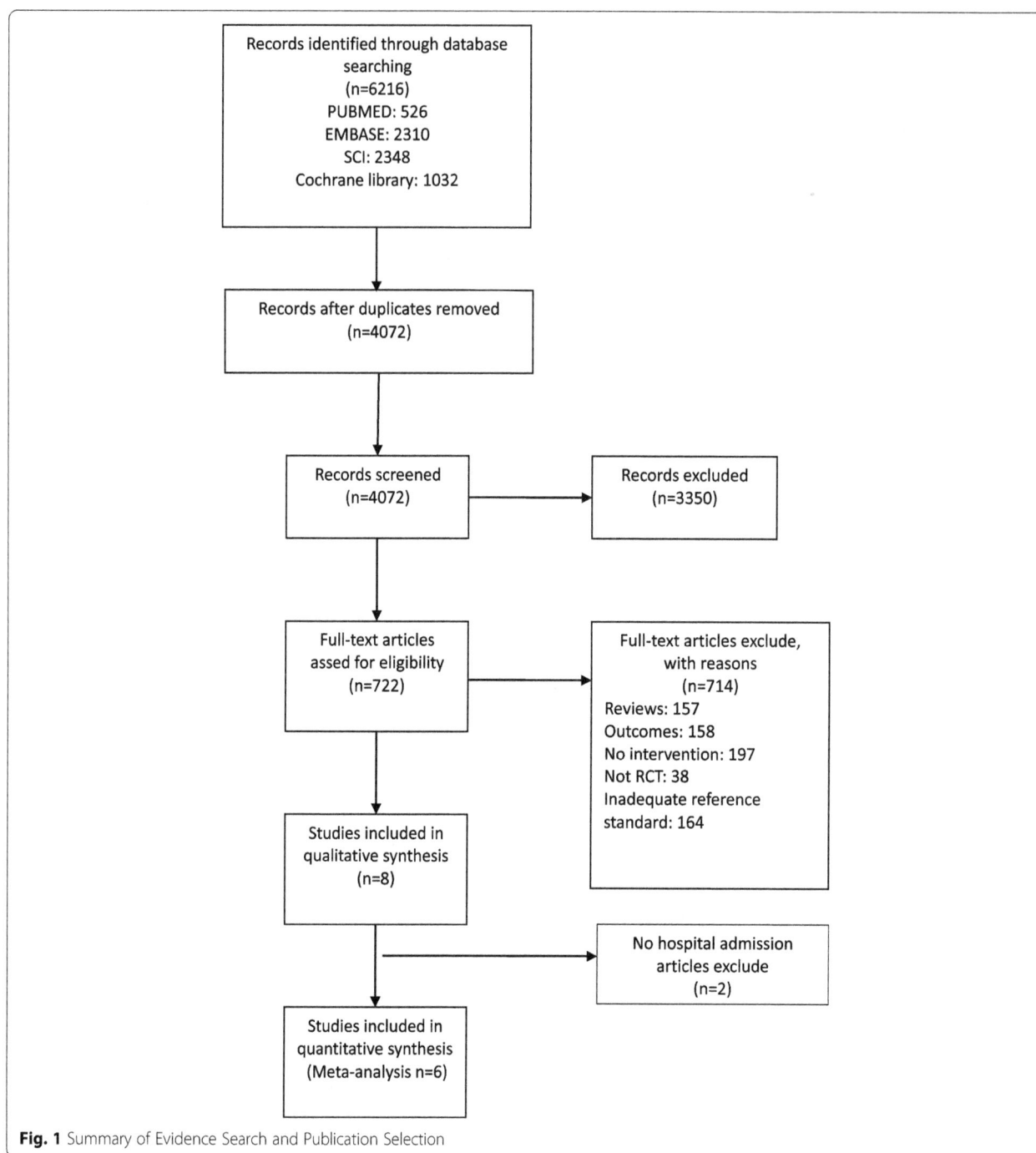

Fig. 1 Summary of Evidence Search and Publication Selection

293 (74.9%) of whom were men. The participants in one study had additional heart failures [27]. The sample sizes of subjects ranged from 24 to 99. There were six studies reporting the duration of the intervention equal or more than 6 months. The age of participants ranged from 63.5 to 81.0 years. The lung dysfunction was indicated by FEV1 (% predicted) that ranged from 37.9 to 58.9%. BMI ranged from 23.2 to 28.8 kg/m^2. Follow-ups were conducted for a range of 1 to 12 months and a mean of 6.9 months.

The intervention of the five studies included mobile/ smartphones with different software (Phone-personal digital assistant, MMA400, HTC P3600/3700, Sony Ericsson K600i, and HTC Desire S) and measuring devices. Applications were installed on smartphones to support patients in recording and monitoring their own physiological status, such as oxygen saturation levels, pulse rates, pedometers, or blood pressure monitors; or health behaviors, such as medications and dietary intake and exercise levels. Patients uploaded the data to their phones and sent

Table 1 Description of included trails

Source	Country	Mean (Age, y)	N	Setting	Male (%)	FEV1%	BMI (kg/m²)	Months of follow-up	Intervention
Liu WT et al., 2008 [26]	China	72.1	IG:24;CG:24	Single-center	48(100.0)	45.6	23.2	12	Patients were asked to complete respiratory symptoms by a cell phone using a Java application software, before they started daily endurance walking training.
Chau JP et al., 2012 [25]	China	72.9	IG:22;CG:18	single-center	39(97.5)	37.9	NR	2	The ASTRI telecare system (AST): a device kit which includes a mobile phone, a respiratory rate sensor and a pulse oximeter, an online network platform, a call center and a networking system. Participants in the intervention group measured their oxygen saturation, pulse rate and respiration rate at home and sent the results to the online network platform by mobile phone.
Jehn M et al., 2013 [24]	Germany	66.6	IG:32;CG:30	single-center	48(74.4)	51.4	27.3	9	Tele-monitoring: COPD Assessment Test (CAT), daily lung function and weekly 6-minute walk test (6MWT). The patients entered CAT by mobile phone (PDA system, MMA400).
Martin-Lesende I et al., 2013 [27]	Spain	81.0	IG:28;CG:30	Multicenter	34(58.6)	NA	NR	3, 6, 12	Tele-monitoring: daily transmissions from the patients' homes of the following self-measured clinical parameters (such as blood oxygen saturation, blood pressure, heart and respiratory rates, body weight and temperature) using a smart phone- personal digital assistant (PDA).
Pedone C et al., 2013 [28]	Italy	74.8	IG:50;CG:49	Single-center	67(67.7)	54.0	NR	9	"SweetAge" monitoring system: A commercial cellular telephone was equipped with a software that allowed the reception of the data(oxygen saturation, heart rate, near-body temperature, overall physical activity) transmitted by the wristband and sent the data to the monitoring system.
Tabak M et al., 2014 [29, 30]	the Netherlands	63.5	IG:12;CG:12	Single-center	12(50.0)	43.0	26.8	9	Condition Coach: teleconsultation (module for comments and asking questions of the patient's primary care physiotherapist and vice versa), Web-based exercising (including breathing exercises, relaxation, mobilization, resistance and endurance training, and mucus clearance), self-management and activity coach(A smartphone shows the measured activity cumulatively in a graph).
Tabak M et al., 2014 [29, 30]	the Netherlands	66.6	IG:14;CG:16	Single-center	19(63.3)	52.6	28.8	1	Tele-rehabilitation: (1) a smartphone (HTC P3600/3700) was used for activity coach; (2) web portal with a symptom diary for self-treatment of exacerbations and an overview of the measured activity levels.
Wang CH et al., 2014 [31]	China	71.7	IG:14;CG:16	Single-center	26(86.7)	58.9	23.5	6	Patients in the intervention group performed daily endurance exercise training under mobile phone guidance, and adherence was reported back to the central server.

NR not reported, IG Intervention Group, CG Control Group

the data to the networking/monitoring systems for health-care providers to follow up and personalize feedbacks. The aim of the intervention was to train patients and promote self-monitoring and healthy lifestyle behaviors. In three of all the trials, the mobile/smartphone was used to coach activities. The patients in control groups received usual care.

Study quality and publication Bias
The overall quality of the studies (Table 2) was moderate to high (4–7 scores). Five studies scored less than or equal to 6, and three studies scored less than 9. The most common reason for lower scores was the absence of a double–blind procedure, which was impossible due to the nature of the intervention. The assessors were not blinded to the outcomes in all the studies (100.0%) and researchers/participants were not blinded in 6 studies (75.0%). Only one study (12.5%) did not report the characteristics of participants lost for follow-ups. Begg's plot that was used to examine publication bias showed that there was no evident publication bias ($p = 1.00$).

Hospital admission rates
Figure 2 presented our meta-analyses and RR calculations of RCTs reported hospital admission. Six studies [24–29] assessed the effect of mobile health applications on hospital admission. As Martín-Lesende [27] reported the data of patients at the follow-up of 3 months, 6 months, and 12 months, we treated it as three separate experiments in our meta-analysis. We found that a lower risk for hospital admission among patients using mobile phone applications than that of the usual care group (RR = 0.73 [95% CI, 0.52 to 1.04]). The study by Jehn M [24] found that the hospital admission rates decreased significantly (RR, 0.30 [95% CI, 0.15 to 0.59]). But the heterogeneity in the overall pooled effect is 51.4% (I^2 = 51.4%, $p = 0.04$), implying that effect sizes varied across studies.

Average days of hospitalization
As shown in Fig. 3, six studies reported the average days of hospital stays. No significant difference was found between the intervention group and control group (SMD -0.06 [95% CI, – 0.31 to 0.18]).

Other results
Five articles reported that phone-based system could significantly improve exercise capacity and activity levels [24, 26, 29–31]. One study showed a significant reduction (lower predicted FEV1 percentage) in lung function of tele-monitoring intervention groups [24]. However, there was no significant differences found in another study [26].

Sensitivity analysis
A sensitivity analysis was performed for the primary outcome to test an overall pooled effect. The results were no different between fixed and random statistical effects (RR = 0.73; $P = 0.000$). The effect of sequentially omitting a low-quality study [24] and recalculating the pooled estimates for the remaining studies did not significantly alter the effect on all cause readmission (RR = 0.73 vs. 0.83; $P = 0.000$).

Discussion
Our results showed that mobile phone-based health applications in self-management currently could reduce hospital admissions of patients with COPD and could improve exercise capacity and activity levels, but could not reduce the average days of hospitalization.

Our findings were slightly different from another telemonitoring study which used a touch screen telemonitoring equipment to record and transmit a daily questionnaire about symptoms and corresponding treatment, and did not provide any convincing evidence of effectiveness on hospital admission and the duration of admissions [34]. The inconsistence may be due to the difference between screen telemonitoring and mobile phone. Mobile phone-based applications were found easy to learn and use by the participants as well as the patients with COPD. Mobile phone-based health applications could be practically more feasible as an intervention. Some studies reported they were a simple, reliable, easy to perform, and cost-saving intervention in behavior-changes, with advantages like adherence and intensity of the interventions, and more willingness of patients to use than other electronic devices [35, 36]. In addition, the virtual link created by sending self-monitoring data to a research nurse provided patients with a sense of continuity of care [37].

Mobile-phone-based system provides a feasible, efficient exercise training in improving exercise capacity, which was similar with other studies [38, 39]. Patients with COPD have decreased exercise capacity in their daily activities and they may have an inactive lifestyle [40–43]. Mobile phone applications, as a feasible and acceptable method for patients with COPD, can increase the capacity of self-management and the exercise adherence [44]. This result was similar with another review which evaluated the effectiveness of interventions delivered by computer and by mobile technology versus face-to-face or hard copy/digital documentary-delivered interventions [45]. A recent systematic review reported that mobile-based exercise programs could improve exercise capacity in patients with COPD in short and long term [30].

There are several limitations of our study. First, most RCTs compared an intervention with "usual care" whose details were not reported. Second, we only selected studies that reported the proportion of hospital admitted

Table 2 Quality assessment of included studies

Study	Randomization	Concealing Allocation	Baseline Similarity	Inclusion/Exclusion Criteria	Blinded Researchers/ Participants	Blinded Assessors	Attrition Rate Reported	Describing Lost Participants	Intention-to- Treat Analysis	Power Analysis	Total
Liu WT et al., 2008 [26]	Yes	No	Yes	Yes	No	No	Yes	Yes	No	Yes	6
Chau JP et al., 2012 [25]	Yes	No	Yes	Yes	No	No	Yes	Yes	No	No	5
Jehn M et al., 2013 [24]	Yes	No	Yes	Yes	No	No	Yes	No	No	No	4
Martin-Lesende I et al., 2013 [27]	Yes	No	Yes	Yes	No	No	Yes	Yes	No	Yes	6
Pedone C et al., 2013 [28]	Yes	No	Yes	Yes	No	No	Yes	Yes	Yes	Yes	7
Tabak M et al., 2014 [29, 30]	Yes	Yes	Yes	Yes	Yes	No	Yes	Yes	No	No	7
Tabak M et al., 2014 [29, 30]	Yes	Yes	Yes	Yes	Yes	No	Yes	Yes	No	No	7
Wang CH et al., 2014 [31]	Yes	No	Yes	Yes	No	No	No	Yes	No	No	4

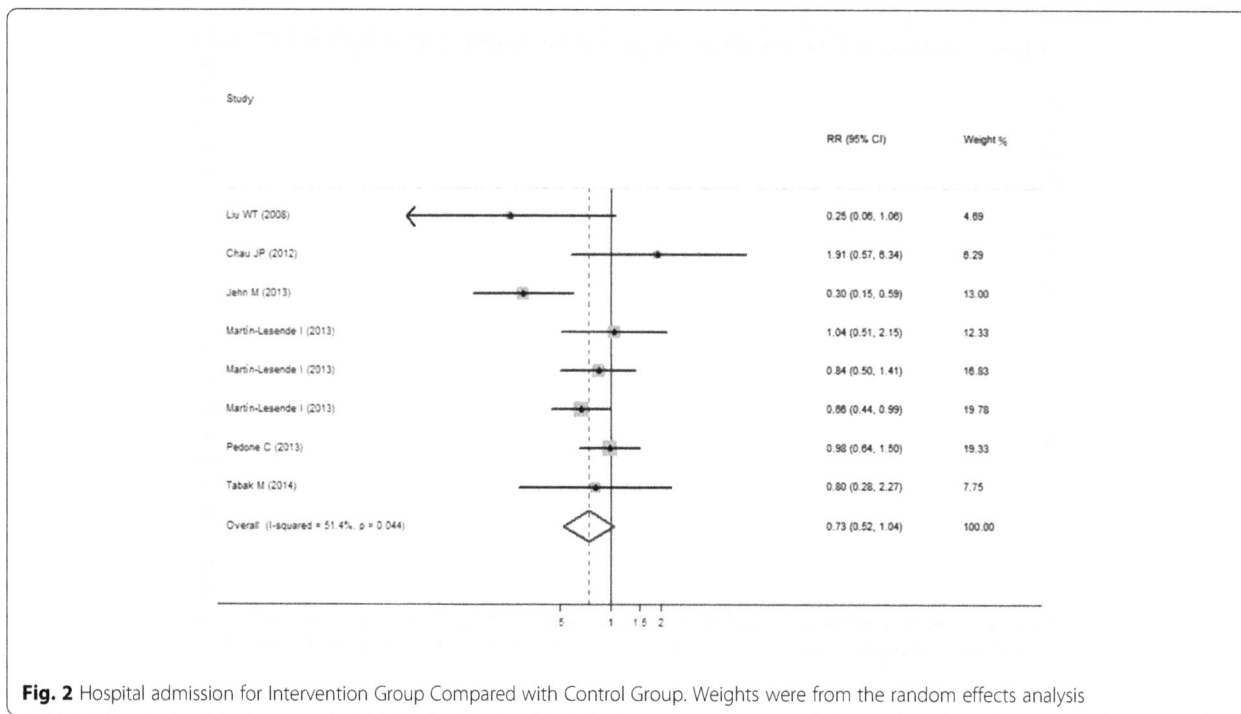

Fig. 2 Hospital admission for Intervention Group Compared with Control Group. Weights were from the random effects analysis

patients, but ignored information about secondary outcomes such as costs. Third, only eight studies were included in this systematic review and 6 studies in meta-analysis, most interventions were performed in short terms which could have influenced the results. Mobile phones will continue to evolve and are expected to be robust ubiquitous devices in the future, and researchers may think about how mobile phones can be used in future self-management of chronic disease. With the development of information technology and the expansion of mobile applications in medicine, we could improve the designs and clarify the effects of mobile health applications interventions for reducing hospital admission in patients with COPD in the future.

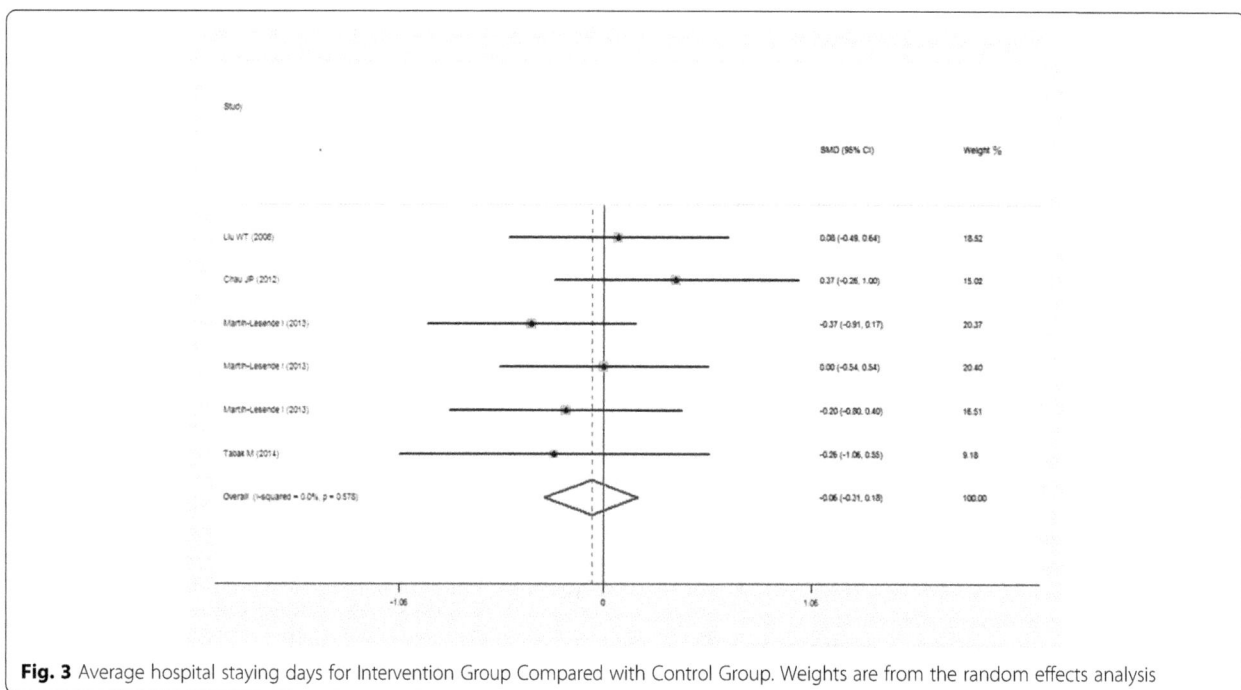

Fig. 3 Average hospital staying days for Intervention Group Compared with Control Group. Weights are from the random effects analysis

Mobile health applications in self-management of patients with chronic obstructive pulmonary...

123

Conclusions

The effectiveness of self-management with mobile or smart phones may help to reduce hospital admissions or improve health status of patients with COPD. Mobile phone with convenient applications have a great potential to minimize health problems and improve healthcare delivery.

Authors' contributions

YF preformed the work of design, acquisition of data and drafting the manuscript; WYC acquitted the data and wrote part of article; YCM and XZF analysed the data; HH conceived the report and wrote the manuscript. All the authors have read and approved the final manuscript.

Consent for publication

Not applicable.

Competing interests

The authors declare that they have no competing interests.

Author details

[1]School of Nursing, Hubei University of Chinese Medicine, Wuhan, China.
[2]Research Support Center, Brigham Young University, Provo, UT, USA.

References

1. Global initial for chronic obstructive lung disease: Gloable strategy for the diagnosis, management, and prevention of chronic obstructive pulmonary disease (2017 report). Retrieved on August 1, 2018 at https://goldcopd.org/gold-2017-global-strategy-diagnosis-management-prevention-copd/.
2. Puhan MA, Scharplatz M, Troosters T, Steurer J. Respiratory rehabilitation after acute exacerbation of COPD may reduce risk for readmission and mortality - a systematic review. Respir Res. 2005;6(1):54.
3. Mannino DM, Buist AS. Global burden of COPD: risk factors, prevalence, and future trends. Lancet. 2007;370(9589):765–73.
4. Lopez AD, Shibuya K, Rao C, Mathers CD, Hansell AL, Held LS, et al. Chronic obstructive pulmonary disease: current burden and future projections. Eur Respir J. 2006;27(2):397–412.
5. Buist AS, McBurnie MA, Vollmer WM, Gillespie S, Burney P, Mannino DM, et al. International variation in the prevalence of COPD (the BOLD study): a population-based prevalence study. Lancet. 2007;370(9589):741–50.
6. Mapel DW, McMillan GP, Frost FJ, Hurley JS, Picchi MA, Lydick E, et al. Predicting the costs of managing patients with chronic obstructive pulmonary disease. Respir Med. 2005;99(10):1325–33.
7. Tynan AJ, Lane SJCOPD. Illness severity, resource utilization and cost. Ir Med J. 2005;98(2):41–2.
8. Efraimsson EO, Hillervik C, Ehrenberg A. Effects of COPD self-care management education at a nurse-led primary health care clinic. Scand J Caring Sci. 2008;22(2):178–85.
9. Bourbeau J, Julien M, Maltais F, Rouleau M, Beaupré A, Bégin R, et al. Reduction of hospital utilization in patients with chronic obstructive pulmonary disease: a disease-specific self-management intervention. Arch Intern Med. 2003;163(5):585–91.
10. Zwerink M, Brusse-Keizer M, Van PD ZGA, Monninkhof EM, van der Palen J, et al. Self-management for patients with chronic obstructive pulmonary disease. Cochrane Database Syst Rev. 2014;3(3):CD002990.
11. Warwick M, Gallagher R, Chenoweth L, Stein-Parbury J. Self-management and symptom monitoring among older adults with chronic obstructive pulmonary disease. J Adv Nurs. 2010;66(4):784–93.
12. Black AD, Car J, Pagliari C, Anandan C, Cresswell K, Bokun T, et al. The impact of eHealth on the quality and safety of health care: a systematic overview. PLoS Med. 2011;8(1):e1000387.
13. Boulos MN, Brewer AC, Karimkhani C, Buller DB, Dellavalle RP. Mobile medical and health apps: state of the art, concerns, regulatory control and certification. Online J Public Health Inform. 2014;5(3):229.
14. Nguyen HQ, Wolpin S, Chiang KC, Cuenco D, Carrieri- Kohlman V. Exercise and symptom monitoring with a mobile device. AMIA Annu Symp Proc. 2006;1047
15. Nour M, Chen J, Allman-Farinelli M. Efficacy and external validity of electronic and mobile phone-based interventions promoting vegetable intake in young adults: systematic review and meta-analysis. J Med Internet Res. 2016;18(4):e58.
16. Devi BR, Syed-Abdul S, Kumar A, Iqbal U, Nguyen PA, Li YC, et al. An updated systematic review with a focus on HIV/AIDS and tuberculosis long term management using mobile phones. Comput Methods Prog Biomed. 2015;122(2):257–65.
17. Cui M, Wu X, Mao J, Wang X, Nie M. T2DM self-management via smartphone applications: a systematic review and meta-analysis. PLoS One. 2016;11(11):e0166718.
18. Hurling R, Catt M, Boni MD, Fairley BW, Hurst T, Murray P, et al. Using internet and mobile phone technology to deliver an automated physical activity program: randomized controlled trial. J Med Internet Res. 2007;9(2):e7.
19. Brendryen H, Drozd F, Kraft P. A digital smoking cessation program delivered through internet and cell phone without nicotine replacement (happy ending): randomized controlled trial. J Med Internet Res. 2008;10(5):e51.
20. Wennberg DE, Marr A, Lang L, O'Malley S, Bennett G. A randomized trial of a telephone care-management strategy. N Engl J Med. 2010;363(13):1245–55.
21. Martínez-García MDM, Ruiz-Cárdenas JD, Rabinovich RA. Effectiveness of smartphone devices in promoting physical activity and exercise in patients with chronic obstructive pulmonary disease: a systematic review. COPD. 2017;14(5):543–51.
22. Polisena J, Tran K, Cimon K, Hutton B, McGill S, Palmer K, et al. Home telehealth for chronic obstructive pulmonary disease: a systematic review and meta-analysis. J Telemed Telecare. 2010;16(3):120–7.
23. Higgins J, Green S. Cochrane Handbook for Systematic Reviews of Interventions. Chichester: J Wiley; 2006.
24. Jehn M, Donaldson G, Kiran B, Liebers U, Mueller K, Scherer D, et al. Tele-monitoring reduces exacerbation of COPD in the context of climate change–a randomized controlled trial. Environ Health. 2013;12:99.
25. Chau JP, Lee DT, Yu DS, Chow AY, Yu WC, Chair SY, et al. A feasibility study to investigate the acceptability and potential effectiveness of a telecare service for older people with chronic obstructive pulmonary disease. Int J Med Inform. 2012;81(10):674–82.
26. Liu WT, Wang CH, Lin HC, Lin SM, Lee KY, Lo YL, et al. Efficacy of a cell phone-based exercise programme for COPD. Eur Respir J. 2008;32(3):651–9.
27. Martín-Lesende I, Orruño E, Bilbao A, Vergara I, Cairo MC, Bayón JC, et al. Impact of telemonitoring home care patients with heart failure or chronic lung disease from primary care on healthcare resource use (the TELBIL study randomised controlled trial). BMC Health Serv Res. 2013;13:118.
28. Pedone C, Chiurco D, Scarlata S, Incalzi RA. Efficacy of multiparametric telemonitoring on respiratory outcomes in elderly people with COPD: a randomized controlled trial. BMC Health Serv Res. 2013;13:82.
29. Tabak M, Brusse-Keizer M, van der Valk P, Hermens H, Vollenbroek-Hutten M. A telehealth program for self-management of COPD exacerbations and promotion of an active lifestyle: a pilot randomized controlled trial. Int J Chron Obstruct Pulmon Dis. 2014;9:935–44.
30. Tabak M, Vollenbroek-Hutten MM, van der Valk PD, van der Palen J, Hermens HJ. A telerehabilitation intervention for patients with chronic obstructive pulmonary disease: a randomized controlled pilot trial. Clin Rehabil. 2014;28(6):582–91.
31. Wang CH, Chou PC, Joa WC, Chen LF, Sheng TF, Ho SC, et al. Mobile-phone-based home exercise training program decreases systemic inflammation in COPD: a pilot study. BMC Pulm Med. 2014;14:142.
32. Borenstein M, Hedges LV, Higgins JP, Rothstein HR. A basic introduction to fixed-effect and random-effects models for meta-analysis. Res Synth Methods. 2010;1(2):97–111.
33. Higgins JP, Thompson SG, Deeks JJ, Altman DG. Measuring inconsistency in meta-analyses. BMJ. 2003;327(7414):557–60.
34. Pinnock H, Hanley J, McCloughan L, Todd A, Krishan A, Lewis S, et al. Effectiveness of telemonitoring integrated into existing clinical services on hospital admission for exacerbation of chronic obstructive pulmonary disease: researcher blind, multicenter, randomized controlled trial. BMJ. 2013;347:f6070.
35. Kobayashi M, Hiyama A, Miura T, Asakawa C, Hirose M, Ifukube T. Elderly user evaluation of mobile touchscreen interactions. Springer Berlin Heidelberg. 2011;6946:83–99.

36. Velardo C, Shah SA, Gibson O, Clifford G, Heneghan C, Rutter H, et al. Digital health system for personalised COPD long-term management. BMC Med Inform Decis Mak. 2017;17(1):19.

37. Abaza H, Marschollek M. mHealth application areas and technology combinations. A comparison of literature from high and low/middle income countries. Methods Inf Med. 2017;56(7):e105–22.

38. Gosselink R, Langer D, Burtin C, Probst V, Hendriks HJM, van der Schans CP, et al. Clinical practice guideline for physical therapy in patients with COPD – practice guidelines. Dutch J Phys Ther. 2008;118(suppl):1–60.

39. Langer D, Hendriks E, Burtin C, Probst V, van der Schans C, Paterson W, et al. A clinical practice guideline for physiotherapists treating patients with chronic obstructive pulmonary disease based on a systematic review of available evidence. Clin Rehabil. 2009;23(5):445–62.

40. Sandland CJ, Singh SJ, Curcio A, Jones PM, Morgan MD. A profile of daily activity in chronic obstructive pulmonary disease. J Cardpulm Rehabil. 2005;25(3):181–3.

41. Pitta F, Troosters T, Spruit MA, Probst VS, Decramer M, Gosselink R. Characteristics of physical activities in daily life in chronic obstructive pulmonary disease. Am J Respir Crit Care Med. 2005;171(9):972–7.

42. Tabak M, Vollenbroek-Hutten M, van der Valk P, van der Palen J, Tönis T, Hermens H. Telemonitoring of daily activity and symptom behavior in patients with COPD. Int J Telemed Appl. 2012;2012:438736.

43. Lores V, Garcia-Rio F, Rojo B, Alcolea S, Mediano O. Recording the daily physical activity of COPD patients with an accelerometer: an analysis of agreement and repeatability. Arch Bronconeumol. 2006;42(12):627–32.

44. Dale J, Connor S, Tolley K. An evaluation of the west surrey telemedicine monitoring project. J Telemed Telecare. 2003;9(Suppl 1):S39–41.

45. McCabe C, McCann M, Brady AM. Computer and mobile technology interventions for self-management in chronic obstructive pulmonary disease. Cochrane Database Syst Rev. 2017;5:CD011425.

16

Stability of gene expression by primary bronchial epithelial cells over increasing passage number

Stephen R. Reeves[1,2†], Kaitlyn A. Barrow[1†], Maria P. White[1], Lucille M. Rich[1], Maryam Naushab[1] and Jason S. Debley[1,2*] ⓘ

Abstract

Background: An increasing number of studies using primary human bronchial epithelial cells (BECs) have reported intrinsic differences in the expression of several genes between cells from asthmatic and non-asthmatic donors. The stability of gene expression by primary BECs with increasing cell passage number has not been well characterized.

Methods: To determine if expression by primary BECs from asthmatic and non-asthmatic children of selected genes associated with airway remodeling, innate immune response, immunomodulatory factors, and markers of differentiated airway epithelium, are stable over increasing cell passage number, we studied gene expression patterns in passages 1, 2, 3, 4, and 5 BECs from asthmatic ($n = 6$) and healthy ($n = 6$) subjects that were differentiated at an air-liquid interface. RNA was harvested from BECs and RT-PCR was performed for TGFβ1, TGFβ2, activin A, FSTL3, MUC5AC, TSLP, IL-33, CXCL10, IFIH1, p63, KT5, TUBB4A, TJP1, OCLN, and FOXJ1.

Results: Expression of TGFβ1, TGFβ2, activin A, FSTL3, MUC5AC, CXCL10, IFIH1, p63, KT5, TUBB4A, TJP1, OCLN, and FOXJ1 by primary BECs from asthmatic and healthy children was stable with no significant differences between passages 1, 2 and 3; however, gene expression at cell passages 4 and 5 was significantly greater and more variable compared to passage 1 BECs for many of these genes. IL-33 and FOXJ1 expression was also stable between passages 1 through 3, however, expression at passages 4 and 5 was significantly lower than by passage 1 BECs. TSLP, p63, and KRT5 expression was stable across BEC passages 1 through 5 for both asthmatic and healthy BECs.

Conclusions: These observations illustrate the importance of using BECs from passage ≤3 when studying gene expression by asthmatic and non-asthmatic primary BECs and characterizing the expression pattern across increasing cell passage number for each new gene studied, as beyond passage 3 genes expressed by primary BECs appear to less accurately model in vivo airway epithelial gene expression.

Keywords: Asthma, Children, Airway remodeling, Epithelial cells

Background

Asthma continues to be one of the most prevalent and costly diseases of childhood throughout the world [1]. In recent years, our understanding of asthma pathogenesis has grown to include a central role for bronchial epithelial cells (BECs) in the establishment and maintenance of

---
* Correspondence: jason.debley@seattlechildrens.org
†Stephen R. Reeves and Kaitlyn A. Barrow contributed equally to this work.
[1]Center for Immunity and Immunotherapies, Seattle Children's Research Institute, Seattle, WA, USA
[2]Pulmonary and Sleep Medicine Division, Department of Pediatrics, University of Washington, Seattle, WA, USA

asthmatic airway disease [2]. Additionally, understanding of the importance of BECs in immune surveillance and coordination of the immune response to infections and environmental antigens has grown to include an important role for BEC-derived cytokines and direct cell-to-cell communication beyond their role in barrier function and innate immunity [3]. As a result, BECs have become the focus of many recent studies aimed to elucidate mechanisms underlying asthma pathogenesis in children [4].

Studying BECs in children with and without asthma presents a unique set of challenges. Unlike studies in adults, obtaining cells via bronchoscopic airway biopsy from children is problematic as most institutional review boards cannot approve such studies in children as the risk of general anesthesia and the lack of direct benefit to the subject precludes such investigations. While transformed and immortalized cell lines exist and are commercially available for in vitro studies, none of the currently available cell lines are derived from pediatric donors, and very little clinical data is provided about the subjects from whom such lines were obtained. Furthermore, immortalized BEC cell lines are variable in their ability to recapitulate the anatomical and physiologic features observed in the in vivo condition [5]. Direct comparisons of airway epithelial behavior in the asthmatic vs. non-asthmatic conditions is critical to furthering our understanding of the pathophysiology of asthma, which therefore requires use of primary airway epithelial cells. In addition, given the recognition that asthma is a complex and heterogeneous disease with multiple endotypes with likely unique aspects driving pathophysiology [6], it is increasingly important that donors of primary epithelial cells used in basic and translational studies be carefully clinically characterized so as to allow investigations of the role of the airway epithelium within unique asthma endotypes.

Given the limitations of in vitro models utilizing cell lines and the difficulty obtaining biopsy specimens in the pediatric population, ex vivo cultures of primary BECs obtained via bronchial brushings have become a useful model in which to perform studies related to the airway epithelium in children [7]. Collection of bronchial epithelial cells using brushings performed through an endotracheal tube while a patient is under general anesthesia (taking advantage of a planned anesthesia for a separate, clinically indicated procedure) have been described and importantly pose minimal additional risk to the subject [7, 8]. While this methodology has been utilized successfully in children and adults for more than a decade and provides a reliable, safe, and relatively non-invasive way to obtain primary BECs [7–10] that can be utilized to support ex vivo studies, the major trade-off is that the number of cells obtained using this methodology is relatively low. In most cases expansion of the cell number in culture is an essential step required to produce sufficient material to conduct experiments.

While the passage of cells in culture poses a theoretical loss of cellular phenotype the further cells are propagated beyond the donor, several studies including work from our lab have demonstrated phenotypic differences in primary cells obtained from children with and without asthma (reviewed by McLellan et al.) suggesting that cell phenotype is preserved at least in the initial 2-3 passages [4]. While there have been anecdotal reports of cells performing poorly in cell cultures at later passages, we are not aware of studies that have rigorously examined gene expression differences that occur in BECs over subsequent passages. In order to better characterize the stability of gene expression by primary BECs over multiple passages, we tested the hypothesis that the expression of a panel of genes involved in airway remodeling, immune regulation, innate immune response, airway epithelial basal cells, ciliogenesis, and epithelial tight junctions would be stable through increasing cell passages in an ex vivo organotypic culture model system using primary BECs obtained from well-phenotyped children with or without asthma that were differentiated at an air-liquid interface (ALI).

Methods

Subjects

For this study, we recruited asthmatic and healthy children ages 6-18 years undergoing an elective surgical procedure that required endotracheal intubation and general anesthesia for a clinically indicated procedure. Children with asthma had at least a 1-year history of physician-diagnosed asthma, used a short-acting beta-agonist ≥ twice a month or were taking a daily maintenance medication (inhaled corticosteroid or montelukast), and were born ≥36 weeks gestation. Additionally, children with asthma had one or more of the following atopic features: history of a positive skin prick test or positive radioallergosorbent testing (RAST) for a common aeroallergen, elevated serum IgE (> 100 IU/mL), history of physician-treated allergic rhinitis, history of physician-treated atopic dermatitis. Healthy subjects were born ≥36 weeks gestation, and lacked a history of asthma, reactive airway disease, chronic cough, chronic lung disease, or past treatment with bronchodilators, systemic or inhaled steroids, or oxygen. A detailed medical history was obtained to ensure the subjects met these inclusion criteria.

At the time of anesthesia, a blood sample was drawn from each subject and used to measure total serum IgE and RAST allergen-specific IgE to dust mites (D. farina and D. pteronyssinus), cat epithelium, dog epithelium, Alternaria tenuis, Aspergillus fumigatus, and timothy grass. At a subsequent follow-up visit the fraction of exhaled nitric oxide (FE_{NO}) was measured according to American Thoracic Society (ATS) guidelines using a NIOX MINO nitric oxide analyzer (Aerocrine®, Sweden) [11]. Spirometry was performed using a VMAX® series 2130 spirometer (VIASYS Healthcare, Hong Kong) to quantify forced vital capacity (FVC), forced expiratory volume in 1 s (FEV_1), and forced expiratory flow between 25 and 75% of FVC (FEF_{25-75}) according to ATS guidelines.

Ethics, consent and permissions

Written consent was obtained from parents of subjects and assent was obtained for children ≥ age 10 years. The work presented in this study was approved by the Seattle Children's Hospital Institutional Review Board.

Establishment of bronchial epithelial cell cultures

Following the induction of anesthesia and securing of the endotracheal tube, three samples of BECs were obtained from each subject using 4 mm Harrell® unsheathed bronchoscope cytology brushes (CONMED® Corporation). The brush was inserted through an endotracheal tube, advanced until resistance was felt, and rubbed against the airway surface for 2-3 s as described previously [7, 8]. Cells were seeded onto type I collagen coated T-25 cell culture flasks and proliferated under submerged culture conditions. Cultures were proliferated in a humidified incubator at 37 °C in an atmosphere of 5% CO_2 in PneumaCult™-Ex bronchial epithelial growth medium (BEGM) (StemCell™ Technologies) containing gentamicin and amphotericin B, and supplemented with penicillin-streptomycin (100 μg/ml; Invitrogen®). Fluconazole (25 μg/mL) was added to P0 medium for the first 96 h, after which medium was aspirated and replaced with medium without fluconazole. Medium was thereafter changed every 48 h until the culture reached ~70-90% confluence. All primary BEC lines were screened for mycoplasma using MycoAlert™ PLUS Mycoplasma Detection Kit (Lonza, Inc) and found to be negative.

Air-liquid Interface (ALI) epithelial cell cultures

BECs were used for these studies at each passage corresponding number. Once cells were ~70-90% confluence in flasks, they were trypsinized with 1 mL of 0.025% Trypsin-EDTA and then seeded onto collagen I pre-coated (Collagen Solution, STEMCELL™ Technologies) Corning Costar 12 mm 0.4 μm Transwells® (Corning® Life Sciences) at a concentration of 100,000 cells per transwell. Cells were then kept in submerged culture using BEGM in both the apical and basolateral well chambers for 7 days or until confluent. Once confluent, cells were then changed to Pneumacult™ ALI Medium (StemCell™ Technologies) in the lower basolateral chamber only and the remaining apical media was aspirated. ALI media in the basolateral compartment was changed every other day and cells were differentiated at an ALI for 21 days.

Study design

BECs seeded into the initial T25 flasks were designated passage 0 (P0) and allowed to proliferate until cells were ~70-90% confluent at which point cells were passaged. One of the three flasks was then passaged into a transwell plate in order to establish P1 ALI cultures for experiments. Another P0 T25 flask was split into 3 additional T25 flasks (also P1) to carry forward into subsequent experiments. The remaining P0 T25 was either preserved in liquid nitrogen or also carried forward for separate studies. This paradigm was carried forward for each passage (P + 1) until reaching ALI cultures up through passage 5 (P5) to conduct experiments (Fig. 1).

RNA extraction and real-time PCR

Total RNA was isolated from BECs differentiated at an ALI. Three wells from each experimental condition were harvested and pooled to isolate RNA using the RNAqueous kit for total RNA purification from Ambion®-Applied Biosystems (Austin, TX). RNA concentration and quality was determined using a NanoDrop ND-1000 spectrophotometer Thermo Fisher Scientific). RNA samples (1 μg) were reverse-transcribed using the SuperScript® VILO cDNA Synthesis Kit (Life Technologies, Grand Island, NY). Samples were diluted up to a final volume of 100 μl (10 ng/μl). Quantitative real-time PCR was performed using validated TaqMan® probes (Life Technologies) for transforming growth factor beta (TGFβ)1 (Hs00998133_m1), TGFβ2 (Hs00234244_m1), activin A (Hs01081598_m1), follistatin-like-3 (FSTL3, Hs00610505_m1), mucin 5 AC (MUC5AC, Hs01365616_m1), thymic stromal lymphopoietin (TSLP, Hs00263639_m1), interleukin-33 (IL-33, Hs01125942_m1), C-X-C motif chemokine 10 (CXCL10, Hs00171042_m1), interferon induced with helicase C domain (1IFIH1, Hs00223420_m1), p63 (TP63, Hs00978340_m1), cytokeratin 5 (KRT5, Hs00361185_m1), beta-tubulin (TUBB4A, Hs00760066_s1), forkhead box J1 (FOXJ1, Hs00230964_m1), zona occluden-1 (TJP1, Hs01551861_m1), occludin (OCLN, Hs05465837_g1), and glyceraldehyde 3-phosphate dehydrogenase (GAPDH, Hs02758991_g1). Assays were performed using the TaqMan® Fast Advanced Master Mix reagents and accompanying protocol and the Applied Biosystems StepOnePlus™ Real-Time PCR System with StepOne Software v2.2.2 (Life Technologies). The primary quantitative PCR datasets used and/or analyzed for this study are provided as a (Additional file 1: Appendix I).

Statistical analysis

For clinical parameters, the paired t-test was used for comparisons that were normally distributed within each subject group. For non-normally distributed data, the Wilcoxon signed-rank test was used. For RT-PCR studies, the relative expression of genes were normalized using glyceraldehyde 3-phosphate dehydrogenase (GAPDH) as a non-regulated reference gene. Gene expression at P2-P5 is reported as fold change compared to the gene expression at P1. Analyses of RT-PCR results were performed using GenEx version 5.0.1 (MultiD Analyses AB, Göteborg, Sweden) based on methods described by Pfaffl [12]. Statistical significance was set at $P < 0.05$. One-way ANOVA (ordinary one-way ANOVA with Sidak's mutltiple comparisons test for normally distributed data; Kruskal-Wallis ANOVA with Dunn's multiple comparisons test for non-normally distributed data) was used to compare expression of genes at P2-P5 to expression at P1 using Prism® 6.0 software (GraphPad Software Inc., San Diego, CA). Two-way ANOVA was used to determine if gene

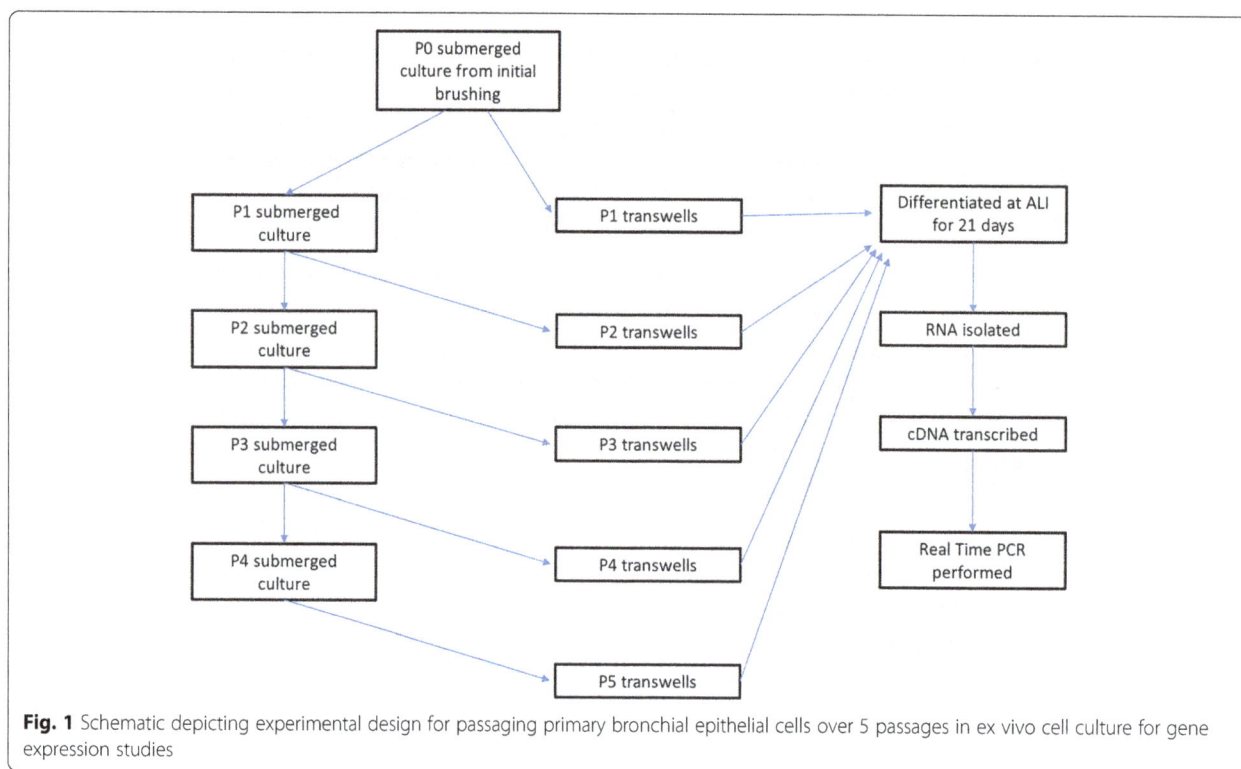

Fig. 1 Schematic depicting experimental design for passaging primary bronchial epithelial cells over 5 passages in ex vivo cell culture for gene expression studies

expression patterns over increasing cell passage were different between BECs from asthmatic and healthy subjects. Statistical analyses of clinical and lung function data were also performed using Prism®.

Results

Bronchial brushings were obtained from both asthmatic ($n = 6$) and healthy donors ($n = 6$) to generate ALI cultures used in this study. Clinical characteristics for each group are shown in Table 1. Asthmatic and healthy donors were similar in age (11.16 ± 3.7 years vs. 11.98 ± 5.1 years, respectively, $p = $ NS). There was a 2/3 male predominance with both groups (no difference between asthma vs. healthy). All asthmatic subjects displayed atopic features including eczema (50%), allergic rhinitis (83%), or positivity to aeroallergen by RAST IgE testing (83%). No history of eczema or allergic rhinitis was reported in the non-asthmatic group. One subject in the healthy group did display a positive RAST result. The majority of asthmatic subjects were using inhaled corticosteroids (83%) at

Table 1 Subject Characteristics

	Asthmatic Subjects $n = 6$	Healthy Subjects $n = 6$	p Value
Age yrs. (mean ± SD)	11.16 (3.7)	11.98 (5.1)	0.76
Sex (female/male)	4/6	4/6	
Currently using daily asthma controller (%)	5 (83%)	N/A	
History of atopy, n; (%)	6 (100%)	1 (17%)	< 0.01
Positive RAST, n; (%)	5 (83%)	1 (17%)	0.02
IgE IU/mL (median ± SD)	306.5 (387.32)	185.83 (403.47)	0.6
FVC % predicted (mean ± SD)	106.4 (13.1)	95.0 (13.9)	0.22
FEV$_1$/FVC Ratio (mean ± SD)	0.78 (0.03)	0.89 (0.07)	0.02
FEV$_1$% predicted (mean ± SD)	94.4 (14.1)	97.25 (13.9)	0.77
FEF$_{25-75}$% predicted (mean ± SD)	78.4 (4.9)	103.9 (5.5)	0.03
FE$_{NO}$ ppb (mean ± SD)	31.2 (24.2)	12.0 (5.1)	0.26

RAST Radioallergosorbent testing, *FVC* Forced vital capacity, *FEV$_1$* Forced expiratory volume in one second, *FEF$_{25-75}$* Forced expiratory flow between 25 and 75% of expiration

the time of enrollment. There was a non-significant trend toward higher FENO levels in asthmatic subjects compared to healthy subjects (31.2 ± 24.2 ppb vs. 12.0 ± 5.1 ppb, $p = 0.26$). Total serum IgE levels were not significantly different between asthmatic and healthy subjects (306.5 ± 387.32 IU/mL vs. 185.83 ± 403.47 IU/mL, $p = 0.6$). Measures of lung function by spirometry demonstrated no differences in FVC or FEV_1 between the groups; however, FEF_{25-75} ($78.4\% \pm 4.9\%$ vs $103.9\% \pm 5.5\%$, $p = 0.03$) and FEV_1/FVC ($0.78\% \pm 0.03\%$ vs. $103.9\% \pm 5.5\%$, $p = 0.02$) were significantly lower in the asthmatic group and consistent with airway obstruction.

Expression of genes associated with airway remodeling by differentiated primary BECs over successive passages (P1-P5) is depicted in Fig. 2. TGFβ1 expression was not significantly different from P1 through P3; however, expression was increased in P4 and P5 compared to P1 BECs from both asthmatic and healthy donors ($p < 0.05$, Fig. 2a), and there was not a difference in the pattern of expression with increasing passage between BECs from asthmatic and healthy subjects ($p = 0.9$). TGFβ2 expression was also not significantly different from P1 through P3, but similar to TGFβ1, expression was significantly increased in both P4 and P5 compared to P1 among both asthmatic and healthy subjects ($p < 0.05$, Fig. 2b), without significant differences in the pattern of gene expression by BECs from the two subject groups ($p = 0.08$). Expression of MUC5AC displayed marked variability beginning with P3, with the greatest variability observed at P4 and P5. However, given the high degree of variability, MUC5AC expression was not significantly different at P2-P5 compared to P1 ($p = 0.3$, Fig. 2c) by BECs, nor was there a difference in the pattern of gene expression by BECs from asthmatic and healthy donors ($p = 0.4$). Gene expression of both activin A and FSTL3 were orders of magnitude greater at P4 and P5 compared to expression at P1 ($p < 0.01$ and $p < 0.001$, respectively) for BECs from both asthmatic and healthy donors, without

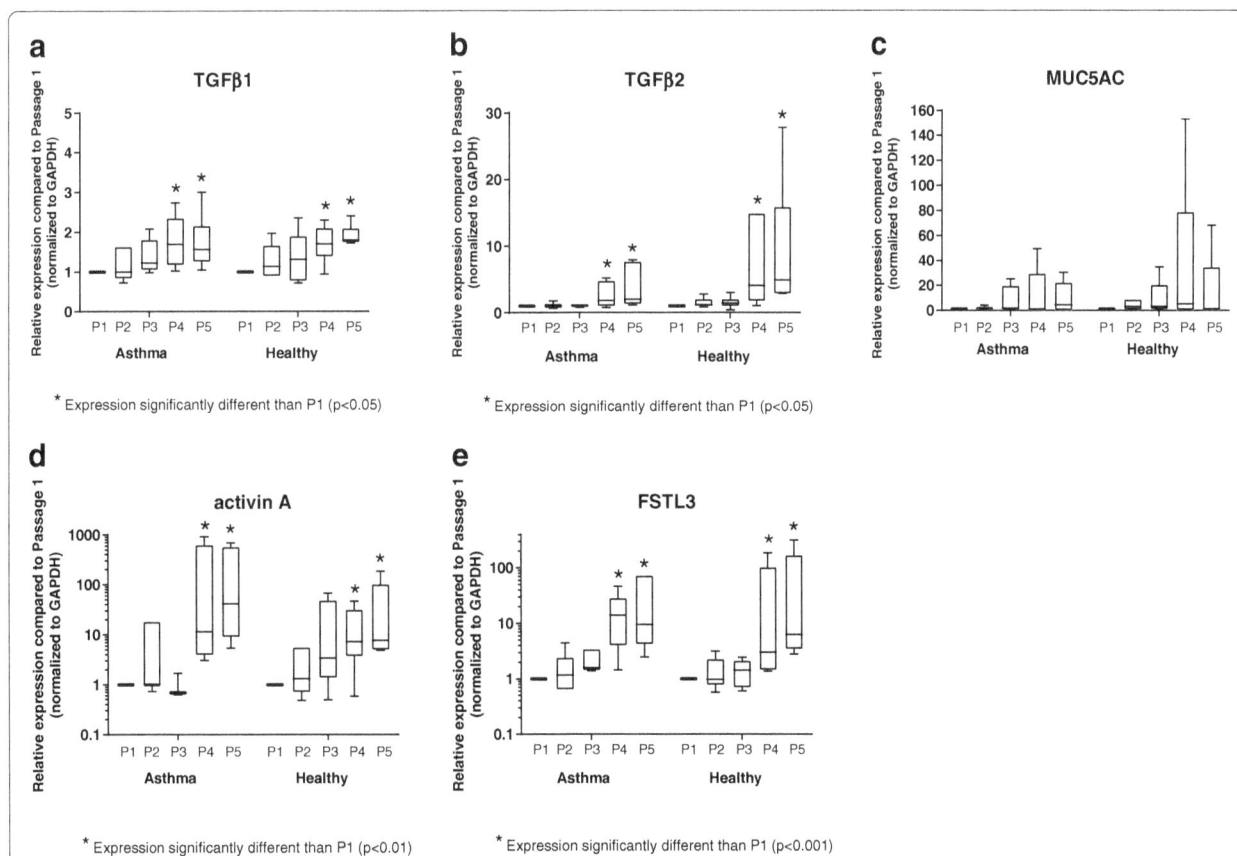

Fig. 2 Expression of genes related to airway remodeling by primary BECs. Expression of TGFβ1 (**a**), TGFβ2 (**b**), MUC5AC (**c**), activin A (**d**), and FSTL3 (**e**) by BECs at P1 ($n = 6$ asthma donors, $n = 6$ healthy donors), P2 ($n = 6$ asthma donors, $n = 6$ healthy donors), P3 ($n = 4$ asthma donors, $n = 6$ healthy donors), P4 ($n = 6$ asthma donors, $n = 6$ healthy donors), and P5 ($n = 6$ asthma donors, $n = 6$ healthy donors) are presented as box-and-whisker plots which depict the interquartile range and median (the ends of each box represent the upper and lower quartiles, error bars represent the maximum and minimum, and the horizontal line within the box represents the median). To compare expression of genes at P2-P5 to expression at P1, and to compare patterns of gene expression between asthmatic and healthy donors, ordinary two-way ANOVA with Dunnett's multiple comparisons test was used for normally distributed data, and Kruskal-Wallis ANOVA with Dunn's multiple comparisons test was used for non-normally distributed data

pattern differences between the two subject groups (activin A: $p = 0.08$; FSTL3: $p = 0.3$); however, expression for both were not significantly different at P2 or P3 compared to P1 (Fig. 2d and e). Although the study was not designed or powered to assess differences in the expression of specific genes between asthmatic and healthy BECs, at P1 expression of TGFβ2 and MUC5AC, normalized to GAPDH, were significantly greater by asthmatic as compared to healthy BECs (Additional file 2: Figure S2).

In addition to genes associated with airway remodeling, expression of several genes involved in innate immune response (IFIH1, CXCL10) and immunomodulation (TSLP, IL-33) were also analyzed over increasing passages by BECs. There was significant variability in CXCL10 expression by BECs from both asthmatic and healthy donors from P2-P4 compared to expression at P1, with significantly increased expression at P4 and P5 compared to P1 by asthmatic BECs and significantly increased expression at P5 by healthy BECs (Fig. 3a), however, there was not a difference in the overall pattern of CXCL10 expression with increasing cell passage between asthmatic and healthy donors ($p = 0.9$). Expression of IFIH1 was significantly elevated at P4 and P5 compared to expression at P1 for BECs from both asthmatic and healthy donors ($p < 0.05$, Fig. 3b), without pattern differences between the subject groups ($p = 0.4$), but was not significantly different at P2 or P3. In contrast, Expression of IL-33 was significantly decreased at P4 and P5 compared to P1 by BECs from both asthmatic and healthy donors ($p < 0.01$; Fig. 3c); however, expression of IL-33 at P2 and P3 were not significantly different compared to P1, and there were no significant differences in IL-33 gene expression patterns with increasing cell passage between BECs from asthmatic and healthy donors ($p = 0.4$). Gene expression of TSLP remained stable throughout all 5 successive passages and was not significantly different compared to P1 by BECs from both asthmatic and health donors (Fig. 3d). Of note, at P1 expression of TSLP, normalized to GAPDH, was significantly greater by asthmatic as compared to healthy BECs (Additional file 2: Figure S2).

To assess the stability of expression of airway epithelial differentiation-associated genes and markers of epithelial basal cells over serial BEC passages, we measured the expression of the basal cell-associated gene TP63, the epithelial marker cytokeratin 5 (KRT5), ciliogenesis-associated genes TUBB4A and FOXJ1, and genes coding for the tight junctional proteins zona occluden-1 (TJP1) and occludin (OCLN). Expression of all of these genes was stable through at least P3 (Fig. 4). Expression of TP63 and KRT5 at passages 4 and 5 were not significantly different from expression at P1 by BECs from both asthmatic and healthy donors, but was more variable between individual cell lines at later passages (Fig. 4a, b). Among BECs from both asthmatic and healthy subjects expression of TJP1 was

significantly greater at P4 and P5 as compared to P1 ($p < 0.01$; Fig. 4d), expression of TUBB4A and OCLN were significantly greater at P5 as compared to P1 ($p = 0.05$; Fig. 4c, e), and there were not significant differences in the overall patterns of expression of these genes with increasing cell passage between the asthmatic and healthy subject groups (TJP1: $p = 0.5$; TUBB4A: $p = 0.6$; OCLN: $p = 0.8$). In contrast to the other studied genes associated with epithelial differentiation, expression of FOXJ1 decreased in later passage ALI cultures, and expression was significantly lower at P4 and P5 compared to expression at P1 by BECs from both asthmatic and healthy BECs ($p < 0.01$; Fig. 4f), without pattern differences between the subject groups ($p = 0.2$). Although the study was not powered to assess differences in the expression of specific differentiation-associated genes or markers of epithelial basal cells between asthmatic and healthy BECs, no significant differences were observed at P1 (Additional file 2: Figure S2).

In order to assure that differences in gene expression patterns were not related to differential expression of housekeeping genes over multiple passages we compared the expression of GAPDH by BECs across the five passages and found no differences in mRNA Ct values (Additional file 3: Figure S1). We also assessed mRNA expression for each of the genes studied prior to normalization by GAPDH to show the natural variation in mRNA levels across asthmatic and healthy donors. For TGFβ1, TGFβ2, MUC5AC, FSTL3, and activin A, mRNA Ct values were significantly lower (greater un-normalized gene expression) at P4 and P5 compared to P1 ($p < 0.05$; Additional file 4: Figure S3) by BECs from both asthmatic and healthy donors, and there were not significant pattern differences in mRNA Ct values between the two subject groups with increasing cell passage for TGFβ1 ($p = 0.4$), FSTL3 ($p = 0.4$), and activin A ($p = 0.6$). However, mRNA Ct values were significantly lower (greater gene expression prior to normalization) by BECs from asthmatic as compared to healthy donors for TGFβ2 ($p = 0.004$) and MUC5AC ($p = 0.04$). Un-normalized mRNA Ct values for CXCL10 and IFIH1 were significantly lower at P4 and P5 compared to P1 among asthmatic and healthy BECs ($p < 0.05$; Additional file 5: Figure S4), whereas IL-33 mRNA Ct values were significant higher at P4 and P5 compared to P1 among asthmatic and healthy BECs ($p < 0.05$). For TP63 and KRT5, there were no significant differences in mRNA Ct values among or between asthmatic and healthy BECs with increasing cell passage (Additional file 6: Figure S5), whereas mRNA Ct values were significantly lower at P4 and P5 compared to P1 for asthmatic and healthy BECs for TUBB4A ($p = 0.03$), TPJ1 ($p < 0.01$), and OCLN ($p < 0.05$) without pattern differences between asthmatic and healthy BECs. Finally, FOXJ1 mRNA Ct values were significantly higher at P4 and P5 compared to P1 for asthmatic and healthy BECs, with a similar pattern between asthmatic and healthy BECs.

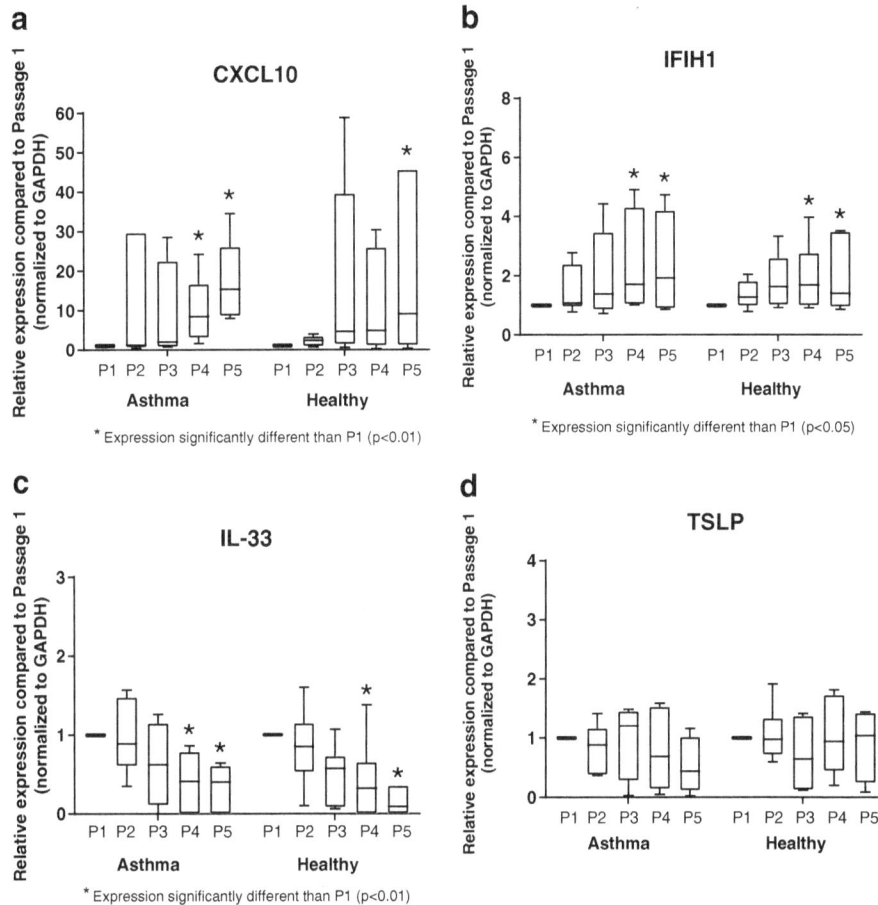

Fig. 3 Expression of innate immunity and immunomodulatory genes by primary BECs. Expression of CXCL10 (**a**), IFIH1 (**b**), IL-33 (**c**), and TSLP (**d**) by BECs at P1 ($n = 6$ asthma donors, $n = 6$ healthy donors), P2 ($n = 6$ asthma donors, $n = 6$ healthy donors), P3 ($n = 4$ asthma donors, $n = 6$ healthy donors), P4 ($n = 6$ asthma donors, $n = 6$ healthy donors), and P5 ($n = 6$ asthma donors, $n = 6$ healthy donors) are presented as box-and-whisker plots which depict the interquartile range and median (the ends of each box represent the upper and lower quartiles, error bars represent the maximum and minimum, and the horizontal line within the box represents the median). To compare expression of genes at P2-P5 to expression at P1, and to compare patterns of gene expression between asthmatic and healthy donors, ordinary two-way ANOVA with Dunnett's multiple comparisons test was used for normally distributed data, and Kruskal-Wallis ANOVA with Dunn's multiple comparisons test was used for non-normally distributed data

Discussion

In the present study, we have demonstrated that primary differentiated BECs obtained from children with or without atopic asthma maintain stable expression of a panel of genes related to airway remodeling, innate immunity, immunomodulation, epithelial differentiation, and epithelial basal cells through passage 3 in ex vivo ALI cell cultures. We further report that in primary BECs beyond passage 3 expression of the studied genes became significantly more variable with expression of most genes increasing (TGFβ1, TGFβ2, activin A, FSTL3, MUC5AC, CXCL10, IFIH1, TUBB4A, TJP1, OCLN) and expression of other genes decreasing (IL-33, FOXJ1). Some genes were also found to be stable throughout the five passages studied (TSLP, TP63, KRT5). While the assumption that primary BECs retain their original phenotype

up to passage 3 has been reported previously [4], those observations were based on a review of the available literature. In the present study, we present for the first time a study designed to compare the stability of gene expression of multiple airway remodeling, innate immunity, immunomodulation, epithelial differentiation, and epithelial basal cells genes by BECs over successive passages. Our findings further support the use of primary BECs obtained from pediatric donors at passage ≤3.

Primary ex vivo cell cultures of BECs obtained by bronchial brushings have been used successfully in children and adults for more than a decade and have become an attractive model to study the airway epithelium in various diseases. This is especially true in the pediatric population where obtaining cells via airway biopsies is problematic given that performing a sedated bronchoscopy in a pediatric subject

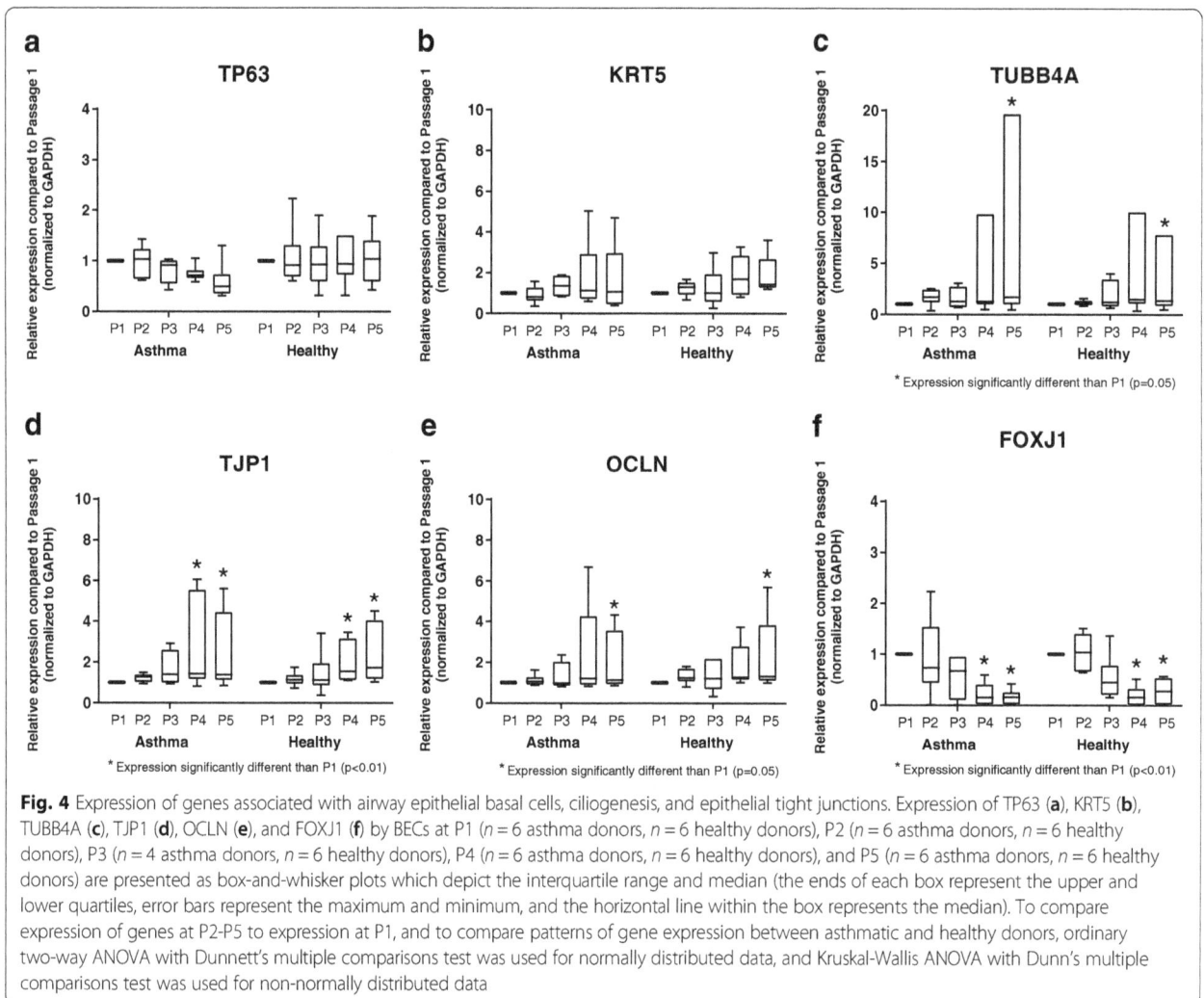

Fig. 4 Expression of genes associated with airway epithelial basal cells, ciliogenesis, and epithelial tight junctions. Expression of TP63 (**a**), KRT5 (**b**), TUBB4A (**c**), TJP1 (**d**), OCLN (**e**), and FOXJ1 (**f**) by BECs at P1 ($n = 6$ asthma donors, $n = 6$ healthy donors), P2 ($n = 6$ asthma donors, $n = 6$ healthy donors), P3 ($n = 4$ asthma donors, $n = 6$ healthy donors), P4 ($n = 6$ asthma donors, $n = 6$ healthy donors), and P5 ($n = 6$ asthma donors, $n = 6$ healthy donors) are presented as box-and-whisker plots which depict the interquartile range and median (the ends of each box represent the upper and lower quartiles, error bars represent the maximum and minimum, and the horizontal line within the box represents the median). To compare expression of genes at P2-P5 to expression at P1, and to compare patterns of gene expression between asthmatic and healthy donors, ordinary two-way ANOVA with Dunnett's multiple comparisons test was used for normally distributed data, and Kruskal-Wallis ANOVA with Dunn's multiple comparisons test was used for non-normally distributed data

for research purposes is ethically challenging. The initial description of the procedure to obtain primary BECs for research purposes from children already under anesthesia for a clinical indication was published by Doherty et al. in 2003 [7]. In that study, the authors compared the yield and viability of cells obtained via non-bronchoscopic airway brushings through an endotracheal tube under general anesthesia in 63 pediatric subjects to brushings obtained from a control population of adult patients undergoing bronchoscopy. Doherty and colleagues reported that a similar number of cells were obtained via the blind bronchial brushing as compared to the brushings obtained during bronchoscopy. Furthermore, the success rate of cell cultures obtained using this methodology was reported to be 82% despite a trend to lower viability of the cells obtained via the blind bronchial brushings, suggesting that this method harvested a sufficient amount of viable basal cells to establish the cell cultures [7]. Importantly, no adverse events where reported following the bronchial brushings and the authors concluded that this method of harvesting primary BECs in

children was both effective and safe. In a separate study, Lane and colleagues reported similar results in a cohort of children with and without mild asthma [8]. In that study, the authors included an additional control group of children who did not undergo bronchial brushings and compared post-operative symptoms between the groups. No significant risk of adverse symptoms was reported with the most frequent symptom reported being a mild cough in less than half of the participants that underwent the bronchial brushings. Similar to the results reported by Doherty et al., Lane and colleagues found that the non-bronchoscopic brushings provided sufficient cells to carry out studies of RNA and protein-based assays, but also contained a sufficient population of basal cells to propagate in ex vivo cell cultures over multiple cell passages. Importantly, the subjects with mild asthma displayed no greater risk of adverse outcomes compared to the healthy control subjects further demonstrating the usefulness of this model in studying the role of BECs in pediatric asthma.

Optimal growth conditions for primary BECs have been extensively studied and have been reported elsewhere in the literature (reviewed by Gruenert et al. [13]). Most protocols utilize a defined, serum-free media that has been optimized to exclude contaminating cells such as fibroblasts. In addition to factors related to the growth media, the phenotype of the BECs grown in cell culture is critically dependent on the culture conditions. For example, cells can either be grown as a confluent monolayer in submerged cell culture or grown in a semi-permeable transwell insert at an air-liquid interface [13]. Cells grown at an ALI differentiate into a mucociliary phenotype that more closely resembles the native human airway epithelium than submerged cultures [14]. Recent studies have emphasized differences in epithelial responses during stimulation experiments based on whether a submerged vs. differentiated ALI culture model was used. For example, Kikuchi and colleagues compared the responses of BECs grown at an ALI to submerged BECs cultures. Following stimulation with IL-4 or IL-13 no differences in STAT6 phosphorylation were observed between BECs grown in submerged culture or at an ALI [15]. Conversely, the downstream effects of GM-CSF and TGFβ2 secretion in these models were found to be markedly different leading the authors to conclude that responses to IL-4 or IL-13 are critically dependent on the cell culture model system utilized in the study. In a separate series of experiments reported by Pezzulo et al., the authors examined the gene expression profile of primary BECs grown in either submerged conditions or differentiated at an ALI and compared their findings to both the in vivo condition as well as to a BEC cell line using genome-wide transcriptional profiling [16]. The authors of that study demonstrated that BECs differentiated at an ALI not only displayed morphological characteristics most similar to the in vivo condition (goblet cells, the presence of cilia, etc.), but also most closely recapitulated the transcriptional profile of the native airway epithelium. Thus, the authors concluded that the primary BECs differentiated at an ALI most closely represented the biology of the airway epithelium.

While primary BECs obtained via bronchial brushes or bronchoscopic biopsy differentiated at an ALI most closely resemble the in vivo airway epithelium, there are several caveats that must also be taken into account that may limit their utility in some experimental models. Given that primary BECs are derived from individual human donors there is a significant degree of variability between BECs from different donors. Furthermore, the findings in the present study would also suggest that cell passage number also contributes to increased phenotypic variability. The need to utilize greater replicates during experiments significantly increases the timeline and expense and may make primary cells less attractive for high-throughput screening studies. With this in mind,

other studies have compared primary BECs differentiated at an ALI to existing transformed or immortalized cell lines. In one such study, Stewart and colleagues compared two different donor-derived primary BECs with three different available bronchial cell lines. In that study, the primary BECs expressed several markers of BEC differentiation and developed measurable trans-epithelial electrical resistance (TEER), albeit with intra-donor and intra-experimental variability [5]. Measurements of TEER were more consistent in Calu-3 cells; however, these cells also displayed distinct disparities in their expression of several markers of epithelial differentiation when compared to the primary BECs. Another cell line examined in that study (BEAS-2B) failed to differentiate at an ALI. These findings underscore the importance of choosing an appropriate model system for a given experimental question. Details regarding characteristics of available transformed cell lines have been reviewed elsewhere by Papazian et al. [17].

In this study we assessed over serial cell passages in ALI cultures the stability of expression of genes associated with airway epithelial basal cells and structural features unique to differentiated airway epithelium. Interestingly, expression of the airway epithelial basal cell associated gene p63 [18, 19] and epithelial marker cytokeratin 5 [20] were overall stable in ALI cultures over 5 consecutive cell passages, although there was a non-significant modest trend toward decreased and more variable p63 expression at P5 and increased variability of cytokeratin 5 expression at P4 and P5. Expression of the cillogenesis-associated genes TUBB4A and FOXJ1 [21, 22] as well as the tight junctional-associated genes TJP1 and OCLN [23] were stable through P3, however, expression of both of these genes become significantly more variable at passages beyond P3. In summary, similar to our observations for the remodeling-associated genes, innate immune response genes, and immunomodulatory genes studied, expression of several genes associated with airway epithelial differentiation were stable through P3, however, for later passages became significantly more variable.

The present study design includes several important strengths, including the use of primary BECs obtained from asthmatic and non-asthmatic children that are differentiated at an ALI. Additionally, our cohort is carefully phenotyped based on medical history and clinical features such as lung function and allergy testing. Despite these strengths our study also has several inherent limitations. In this study, our main outcome is the stability of gene expression over 5 successive passages in cell culture. We included cells obtained from both asthmatic and healthy donors in order to ensure that stability of gene expression was generalizable to both groups. Indeed, we have demonstrated that BECs obtained from both asthmatic and non-asthmatic donors similarly display stable gene expression through passage 3. Variability in gene expression beyond passage 3 was also observed in BECs derived from asthmatic and healthy donors to a similar degree. Although we did not observe statistically significant differences in the stability and variability of gene expression between BECs from asthmatic and healthy donors, our sample size was insufficient to detect subtle differences in patterns of gene expression with increasing passage between BECs from asthmatic and healthy children. Furthermore, this study is also underpowered to perform subgroup analysis of the data such as gender differences. Lung function data demonstrates that our cohort of asthmatic donors have a mild degree of airflow limitation signifying a relatively mild asthma phenotype in our cohort.

Additional limitations of our study include that we did not perform TEER measurements over serial passages and did not perform histological sections and/or immunostaining of our ALI cultures for basal cell markers or proteins associated with airway epithelial cell differentiation. Although beyond the scope of the current study, such outcome measures would be of interest in future studies of primary airway epithelial cells over serial culture passages. We did however study the expression stability of genes associated with airway epithelial basal cells, ciliogenesis, and epithelial tight junctions. Expression of the basal cell-associated gene TP63 as well as cytokeratin 5 were stable through P5, whereas expression of genes associated with ciliogenesis and tight junctions were less stable beyond P3. Of note, several groups have demonstrated over the past several years that airway epithelial basal cells can be expanded in culture and retain their ability to differentiate at the ALI many passages removed from the host [21, 24]. A final limitation of our study is that we did not analyze airway epithelial gene expression across serial passages from submerged undifferentiated cultures.

Conclusions

While ex vivo primary BECs differentiated at an ALI represent one of the best available models to study the role of the airway epithelium in disease processes such as asthma in children, care must be taken to ensure that cell phenotype and gene expression patterns are preserved such that ex vivo studies reflect the in vivo condition as closely as possible. We have provided new evidence that primary BECs from children differentiated at an ALI display stable gene expression patterns over 3 successive passages; however, we have also shown that gene expression becomes significantly more variable at later passages, which could potentially affect study outcomes if later passages are used in experiments. These findings should be carefully considered in future study designs using primary BECs in ex vivo model systems.

Additional files

Additional file 1 Primary quantitative PCR datasets. (XLSX 37 kb)

Additional file 2: Figure S2. Comparison of gene expression between asthmatic and healthy BECs at passage 1 (P1). Expression of genes related to airway remodeling (panel A.; TGFβ1, TGFβ2, MUC5AC, activin A, and FSTL3), innate immunity and immunomodulatory genes (panel B.; CXCL10, IFIH1, IL-33, and TSLP), and expression of genes associated with airway epithelial basal cells, ciliogenesis, and epithelial tight junctions (panel C.; TP63, KRT5, TUBB4A, TJP1, OCLN, and FOXJ1) by primary asthmatic (grey plots) and healthy (white plots) BECs at P1 (n = 6 asthma donors, n = 6 healthy donors). Expression of each gene (normalized to GAPDH) relative to the median of healthy BECs are presented as box-and-whisker plots which depict the interquartile range and median (the ends of each box represent the upper and lower quartiles, error bars represent the maximum and minimum, and the horizontal line within the box represents the median). The Wilcoxon signed rank test was used to test differences in expression of specific genes between asthmatic and healthy BECs. (EMF 109 kb)

Additional file 3: Figure S1. Expression of GAPDH as a reference gene. Ct values for GAPDH were compared for each cell passage. No significant differences were observed from P1 through P5. (TIF 73 kb)

Additional file 4: Figure S3. Un-normalized mRNA expression of genes related to airway remodeling by primary BECs. Un-normalized mRNA Ct values for TGFβ1 (A.), TGFβ2 (B.), MUC5AC (C.), activin A (D.), and FSTL3 (E.) by BECs at P1 (n = 6 asthma donors, n = 6 healthy donors), P2 (n = 6 asthma donors, n = 6 healthy donors), P3 (n = 4 asthma donors, n = 6 healthy donors), P4 (n = 6 asthma donors, n = 6 healthy donors), and P5 (n = 6 asthma donors, n = 6 healthy donors) are presented as individual data points for each donor cell line. To compare expression of genes at P2-P5 to expression at P1, and to compare patterns of gene expression between asthmatic and healthy donors, ordinary two-way ANOVA with Dunnett's multiple comparisons test was used for normally distributed data, and Kruskal-Wallis ANOVA with Dunn's multiple comparisons test was used for non-normally distributed data. (EMF 195 kb)

Additional file 5: Figure S4. Un-normalized mRNA expression of innate immunity and immunomodulatory genes by primary BECs. Un-normalized mRNA Ct values for CXCL10 (A.), IFIH1 (B.), IL-33 (C.), and TSLP (D.) by BECs at P1 (n = 6 asthma donors, n = 6 healthy donors), P2 (n = 6 asthma donors, n = 6 healthy donors), P3 (n = 4 asthma donors, n = 6 healthy donors), P4 (n = 6 asthma donors, n = 6 healthy donors), and P5 (n = 6 asthma donors, n = 6 healthy donors) are presented as individual data points for each donor cell line. To compare expression of genes at P2-P5 to expression at P1, and to compare patterns of gene expression between asthmatic and healthy donors, ordinary two-way ANOVA with Dunnett's multiple comparisons test was used for normally distributed data, and Kruskal-Wallis ANOVA with Dunn's multiple comparisons test was used for non-normally distributed data. (EMF 155 kb)

Additional file 6: Figure S5. Un-normalized mRNA expression of genes associated with airway epithelial basal cells, ciliogenesis, and epithelial tight junctions by primary BECs. Un-normalized mRNA Ct values for TP63 (A.), KRT5 (B.), TUBB4A (C.), TPJ1 (D.), FOXJ1 (E.), and OCLN (F.) by BECs at P1 (n = 6 asthma donors, n = 6 healthy donors), P2 (n = 6 asthma donors, n = 6 healthy donors), P3 (n = 4 asthma donors, n = 6 healthy donors), P4 (n = 6 asthma donors, n = 6 healthy donors), and P5 (n = 6 asthma donors, n = 6 healthy donors) are presented as individual data points for each donor cell line. To compare expression of genes at P2-P5 to expression at P1, and to compare patterns of gene expression between asthmatic and healthy donors, ordinary two-way ANOVA with Dunnett's multiple comparisons test was used for normally distributed data, and Kruskal-Wallis ANOVA with Dunn's multiple comparisons test was used for non-normally distributed data. (EMF 224 kb)

Abbreviations

ALI: Air-liquid interface; BDR: Bronchodilator responsive; BEC: Bronchial epithelial cell; BEGM: Bronchial epithelial growth medium; FEF$_{25-75}$: Forced expiratory flow between 25 and 75% of FVC; FENO: Fraction of exhaled nitric oxide; FEV1: Forced expiratory volume in 1 s; FVC: Forced vital capacity; GAPDH: Glyceraldehyde 3-phosphate dehydrogenase; ICS: Inhaled corticosteroid; IgE: Immunoglobulin E; RAST: Radioallergosorbent testing; RNA: Ribonucleic acid

Funding

National Heart, Lung, and Blood Institute (JD: R01HL128361, SR: K08HL135266), National Institute of Allergy and Infectious Diseases (JD: U19 AI125378), Parker B. Francis Foundation Fellowship (SR).

Authors' contributions

Conception and Design: SR, JD, KB; Conducted Experiments: KB, MW, MN, LR; Drafted the Manuscript, Critical Revision: KB, SR, MW, MN, JD; All authors have read and approved the manuscript.

Competing interests

The authors declare that they have no competing interests, financial or non-financial.

References

1. The global asthma report 2014. Auckland: Global Asthma Network; 2014. www.globalasthmanetwork.org.
2. Holgate ST. The sentinel role of the airway epithelium in asthma pathogenesis. Immunol Rev. 2011;242:205–19.
3. Holtzman MJ, Byers DE, Alexander-Brett J, Wang X. The role of airway epithelial cells and innate immune cells in chronic respiratory disease. Nat Rev Immunol. 2014;14:686–98.
4. McLellan K, Shields M, Power U, Turner S. Primary airway epithelial cell culture and asthma in children-lessons learnt and yet to come. Pediatr Pulmonol. 2015;50:1393–405.
5. Stewart CE, Torr EE, Mohd Jamili NH, Bosquillon C, Sayers I. Evaluation of differentiated human bronchial epithelial cell culture systems for asthma research. J Allergy (Cairo). 2012;2012:943982.
6. Lotvall J, Akdis CA, Bacharier LB, Bjermer L, Casale TB, Custovic A, Lemanske RF Jr, Wardlaw AJ, Wenzel SE, Greenberger PA. Asthma endotypes: a new approach to classification of disease entities within the asthma syndrome. J Allergy Clin Immunol. 2011;127:355–60.
7. Doherty GM, Christie SN, Skibinski G, Puddicombe SM, Warke TJ, de Courcey F, Cross AL, Lyons JD, Ennis M, Shields MD, Heaney LG. Non-bronchoscopic sampling and culture of bronchial epithelial cells in children. Clin Exp Allergy. 2003;33:1221–5.
8. Lane C, Burgess S, Kicic A, Knight D, Stick S. The use of non-bronchoscopic brushings to study the paediatric airway. Respir Res. 2005;6:53.
9. Pierrou S, Broberg P, O'Donnell RA, Pawlowski K, Virtala R, Lindqvist E, Richter A, Wilson SJ, Angco G, Moller S, et al. Expression of genes involved in oxidative stress responses in airway epithelial cells of smokers with chronic obstructive pulmonary disease. Am J Respir Crit Care Med. 2007;175:577–86.
10. Gras D, Petit A, Charriot J, Knabe L, Alagha K, Gamez AS, Garulli C, Bourdin A, Chanez P, Molinari N, Vachier I. Epithelial ciliated beating cells essential for ex vivo ALI culture growth. BMC Pulm Med. 2017;17:80.
11. Dweik RA, Boggs PB, Erzurum SC, Irvin CG, Leigh MW, Lundberg JO, Olin AC, Plummer AL, Taylor DR, American Thoracic Society Committee on Interpretation of Exhaled Nitric Oxide Levels for Clinical A. An official ATS clinical practice guideline: interpretation of exhaled nitric oxide levels (FENO) for clinical applications. Am J Respir Crit Care Med. 2011;184:602–15.
12. Pfaffl MW. A new mathematical model for relative quantification in real-time RT-PCR. Nucleic Acids Res. 2001;29:e45.
13. Gruenert DC, Finkbeiner WE, Widdicombe JH. Culture and transformation of human airway epithelial cells. Am J Phys. 1995;268:L347–60.
14. Karp PH, Moninger TO, Weber SP, Nesselhauf TS, Launspach JL, Zabner J, Welsh MJ. An in vitro model of differentiated human airway epithelia. Methods for establishing primary cultures. Methods Mol Biol. 2002;188:115–37.
15. Kikuchi T, Shively JD, Foley JS, Drazen JM, Tschumperlin DJ. Differentiation-dependent responsiveness of bronchial epithelial cells to IL-4/13 stimulation. Am J Physiol Lung Cell Mol Physiol. 2004;287:L119–26.
16. Pezzulo AA, Starner TD, Scheetz TE, Traver GL, Tilley AE, Harvey BG, Crystal RG, McCray PB Jr, Zabner J. The air-liquid interface and use of primary cell cultures are important to recapitulate the transcriptional profile of in vivo airway epithelia. Am J Physiol Lung Cell Mol Physiol. 2011;300:L25–31.
17. Papazian D, Wurtzen PA, Hansen SW. Polarized airway epithelial models for immunological co-culture studies. Int Arch Allergy Immunol. 2016;170:1–21.
18. Hackett TL, Singhera GK, Shaheen F, Hayden P, Jackson GR, Hegele RG, Van Eeden S, Bai TR, Dorscheid DR, Knight DA. Intrinsic phenotypic differences of asthmatic epithelium and its inflammatory responses to respiratory syncytial virus and air pollution. Am J Respir Cell Mol Biol. 2011;45:1090-1100.
19. Warner SM, Hackett TL, Shaheen F, Hallstrand TS, Kicic A, Stick SM, Knight DA. Transcription factor p63 regulates key genes and wound repair in human airway epithelial basal cells. Am J Respir Cell Mol Biol. 2013;49:978-988.
20. Hackett TL, Shaheen F, Johnson A, Wadsworth S, Pechkovsky DV, Jacoby DB, Kicic A, Stick SM, Knight DA. Characterization of side population cells from human airway epithelium. Stem Cells. 2008;26:2576-2585.
21. Walters MS, Gomi K, Ashbridge B, Moore MA, Arbelaez V, Heldrich J, Ding BS, Rafii S, Staudt MR, Crystal RG. Generation of a human airway epithelium derived basal cell line with multipotent differentiation capacity. Respir Res. 2013;14:135.
22. LeSimple P, van Seuningen I, Buisine MP, Copin MC, Hinz M, Hoffmann W, Hajj R, Brody SL, Coraux C, Puchelle E. Trefoil factor family 3 peptide promotes human airway epithelial ciliated cell differentiation. Am J Respir Cell Mol Biol. 2007;36:296-303.
23. Coyne CB, Vanhook MK, Gambling TM, Carson JL, Boucher RC, Johnson LG. Regulation of airway tight junctions by proinflammatory cytokines. Mol Biol Cell. 2002;13:3218-3234.
24. Butler CR, Hynds RE, Gowers KH, Lee Ddo H, Brown JM, Crowley C, Teixeira VH, Smith CM, Urbani L, Hamilton NJ, et al. Rapid Expansion of Human Epithelial Stem Cells Suitable for Airway Tissue Engineering. Am J Respir Crit Care Med. 2016;194:156-168.

17

The features of AECOPD with carbon dioxide retention

Xia Wei[1,2], Nan Yu[3], Qi Ding[2], Jingting Ren[2], Jiuyun Mi[2], Lu Bai[1], Jianying Li[4], Min Qi[5] and Youmin Guo[1*]

Abstract

Background: Chronic obstructive pulmonary disease (COPD) with carbon dioxide retention is associated with a worsening clinical condition and the beginning of pulmonary ventilation decompensation. This study aimed to identify the factors associated with carbon dioxide retention.

Methods: This was a retrospective study of consecutive patients with COPD (meeting the Global Initiative for Chronic Obstructive Lung Disease diagnostic criteria) hospitalized at The Ninth Hospital of Xi'an Affiliated Hospital of Xi'an Jiaotong University between October 2014 and September 2017. The baseline demographic, clinical, laboratory, pulmonary function, and imaging data were compared between the 86 cases with carbon dioxide retention and the 144 cases without carbon dioxide retention.

Results: Compared with the non-carbon dioxide retention group, the group with carbon dioxide retention had a higher number of hospitalizations in the previous 12 months ($p = 0.013$), higher modified Medical Research Council (mMRC) dyspnea scores ($p = 0.034$), lower arterial oxygen pressure ($p = 0.018$), worse pulmonary function (forced expiratory volume in one second/forced vital capacity [FEV_1/FVC; $p < 0.001$], FEV_1%pred [$p < 0.001$], Z5%pred [$p = 0.004$], R5%pred [$p = 0.008$], R5-R20 [$p = 0.009$], X5 [$p = 0.022$], and Ax [$p = 0.011$]), more severe lung damage (such as increased lung volume [$p = 0.011$], more emphysema range [$p = 0.007$], and lower mean lung density [$p = 0.043$]). $FEV_1 < 1$ L (odds ratio [OR] = 4.011, 95% confidence interval [CI]: 2.216–7.262) and emphysema index (EI) > 20% (OR = 1.926, 95% CI: 1.080–3.432) were independently associated with carbon dioxide retention in COPD.

Conclusion: Compared with the non-carbon dioxide retention group, the group with carbon dioxide retention had different clinical, pulmonary function, and imaging features. $FEV_1 < 1$ L and EI > 20% were independently associated with carbon dioxide retention in AECOPD.

Keywords: Acute exacerbation, Chronic obstructive pulmonary disease, Pulmonary function test, Emphysema index, Carbon dioxide retention

Background

Chronic obstructive pulmonary disease (COPD) is the fourth leading cause of death worldwide and is expected to be the third leading cause of death by 2020 [1]. COPD is also a major chronic disease that produces a large economic and social burden worldwide [2]. In China, COPD is a major contributor to the overall morbidity and mortality burden owing to the relatively high prevalence of smoking and rising environmental pollution [3, 4]. There are limited treatments available for the effective prevention of COPD progression. Respiratory failure secondary to AECOPD can lead to disease progression. Therefore, distinguishing patients with a risk of carbon dioxide retention is of clinical importance in the management of acute exacerbation of chronic obstructive pulmonary disease (AECOPD).

Since COPD is a heterogeneous disease, it is difficult for a single indicator to reflect all features of the disease. Pulmonary function indicators, especially FEV_1 (forced expiratory volume in 1 s), are recognized as important

* Correspondence: guoyoumin163@sina.com
[1]Department of Radiology, Xi'an Jiaotong University Medical College First Affiliated Hospital, Xi'an, China
Full list of author information is available at the end of the article

because they can reflect one of the key characteristics of COPD - airflow limitation, but according to the Global Initiative for Chronic Obstructive Lung Disease (GOLD) update in 2017 [5], FEV_1 was used for grading of disease severity but was not a variable used to guide treatment. Other well accepted indicators include 64-detector computed tomography (CT) parameters such as bronchial wall thickness and emphysema index (EI), which reflect COPD pathological changes [6, 7], airway wall thickening, and airway remodeling response. Emphysema index refers to the proportion of low-density areas less than – 950 HU occupying the lung volume. An increase in the emphysema index reflects an increase in the extent of parenchymal destruction of the lungs. Yamasawa [8] reported that CT could be used as a non-invasive tool to predict aerobic capacity in COPD.

Another indicator that holds promise for assessing the severity of COPD is carbon dioxide retention. Carbon dioxide retention indicates the exhaustion of lung reserve, loss of ventilatory function, worsening of clinical symptoms, respiratory failure, and secondary damage. But actually we don't know the complete long term consequences of hypercapnia [9]. Tsuboi [10] reported that persistent carbon dioxide retention in chronic ventilatory deficient subjects may reflect an adaptive mechanism that allows for lower levels of alveolar ventilation so as not to overload the respiratory muscles. In summary, carbon dioxide retention is involved in the respiratory center drive capacity, respiratory muscle strength, airway obstruction, pulmonary parenchymal damage, and many other complex processes. The gold standard for carbon dioxide retention is arterial blood gas analysis, but arterial blood gas analysis only reflects the instantaneous partial pressure of carbon dioxide in the blood. Therefore, checking blood gas at different times will produce different results, and the overall extent of COPD disease leading to carbon dioxide retention (or even respiratory failure) cannot be determined accurately. Accurate prediction of COPD carbon dioxide retention from pathological changes level would be of great help in disease monitoring.

What is the relationship between carbon dioxide retention and pulmonary function and imaging parameters? To date, this relationship has not been clear. For this study, we were interested in the ability to predict and estimate carbon dioxide retention using pulmonary function parameters and imaging parameters. Therefore, the aims of the present study were: 1) to compare the differences in clinical symptom scores, inflammatory markers, pulmonary function indicators, and CT parameters between patients with carbon dioxide retention in COPD vs those without carbon dioxide retention; and 2) to identify the factors associated with carbon dioxide retention in AECOPD.

Methods

Study design and subjects

This study was a retrospective study of consecutive AECOPD patients admitted to the Department of Respiratory Medicine of The Ninth Hospital of Xi'an Affiliated Hospital of Xi'an Jiaotong University from October 2014 to September 2017, meeting the GOLD diagnostic criteria (FEV_1 / FVC < 70% bronchodilators inhaled). AECOPD refers to patients who have COPD symptoms (cough, sputum, shortness of breath, etc.) exacerbating the need for hospitalization. These patients are typically treated with a short acting bronchodilator, antibiotics, and / or a glucocorticoid. Exclusion criteria were as follows: 1) < 40 years of age; 2) pregnant women; 3) lung diseases such as lung cancer, pneumonia, active tuberculosis, pulmonary embolism, or interstitial lung disease; 4) previous pulmonary surgery; 5) unable to complete the pulmonary function test; 6) asthma, severe heart, liver, or kidney dysfunction; 7) CT images of insufficient quality for analysis; 8) other causes of respiratory failure such as obstructive sleep apnea syndrome; 9) Inclusion of AECOPD patients did not use NIV before blood gas analysis; and 10) prehospital treatment that included glucocorticoids or antibiotics.

This is a subgroup of the "Digital Lung" disease assessment system and diagnostic criteria (201402013) approved by the Chinese Society for Clinical Research (Grant No.: ChiCTR-OCH-14004904). The study was approved by the Ninth Hospital of Xi'an ethics committee (No.2014001). Written informed consent was obtained from all patients.

Grouping

Among the included patients with AECOPD, those with arterial carbon dioxide partial pressure greater than 45 mmHg were assigned to the carbon dioxide retention group. Patients with arterial carbon dioxide partial pressure less than 45 mmHg were assigned to the non-carbon dioxide retention group (control group). The 45 mmHg was chosen as the threshold, rather than the diagnostic threshold of 50 mmHg for type II respiratory failure, because our interest was to study the differences in the characteristics of people with carbon dioxide retention and those without carbon dioxide retention. Of course, for treatment, this threshold is low, but for the study of carbon dioxide retention, we believe that the key point of ventilatory decompensation is more suitable, that is, arterial blood gas carbon dioxide partial pressure 45 mmHg. In addition, according to AECOPD treatment recommendations [11], $PaCO2 \geq 45$ mmHg can also be used as a threshold for non-invasive ventilation treatment.

Clinic and biochemistry data collection

A questionnaire was used to collect data on the participants' sex, age, smoking status, body mass index (BMI), number of hospitalizations caused by AECOPD during the previous 12 months, the COPD Assessment Test (CAT), and the modified Medical Research Council (mMRC) dyspnea index at admission. Blood gas analysis was performed within 1 day of admission using a RADIOMETER ABL automatic blood gas analyzer (ABL800, RADIOMETER, Copenhagen, Denmark).

Pulmonary function test (PFT)

Spirometry and impulse oscillometry (IOS) (MasterScreen, JAEGER, Germany) were performed before discharge. The maximum expiratory flow-volume curve, forced vital capacity, pulmonary diffusion function in one breath, and bronchial diastolic function were evaluated after administration of 200 μg of salbutamol (GlaxoSmithKline Pharmaceuticals Ltd.). The procedure was performed according to the ATS/ESR guidelines [12].

64-detector CT examination

Imaging examinations were performed using a 64-detector CT scanner (SOMATOM Definition AS, Siemens, Erlangen, Germany) with subjects holding their breath at full inspiration in the supine position. Technical parameters were based on our prior study [13] .

All CT images were automatically analyzed using the FACT-Digital Lung software [14, 15]. The percentage of the wall area (%WA) of different generations of bronchi in each lobe, the extent of emphysema in the whole lung, right lung, left lung, and emphysema heterogeneity index (HI) were expressed according to our prior study [13, 15, 16].

Statistical analysis

Statistical analysis was performed with SPSS 19.0 (IBM, Armonk, NY, USA). Two-sided P-values < 0.05 were deemed statistically significant. Continuous data were tested for normality using the Kolmogorov-Smirnov test. Data meeting the normal distribution were expressed as mean ± standard deviation and were analyzed using Student's test. Non-normally distributed data were expressed as median (range of 25th to 75th) and analyzed using the Mann-Whitney U test. Binary logistic regression models were used to identify predictive factors for the carbon dioxide retention group using a backward stepwise method, with a probability value for entry of $P = 0.10$ and removal of $P = 0.05$.

Results

Comparison of blood gas analysis data and other clinical parameters between the groups

Blood gas analysis showed that $PaCO_2$ in the carbon dioxide retention group was 49.5 (46–57.75) mmHg, higher than 38 (35–41) mmHg in the non-retention group ($P < 0.001$). The pH in the carbon dioxide retention group

was 7.39 (7.36–7.40), lower than 7.43 (7.41–7.45) in the non-retention group ($P < 0.001$), while PaO_2 was 69 (58–89) mmHg in the carbon dioxide retention group, lower than 76.5 (67–85.5) mmHg in the non-retention group ($P = 0.018$).

Compared with the non-carbon dioxide retention group, the number of hospitalizations for the carbon dioxide retention group increased significantly during the 12 months prior to the study ($P = 0.013$); mMRC also increased ($P = 0.034$); There was no significant statistical difference between the groups for age, smoking, number of comorbidities, body mass index, CAT score ($P > 0.05$) (Table 1).

Comparison of traditional lung function and IOS parameters between the groups

In traditional lung function tests, compared with the non-carbon dioxide retention group, the carbon dioxide retention group had lower FEV_1, $FEV_1\%pred$, FEV_1 / FVC, and $MMEF_{25-75\%}$ ($P < 0.001$), and higher RV/TLC ($P = 0.017$).

In the IOS test, compared with the non-carbon dioxide retention group, the carbon dioxide retention group possessed higher total airway resistance $Z_{5\%pred}$ and $R_{5\%pred}$ ($P = 0.004$ and 0.008, respectively), and higher peripheral airway resistance parameters R_5-R_{20} and Ax ($P = 0.009$ and $P = 0.011$, respectively). X_5 negative increase was more pronounced in the carbon dioxide retention group than the non-retention group ($P = 0.022$; Table 2).

The above results show that the airflow restriction in the retention group was more obvious; total airway resistance and peripheral airway resistance were higher.

Comparison of CT parameters between the groups

There was a statistical difference in total lung capacity, emphysematous index, and mean lung density between the groups. Compared to the non-carbon dioxide retention group, the carbon dioxide retention group had increased total lung volume [6106.56 (5113.8–6767.43) vs 5578.61 (4512.44–6459.67), $P = 0.011$], increased %LAA_{whole} [23.23 (15.43–29.51) vs 18.02 (11.83–25.83), $P = 0.007$], and lower mean lung density [− 861.37 (− 878.99--834.07) vs − 851.21 (− 867.76--829.83), $P = 0.043$] (Table 3). The above results show that the carbon dioxide retention group had more obvious increased lung volume and emphysema, and that pulmonary parenchyma damage was more pronounced (Figs. 1 and 2).

There were no statistical differences in %WA_{RUL4-7}, %WA_{RML4-7}, %WA_{RLL4-9}, %WA_{LUL4-7}, and %WA_{LLL4-9} between the groups ($P > 0.05$; Additional file 1: Table S1).

Factors influencing carbon dioxide retention

Based on the results of the univariate analysis and their clinical significance, 6 parameters were entered into the

Table 1 Demographic and clinical datas between the carbon dioxide retention and non-carbon dioxide retention COPD

Varias	Carbon dioxide retention	Non-carbon dioxide retention	p value
	n = 86	n = 144	
Age, years	65.3 ± 9.43	67.53 ± 10.24	0.102
pack years	46.55 ± 32.49	41.62 ± 26.96	0.318
Number of hospitalizations in the past 12 months	0 (0–1.25)	0 (0–1)	0.013*
Comorbidities	1 (0–1)	1 (0–2)	0.369
BMI, kg/m²	22.97 ± 3.61	23.40 ± 3.80	0.449
CAT	21 (14–25)	18.5 (12.5–25)	0.18
mMRC	2 (1–3)	1 (0–2)	0.034*
WBC,*109/L	6.55 (5.24–8.07)	7.15 (5.5–9.12)	0.088
N,%	72.8 (63.7–80.5)	73 (62.75–81.2)	0.972
E,%	1.2 (0.5–2.4)	1.6 (0.6–3.2)	0.241
HB, g/L	144 (135–152)	142 (129.5–151)	0.142
PLT*109/L	155.5 (125–202)	169 (135–218)	0.057
FIB, g/L	3.64 (2.91–4.47)	4.06 (3.25–5.1)	0.02*
D-Dimer	0.89 (0.58–1.1)	0.87 (0.59–1.24)	0.843
CRP, mg/L	3.29 (3.28–13.15)	11.3 (3.28–36.3)	0.001**
PCT	0.05 (0.05–0.05)	0.05 (0.05–0.05)	0.203
PH	7.39 (7.36–7.40)	7.43 (7.41–7.45)	< 0.001***
PaO2, mmHg	69 (58–89)	76.5 (67–85.5)	0.018*
PaCO2, mmHg	49.5(46–57.75)	38 (35–41)	< 0.001***

Abbreviations: *BMI* body mass index, *GOLD* Global Initiative for Chronic Obstructive Lung Disease, *COPD* chronic obstructive pulmonary disease, *WBC* white blood cell count, *N* neutrophil, *E* Eosinophils, *HB* Hemoglobin, *PLT* blood platelet count, *FIB* fibrinogen, *CRP* C-reactive protein, *PCT* Procalcitonin
Note:*$p < 0.05$; **$p < 0.01$; ***$p < 0.001$

Table 2 Comparison of traditional pulmonary function tests and pulsed oscillatory resistance determination between the carbon dioxide retention and non-carbon dioxide retention COPD

	Carbon dioxide retention (n = 86)	Non-carbon dioxide retention (n = 144)	p value
Z5%pred	185.9 (154–216.65)	162.4 (131.35–199.6)	0.004
R5%pred	168 (138.85–197.7)	148 (126.75–182.75)	0.008
R5	0.52 (0.43–0.61)	0.49 (0.39–0.57)	0.057
R20%pred	123.4 (105.75–139.55)	117.2 (104.3–135.6)	0.236
R20	0.32 (0.29–0.375)	0.33 (0.29–0.37)	0.764
R5-R20	0.18 (0.125–0.23)	0.14 (0.09–0.205)	0.009
X5	−0.24 (−0.31–−0.16)	−0.19 (−0.32–−0.13)	0.022
Fres	22 (18.26–26.19)	21.2 (17.48–24.61)	0.173
Ax	1.89 (1.27–2.57)	1.54 (0.74–2.44)	0.011
FEV1	0.95 (0.77–1.42)	1.39 (1.06–1.74)	< 0.001
FEV1%pred	34.25 (25.4–47.8)	51.45 (40–61.7)	< 0.001
FEV1/FVC	48.14 (42.08–56.71)	56.26 (46.55–62.79)	< 0.001
MMEF75–25%pred	14.25 (9.7–19.9)	21.5 (16.1–27.75)	< 0.001
DLCO/VA	75.47 ± 24.29	80.13 ± 24.34	0.169
RV/TLC	59.44 ± 10.11	55.98 ± 10.63	0.017

Abbreviations: *PFT* Pulmonary function test, *FEV1* forced expiratory volume in 1 sec, *FVC* forced vital capacity, *FEV1/FVC* forced expiratory volume in 1 sec/forced vital capacity, *MMEF$_{25-75\%}$* maximal mid expiratory flow, *RV/TLC* residual volume/total lung capacity, *DLCO/VA* ratio of carbon monoxide diffusion capacity to alveolar ventilation, *%Pred*, of the predicted value, *Z$_5$* Total respiratory impedance, *R5* resistance at 5 Hz, *R$_{20}$* resistance at 20 Hz, *X$_5$* reactance at 5 Hz, *Fres* response frequency, *Ax* reactance area

Table 3 Comparison of Emphysema variables between the carbon dioxide retention and non-carbon dioxide retention COPD

Emphysema variables	Carbon dioxide retention	Non-carbon dioxide retention	p value
Volume $_{whole}$	6106.56 (5113.8–6767.43)	5578.61 (4512.44–6459.67)	0.011
%LAA $_{whole}$	23.23 (15.43–29.51)	18.02 (11.83–25.83)	0.007
Mean lung density $_{whole}$	−861.37(−878.99--834.07)	−851.21 (−867.76--829.83)	0.043
Volume $_{Right\ lung}$	3180.79 (2756.52–3578.41)	3014.42 (2482.47–3488.95)	0.047
%LAA $_{Right\ lung}$	23.4 (15.24–30.08)	17.65 (12.28–25.68)	0.006
Mean lung density $_{Right}$	−859.2 (− 879.56--835.39)	−851.14 (− 866.61--829.63)	0.032
Volume $_{Left\ lung}$	2878.78 (2319.57–3221.92)	2599.85 (2039.45–3039.15)	0.003
%LAA $_{Left\ lung}$	23.39 (14.8–29.1)	18.83 (11.65–26.32)	0.008
Mean lung density $_{Left}$	− 862.98 (−876.01--837.3)	− 847.85 (− 870.33--826.79)	0.039
HI $_{whole}$	0.09 (−0.08–0.29)	0.16 (−0.02–0.32)	0.169
HI $_{Right\ lung}$	0.15 (−0.06–0.35)	0.18 (− 0.02–0.38)	0.458
HI $_{Right\ lung}$	− 0.17 (− 0.41–0.05)	−0.08 (− 0.28–0.11)	0.079

Abbreviations: *%LAA* the extent of emphysema of CT attenuation value below −950 HU;MDE:Mean density of emphysema;HI:emphysema heterogeneity index, when emphysemais equally distributed among the lobes or the full extent in the whole lung is < 1%, HI is near zero; otherwise,HI = (%LAAupper -%LAAlower)/(%LAAupper+%LAAlower)*100

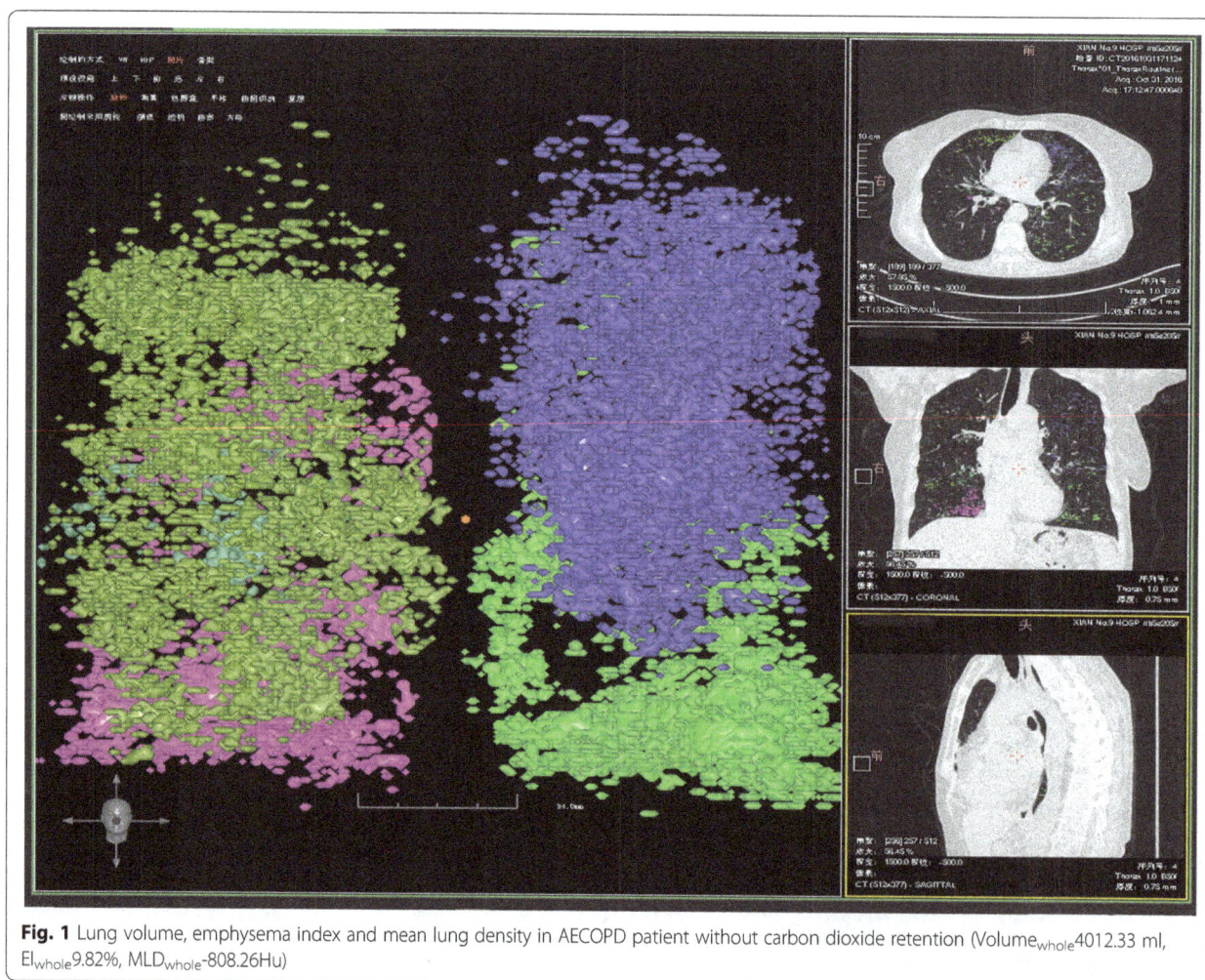

Fig. 1 Lung volume, emphysema index and mean lung density in AECOPD patient without carbon dioxide retention (Volume$_{whole}$4012.33 ml, EI$_{whole}$9.82%, MLD$_{whole}$-808.26Hu)

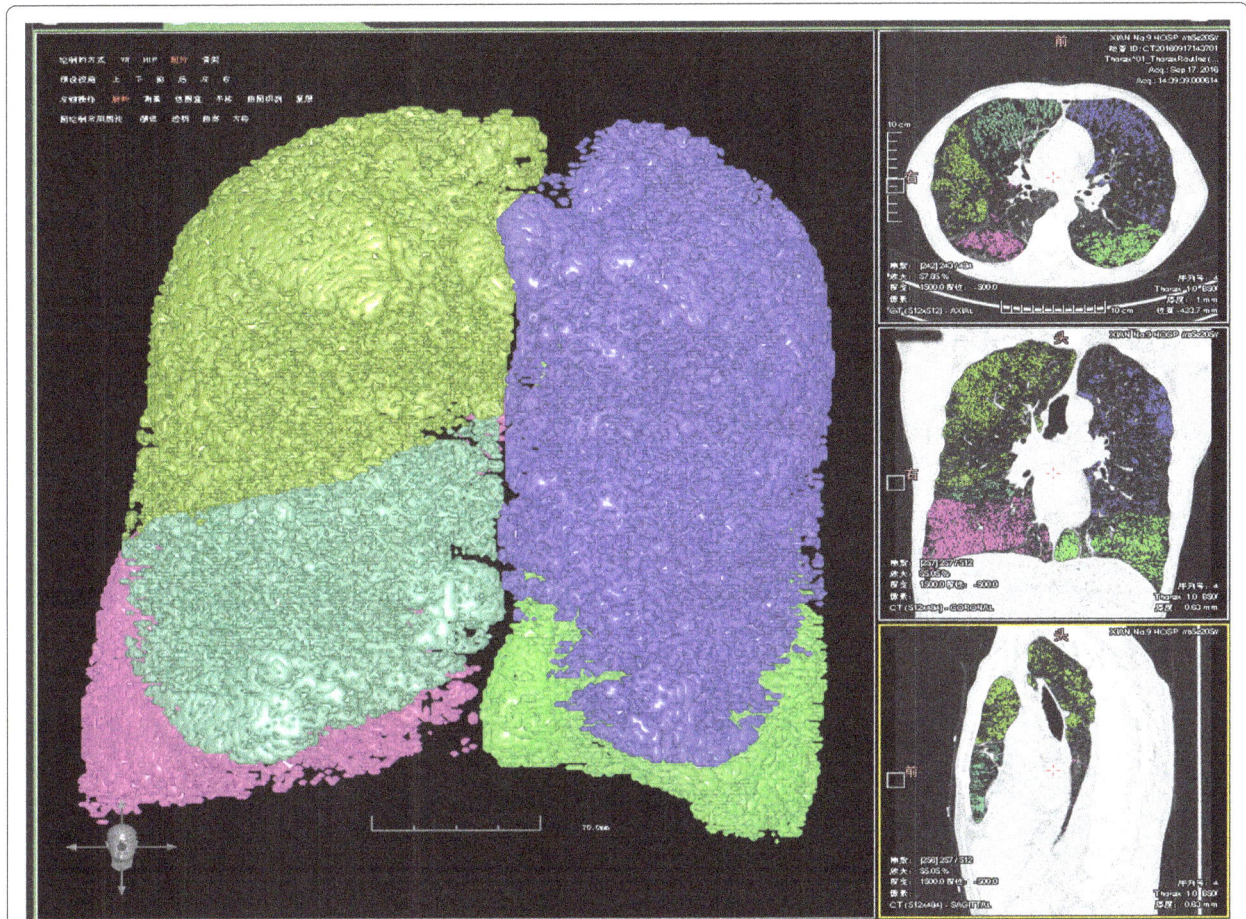

Fig. 2 Lung volume, emphysema index and mean lung density in AECOPD patient with carbon dioxide retention (Volume$_{whole}$6187.62 ml, EI$_{whole}$15.17%, MLD$_{whole}$-851.18Hu)

logistics analysis: the number of hospitalizations because of AECOPD in the previous 12 months (≥1), mMRC (≥2), neutrophil ratio (≥70%), X5 negative increase (< 0), whole lung emphysema index (EI > 20%) and FEV$_1$ (< 1 L). Logistic regression analysis, using the back stepwise method, showed that FEV$_1$ < 1 L and %LAA$_{-950HU}$ > 20% were independent risk factors for carbon dioxide retention (Table 4). The predictive value of these two parameters for carbon dioxide retention was 69.4%.

Discussion

COPD is a heterogeneous disease, and for the specific population included in this study, carbon dioxide retention indicates that the disease has progressed to the

Table 4 Logistic regression analysis of factors associated with carbon dioxide retention

	P	OR (95% CI)
FEV1 < 1 L	< 0.001	4.011 (2.216–7.262)
%LAA-950Hu > 20%	0.026	1.926 (1.080–3.432)

decompensation phase of respiratory dysfunction. In terms of COPD treatment, this population therefore requires the most medical resources and tends to respond poorly to clinical treatment. Our study revealed the clinical, pulmonary function, and imaging features of patients who have carbon dioxide retention. The carbon dioxide retention group had more frequent hospital admissions for acute exacerbations in the 12 months prior to the study, more pronounced dyspnea symptoms, and lower arterial partial pressure of oxygen. Regardless of the traditional lung function or IOS test, the carbon dioxide retention group had poorer parameters, more obstructive airflow, and higher residual volume. In imaging, the carbon dioxide retention group had higher lung volume and emphysema index, and lower mean lung density. However, there was no difference in emphysematous distribution and multi-stage bronchial wall area. Our results showed that FEV$_1$ < 1 L and EI > 20% can help predict the increased risk of COPD with carbon dioxide retention.

Studies from ECLIPSE suggest that the clinical manifestations of COPD vary widely, and the extent of airflow limitation cannot capture the heterogeneity of the disease [17]. FEV_1 is not believed to reflect the whole picture of COPD and is not a reliable predictor of disease stage for specific individuals [18]. However, there is also the opinion [19] that $FEV_1 < 1$ L is an independent prognostic factor. Although FEV1 is generally expressed more accurately as a percentage of the predicted value, a fixed cutoff is assessed for limited airflow severity when FEV1 is much lower than normal, and we believe it to be reliable for clinical use. Our study also showed that $FEV_1 < 1$ L predicts the presence of carbon dioxide, which is especially useful for assessing COPD with chronic long-term carbon dioxide retention and to provide a reference for deciding on treatments like adjuvant ventilation, or for parameter selection as a follow-up step. Emphysema index is currently a more accepted imaging parameter for the assessment of COPD [20, 21] because of its reflection of both pathological and functional impairments. Our regression analysis showed that EI > 20% and $FEV_1 < 1$ L can be used to predict carbon dioxide retention, reflecting both pathological and functional impairments. O'Donnell [22] conducted a similar study using discriminant analysis and found that FEV_1 / FVC rates, as well as vital capacity (% predicted) or FVC (% predicted), differentiated patients requiring mechanical ventilation from those who did not.

There are many phenotypes based on COPD [23], however, COPD with carbon dioxide retention has rarely been studied. Gas exchange in COPD is very complicated; the mechanism of carbon dioxide retention induced hypercapnia is the result of multiple pathological processes that are interwoven at varying degrees and affected by the disease process itself. In addition, the cellular and molecular details of lung tissue destruction are not completely understood [24]. The destruction of lung parenchyma mainly manifested as emphysema, accompanied by pulmonary vascular bed damage. Small airway remodeling and occlusion are other important outcomes of pathological damage. In acute exacerbation events, airway spasms, mucosal edema, and sputum cause increased airway obstruction and inflammation.

Chronic respiratory failure results in carbon dioxide retention due to respiratory insufficiency [25, 26], We found that there was a more severe airflow limitation in the carbon dioxide retention group. In the image data for this group, we found a more obvious increase in the lung volume and the emphysema index, and that the mean lung density was lower, suggesting that there was not only excessive expansion of dynamic lung, but also more physical damage to the lung involved in the pathological process.

Clinical strategies for AECOPD include: treatment of the primary disease, controlled oxygen therapy, and the use of an invasive or non-invasive ventilator to improve lung ventilation. Current clinical treatment is partial to improving lung ventilation, while putting less emphasis on changes in the pulmonary parenchyma. However, better carbon dioxide removal has been a topic of growing interest in recent years, and a new approach involves extracorporeal venous CO_2 removal [27–29].

Carbon dioxide retention in the body can cause harm that is multi-system and widespread. Clinical emphasis is on the treatment of hypoxia, but there is an attitude of tolerance to carbon dioxide retention. Clinicians should recognize that carbon dioxide retention will increase the hypoxic damage to multiple tissues [30, 31]. Hypervolemic respiratory failure noninvasive ventilation (NIV) treatment is the primary method of clinical management and, based several large studies [32, 33], it is reasonable to use a higher level of partial pressure of carbon dioxide to determine NIV use. Our study focused on the parameters of pulmonary function and imaging that would be valuable when carbon dioxide retention was elevated, so the cutoff partial pressure of carbon dioxide was chosen as 45 mmHg.

The characteristics of COPD populations with carbon dioxide retention are typically not of concern. Most studies focus on the COPD populations based on pulmonary function grading. In contrast, our research is novel because we focused on a particular population with specific clinical features, and so were able to obtain some valuable results. However, the present study is not without limitations. It is only assumed that persistent carbon dioxide retention and transient carbon dioxide retention are different, but there are no observations for the longitudinal outcomes of these conditions. Secondly, the sample size was small. To address these issues, more research is needed to explore the features of carbon dioxide retention in patients with AECOPD.

Conclusion

The carbon dioxide retention COPD group had more airflow obstruction and higher residual volume, lung volume, and emphysema index, as well as lower mean lung density compared to the COPD group without carbon dioxide retention. FEV1 < 1 L and EI > 20% may be predictors of an increased risk of carbon dioxide retention.

Funding

This research was supported by the Social Development Science Research Project of Shaanxi Province (No. 2016SF-151) and Xi'an Science and Technology Project (No. 2016045SF / YX01). Funders had no role in the study design, data collection and analysis, decision to publish, or in the preparation of the manuscript.

Authors' contributions

XW conceived and designed the study, designed, performed and analyzed the experiments, and wrote the paper. QD, JTR, JYM, LB, JYL, and MQ carried out the data collection, data analysis, and revised the paper. YN and YMG designed the study and revised the paper. All authors read and approved the final manuscript.

Competing interest

The authors declare that they have no competing interests.

Author details

[1]Department of Radiology, Xi'an Jiaotong University Medical College First Affiliated Hospital, Xi'an, China. [2]Department of Respiratory Medicine, The Ninth Hospital of Xi'an Affiliated Hospital of Xi'an Jiaotong University, Xi'an, China. [3]Department of Radiology, The Affiliated Hospital of Shaanxi University of Traditional Chinese Medicine, Xianyang, Shaanxi, China. [4]Department of Respiratory Medicine, Central Hospital of Xi'an Affiliated Hospital of Xi'an Jiaotong University, Xi'an, Shaanxi, China. [5]Department of Radiology, Shaanxi Provincial People's Hospital, Xi'an, China.

References

1. Lozano R, Naghavi M, Foreman K, Lim S, Shibuya K, Aboyans V, Abraham J, Adair T, Aggarwal R, Ahn SY, et al. Global and regional mortality from 235 causes of death for 20 age groups in 1990 and 2010: a systematic analysis for the global burden of disease study 2010. Lancet. 2012;380(9859):2095–128.
2. Vos T, Flaxman AD, Naghavi M, Lozano R, Michaud C, Ezzati M, Shibuya K, Salomon JA, Abdalla S, Aboyans V, et al. Years lived with disability (YLDs) for 1160 sequelae of 289 diseases and injuries 1990-2010: a systematic analysis for the global burden of disease study 2010. Lancet. 2012;380(9859):2163–96.
3. Yin P, Wang H, Vos T, Li Y, Liu S, Liu Y, Liu J, Wang L, Naghavi M, Murray CJ, et al. A subnational analysis of mortality and prevalence of COPD in China from 1990 to 2013: findings from the global burden of disease study 2013. Chest. 2016;150(6):1269–80.
4. Liu S, Zhou Y, Liu S, Chen X, Zou W, Zhao D, Li X, Pu J, Huang L, Chen J, et al. Association between exposure to ambient particulate matter and chronic obstructive pulmonary disease: results from a cross-sectional study in China. Thorax. 2017;72(9):788–95.
5. From the Global Strategy for the Diagnosis, Management and Prevention of COPD, Global Initiative for Chronic Obstructive Lung Disease (GOLD) [http://goldcopd.org/gold-2017-global-strategy-diagnosis-management-prevention-copd/]. Accessed 12 Feb 2017.
6. Chae EJ, Seo JB, Song J-W, Kim N, Park B-W, Lee YK, Oh Y-M, Lee SD, Lim SY. Slope of emphysema index: an objective descriptor of regional heterogeneity of emphysema and an independent determinant of pulmonary function. Am J Roentgenol. 2010;194(3):W248–55.
7. Choromanska A, Macura KJ. Role of computed tomography in quantitative assessment of emphysema. Pol J Radiol. 2012;77(1):28–36.
8. Yamasawa W, Tasaka S, Betsuyaku T, Yamaguchi K. Correlation of a decline in aerobic capacity with development of emphysema in patients with chronic obstructive pulmonary disease: a prospective observational study. PLoS One. 2015;10(4):17.
9. Costello R, Deegan P, Fitzpatrick M, McNicholas WT. Reversible hypercapnia in chronic obstructive pulmonary disease: a distinct pattern of respiratory failure with a favorable prognosis. Am J Med. 1997;102(3):239–44.
10. Tsuboi T, Oga T, Sumi K, Machida K, Ohi M, Chin K. The importance of stabilizing PaCO2 during long-term non-invasive ventilation in subjects with COPD. Intern Med. 2015;54(10):1193–8.
11. Cai BQ, Cai SX, Chen RC, Cui LY, Feng YL, Gu YT, Huang SG, Liu RY, Liu GN, Shi HZ, et al. Expert consensus on acute exacerbation of chronic obstructive pulmonary disease in the People's Republic of China. Int J Chron Obstruct Pulmon Dis. 2014;9:381–95.
12. M MR, H J, B V. ATS/ERS task force: standardisation of spirometry. Eur Respir J. 2005;26(2):319–38.
13. Wei X, Ma Z, Yu N, Ren J, Jin C, Mi J, Shi M, Tian L, Gao Y, Guo Y. Risk factors predict frequent hospitalization in patients with acute exacerbation of COPD. Int J Chron Obstruct Pulmon Dis. 2018;13:121–9.
14. Pu J, Fuhrman C, Good WF, Sciurba FC, Gur D. A differential geometric approach to automated segmentation of human airway tree. IEEE Trans Med Imaging. 2011;30(2):266–78.
15. Yu N, Xin X-M, Li Y, Ma J-C, Gao J-G, Jin C-W, Guo Y-M. Effect of computed tomography dose on quantitative measurement and automated segmentation of airway tree. J Med Imaging and Health Informatics. 2015;5(7):1519–23.
16. Yu N, Wei X, Li Y, Deng L, Jin C-W, Guo Y. Computed tomography quantification of pulmonary vessels in chronic obstructive pulmonary disease as identified by 3D automated approach. Medicine. 2016;95(40):e5095.
17. Agusti A, Calverley PM, Celli B, Coxson HO, Edwards LD, Lomas DA, MacNee W, Miller BE, Rennard S, Silverman EK, et al. Characterisation of COPD heterogeneity in the ECLIPSE cohort. Respir Res. 2010;11:122.
18. Han MK, Agusti A, Calverley PM, Celli BR, Criner G, Curtis JL, Fabbri LM, Goldin JG, Jones PW, MacNee W, et al. Chronic obstructive pulmonary disease phenotypes the future of COPD. Am J Respir Crit Care Med. 2010; 182(5):598–604.
19. Gorzelak K, Sliwinski P, Tobiasz M, Gorecka D. Zielinski J: [predictors of survival in patients with chronic obstructive pulmonary disease with moderate hypoxemia]. Pol Arch Med Wewn. 1995;93(6):491–7.
20. Mohamed Hoesein FA, de Hoop B, Zanen P, Gietema H, Kruitwagen CL, van Ginneken B, Isgum I, Mol C, van Klaveren RJ, Dijkstra AE, et al. CT-quantified emphysema in male heavy smokers: association with lung function decline. Thorax. 2011;66(9):782–7.
21. Xie M, Wang W, Dou S, Cui L, Xiao W. Quantitative computed tomography measurements of emphysema for diagnosing asthma-chronic obstructive pulmonary disease overlap syndrome. Int J Chron Obstruct. Pulmon Dis. 2016;11:953–61.
22. O'Donnell DE, Parker CM. COPD exacerbations center dot 3: pathophysiology. Thorax. 2006;61(4):354–61.
23. Chen Y. Heterogeneity of acute exacerbation of chronic obstructive pulmonary disease in clinical manifestations. *Zhonghua jie he he hu xi za zhi = Zhonghua jiehe he huxi zazhi =*. Chinese J Tuberculosis and Respiratory Dis. 2014;37(4):244–6.
24. Taraseviciene-Stewart L, Voelkel NF. Molecular pathogenesis of emphysema. J Clin Investig. 2008;118(2):394–402.
25. Schonhofer B. Noninvasive ventilation in patients with persistent hypercapnia. Medizinische Klinik, Intensivmedizin und Notfallmedizin. 2015; 110(3):182–7.
26. Brill SE, Wedzicha JA. Oxygen therapy in acute exacerbations of chronic obstructive pulmonary disease. Int J Chron Obstruct Pulmon Dis. 2014;9: 1241–52.
27. Kreppein U, Litterst P, Westhoff M. Hypercapnic respiratory failure. Pathophysiology, indications for mechanical ventilation and management. Medizinische Klinik-Intensivmedizin Und Notfallmedizin. 2016;111(3):196–201.
28. Burki NK, Mani RK, Herth FJF, Schmidt W, Teschler H, Bonin F, Becker H, Randerath WJ, Stieglitz S, Hagmeyer L, et al. A novel extracorporeal CO(2) removal system: results of a pilot study of hypercapnic respiratory failure in patients with COPD. Chest. 2013;143(3):678–86.
29. Cove ME, MacLaren G, Federspiel WJ, Kellum JA. Bench to bedside review: Extracorporeal carbon dioxide removal, past present and future. Crit Care. 2012;16(5):232.
30. Yasuo M, Mizuno S, Kraskauskas D, Bogaard HJ, Natarajan R, Cool CD, Zamora M, Voelkel NF. Hypoxia inducible factor-1 alpha in human emphysema lung tissue. Eur Respir J. 2011;37(4):775–83.
31. Selfridge AC, Cavadas MAS, Scholz CC, Campbell EL, Welch LC, Lecuona E, Colgan SP, Barrett KE, Sporn PHS, Sznajder JI, et al. Hypercapnia suppresses the HIF-dependent adaptive response to hypoxia. J Biol Chem. 2016;291(22): 11800–8.
32. Kohnlein T, Windisch W, Kohler D, Drabik A, Geiseler J, Hartl S, Karg O, Laier-Groeneveld G, Nava S, Schonhofer B, et al. Non-invasive positive pressure ventilation for the treatment of severe stable chronic obstructive pulmonary disease: a prospective, multicentre, randomised, controlled clinical trial. Lancet Respir Med. 2014;2(9):698–705.

18

Interleukin-3 plays a vital role in hyperoxic acute lung injury in mice via mediating inflammation

Zhijian Huang[1†], Wei Zhang[2†], Jian Yang[2], Feiyu Sun[1] and Hongwei Zhou[3*]

Abstract

Background: Interleukin (IL)-3 amplifies inflammation. However, the effect of IL-3 in acute lung injury (ALI), an acute inflammatory disease, is unclear. The aim of this study was to test the hypothesis that IL-3 plays an important role in hyperoxia-induced ALI.

Methods: Hyperoxic ALI was induced in wild-type (WT) and IL-3 gene disrupted (IL-3$^{-/-}$) mice by exposure to 100% O_2 for 72 h.

Results: Hyperoxia increased IL-3 levels in plasma and lung tissues in WT mice. Pulmonary inflammation and edema were detected by histological assay in WT mice exposed to 100% O_2 for 72 h. However, the hyperoxia-induced lung histological changes were improved in IL-3$^{-/-}$ mice. The hyperoxia-induced elevation of neutrophils in bronchoalveolar lavage fluids and circulation were reduced in IL-3$^{-/-}$ mice. Meanwhile, the levels of tumor necrosis factor-α and IL-6 were suppressed in IL-3$^{-/-}$ mice compared with WT mice. Moreover, the hyperoxia-induced the activation of IκBα kinase (IKK) β, IκBα phosphorylation, and nuclear factor-κB translocation were inhibited in IL-3$^{-/-}$ mice compared with WT mice.

Conclusions: Our results suggest IL-3 is a potential therapeutic target for hyperoxia-induced ALI.

Keywords: Interleukin-3, Acute lung injury, Inflammation, Hyperoxia

Background

Acute respiratory distress syndrome (ARDS) remains a major challenge in intensive care medicine [1, 2]. Acute lung injury (ALI) is a mild form of ARDS. Inflammation is thought to contribute to the pathogenesis of ALI/ARDS [1–5], as ALI/ARDS is characterized by increased vascular permeability, extravasation of plasma, and neutrophil infiltration in the lung [1–4]. Thus, it is rational to explore anti-inflammatory therapies for this disorder [1, 5, 6]. However, it is bewildering that the results from clinical trials of novel anti-inflammatory strategies for ALI/ARDS have been disappointingly negative [1, 2, 4, 7]. These results reflect an incomplete understanding of ALI/ARDS pathogenesis. Therefore, the complicated cellular and molecular mechanisms contributing to the pathogenesis of ALI/ARDS needs to be further elucidated.

A recent study showed that interleukin (IL)-3 and its specific receptor α chain (IL-3Rα, also know as CD123) axis is responsible for cytokine storm during the pathogenesis of cecal ligation and puncture induced sepsis [8]. IL-3/CD123 axis is suggested as a potential therapeutic target for sepsis [8]. However, the underlying mechanism has not been adequately defined. Excessive cytokine-mediated inflammation plays a fundamental role in the pathogenesis of ALI/ARDS [9, 10], one of the most feared complications of sepsis [9, 11]. Nuclear factor (NF)-κB is known as a pivotal inducer of proinflammatory cytokines and highly activated in various inflammation-related diseases such as ALI [10, 12, 13]. A previous in vitro study reported IL-3 has potential effect on induction of IκBα kinase (IKK) β activation [14]. IKK plays a key role on regulation of NF-κB activation [15]. In the present study, we investigated the role of IL-3 in hyperoxia-induced ALI.

* Correspondence: 2545419172@qq.com
†Zhijian Huang and Wei Zhang contributed equally to this work.
³Department of Intensive Care Unit, Xia'men Traditional Chinese Medicine Hospital affiliated to Beijing University of Traditional Chinese Medicine, No.1739 Xianyue Road, Xia'men 361009, Fujian, China
Full list of author information is available at the end of the article

Our findings may suggest new therapeutic target to prevent the onset of hyperoxic lung injury.

Methods

Animals

All animal experiments were performed in accordance with the National Institutes of Health guidelines for the use of experimental animals. All animal care and experimental procedures used in the present study were approved by the Ethics committee of Beijing University of Traditional Chinese Medicine. Healthy wild-type (WT) C57BL/6 mice (6–8 weeks old, body weight 16–20 g) were obtained from Beijing University of Traditional Chinese Medicine. IL-3 gene disrupted (IL-3$^{-/-}$) mice on a C57BL/6 background were obtained from The Jackson Laboratory (Bar Harbor, ME). All of our current studies were performed using male mice. The animals were housed in individually ventilated cages under a 12 h light/dark cycle. Before the experiment, mice were habituated to the environment for at least 1 week. Standard chow and water were provided ad libitum. All procedures were performed as humanely as possible to minimize animal suffering.

Experimental protocol

Mice were assigned to four groups ($n = 8$): sham+WT mice, sham+IL-3$^{-/-}$ mice, hyperoxia+WT mice, and hyperoxia+IL-3$^{-/-}$ mice. In brief, the mice were exposed to 100% O_2 in a specially constructed plexiglas chamber to induce hyperoxic ALI [16]. Mice in sham group were exposed in room air. Seventy-two hours after hyperoxia or room air challenge, mice were sacrificed after anesthesia by pentobarbitone (50 mg/kg intraperitoneal injection) and were exsanguinated through the vena cava. Then, lung tissue sampling (for lung histology, and lung wet to dry weight ratio) was collected. Bronchoalveolar lavage fluids (BALF) and pulmonary tissue samples (for preparation of lung tissue homogenates) were collected in separate experiments.

Lung histology

The lungs were fixed with formalin overnight. Five micrometer sections were deparaffinized. The sections were stained by haematoxylin/eosin (H&E). Lung injury scores were performed according to the following histological features: pulmonary edema, neutrophil infiltration, hyperemia, hemorrhage, and cellular hyperplasia. A score of 0 represented absent damage; 1 represented mild damage; 2 represented moderate damage; 3 represented severe damage [17].

Lung water content

To quantify the magnitude of pulmonary edema, we evaluated the dry to wet (D/W) ratio of the lung. The left main bronchi were clamped, and the wet left lung was harvested. They were then placed in an oven for 48 h at 80 °C. Lung water content was calculated as (1-D/W) × 100%.

Collection of BALF

The trachea was cannulated, and the lung was lavaged with 0.5 mL PBS for six times. The recovery rate of BALF was > 90% in all samples. Collected BALF was centrifuged at 1,200 rpm for 3 min. The supernatant was collected for further study.

Enzyme linked immunosorbent assay (ELISA)

The concentrations of tumor necrosis factor (TNF)-α, IL-6, and IL-3 were measured by ELISA according to the manufacturer's instructions (R&D Systems Inc., Minneapolis, MN, USA). The DNA-binding activity of NF-κB p65 was determined using an ELISA NF-κB p65 transcription factor assay kit according to the manufacturer's instructions (Chemicon, Temecula, CA, USA).

Western blotting analysis

Cytoplasmic and nuclear proteins were extracted from frozen lung tissue with the Nuclear/Cytosol Extraction kit (BioVision, Inc., Mountain View, CA, USA) according to the manufacturer's instructions. Protein concentrations were determined using the bicinchoninic acid protein assay (Pierce, Rockford, IL, USA). 50 μg of total protein were subjected to SDS-PAGE and transferred onto PVDF membranes. Membranes were blocked with 5% non-fat milk at room temperature for 3 h, incubated with primary antibodies (Anti-NF-κB p65 (sc-7151) and phosphorylated IκBα antibodies (sc-7977), diluted 1:500, Santa Cruz Biotechnology, Santa Cruz, CA, USA; Anti-phosphorylated IKKα/IKKβ antibody (2078), diluted 1:500, Cell Signaling, Boston, MA, USA; Anti-IL-3 antibody (AF-403-NA), diluted 1:200, R&D Systems Inc., Minneapolis, MN, USA; Anti-CD123 antibody (106002), diluted 1:200, Biolegend, San Diego, CA, USA) at 4 °C overnight. β-actin (3700) and Lamin B (12586) (Cell Signaling, Boston, MA, USA) were used as an internal control for cytoplasmic and nuclear protein, respectively. On the next day, membranes were incubated with HRP-conjugated secondary antibodies (Cell Signaling, Boston, MA, USA) at 37 °C for 1 h. Protein bands on the membrane were visualized with ECL Kit (Biovision, Milpitas, CA, USA) using FluorChem FC3 system (ProteinSimple, San Jose, CA, USA). Results were presented as densitometric ratio between the protein of interest and the loading control.

Survival study

The survival rate was observed at 24-h intervals. Observation was continued 72 h.

Statistical analysis

All data were analyzed with GraphPad Prism 6.0 (GraphPad Software, CA, USA) and were presented as mean ± SEM. Two-way ANOVA with Bonferroni's multiple-comparisons test was used for multiple group analysis. Histopathologic scores were compared using the Mann-Whitney U test. The survival rate was estimated by the Kaplan-Meier method and compared by log-rank test. $P < 0.05$ was accepted as statistically significant.

Results

Effect of hyperoxia on IL-3 and IL-3Rα

The levels of IL-3 and IL-3Rα in the lung were detected by Western Blotting in additional groups of animals (Fig. 1a and Additional file 1: Figure S1). Hyperoxia caused significant increase of IL-3 in the lung (Fig. 1a). It was simultaneously associated with an increase in expression of IL-3Rα in the lung 72 h after hyperoxia challenge (Fig. 1a). Moreover, the concentration of IL-3 in plasma was significantly elevated in hyperoxia exposure group compared with sham (Fig. 1a).

Effects of IL-3 on lung injury and mortality in hyperoxia-induced ALI

Hyperoxia caused significant neutrophil infiltration, alveolar capillary protein leak, and lung edema after 72 h, which could be dampened in IL-3$^{-/-}$ mice (Fig. 1b, c, d, and e). When IL-3$^{-/-}$ mice were treated with hyperoxia, the lung histological changes were reduced compared with WT mice (Fig.1f; Fig. 2). All mice died within 3 days in hyperoxia+WT group. In contrast, mice were more resistant to hyperoxia in IL-3$^{-/-}$ mice. A total of 50% of the mice in the WT mice treated hyperoxia group died within 24 h, and an additional 50% died within 72 h, while 60% of the mice in the IL-3$^{-/-}$ mice treated hyperoxia group survived.

Effects of IL-3 on proinflammatory mediators in hyperoxia-induced ALI

As proinflammatory cytokines have a key role in ALI [10, 12], the IL-6 and TNF-α in BALF were studied in our study. Seventy-two hours after hyperoxia challenge, there was a significant reduction in TNF-α and IL-6 concentrations in IL-3$^{-/-}$ mice versus WT mice (Fig. 3a).

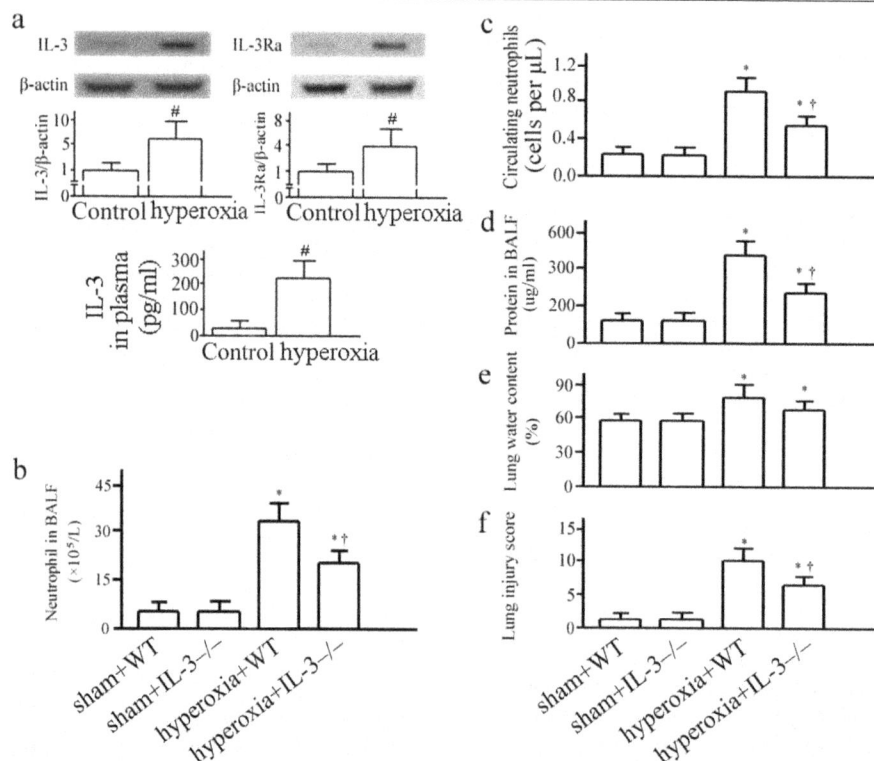

Fig. 1 Effect of hyperoxia on interleukin (IL)-3 and IL-3-specific receptor α chain (IL-3Rα). C57BL/6 mice were challenged with room air (control) or hyperoxia for 72 h and pulmonary protein of IL-3 and IL-3Rα were assessed by western blotting, and IL-3 levels in plasma was measured by enzyme linked immunosorbent assay (ELISA) (**a**). Neutrophils in bronchoalveolar lavage fluids (BALF) (**b**) and circulation (**c**), protein in BALF (**d**), lung edema (**e**), and lung injury score (**f**) were assessed 72 h after hyperoxia or room air challenge. Data represent assessments in a minimum of $n = 5$ mice. #$P < 0.05$ vs. control; *$P < 0.05$ vs. sham+wild type (WT) group; † $P < 0.05$ vs. hyperoxia +WT group. IL-3$^{-/-}$, IL-3 gene disrupted mice

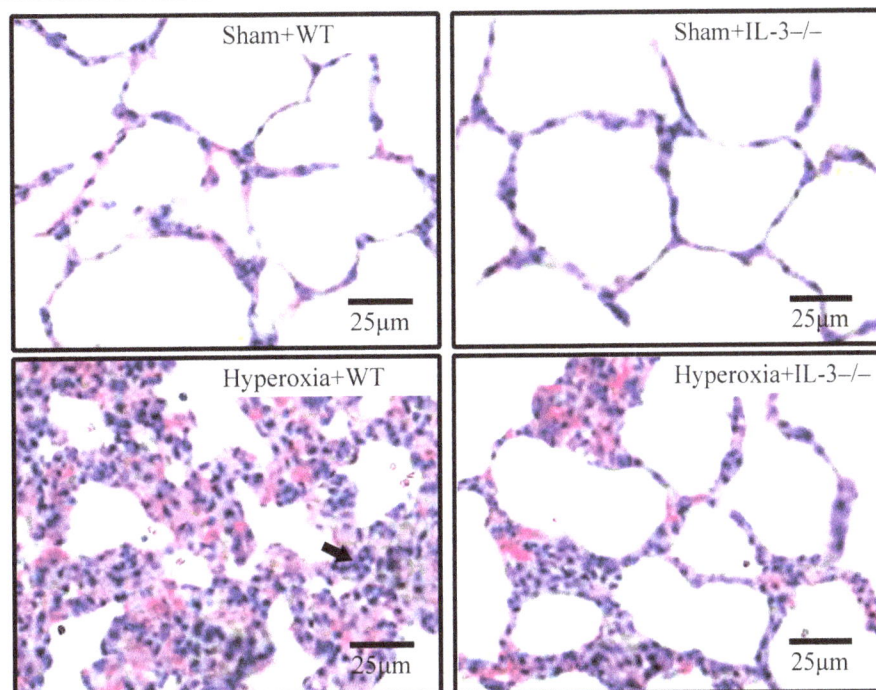

Fig. 2 Lung histological features were assessed 72 h after hyperoxia or room air challenge by light microscopy, hematoxylin and eosin stain in wild-type mice (WT) and interleukin-3 gene disrupted mice (IL-3$^{-/-}$). Original magnification, × 400

Effects of IL-3 on IKK/NF-κB pathway

Hyperoxia exposure induced IκB phosphorylation and NF-κB p65 nuclear translocation in the lung (Fig. 3b, and c). NF-κB p65 levels in the nucleus and phosphorylated IκBα levels in the cytoplasm were reduced in IL-3$^{-/-}$ mice (Fig. 3b, and c). The hyperoxia-induced IKKβ activation was dampened in IL-3$^{-/-}$ mice (Fig. 3d). Hyperoxia exposure induced activation of NF-κB was reduced in IL-3$^{-/-}$ mice (Fig. 3e).

Discussion

IL-3 was first reported to be a potential new therapeutic target for sepsis in 2015 [8]. However, the effect of IL-3 in ALI has been generally understudied. Our results showed that IL-3 gene deleted mice have improved lung inflammation and edema in hyperoxia-induced ALI. Moreover, hyperoxia-induced the activation of IKK/NF-κB signaling pathways and upregulation of proinflammatory mediators were reduced in IL-3$^{-/-}$ mice.

Lines of evidence have shown that IL-3 is released by activated Th2 lymphocytes which play crucial roles in allergic disorders [8, 18]. IL-3 is also known as multi-potential colony-stimulating factor which stimulating proliferation of pluripotent hematopoietic stem cells and progenitor cells [19–21]. A recent study suggests that IL-3 plays a vital role in sepsis [8], an infectious disorder [9, 11]. IL-3 plays its effect via combining with its receptor. The IL-3 receptor is a heterodimer which composed of one α chain and oneβchain [19, 22]. The α chain is IL-3 specific receptor also known as CD123. IL-3Rα is expressed in hematopoietic stem and progenitor cells, dendritic progenitors, and macrophage [8, 19]. These cells were infiltrated in the lung in the pathogenesis of ALI. In the present study, a significant increase in IL-3 and IL-3Rα levels in the lung homogenates 72 h after hyperoxia stimulation was detected by Western Blotting.

Over released proinflammatory mediators are crucial to the initiation of inflammatory tissue injury [9]. The influence of IL-3 and it receptor on proinflammatory mediators has been reported [8, 14, 23, 24]. A previous in vitro study suggests a potential posttranscriptional regulation effect of IL-3 on TNF-α via a p38-mitogen-activated protein kinase and silent information regulator type-2-dependent manner [23]. The limiting role of anti-CD123 in cytokine secretion has been recognized previously [8]. Our data showed that TNF-α and IL-6 were reduced in IL-3 gene deleted mice compared with WT mice at 72 h after hyperoxia stimulation. However, little is known regarding the underlying mechanisms. IKK/NF-κB pathway is one critical transcriptional mechanism required for maximal expression of many cytokines involved in the pathogenesis of ALI [10, 12]. A previous in vitro study reported IL-3 induces the activation of IKKβ in mast cell via a Src family kinase and Ca^{2+} dependent manner [14]. Activation

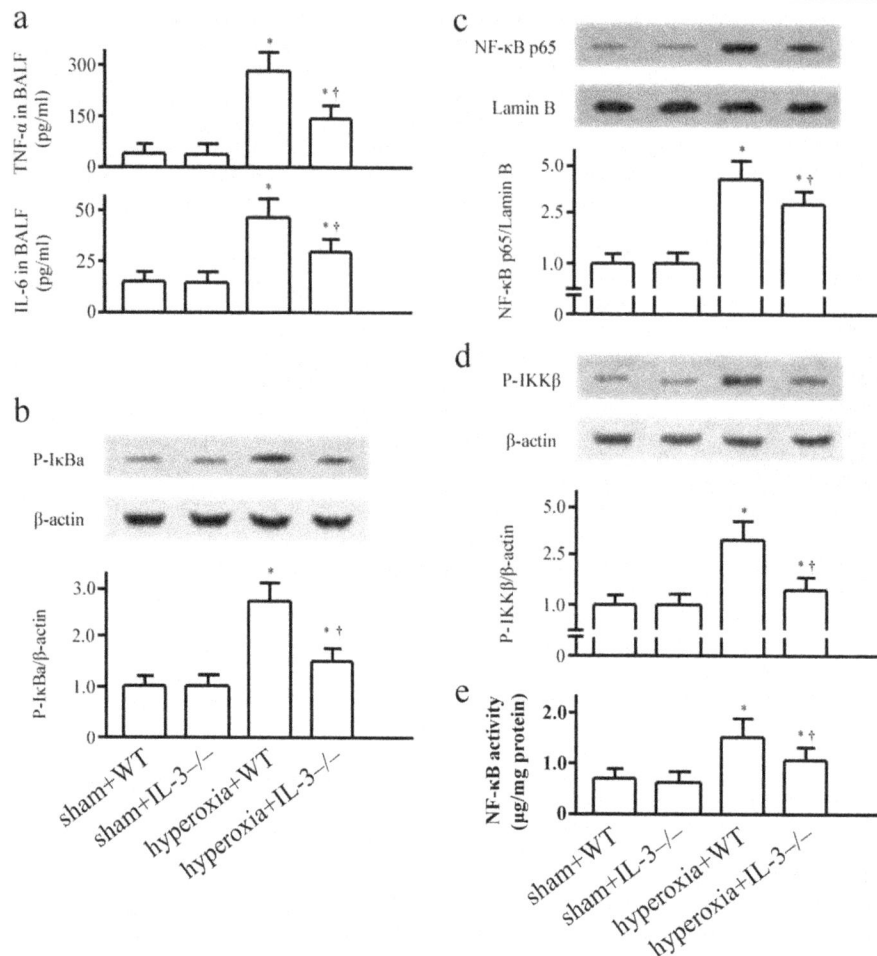

Fig. 3 Effect of IL-3 on proinflammatory mediators and nuclear factor (NF)-κB activation in mice. Tumor necrosis factor (TNF)-α and interleukin (IL)-6 (**a**) in bronchoalveolar lavage fluids (BALF), phosphorylated (p)-IκBα in the cytoplasm (**b**), nuclear factor (NF)-κB p65 in the nucleus (**c**), p-IκBα kinase (IKK) β (**d**), and NF-κB activity (**e**) in lung tissues were assessed 72 hours after hyperoxia or room air challenge by enzyme linked immunosorbent assay (ELISA) or western blotting. Data represent assessments in a minimum of n = 5 mice. *P <0.05 vs. sham+wild type (WT) group; † P <0.05 vs. hyperoxia+WT group. IL-3−/−, IL-3 gene disrupted mice

of IKK induces phosphorylation and degradation of IκB, leading to the nuclear translocation of NF-κB and transcriptional activation [15]. Our results showed that the IL-3 levels in the lung and plasma were significantly elevated in hyperoxia exposure group compared with sham. Meanwhile, the IKK/NF-κB pathway was activated by hyperoxia exposure. However, when the IL-3 gene was deleted in mice, the hyperoxia-induced the activation of IKK/NF-κB pathway and cytokine productions were dampened. Our results suggest that IL-3 is associated with the activation of IKK/NF-κB pathway. However, the precise mechanism responsible for the effect of IL-3 on the IKK/NF-κB pathway and cytokine productions warrants further investigation.

Overall, our data suggest that IL-3 and its receptor IL-3Rα are induced during hyperoxia-induced lung injury, and thus further mediate inflammation via IKK/NF-κB axis to promote proinflammatory cytokine production and elevate inflammation.

Conclusions

In summary, our findings show that IL-3 and IL-3Rα are stimulated in mice hyperoxia-induced ALI. Deletion of IL-3 reduced hyperoxia-induced ALI. Our results suggest IL-3 is a potential therapeutic target for hyperoxia-induced ALI.

Acknowledgments

We thank M.Y. Xiao and X. Chen for help with the lung histology evaluation. We thank M. Luo, Ph. D, C. Zhu and J. Lu for their help with the experiment. All authors have read and approved the manuscript.

Authors' contributions

ZJH, WZ and HWZ had full access to all of the data in the study and take responsibility for the integrity of the data and the accuracy of the data analysis. JY and FYS contributed to the coordination of the study and review of the manuscript. All authors read and approved the final manuscript.

Competing interests

The authors declare that they have no competing interests.

Author details

[1]Department of Emergency, Xia'men Traditional Chinese Medicine Hospital affiliated to Beijing University of Traditional Chinese Medicine, Xia'men, Fujian, China. [2]Department of Respiratory, Jiangning Hospital affiliated to Nanjing Medical University, Nanjing, Jiangsu, China. [3]Department of Intensive Care Unit, Xia'men Traditional Chinese Medicine Hospital affiliated to Beijing University of Traditional Chinese Medicine, No.1739 Xianyue Road, Xia'men 361009, Fujian, China.

References

1. Sweeney RM, McAuley DF. Acute respiratory distress syndrome. Lancet. 2016;388(10058):2416–30.
2. Leaver SK, Evans TW. Acute respiratory distress syndrome. Bmj. 2007; 335(7616):389–94.
3. Aschner Y, Zemans RL, Yamashita CM, Downey GP. Matrix metalloproteinases and protein tyrosine kinases: potential novel targets in acute lung injury and ARDS. Chest. 2014;146(4):1081–91.
4. Matthay MA, Idell S. Update on acute lung injury and critical care medicine 2009. Am J Respir Crit Care Med. 2010;181(10):1027–32.
5. Tao W, Li PS, Xu G, Luo Y, Shu YS, Tao YZ, Yang LQ. Soluble Epoxide Hydrolase Plays a Vital role In Angiotensin II-Induced Lung Injury in Mice. Shock (Augusta, Ga). 2017.
6. Tao W, Li PS, Yang LQ, Ma YB. Effects of a soluble epoxide hydrolase inhibitor on lipopolysaccharide-induced acute lung injury in mice. PLoS One. 2016;11(8):e0160359.
7. Wheeler AP, Bernard GR. Acute lung injury and the acute respiratory distress syndrome: a clinical review. Lancet. 2007;369(9572):1553–64.
8. Weber GF, Chousterman BG, He S, Fenn AM, Nairz M, Anzai A, Brenner T, Uhle F, Iwamoto Y, Robbins CS, et al. Interleukin-3 amplifies acute inflammation and is a potential therapeutic target in sepsis. Science. 2015; 347(6227):1260–5.
9. Gotts JE, Matthay MA. Sepsis: pathophysiology and clinical management. BMJ. 2016;353:i1585.
10. Meduri GU, Annane D, Chrousos GP, Marik PE, Sinclair SE. Activation and regulation of systemic inflammation in ARDS: rationale for prolonged glucocorticoid therapy. Chest. 2009;136(6):1631–43.
11. Tao W, Li PS, Shen Z, Shu YS, Liu S. Effects of omega-3 fatty acid nutrition on mortality in septic patients: a meta-analysis of randomized controlled trials. BMC Anesthesiol. 2016;16(1):39.
12. Wright JG, Christman JW. The role of nuclear factor kappa B in the pathogenesis of pulmonary diseases: implications for therapy. Am J Respir Med. 2003;2(3):211–9.
13. Masterson C, O'Toole D, Leo A, McHale P, Horie S, Devaney J, Laffey JG. Effects and mechanisms by which Hypercapnic acidosis inhibits Sepsis-induced canonical nuclear factor-kappaB signaling in the lung. Crit Care Med. 2016;44(4):e207–17.
14. Drube S, Weber F, Loschinski R, Beyer M, Rothe M, Rabenhorst A, Gopfert C, Meininger I, Diamanti MA, Stegner D, et al. Subthreshold IKK activation modulates the effector functions of primary mast cells and allows specific targeting of transformed mast cells. Oncotarget. 2015;6(7):5354–68.
15. Hinz M, Scheidereit C. The IkappaB kinase complex in NF-kappaB regulation and beyond. EMBO Rep. 2014;15(1):46–61.
16. Tao W, Shu YS, Miao QB, Zhu YB. Attenuation of hyperoxia-induced lung injury in rats by adrenomedullin. Inflammation. 2012;35(1):150–7.
17. Bachofen M, Weibel ER. Structural alterations of lung parenchyma in the adult respiratory distress syndrome. Clin Chest Med. 1982;3(1):35–56.
18. Schroeder JT, Chichester KL, Bieneman AP. Human basophils secrete IL-3: evidence of autocrine priming for phenotypic and functional responses in allergic disease. J Immunol. 2009;182(4):2432–8.
19. Hara T, Miyajima A. Function and signal transduction mediated by the interleukin 3 receptor system in hematopoiesis. Stem Cells. 1996;14(6):605–18.
20. Hapel AJ, Fung MC, Johnson RM, Young IG, Johnson G, Metcalf D. Biologic properties of molecularly cloned and expressed murine interleukin-3. Blood. 1985;65(6):1453–9.
21. Metcalf D, Begley CG, Johnson GR, Nicola NA, Lopez AF, Williamson DJ. Effects of purified bacterially synthesized murine multi-CSF (IL-3) on hematopoiesis in normal adult mice. Blood. 1986;68(1):46–57.
22. Williams GT, Smith CA, Spooncer E, Dexter TM, Taylor DR. Haemopoietic colony stimulating factors promote cell survival by suppressing apoptosis. Nature. 1990;343(6253):76–9.
23. Borriello F, Iannone R, Di Somma S, Loffredo S, Scamardella E, Galdiero MR, Varricchi G, Granata F, Portella G, Marone G. GM-CSF and IL-3 modulate human monocyte TNF-alpha production and renewal in in vitro models of trained immunity. Front Immunol. 2016;7:680.
24. Singha AK, Bhattacharjee B, Saha B, Maiti D. IL-3 and GM-CSF modulate functions of splenic macrophages in ENU induced leukemia. Cytokine. 2017; 91:89–95.

19

Survival after repeated surgery for lung cancer with idiopathic pulmonary fibrosis: a retrospective study

Seijiro Sato[1]*, Yuki Shimizu[1], Tatsuya Goto[1], Akihiko Kitahara[1], Terumoto Koike[1], Hiroyuki Ishikawa[2], Takehiro Watanabe[3] and Masanori Tsuchida[1]

Abstract

Background: Patients with idiopathic pulmonary fibrosis (IPF) have a high risk of developing lung cancer, but few studies have investigated the long-term outcomes of repeated surgery in such patients. The purpose of this study was to evaluate the surgical outcomes of repeated lung cancer surgery in patients with IPF.

Methods: From January 2001 to December 2015, 108 lung cancer patients with IPF underwent pulmonary resection at two institutions; 13 of these patients underwent repeated surgery for lung cancer, and their data were reviewed.

Results: The initial procedures of the 13 patients were lobectomy in 8, segmentectomy in 2, and wedge resection in 3. The subsequent procedures were wedge resection in 10 and segmentectomy in 3. The clinical stage of the second tumor was stage IA in 12 and stage IB in 1. Postoperatively, 3 patients (23.1%) developed acute exacerbation (AE) of IPF and died. The rate of decrease in percent vital capacity was significantly higher in patients with AE than in those without AE ($p = 0.011$). The 3-year overall survival rate was 34.6%. The causes of death were cancer-related in 7, AE of IPF in 3, and metachronous lung cancer in 1.

Conclusions: Despite limited resection, a high incidence of AE was identified. The early and long-term outcomes of repeated surgery in lung cancer patients with IPF were poor because of the high risk of AE of IPF and lung cancer recurrence. Long-term intensive surveillance will be required to determine whether surgical intervention is justified in patients with multiple primary lung cancers and IPF.

Keywords: Lung cancer, Idiopathic pulmonary fibrosis, Repeated surgery, Acute exacerbation, Percent vital capacity

Background

The incidence of lung cancer is higher in patients with idiopathic pulmonary fibrosis (IPF) than in the general population; the relative risk of lung cancer in such patients ranges from 6 to 17% [1, 2]. In the general population, the likelihood of a new primary lung cancer developing after complete resection for an initial lung cancer has been reported to be 1% to 2% per patient per year [3, 4]. On the other hand, in patients with IPF, the cumulative rate of developing lung cancer has been reported to increase as the duration of follow-up increased (3.3%, 15.4%, and 54.7% at 1, 5, and 10 years, respectively) [5].

Thoracic surgeons, as well as medical and radiation oncologists, must often make difficult decisions in treating lung cancer patients with IPF because of the poor prognosis of IPF itself and the complications, such as acute exacerbation (AE), which arise after each intervention [5–9]. Several previous studies demonstrated a median survival time of 2 to 3 years after diagnosis in patients with IPF [10–14]. Sato and colleagues [15] reported that 9.3% of lung cancer patients with IPF developed AE after pulmonary resection. To estimate the risk of surgery, they proposed a risk score using clinical characteristics and surgical procedures. However, repeated surgical intervention was not included as a risk factor. With regard to the outcome of surgical intervention,

---
* Correspondence: seisato@med.niigata-u.ac.jp
[1]Division of Thoracic and Cardiovascular Surgery, Niigata University Graduate School of Medical and Dental Sciences, 1-757 Asahimachi-dori, Chuo-ku, Niigata-shi, Niigata 951-8510, Japan
Full list of author information is available at the end of the article

several studies [9, 16, 17] reported 5-year survival rates of about 40% to 60% for stage I patients; therefore, surgical treatment for lung cancer with concomitant IPF might not be an absolute contraindication, as long as the patients are carefully selected. For lung cancer patients with IPF who undergo surgical interventions, many challenging problems, such as AE of IPF and high rates of second and third primary cancers, have been cited; however, to the best of our knowledge, there have been no studies focusing on the incidence of postoperative AE of IPF and the long-term outcome after a second pulmonary resection. Thus, the purpose of this study was to evaluate the outcomes and risks after a second pulmonary resection and to elucidate the implications of surgical interventions in lung cancer patients with IPF.

Methods

The medical records of all lung cancer patients admitted from 2001 to 2015 to the Division of Thoracic and Cardiovascular Surgery at Niigata University Hospital and the Department of Thoracic Surgery at Nishi-Niigata Chuo National Hospital were retrospectively reviewed; patients diagnosed with IPF before surgical treatment for lung cancer were identified. The eligibility criteria for surgical resection of lung cancer with IPF were: a resting partial pressure of arterial oxygen > 60 mmHg; predicted postoperative forced expiratory volume in 1 s > 1.0 L; clinically stable and symptomless IPF; and complete resection possible. Of a total of 108 patients enrolled in this study, 17 (15.7%) with IPF developed second primary lung cancers. Thirteen of these patients underwent a second pulmonary resection, 2 patients received radiotherapy, 1 patient received chemotherapy, and 1 patient had best supportive care. The institutional review board approved this study (Niigata University, 2302) and waived the requirement for informed consent because the study was a retrospective review.

Radiologic assessment of the preoperative conventional chest computed tomography (CT) or high-resolution CT (HRCT) of all patients was performed to confirm the following criteria for IPF: 1) CT patterns compatible with IPF, as proposed by the American Thoracic Society and the European Respiratory Society [18], with bilateral reticular opacities and/or honeycombing predominant in the peripheral, subpleural, and basal locations; and 2) absence of known causes of pulmonary fibrosis, such as hypersensitivity pneumonitis, pneumoconiosis, sarcoidosis, eosinophilic pneumonia, lymphangioleiomyomatosis, drug-induced lung disease, and collagen vascular disease. One thoracic radiologist (HI) and one thoracic surgeon (SS) who were blinded to the clinical data evaluated the preoperative chest CT scans.

The medical records were reviewed to obtain the: demographic and clinical characteristics; chest CT scan findings; pulmonary function test results, including percent vital capacity (%VC) and percent forced expiratory volume in one second (FEV1%); surgical procedure; histologic findings; morbidity within 30 days of surgery; postoperative AE of IPF; and survival. AE was defined as: 1) onset within 30 days after pulmonary resection; 2) increasing respiratory distress; 3) newly developed fibrosis, ground glass opacity, or infiltrates on chest radiograph; 4) decrease in the resting partial pressure of arterial oxygen > 10 mmHg; and 5) the absence of heart failure or infectious lung disease [19]. A recently reported scoring system was used to assess the 30-day risk of AE onset after pulmonary resection in lung cancer patients with interstitial lung disease (ILD) based on seven risk factors, including a history of AE of ILD, preoperative steroid use, elevated serum sialylated carbohydrate antigen, KL-6 level, surgical procedure, usual interstitial pneumonia (UIP) pattern on CT scan, male sex, and low %VC [15].

Pathologic cancer stage was determined using the 7th edition of the International Union Against Cancer tumor-node-metastasis staging system [20]. Information was obtained for all survivors, either during office visits or by telephone interviews with the patient or a relative. The criteria for the diagnosis of multiple primary lung cancers were those described by Martini and Melamed [21] in 1975: 1) different histology or 2) same histology, if the disease-free interval between the two lesions was at least 2 years or development of a new neoplasm from an in situ carcinoma and occurrence of the second tumor in a different lobe or lung, provided that extrapulmonary metastases and lymphatic involvement common to both tumors were excluded. Tumors were designated as 'synchronous' when detected or resected simultaneously and as 'metachronous' when the second tumor was found some time later.

Statistical analyses

The patients' characteristics are expressed as counts and proportions; categorical variables were compared using the chi-squared test or Fisher's exact test if there were 5 or fewer observations in a cohort. The Mann–Whitney U-test was used to compare quantitative parameters. Disease-free survival (DFS) was defined as the time from surgery to documented clinical progression or death. Overall survival (OS) was defined as the time from surgery to death. Prognosis was analyzed using the Kaplan–Meier method with the log-rank test. Differences were considered significant if the P-value was less than 0.05. All statistical analyses were performed using SPSS for Windows Version 22.0 (SPSS, Inc., Chicago, IL, USA).

Results

Patients' characteristics

A total of 108 patients were diagnosed as having IPF based on conventional CT or HRCT findings, and, of them, 17 developed second primary lung cancers. Thirteen patients underwent repeated surgery, and 4 patients did not. The characteristics of the 13 patients are shown in Table 1, and those of the 4 patients are in Additional file 1: Table S1. The median interval between the initial surgery and the second surgery was 2 months (range, 1–3 months) in synchronous tumors, and 26 months (range, 8–68 months) in metachronous tumors. The study group included 11 men and 2 women. The mean age of the patients at the second surgery was 71.6 ± 8.6 years (range, 55–80 years). Six patients had synchronous tumors, and 7 patients had metachronous tumors. A total of 11 of 13 patients (84.6%) were heavy smokers (≥30 pack years). The mean %VC was 104.4% ± 16.1% before the initial surgery and 76.4% ± 19.7% before the second surgery. Regarding the AE risk score [15], 9 patients had intermediate risk and 4 patients had low risk at the initial surgery, but only 2 patients had intermediate risk at the second surgery. During both perioperative periods, IPF prophylaxis, such as steroids, sivelestat sodium hydrate, pirfenidone, and so on, was not given.

Tumor location and type of surgical procedure

The location of the tumors was in the lower lobe in 9 patients at the initial surgery and in 8 patients at the second surgery. Of the 13 patients, 8 patients (61.5%) underwent lobectomy, 2 patients (15.4%) underwent segmentectomy, and 3 patients (23.1%) underwent wedge resection at the initial surgery. At the second surgery, 10 patients (76.9%) underwent wedge resection, and 3 patients (23.1%) underwent segmentectomy; none of the patients underwent lobectomy (Table 2).

Table 1 Characteristics of patients

Variable[a]	Total = 13
Age, years	
at initial surgery	70.2 ± 8.4
at second surgery	71.6 ± 8.6
Sex	
male	11
female	2
Time interval in months, median (range)	
synchronous	2 (1–3)
metachronous	26 (8–68)
Type of multiple cancers	
synchronous	6
metachronous	7
Smoking history	
PY < 30	2
PY ≥30	11
FEV1%, mean	
at initial surgery	79.2 ± 6.8
at second surgery	84.5 ± 7.7
%VC, mean	
at initial surgery	104.4 ± 16.1
at second surgery	76.4 ± 19.7
KL-6 (U/ml), mean	
at initial surgery	693.8 ± 318.4
at second surgery	706.8 ± 377.2
AE risk score (initial/second)	
Low risk/Low risk	3
Low risk/Intermediate risk	1
Intermediate risk/Low risk	8
Intermediate risk/Intermediate risk	1

[a]Categorical data are expressed as numbers, and continuous data are expressed as means ± standard deviation

PY pack years, FEV1 forced expiratory volume in 1 s, VC vital capacity, KL-6 sialylated carbohydrate antigen KL-6, AE acute exacerbation

Table 2 Location, surgical procedure, histology, and stage at initial and second surgeries

Variable	Initial No. (%)	Second No. (%)
Tumor location		
Upper	4 (30.8)	5 (38.5)
Lower	9 (69.2)	8 (61.5)
Surgical procedure		
Wedge	3 (23.1)	10 (76.9)
Segmentectomy	2 (15.4)	3 (23.1)
Lobectomy	8 (61.5)	0 (0)
Lymph node dissection		
None	3 (23.1)	12 (92.3)
Hilum	1 (7.7)	0 (0)
Mediastinum	9 (69.2)	1 (7.7)
Histology		
Ad	3 (23.1)	3 (23.1)
Sq	8 (61.5)	8 (61.5)
Ad-Sq	1 (7.7)	2 (15.4)
Sm	1 (7.7)	0 (0)
Pathological stage		
IA	3 (23.1)	4 (30.8)
IB	5 (38.5)	9 (69.2)
IIA	2 (15.4)	0 (0)
IIB	1 (7.7)	0 (0)
IIIA	2 (15.)	0 (0)

ND node dissection, Ad adenocarcinoma, Sq squamous cell carcinoma, Ad-Sq adenosquamous cell carcinoma, Sm small cell carcinoma

Histologic diagnoses and tumor staging

As shown in Table 2, squamous cell carcinoma was the most common finding at the initial and second surgeries ($n = 8$, 61.5%, for both). Both initial and second tumors were squamous cell carcinoma in 4 patients and adenocarcinoma in 1 patient.

The pathologic stage of the initial tumor was stage I in 8 patients (61.5%), stage II in 3 patients (23.1%), and stage IIIA in 2 patients (15.4%). Ten patients underwent lymph node dissection.

At the second surgery, the clinical stage of the second tumor was stage IA in 12 patients and stage IB in only 1 patient. However, the pathologic stage of the second tumor was stage IA in 4 patients and stage IB in 9 patients. In all 8 cases, the reason for upstaging from IA to IB was pleural invasion. However, 12 patients (92.3%) underwent only sublobar resection without lymph node dissection.

Postoperative acute exacerbation

At initial surgery, 6 (5.6%) of 108 patients developed postoperative AE of IPF (Fig. 1). Table 3 shows the patients who developed postoperative AE of IPF at the initial or second surgery. Comparing the 6 patients at the

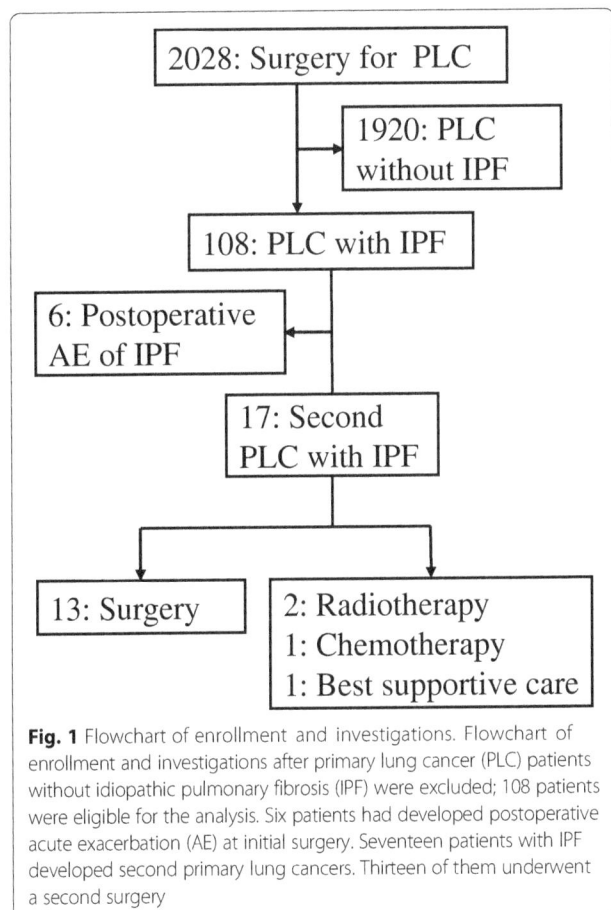

Fig. 1 Flowchart of enrollment and investigations. Flowchart of enrollment and investigations after primary lung cancer (PLC) patients without idiopathic pulmonary fibrosis (IPF) were excluded; 108 patients were eligible for the analysis. Six patients had developed postoperative acute exacerbation (AE) at initial surgery. Seventeen patients with IPF developed second primary lung cancers. Thirteen of them underwent a second surgery

Table 3 Clinical characteristics of patients with postoperative acute exacerbation after initial and second surgeries

Variable[a]	Initial $N = 6$	Second $N = 3$	p Value[b]
Age, years	71.3 ± 8.2	72.7 ± 8.4	1.000
Sex			
Male	6	3	NA
Female	0	0	
Smoking history (PY), mean	50.8 ± 8.3	78.7 ± 43.6	0.381
FEV1%, mean	81.9 ± 5.2	87.5 ± 11.2	0.393
%VC, mean	78.5 ± 9.8	64.4 ± 19.7	0.262
KL-6 (U/ml), mean	1204.4 ± 638.4	606.3 ± 279.2	0.143
AE risk score, mean	12.8 ± 1.2	9.0 ± 1.7	0.024
Low risk	0	2	
Intermediate risk	6	1	
Tumor location			
Upper	2	0	0.417
Lower	4	3	
Surgical procedure			
Wedge	0	1	0.333[c]
Segmentectomy	1	2	
Lobectomy	5	0	
Histology			
Ad	2	1	0.301
Sq	4	1	
Ad-Sq	0	1	
Pathological stage			
IA	0	1	0.392
IB	4	2	
IIA	1	0	
IIB	1	0	

[a]Categorical data are expressed as numbers, and continuous data are expressed as means ± standard deviation
[b]Values of $p < 0.05$ are significant
[c]Value is a comparison between wedge vs. segmentectomy and lobectomy
NA not available, *PY* pack year, *FEV1* forced expiratory volume in 1 s, *VC* vital capacity, *KL-6* sialylated carbohydrate antigen KL-6, *AE* acute exacerbation, *Ad* adenocarcinoma, *Sq* squamous cell carcinoma, *Ad-Sq* adenosquamous cell carcinoma

initial surgery and the 3 patients at the second surgery, the AE risk score was significantly lower for the second surgery cohort than for the initial surgery cohort ($p = 0.024$).

Comparison of the patients according to the presence or absence of postoperative AE of IPF at the second surgery is shown in Table 4. In this series, 3 patients developed and died of AE in the postoperative period (Table 5). The rate of %VC decrease was significantly higher in patients with AE than in patients without AE ($p = 0.011$). In all 3 patients with AE, tumor location was the lower lobe at the initial and second surgeries. On the

Table 4 Clinical characteristics of patients with and without acute exacerbation after the second surgery

Variable[a]	With AE (n = 3)	Without AE (n = 10)	p Value[b]
Sex			
Male	3	8	0.577
Female	0	2	
Type of multiple cancer			
Synchronous	1	5	0.563
Metachronous	2	5	
Smoking history			
PY < 30	0	2	0.577
PY ≥30	3	8	
FEV1%, mean	87.5 ± 11.2	83.3 ± 6.6	0.455
%VC, mean	64.4 ± 19.7	80.9 ± 19.0	0.234
Rate of %VC decrease from initial surgery, mean	35.9 ± 11.7	20.1 ± 5.6	0.011
KL-6 (U/ml), mean	596.3 ± 270.8	743.5 ± 413.8	0.583
AE risk score			
Low risk	2	9	0.423
Intermediate risk	1	1	
Combination of tumor location (initial/second)			
Lower/Lower	3	3	0.070
Other	0	7	
Combination of surgical procedure (initial/second)			
Wedge/Wedge	0	2	0.296
Lobectomy/Sublobar	3	5	
Other	0	3	

[a]Categorical data are expressed as numbers, and continuous data are expressed as means ± standard deviation
[b]Values of $p < 0.05$ are significant
AE acute exacerbation, PY pack years, FEV1 forced expiratory volume in 1 s, VC vital capacity, KL-6 sialylated carbohydrate antigen KL-6

other hand, development of AE was not significantly correlated with sex, types of multiple cancers, smoking history, KL-6, and combination of surgical procedures. Regarding the AE risk score that was proposed by Sato and colleagues at the second surgery [15], there was no significant difference between patients with and without AE. The risk of developing AE after the second surgery was low in 2 of 11 (18.2%) patients and intermediate in 1 of 2 (50%) patients. Over the same time period, the development of AE of IPF in 4 patients who did not undergo surgical treatment for second primary lung cancer was investigated, and it was found that no patients developed AE of IPF.

Survival

The median follow-up period after the second surgery was 24.9 months (range, 1.5–54.0 months). The disease-free survival (DFS) rates were 60.6% at 1 year and 8.7% at

3 years (Fig. 2a). Overall survival (OS) was 69.2% at 1 year and 34.6% at 3 years (Fig. 2b). Regarding the pattern of lung cancer recurrence in 8 patients, 4 patients developed intrathoracic disease (local), and 4 patients developed extrathoracic spread (distant). During the follow-up period, 11 patients (84.6%) died, and the most common cause was cancer-related; 7 patients died of recurrent lung cancer, and 1 patient died of additional metachronous lung cancer. The 3 other patients died of AE of IPF. Only 2 patients remained alive; one was free of relapse, while the other had local recurrence. Adjuvant therapy with oral tegafur-uracil after the second surgery was administered in 1 patient with stage IB adenocarcinoma.

Discussion

The incidence of lung cancer is higher in patients with IPF than in those without IPF. Notably, Fujimoto and colleagues [22] reported a high incidence of second primary lung cancer in patients with IPF.

Lung cancer patients with IPF are more likely to develop severe morbidity and have poor outcomes after pulmonary resection. Considering the high recurrence rate and the poor prognosis for this patient population, operative indicators for major pulmonary resection in patients with lung cancer with IPF remain unclear. Kushibe and colleagues [23] reported that patients with IPF who had postoperative acute lung injury/acute respiratory distress syndrome had a significantly lower preoperative percent forced VC (%FVC) than those without such complications. IPF patients with a preoperative %FVC < 80% may not have an operative indication for lung cancer, and those with a preoperative %FVC ≥90% could have a good operative indication. Fujimoto and colleagues [22] suggested that patients with lung cancer invading the chest wall were excluded from surgery because chest wall resection is associated with major morbidity [24]. Pneumonectomy should be avoided for the same reason.

There have been several reports on the surgical outcomes of lung cancer patients with IPF [1, 7, 9, 15–17, 22, 23, 25]; however, to the best of our knowledge, the implications of repeated surgery in such patients have not been reported. The present study found a poor prognosis for patients with IPF even after complete repeated resection of lung cancer, with 3-year DFS and OS rates of 8.7% and 34.6%, respectively.

Recently, a large cohort study by Sato and colleagues [15] reported their derived scoring system for the 30-day risk of developing AE of IPF after pulmonary resection and classified patients into three risk groups (i.e., low, intermediate, and high). In the present study, higher rates of developing postoperative AE were found than cited in the previous report. According to Sato and colleagues, the predicted AE

Table 5 Clinical characteristics of patients with acute exacerbation after the second surgery

Variable	Case 1	Case 2	Case 3
Sex	Male	Male	Male
Age (years)	77	78	63
Time interval (months)	34	14	3
Type of multiple cancer	Metachronous	Metachronous	Synchronous
Smoking history (PY)	54	53	129
%VC at second surgery	87.1	52.6	53.4
Rate of %VC decrease	24.3	47.6	35.7
KL-6 (U/ml)	284	766	739
AE risk score	11	8	8
Tumor location (initial/second)	Lower/Lower	Lower/Lower	Lower/Lower
Surgical procedure (initial/second)	Lobectomy/Segmentectomy	Lobectomy/Wedge	Lobectomy/Wedge
Histology (initial/second)	Sq/Ad	Sq/Ad-Sq	Sq/Sq
Pathological stage	IA/IB	IB/IB	IA/IA

PY pack years, *VC* vital capacity, *KL-6* sialylated carbohydrate antigen KL-6, *AE* acute exacerbation, *Sq* squamous cell carcinoma, *Ad-Sq* adenosquamous cell carcinoma

incidence was < 10% [95% confidence interval (CI): 0–10] in the low risk group and 10–25% (95% CI: 8.8–29.7) in the intermediate risk group, though 2 of 11 (18.2%) patients at low risk and 1 of 2 (50%) patients at intermediate risk developed and died of AE in the present study. The patients who developed postoperative AE at the initial surgery were compared with those who developed postoperative AE at the second surgery, and AE in the second surgery cohort developed with a significantly lower risk score than in the initial surgery cohort. The patients who did not undergo surgical treatment for second primary lung cancers were also examined, and no patients developed AE of IPF. Although the present study sample was very small, repeated surgery for lung cancer in patients with IPF could be a risk factor for AE.

The etiologic agents of AE of IPF after pulmonary resection remain unclear. Sakamoto and colleagues [26] reported the possible factors contributing to AE after surgery in patients with IPF: 1) high activity of the disease prior to the surgery; 2) oxygen supplementation at a high concentration during surgery; 3) surgical stress including mechanical ventilation-related lung injury; 4) complicating respiratory infections; 5) postoperative reduction of steroid dose; and 6) medications (anesthesia, anticancer drugs, and so on). Misthos and colleagues [27] investigated the possibility of an association between oxygen radical toxicity and the occurrence of AE of IPF. They found the following: 1) lung re-expansion after one-lung ventilation (OLV) provoked severe oxidative stress; 2) the degree of oxygen-derived free radicals

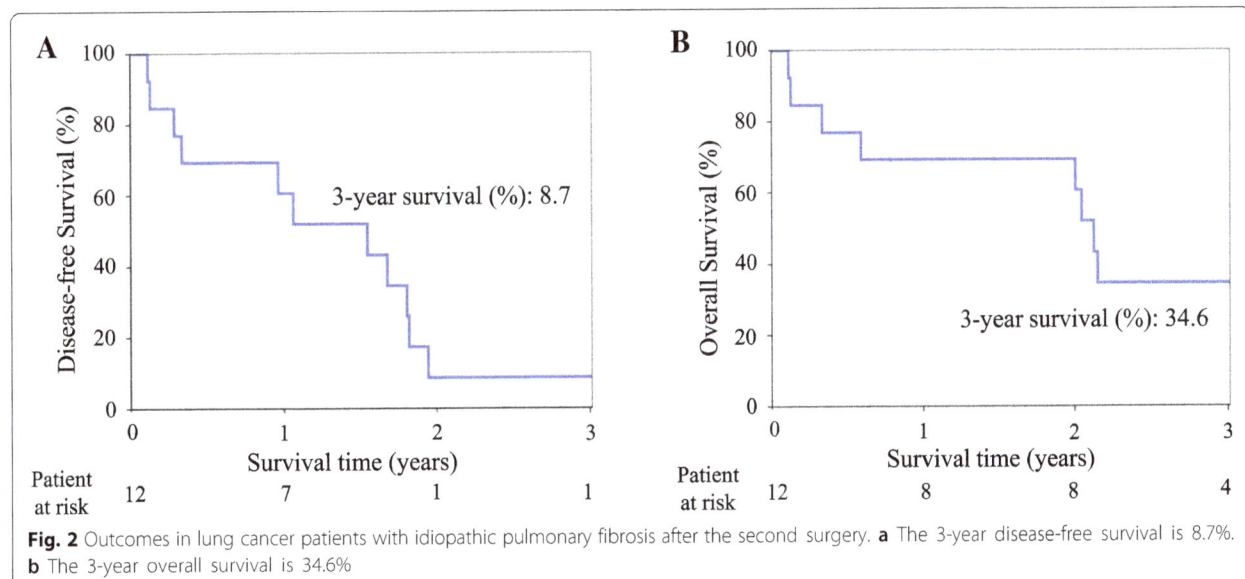

Fig. 2 Outcomes in lung cancer patients with idiopathic pulmonary fibrosis after the second surgery. **a** The 3-year disease-free survival is 8.7%. **b** The 3-year overall survival is 34.6%

generated was associated with the duration of OLV; 3) patients with lung cancer had higher production of oxygen-derived free radicals than the normal population; 4) tumor resection removes a large oxidative burden from the organism; 5) mechanical ventilation and surgical trauma are weak free radical generators; and 6) manipulated lung tissue is also a source of oxygen-derived free radicals, not only intraoperatively, but also for several hours later.

The present analysis showed that the rate of %VC decrease was significantly higher in patients with AE than in those without AE. %VC has been considered a reliable marker of fibrotic change [11, 13], and some previous studies [23, 25] reported that %VC had a significant and independent association with the development of AE. In the present study, the %VC of 1 patient with AE was not lower than 80%, but the rate of %VC decrease was 24.3%. Therefore, the AE incidence at the second surgery for lung cancer in patients with IPF is associated not only with a low %VC, but also with a high rate of %VC decrease. Also, among the pulmonary function tests, %DLCO has been considered a survival predictor [7, 28] and a reliable indicator of fibrotic change [12, 13, 29]. However, it was not included in the present study because the values of only 3 of 13 patients were available.

In the present study, the reason for the poor prognosis was a high rate of cancer recurrence, aside from development of AE. Although all patients were clinical stage IA or IB at the second surgery, 8 of 10 patients had cancer recurrence, except those who died of AE. Saito and colleagues [16] reported that the 5-year survival of lung cancer stage IA patients with IPF was 54.2%. Watanabe and colleagues [9] reported a 5-year survival of 61.6% after pulmonary resection for patients with stage I. Sato and colleagues [17] reported that the 5-year survival rates were 59% and 42% for pathologic stages IA and IB, respectively. Watanabe and colleagues [9] and Okamoto and colleagues [7] suggested that the frequency of cancer recurrence was higher in patients with IPF than in those without. Sato and colleagues [17] reported that recurrence was the main cause of death and posed a risk that was about twice as high as that of respiratory disorders; they underscored the importance of oncologic control for survival. In the present study, sublobar resection was performed in all patients, and lymph node dissection was performed in only 1 patient at the second surgery. Sato and colleagues [17] noted that stage IA patients who underwent wedge resection had a prolonged survival and were less likely to develop AE of IPF, but they had a higher cancer recurrence rate than patients who underwent lobectomy. Furthermore, patients who underwent segmentectomy had less favorable oncologic outcomes than patients who underwent lobectomy. At the second surgery, accurate pathologic staging might not be possible because lymph node dissection was not performed in almost all patients. Needless to say, it was necessary to consider the

influence of lung cancer recurrence not only in the second surgery, but also at the initial surgery. Actually, of the 5 of 8 patients who developed recurrence, 3 were stage II and 2 were stage III at the time of the initial surgery.

With regard to distinguishing multiple primary lung cancers from primary lung cancer with intrapulmonary metastasis, the possible effects of multiple lung tumors, as defined by Martini and Melamed [21], were considered. Although it is important to distinguish a second primary cancer from local recurrence or metastatic disease, this is sometimes difficult and even impossible. Girard and colleagues [30] considered that biologic examinations could be performed, assuming that the independent tumor clones harbor distinct mutations. In the present study, the same histologic diagnoses at the initial and second surgeries were seen in 4 patients with squamous cell carcinoma and in 1 patient with adenocarcinoma. Among them, 2 patients with squamous cell carcinoma and the patient with adenocarcinoma were investigated, but they were negative for epidermal growth factor receptor mutation at both the initial and second surgeries.

Squamous cell carcinoma had a higher prevalence than the other histopathological types among the patients with IPF in the present study, consistent with the previous reports. The cause of the high prevalence of squamous cell carcinoma in IPF patients remains unclear. Song and colleagues [31] found many foci of squamous metaplasia in honeycombing epithelium, and Hironaka and Fukuyama [32] reported that IPF patients with lung cancer showed more frequent foci of squamous metaplasia than IPF patients without lung cancer. Calabrese and colleagues [33] reported the overexpression of squamous cell antigen, a serine protease inhibitor typically expressed by dysplastic and neoplastic cells of epithelial origin, more often in squamous cell tumors, in IPF. These pathological findings support the notion that IPF may be a precursor to the development of squamous cell carcinoma.

Limitations

The present study had some limitations. First, only 3 patients developed AE of IPF at the second surgery; this number could be insufficient to predict the tendency for developing AE. Second, the present study included only IPF patients who underwent surgical procedures for multiple primary lung cancers and did not include IPF patients with multiple primary lung cancers who did not undergo surgical intervention. Therefore, the implications of a second surgery for lung cancer patients with IPF remain unclear. Third, this was a retrospective, two-institution study with a limited sample size. Further studies should be conducted to identify who among the patients with IPF who had undergone a first pulmonary resection for lung cancer could benefit from interventions, including surgery, chemotherapy, and radiotherapy, for the multiple primary lung cancers.

Conclusions

Postoperative development of AE and the long-term survival of patients with a second primary lung cancer with IPF who underwent repeated surgery were investigated. The main cause of their poor prognosis was cancer death, possibly related to sublobar resection. Repeated surgery for patients with lung cancer and concomitant IPF could increase the risk of AE development despite limited surgery. The rate of %VC decrease might be correlated with the incidence of AE. Although these results demonstrated that surgical intervention for multiple primary lung cancers might be contraindicated in patients with IPF, selection of patients who may benefit from such treatment is very important. To confirm these findings, a large, long-term, multi-center surveillance study will be required.

Authors' contributions

SS: contributed to development of the study concept, data collection, data analysis, manuscript drafting including revision, and final manuscript approval. YS, TG, AK, TK, and TW: contributed to performing data collection, data analysis, and final manuscript approval. HI and SS: contributed to the analysis of the CT examination findings. TM: contributed to development of the study concept, data analysis, manuscript drafting including revision, and final manuscript approval. All authors read and approved the final manuscript.

Competing interests

The authors declare that they have no competing interests.

Author details

[1]Division of Thoracic and Cardiovascular Surgery, Niigata University Graduate School of Medical and Dental Sciences, 1-757 Asahimachi-dori, Chuo-ku, Niigata-shi, Niigata 951-8510, Japan. [2]Department of Radiology and Radiation Oncology, Niigata University Graduate School of Medical and Dental Sciences, Niigata, Japan. [3]Department of Thoracic Surgery, National Hospital Organization Nishi-Niigata Chuo National Hospital, Niigata, Japan.

References

1. Kumar P, Goldstraw P, Yamada K, Nicholson AG, Wells AU, Hansell DM, Dubois RM, Ladas G. Pulmonary fibrosis and lung cancer: risk and benefit analysis of pulmonary resection. J Thorac Cardiovasc Surg. 2003;125(6):1321–7.
2. Raghu G, Nyberg F, Morgan G. The epidemiology of interstitial lung disease and its association with lung cancer. Br J Cancer. 2004;91(Suppl 2):S3–10.
3. Johnson BE. Second lung cancers in patients after treatment for an initial lung cancer. J Natl Cancer Inst. 1998;90(18):1335–45.
4. Rubins J, Unger M, Colice GL, American College of Chest P. Follow-up and surveillance of the lung cancer patient following curative intent therapy: ACCP evidence-based clinical practice guideline (2nd edition). Chest. 2007; 132(3 Suppl):355S–67S.
5. Ozawa Y, Suda T, Naito T, Enomoto N, Hashimoto D, Fujisawa T, Nakamura Y, Inui N, Nakamura H, Chida K. Cumulative incidence of and predictive factors for lung cancer in IPF. Respirology. 2009;14(5):723–8.
6. Isobe K, Hata Y, Sakamoto S, Takai Y, Shibuya K, Homma S. Clinical characteristics of acute respiratory deterioration in pulmonary fibrosis associated with lung cancer following anti-cancer therapy. Respirology. 2010;15(1):88–92.
7. Okamoto T, Gotoh M, Masuya D, Nakashima T, Liu D, Kameyama K, Ishikawa S, Yamamoto Y, Huang CL, Yokomise H. Clinical analysis of interstitial pneumonia after surgery for lung cancer. Jpn J Thorac Cardiovasc Surg. 2004;52(7):323–9.
8. Turner-Warwick M, Lebowitz M, Burrows B, Johnson A. Cryptogenic fibrosing alveolitis and lung cancer. Thorax. 1980;35(7):496–9.
9. Watanabe A, Higami T, Ohori S, Koyanagi T, Nakashima S, Mawatari T. Is lung cancer resection indicated in patients with idiopathic pulmonary fibrosis? J Thorac Cardiovasc Surg. 2008;136(5):1357–63. 1363 e1351–1352
10. Bjoraker JA, Ryu JH, Edwin MK, Myers JL, Tazelaar HD, Schroeder DR, Offord KP. Prognostic significance of histopathologic subsets in idiopathic pulmonary fibrosis. Am J Respir Crit Care Med. 1998;157(1):199–203.
11. Ley B, Collard HR, King TE Jr. Clinical course and prediction of survival in idiopathic pulmonary fibrosis. Am J Respir Crit Care Med. 2011;183(4):431–40.
12. Nicholson AG, Colby TV, du Bois RM, Hansell DM, Wells AU. The prognostic significance of the histologic pattern of interstitial pneumonia in patients presenting with the clinical entity of cryptogenic fibrosing alveolitis. Am J Respir Crit Care Med. 2000;162(6):2213–7.
13. Raghu G, Collard HR, Egan JJ, Martinez FJ, Behr J, Brown KK, Colby TV, Cordier JF, Flaherty KR, Lasky JA, et al. An official ATS/ERS/JRS/ALAT statement: idiopathic pulmonary fibrosis: evidence-based guidelines for diagnosis and management. Am J Respir Crit Care Med. 2011;183(6):788–824.
14. Rudd RM, Prescott RJ, Chalmers JC, Johnston ID, Fibrosing Alveolitis Subcommittee of the Research Committee of the British thoracic S. British Thoracic Society study on cryptogenic fibrosing alveolitis: response to treatment and survival. Thorax. 2007;62(1):62–6.
15. Sato T, Teramukai S, Kondo H, Watanabe A, Ebina M, Kishi K, Fujii Y, Mitsudomi T, Yoshimura M, Maniwa T, et al. Impact and predictors of acute exacerbation of interstitial lung diseases after pulmonary resection for lung cancer. J Thorac Cardiovasc Surg. 2014;147(5):1604–11. e1603
16. Saito Y, Kawai Y, Takahashi N, Ikeya T, Murai K, Kawabata Y, Hoshi E. Survival after surgery for pathologic stage IA non-small cell lung cancer associated with idiopathic pulmonary fibrosis. Ann Thorac Surg. 2011;92(5):1812–7.
17. Sato T, Watanabe A, Kondo H, Kanzaki M, Okubo K, Yokoi K, Matsumoto K, Marutsuka T, Shinohara H, Teramukai S, et al. Long-term results and predictors of survival after surgical resection of patients with lung cancer and interstitial lung diseases. J Thorac Cardiovasc Surg. 2015;149(1):64–9. 70 e61–62
18. American Thoracic S, European Respiratory S. American Thoracic Society/ European Respiratory Society international multidisciplinary consensus classification of the idiopathic interstitial pneumonias. This joint statement of the American Thoracic Society (ATS), and the European Respiratory Society (ERS) was adopted by the ATS board of directors, June 2001 and by the ERS executive committee, June 2001. Am J Respir Crit Care Med. 2002; 165(2):277–304.
19. Akira M, Hamada H, Sakatani M, Kobayashi C, Nishioka M, Yamamoto S. CT findings during phase of accelerated deterioration in patients with idiopathic pulmonary fibrosis. AJR Am J Roentgenol. 1997;168(1):79–83.
20. Goldstraw P, Crowley J, Chansky K, Giroux DJ, Groome PA, Rami-Porta R, Postmus PE, Rusch V, Sobin L, International Association for the Study of Lung Cancer international staging C, et al. The IASLC lung Cancer staging project: proposals for the revision of the TNM stage groupings in the forthcoming (seventh) edition of the TNM classification of malignant tumours. J Thorac Oncol. 2007;2(8):706–14.
21. Martini N, Melamed MR. Multiple primary lung cancers. J Thorac Cardiovasc Surg. 1975;70(4):606–12.
22. Fujimoto T, Okazaki T, Matsukura T, Hanawa T, Yamashita N, Nishimura K, Kuwabara M, Matsubara Y. Operation for lung cancer in patients with idiopathic pulmonary fibrosis: surgical contraindication? Ann Thorac Surg. 2003;76(5):1674–8. discussion 1679
23. Kushibe K, Kawaguchi T, Takahama M, Kimura M, Tojo T, Taniguchi S. Operative indications for lung cancer with idiopathic pulmonary fibrosis. Thorac Cardiovasc Surg. 2007;55(8):505–8.
24. Burkhart HM, Allen MS, Nichols FC 3rd, Deschamps C, Miller DL, Trastek VF, Pairolero PC. Results of en bloc resection for bronchogenic carcinoma with chest wall invasion. J Thorac Cardiovasc Surg. 2002;123(4):670–5.
25. Shintani Y, Ohta M, Iwasaki T, Ikeda N, Tomita E, Kawahara K, Ohno Y. Predictive factors for postoperative acute exacerbation of interstitial pneumonia combined with lung cancer. Gen Thorac Cardiovasc Surg. 2010;58(4):182–5.
26. Sakamoto S, Homma S, Mun M, Fujii T, Kurosaki A, Yoshimura K. Acute exacerbation of idiopathic interstitial pneumonia following lung surgery in 3 of 68 consecutive patients: a retrospective study. Intern Med. 2011; 50(2):77–85.
28. Ferguson MK, Reeder LB, Mick R. Optimizing selection of patients for major lung resection. J Thorac Cardiovasc Surg. 1995;109(2):275–81. discussion 281–273

29. Cherniack RM, Colby TV, Flint A, Thurlbeck WM, Waldron JA Jr, Ackerson L, Schwarz MI, King TE Jr. Correlation of structure and function in idiopathic pulmonary fibrosis. Am J Respir Crit Care Med. 1995;151(4):1180–8.

30. Girard N, Deshpande C, Azzoli CG, Rusch VW, Travis WD, Ladanyi M, Pao W. Use of epidermal growth factor receptor/Kirsten rat sarcoma 2 viral oncogene homolog mutation testing to define clonal relationships among multiple lung adenocarcinomas: comparison with clinical guidelines. Chest. 2010;137(1):46–52.

31. Song DH, Choi IH, Ha SY, Han KM, Lee JJ, Hong ME, Jeon K, Chung MP, Kim J, Han J. Usual interstitial pneumonia with lung cancer: clinicopathological analysis of 43 cases. Korean J Pathol. 2014;48(1):10–6.

32. Hironaka M, Fukayama M. Pulmonary fibrosis and lung carcinoma: a comparative study of metaplastic epithelia in honeycombed areas of usual interstitial pneumonia with or without lung carcinoma. Pathol Int. 1999;49(12): 1060–6.

33. Calabrese F, Lunardi F, Giacometti C, Marulli G, Gnoato M, Pontisso P, Saetta M, Valente M, Rea F, Perissinotto E, et al. Overexpression of squamous cell carcinoma antigen in idiopathic pulmonary fibrosis: clinicopathological correlations. Thorax. 2008;63(9):795–802.

20

Acute effects of ambient air pollution on outpatient children with respiratory diseases in Shijiazhuang, China

Jie Song[1,2*], Mengxue Lu[3], Liheng Zheng[4], Yue Liu[5], Pengwei Xu[1], Yuchun Li[1], Dongqun Xu[5] and Weidong Wu[1,2]

Abstract

Background: Associations between ambient air pollution and child health outcomes have been well documented in developed countries such as the United States; however, only a limited number of studies have been conducted in developing countries. This study aimed to explore the acute effects of five ambient air pollutants (inhalable particles [PM_{10}], fine particles [$PM_{2.5}$], sulfur dioxide [SO_2], nitrogen dioxide [NO_2] and 0zone [O_3]) on children hospital outpatients with respiratory diseases in Shijiazhuang, China.

Methods: Three years (2013–2015) of daily data, including cause-specific respiratory outpatient records and the concentrations of five air pollutants, were collected to examine the short-term association between air pollution and children's respiratory diseases; using a quasi-Poisson regression generalized additive model. Stratified analyses by season and age were also performed.

Results: From 2013 to 2015, a total of 551,678 hospital outpatient records for children with respiratory diseases were collected in Shijiazhuang, China. A 10 μg/m³ increase in a two-day average concentration (lag01) of NO_2, $PM_{2.5}$, and SO_2 corresponded to an increase of 0.66% (95% confidence interval [CI]: 0.30–1.03%), 0.13% (95% CI: 0.02–0.24%), and 0.33% (95% CI: 0.10–0.56%) in daily hospital outpatient visits for children with respiratory diseases, respectively. The effects were stronger in the transition season (April, May, September and October) than in other seasons (the hot season [June to August] and the cool season [November to March]). Furthermore, results indicated a generally stronger association in older (7–14 years of age) than younger children (< 7 years of age).

Conclusions: This research found a significant association between ambient NO_2, $PM_{2.5}$, and SO_2 levels and hospital outpatient visits in child with respiratory diseases in Shijiazhuang, China.

Keywords: Air pollution, Respiratory disease, Children, Outpatients, Time-series study

Background

Many epidemiological studies have reported that exposure to air pollution is associated with an increased risk for cardiovascular and respiratory diseases [1–5], even at concentrations less than the current health-based guidelines [6–8]. The Global Burden of Disease study identified air pollution as a leading cause of global disease burden, especially in developing countries [9, 10]. Lelieveld reported that ambient air pollution leads to more than 3 million

premature deaths globally each year, and that China had the most premature deaths (1.36 million) [11].

As a result of rapid industrialization and urbanization in the past two decades, China is experiencing one of its worst air pollution situations. In the first quarter of 2013, China experienced extremely severe and persistent haze pollution, affecting an area > 1.3 million km² and approximately 800 million individuals [12]. The annual average particulate matter < 2.5 μm in aerodynamic diameter ($PM_{2.5}$) and particulate matter < 10 μm in aerodynamic diameter (PM_{10}) concentrations were 141 μg/m³ and 303 μg/m³, respectively [13]. Shijiazhuang has been listed as the second-worst polluted city, with record-breaking daily average concentrations on January 12, 2013, of

* Correspondence: songjie231@126.com
[1]School of Public Health, Xinxiang Medical University, Xinxiang 453003, China
[2]Henan International Collaborative Laboratory for Health Effects and Intervention of Air Pollution, Xinxiang 453003, China
Full list of author information is available at the end of the article

771 µg/m^3 of fine particles (PM$_{2.5}$) and 800 µg/m^3 of inhalable particles (PM$_{10}$). However, only a limited number of studies have investigated the health effects of such levels of air pollution.

It has been established that children are vulnerable to the effects of air pollution [14, 15]. Evidence suggests that ambient air pollution has the potential to increase the severity of respiratory diseases, particularly in children. Nhung [16] observed that all ambient air pollutants (PM$_{2.5}$, PM$_{10}$, PM$_1$, SO$_2$, NO$_2$, NO$_x$, O$_3$, and CO) were positively associated with pneumonia hospitalizations in children. Statistically significant associations were observed for most pollutants, except for O$_3$ and SO$_2$. Moreover, stronger associations were observed in infants than in older children [16]. Another study found that four pollutants (PM$_{2.5}$, PM$_{10}$, NO$_2$, and SO$_2$) were significantly associated with hospital visits for acute upper and lower respiratory infections. A time-series analyses from Shanghai (China) found that an increase of 2.49 µg/m^3 in black carbon was associated with a 7% (95% CI: 5–8%) increase in asthma admission [17]. Moreover, contrary to the study by Nhung, stronger associations were observed among older children [17]. Another study from China also found stronger associations in older children [18]. Despite mounting literature suggesting that air pollution may be associated with respiratory disease in children, information regarding the association remains limited. It is important, therefore, to determine the reasons for these inconsistent data, and to study the exact respiratory effects of air pollution on children, particularly in severely polluted cities.

In the present study, we conducted a time-series study to investigate the association between five ambient air pollutants (PM$_{2.5}$, PM$_{10}$, sulphur dioxide [SO$_2$], nitrogen dioxide [NO$_2$] and Ozone [O$_3$]) and child respiratory outpatients in children in Shijiazhuang, China.

Methods

Shijiazhuang, the capital of Hebei province, comprises eight urban and suburban districts, with a total area of 2206 km^2 and a population of 4.55 million at the end of 2013. The study area was limited to the traditional four urban districts (469 km^2). Approximately 2.19 million permanent residents include 0.31 million children (< 15 years of age) residing in these four districts in 2015.

Hospital outpatient data

The Children's Hospital of Hebei Province is the sole paediatric hospital in Shijiazhuang. Daily hospital outpatient visit data from January 1, 2013 to December 31, 2015 were collected from a database located at this hospital. All disease diagnoses were completed by computer coders. To validate health data, duplicate records were deleted and International Classification of Diseases, 10th Revision (ICD-10) codes were re-matched as reported in the authors' previous research using MySQL server (version 5.6.26) [19]. The data cleaning strategy is described in Fig. 1. When there was a difference between the newly matched and original codes, this record would be picked up and discussed by a doctor's team. Some errors, such as the wrong word, acronym or non-standard name, in the

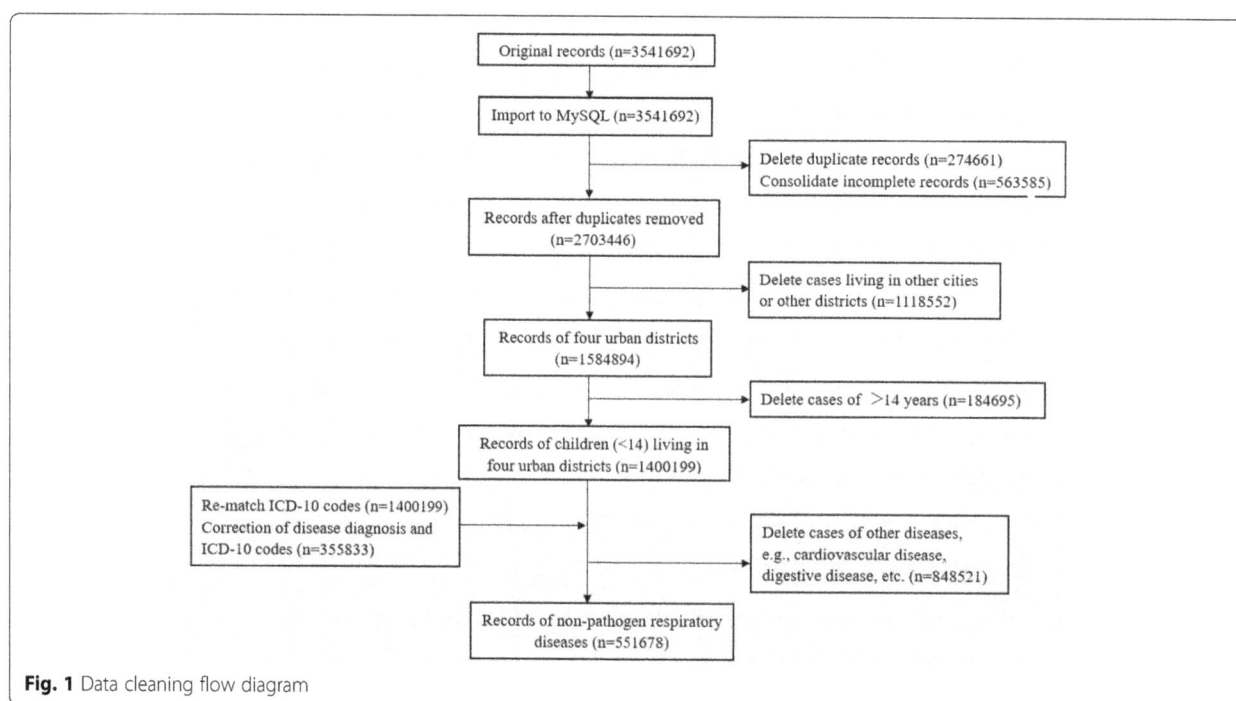

Fig. 1 Data cleaning flow diagram

disease diagnosis would be changed to standard names and subsequently re-matched to an accurate ICD-10 code.

The respiratory outpatients' data (ICD-10 codes J00-J99) were selected and targeted in the database. Patients residing outside of the four urban districts and those >14 years of age were excluded from the analysis. Outpatient visits caused by infection, suppuration, or ulceration were also excluded from this study. Finally, hospital respiratory outpatients' visits (ICD-10 codes J00-J99, excluding pathogenic infections, abscess, suppuration, gangrenous and ulcerative diseases) and six specific or classified diseases (acute upper respiratory infections, ICD-10 codes J02-J06; pneumonia, J18; other acute lower respiratory infection, J20-J22; other diseases of upper respiratory tract, J30-J39; chronic lower respiratory diseases, J40-J47; and other respiratory diseases, J60-J99) were identified as health outcomes.

Air pollution and meteorological data

Daily air pollution data, including $PM_{2.5}$, PM_{10}, SO_2, NO_2 and O_3, were obtained from the website of China's National Urban Air Quality Real Time Publishing Platform (http://106.37.208.233:20035/). The platform is administered by China's Ministry of Environmental Protection. Hourly concentrations of each pollutant were measured from seven fixed site stations distributed in the four urban districts. These stations are mandated to be located away from major roads, industrial sources, buildings, and residential sources of emission from the burning of coal, oil or waste. This ensures that monitoring results reflect the urban air pollution level in the city rather than local sources of traffic or industrial combustion. The methods were based on the tapered element oscillating microbalance, ultraviolet fluorescence, chemiluminescence, ultraviolet fluorescence were used to measure PM ($PM_{2.5}$ and PM_{10}), SO_2, NO_2, and O_3, respectively. For $PM_{2.5}$, PM_{10}, SO_2, and NO_2, daily concentrations were represented 24 h averages, and the O_3 concentration was the maximal 8 h average from all valid monitoring sites in this study.

Daily mean temperature and humidity data were retrieved to adjust the effects of weather on hospital outpatients. Meteorological data were measured at a fixed site station and obtained from the Meteorological Bureau of Shijiazhuang.

Statistical analysis

Time-series analysis is a regular analytic method to explore the acute effects of air pollution based on the daily aggregate date, and can control for both time-invariant and time-varying confounders by design [20].

The statistical analysis used a generalized additive model (GAM) to analyse the data. Because daily hospital visits typically followed an over-dispersed Poisson distribution, quasi-Poisson regression was used in the GAM [21]. Several covariates, including natural splines, were introduced to control for their potential confounding effects. First, a natural cubic regression smoothing function of calendar time with 7 degrees of freedom (df) per year excluded unmeasured long-term and seasonal trends longer than two months [20]. Second, a natural smooth functions of the mean temperature (6 df) and relative humidity (3 df) controlled for the nonlinear confounding effects of weather conditions [20]. Third, indicator variables were implemented for "day of the week" and public holidays. Briefly, the following log-linear GAM was fit to obtain the estimated pollution log-relative rate β in the selected city:

$$logE(Y_t) = \beta Z_t + DOW + ns(time, df)$$
$$+ ns(temperature, 6)$$
$$+ ns(humidity, 3) + intercept,$$

in which $E(Y_t)$ represents the expected number of respiratory disease outpatients at day t; β represents the log-related rate of respiratory diseases associated with a unit increase of air pollutants; Z_t represents the pollutant concentrations at day t; DOW is a dummy variable for day of the week; And ns indicates the natural cubic regression smooth function [22].

After establishing the basic model, single-pollutant models were initially used and introduced, a priori, in turn each air pollutant concentration on the concurrent day (lag0). To verify the stability of the model, three sensitivity analyses were conducted. First, alternative df were selected with 4–10 per year for the smoothness of time trends. Second, given that the health effects of ambient air pollutants could last for multiple days, more single lag days were used (lag1, lag2, lag3, lag4, lag5, lag6, and lag7) and moving average exposure of multiple days (lag01, lag02, lag03, lag04, lag05, lag06, and lag07). Third, two-pollutant models were built to examine the stability of the effect estimates after adjustment for co-pollutants. Co-pollutants with a correlation coefficient < 0.7 would be added to the two-pollutant model.

Both the total respiratory outpatients with non-pathogenic disease and cause-specific respiratory outpatients were assessed. Because behaviour patterns and common diseases may be different in children of different ages, all of these outpatients were stratified by age (0–3, 4–6, and 7–14 years). Because both air pollution levels and the incidence of respiratory disease events are known to vary by season, the analysis was stratified by cool season (November to March), hot season (June to August) and transition season (April, May, September and October), and reduced the df per year to 3, 2, and 3 respectively. The statistical significance of the differences between the effect estimates of the strata of a potential effect modifier (e.g., the difference between age or season) was tested by calculating the 95% confidence interval (CI) as $(\hat{Q}_1 - \hat{Q}_2) \pm 1.96\sqrt{(\hat{SE}_1)^2 + (\hat{SE}_2)^2}$, in which $\hat{Q}_1$ and $\hat{Q}_2$ are the estimates for two categories, and $\hat{SE}_1$ and $\hat{SE}_2$ are their respective SEs [23]. Regardless of significance, modification of effect by a factor ≥ 2 was considered to be important and worthy of attention [23].

The statistical tests were two-sided, and effects with $p < 0.05$ were considered to be statistically significant. All statistical models were constructed using R software version 3.2.1 (R Foundation for Statistical Computing, Vienna, Austria) using the MGCV package. The effects are expressed as the percentage of change and 95% CI in daily hospital child respiratory outpatient visits per 10 µg/m³ increase in pollutant concentrations.

Results

Data description

A total of 3,541,692 total hospital outpatient records were retrieved for the period 2013 to 2015, from the Children's Hospital of Hebei Province. A total of 1,400,199 records remained after deleting duplicate data, the records of cases residing outside of Shijiazhuang, and cases>14 years of age. After ICD-10 code re-matching, approximately 355,833 (25.4%) recodes were mismatched. Finally, 551,678 records of hospital outpatients caused by non-pathogen respiratory diseases were extracted. The percentages of total non-pathogen respiratory hospital outpatients according to age group were 72.2% for 0–3, 18.5% for 4–6 and 9.3% for 7–14 years of age, respectively. Acute upper respiratory infections (ICD-10 codes J00-J06) accounted for 37.4% of the total of non-pathogen respiratory diseases. Other acute lower respiratory infections (ICD-10 codes J20-J22) accounted for 36.7%, while pneumonia (ICD-10 codes J18) accounted for 12.1%. Other diseases of upper respiratory tract (ICD-10 codes J30-J39) accounted for 10.2%, chronic lower respiratory diseases (ICD-10 codes J40-J47) accounted for 3.0%, and other respiratory diseases (ICD-10 codes J60-J99) accounted for 0.7%.

During the study period, there were no missing value days for air pollutant measurements, meteorological variables, or health data. According to the results of the Shapiro-Wilk test, all of these data were skewed (i.e., non-normally distributed); therefore, median and quartile values were used to describe their distribution. Descriptive statistics from this study are summarized in Table 1. There was serious air pollution in Shijiazhuang, especially from PM$_{2.5}$ and PM$_{10}$, and on most days, these two pollutant concentrations exceeded the National Ambient Air Quality Standards (24 h average standards for PM$_{2.5}$ is 75 µg/m³, PM$_{10}$ is 150 µg/m³, SO$_2$ is 150 µg/m³, NO$_2$ is 80 µg/m³, and O$_{3\text{-}8h}$ is 160 µg/m³). The highest daily average concentrations were 10.3 and 5.6

times the limit values, respectively, confirming that the main air pollutants in the selected city are, in fact, PM$_{2.5}$ and PM$_{10}$. The minimal, mean, and maximal daily average temperature and relative humidity were – 7.7 °C, 14.5 °C, 34.7 °C and 11.5%, 57%, 98%, respectively, reflecting the warm temperate continental monsoon climate in Shijiazhuang.

As shown in Fig. 2, daily air pollution concentrations (except for O$_3$) and total respiratory outpatients were highest in the cool season and lowest in the hot season. The interquartile range of PM$_{2.5}$, PM$_{10}$, SO$_2$ and NO$_2$ concentrations in the cool season (158, 272.7, 117.1 and 43.8, respectively) were significantly higher than in the hot season (65.2, 110.8, 22.6 and 19.6, respectively).

Generally, there were strong correlations among PM$_{2.5}$, PM$_{10}$, SO$_2$ and NO$_2$ pollutants with the Spearman correlation coefficients, ranging from 0.50 to 0.75. PM$_{2.5}$, PM$_{10}$, SO$_2$ and NO$_2$ concentrations were negatively or weakly correlated with temperature and relative humidity. Maximal 8 h mean O$_3$ concentrarion was negatively correlated with PM$_{2.5}$, PM$_{10}$, SO$_2$ and NO$_2$ (Spearman correlation coefficients ranged from – 0.31 to – 0.50), weakly correlated with relative humidity, and strongly correlated with temperature ($r = 0.82$, $p < 0.05$).

In the whole-season analysis, SO$_2$, NO$_2$ and PM$_{2.5}$ were significantly associated with increased total respiratory outpatient visits. An increase of 10 µg/m³ in two-day average concentrations of SO$_2$, NO$_2$ and PM$_{2.5}$ corresponded to a 0.33% (95% CI: 0.10–0.56), 0.66% (95% CI: 0.30–1.03), and 0.13% (95% CI: 0.02–0.24) increase in total respiratory outpatient visits (Table 2). The associations between O$_3$, PM$_{10}$ and total respiratory outpatients were positive but non-significant. For cause-specific diseases, positive associations were observed except for correlations between O$_3$ and chronic lower respiratory diseases (ICD-10 codes J40-J47) and other respiratory diseases (ICD-10 codes J60-J99).

Effects by season

The effect estimates of ambient air pollution on total respiratory outpatients showed significant differences among three seasons. Effect estimates of all five pollutants were significant in the transition season, and non-significant in both the cool and hot seasons, except for SO$_2$ in the hot season. NO$_2$, PM$_{2.5}$, PM$_{10}$ and O$_3$ exhibited highest effects in the transition season. The magnitudes of SO$_2$-associated increase were approximately 2 times higher in the hot season than in the transition season. Significant differences were observed for SO$_2$ and O$_3$ between the cool season and the hot, transition season, for PM$_{10}$ in the transition season and the cool and warm season, for NO$_2$ in the cool season and the transition season.

Table 1 Summary statistics of daily air pollutants, weather conditions, and children hospital outpatients caused by respiratory diseases (N = 551,678) in Shijiazhuang from 2013 to 2015

	Min	P25	P50	P75	Max
Air pollutant concentration (μg/m³)[a]					
NO$_2$	13	36.8	51.9	71.6	176.8
O$_3$	3.3	34.1	69.0	115.8	262.4
PM$_{10}$	22.3	146.6	226.7	334.5	842.1
PM$_{2.5}$	9.8	65.2	109.6	166.6	771.3
SO$_2$	5.3	31.5	56.7	118.3	319.3
Meteorological measures					
Temperature (°C)	−7.7	5.0	16.0	24.2	34.7
Humidity (%)	11.5	43.0	58.4	72.3	98.0
No. of daily respiratory outpatients (J00-J98)[b]	243	389	442	527	915
Acute upper respiratory infections (J00-J06)	67	159	183	206	294
Pneumonia (J18)	7	33	45	71	180
Other acute lower respiratory infections (J20-J22)	68	124	149	216	400
Other diseases of upper respiratory tract (J30-J39)	6	35	47	59	150
Chronic lower respiratory diseases (J40-J47)	1	10	14	18	47
Other respiratory diseases (J60-J99)	0	2	3	5	13
Age (N)					
0–3	201	281	315	377	703
4–6	14	66	86	109	194
7–14	13	33	42	55	107
Season (N)					
hot (Jun to Aug)	285	366	407	437	551
Transition (Apr, May, Sep and Oct)	263	403	443	476	690
Cool (Nov to Mar)	243	408	562	700	915

[a]24-hour average for PM$_{2.5}$, PM$_{10}$, SO$_2$, and NO$_2$; maximal 8-h average for O$_3$
[b]respiratory diseases except for pathogen infectious, abscess, suppuration, gangrenous and ulcerative diseases

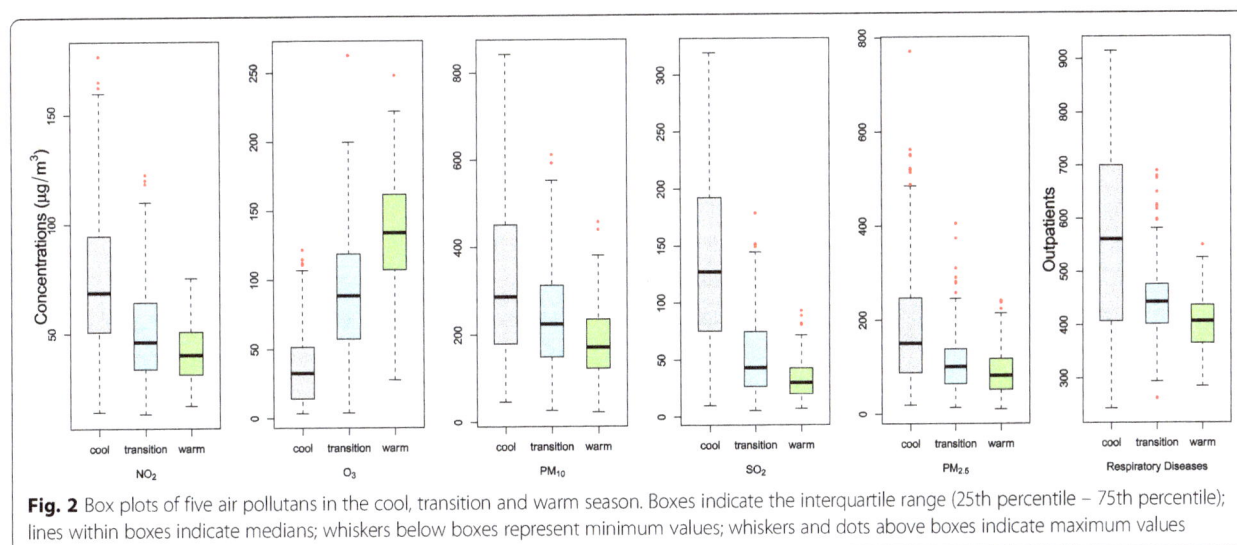

Fig. 2 Box plots of five air pollutans in the cool, transition and warm season. Boxes indicate the interquartile range (25th percentile – 75th percentile); lines within boxes indicate medians; whiskers below boxes represent minimum values; whiskers and dots above boxes indicate maximum values

Table 2 Percent change (95% CI) in children hospital outpatients caused by total and cause-specific respiratory diseases per 10 µg/m³ increase in concentrations of five air pollutants in Shijiazhuang, China, 2013–2015

	Total	Acute upper respiratory infections (J00-J06)	Pneumonia (J18)	Other acute lower respiratory infections (J20-J22)	Other diseases of upper respiratory tract (J30-J39)	Chronic lower respiratory diseases (J40-J47)	Other respiratory diseases (J60-J99)
NO_2	**0.66 (0.30,1.03)**	0.18(−0.3,0.67)	**0.78 (0.2,1.36)**	**0.57 (0.09,1.05)**	**2.25 (1.21,3.3)**	0.62(−0.66,1.91)	1.66(−0.97,4.3)
O_3	0.20(−0.12,0.51)	0.24(−0.13,0.62)	0.08(−0.53,0.68)	0.14(−0.31,0.59)	0.72(−0.16,1.59)	−0.4(−1.49,0.68)	−1.32(−3.35,0.7)
PM_{10}	0.04(−0.04,0.11)	0.01(−0.08,0.11)	0.08(−0.04,0.19)	0.04(−0.05,0.13)	0.07(−0.14,0.27)	0.07(−0.18,0.31)	0.34(−0.16,0.83)
$PM_{2.5}$	**0.13 (0.02,0.24)**	0.12(−0.02,0.27)	**0.19 (0.02,0.36)**	0.12(−0.02,0.26)	0.11(−0.2,0.42)	0.24(−0.14,0.62)	0.51(−0.23,1.24)
SO_2	**0.33 (0.10,0.56)**	0.18(−0.14,0.49)	0.34(−0.02,0.7)	0.22(−0.08,0.52)	**1.14 (0.5,1.79)**	0.11(−0.7,0.92)	0.81(−0.81,2.43)

Significant statistical estimates are highlighted in bold

Effects by age

The percent increase in associations between air pollutants and total respiratory hospital outpatients varied by age group. For NO_2, $PM_{2.5}$ and PM_{10} pollutants, the older the child was, the higher the effect estimates. O_3 had significant influence on children 4–6 years of age, then on those 7–14 years, and the smallest on those 0–3 years of age. There were no significant effects of air pollutants on children 0–3 years of age, except for SO_2. Meanwhile, significant effects were observed in children 4–6 and 7–14 years of age, except for SO_2 and O_3, respectively. Three pollutants (NO_2, PM_{10} and O_3) present significant differences between the 0–3 years of age group and the 4–6/7–14 years group, while differences in the other two pollutants were non-significant among the three groups (Table 3).

Sensitivity results

The results of sensitivity analyses, adjusted for different *df* are shown in Fig. 3. The effect estimates remained stable. The results demonstrated that the acute effects of air pollution did not change substantially with the adjustment of smoothness of time using alternative *df* from 4 to 10 per year.

The results from the single-lag day (lag0-lag7) and cumulative exposure models (lag01-lag07) for the percent increase in children respiratory outpatients per 10 µg/m³ increase in pollutants are shown in Fig. 4. Statistically significant results were observed at lag 0, 1 and 01–07 day for NO_2. Lag 0 and 01 day for $PM_{2.5}$. Lag 0 and 01–07 day for SO_2. respectively. For all five pollutants, the effects on cumulative days were higher than single-lag days. According to previous studies, lag0 day or lag01 air pollution was most closely correlated with child hospital outpatient visits. Therefore, a two-day average (lag01) exposure model was used for modifying effects analyses.

The results of the two-pollutant models using exposure at lag 01 are provided in Table 4. The magnitudes of all five pollutants were stable. Effect estimates of NO_2, SO_2 and $PM_{2.5}$ pollutants remained statistically significant when adjusting for co-pollutants.

Discussion

Although the associations between ambient air pollution and daily hospital child outpatient visits have been well described in developed countries, studies in developing countries, especially in severely pollution haze Chinese cities, remain limited. The present study demonstrated that season and age may modify the health effects of air pollution in Shijiazhuang. Unlike other study results, the association between air pollution and daily children

Table 3 Percent change (95% CI) in children hospital outpatients caused by respiratory diseases per 10 µg/m3 increase in concentrations of five air pollutants stratified by season and age in Shijiazhuang, China, 2013–2015

	Season			Age		
	Cool season	Hot season	Transition season	0–3	4–6	7–14
NO_2	0.17(−0.44, 0.78)[b]	0.71(−0.65, 2.06)	**1.47 (0.69, 2.25)[b]**	0.22(−0.14, 0.59)[d,e]	**1.59 (0.86, 2.31)[d]**	**2.39 (1.38, 3.39)[e]**
O_3	−3.47(−4.38, −2.55)[a,b]	0.26(−0.16, 0.67)[a]	**0.54 (0, 1.07)[b]**	0.05(−0.27, 0.37)[d]	**0.78 (0.16, 1.40)[d]**	0.11(−0.75, 0.98)
PM_{10}	0.02(−0.09, 0.14)[b]	−0.08(−0.36, 0.2)[c]	**0.24 (0.09, 0.39)[b,c]**	−0.03(−0.10, 0.04)[d,e]	**0.19 (0.05, 0.34)[d]**	**0.27 (0.07, 0.47)[e]**
$PM_{2.5}$	0.16(−0.01, 0.33)	−0.1(−0.54, 0.35)	**0.32 (0.02, 0.62)**	0.06(−0.05, 0.17)	**0.30 (0.08, 0.53)**	**0.38 (0.07, 0.68)**
SO_2	−0.05(−0.39, 0.29)[a,b]	**2.09 (0.99, 3.2)[a]**	**1.05 (0.42, 1.68)[b]**	**0.26 (0.03, 0.49)**	0.38(−0.08, 0.84)	**0.83 (0.19, 1.47)**

We used current day temperature and humidity (lag0) and 2-day moving average of air pollutant concentrations (lag01). Significant statistical estimates are highlighted in bold
[a]The difference between cool season and hot season was significant at α = 0.05. [b]The difference between cool season and transition season was significant at α = 0.05. [c]The difference between hot season and transition season was significant at α = 0.05. [d]The difference between 0 and 3 years of age and 4–6 years of age was significant at α = 0.05. [e]The difference between 0 and 3 years of age and 7–14 years of age was significant at α = 0.05. f The difference between 4 and 6 years of age and 7–14 years of age was significant at α = 0.05

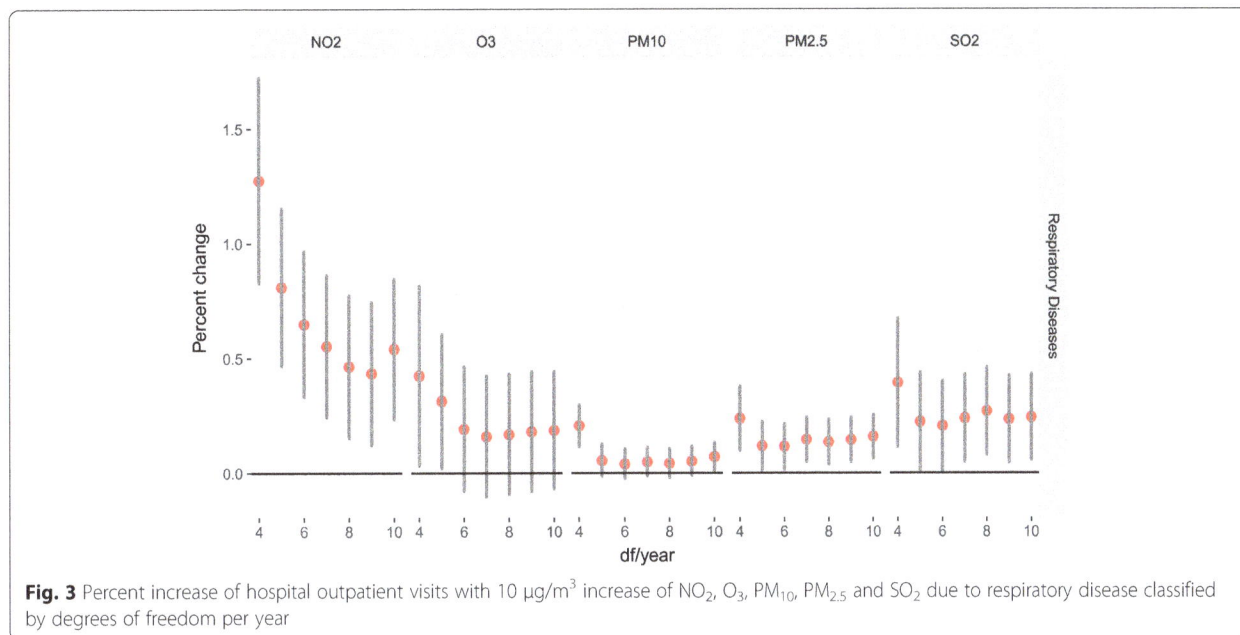

Fig. 3 Percent increase of hospital outpatient visits with 10 µg/m³ increase of NO_2, O_3, PM_{10}, $PM_{2.5}$ and SO_2 due to respiratory disease classified by degrees of freedom per year

outpatient visits was generally more evident in the transition season than the hot or cool seasons.

The effect estimates of our results are lower than reported in previous studies [16, 24–26]. There are several potential reasons for this heterogeneity. First, the lower estimates may reflect the fact that Shijiazhuang's air pollution was significantly more severe than in developed countries and other developing cities in China, which may reflect the shape of the concentration-response curves where there may be a flattening (saturation) at the higher end [27]. Second, the chemical components of PM pollution are very important to their effects on health, which may partially explain the reason for different effects among cities [21]. Third, the varying magnitude of misclassification of clinical diagnosis, as well as other factors such as statistical models and population characteristics, may explain the differences between our results and previous studies [28].

For the first time, the present study observed that the association between air pollution and daily child respiratory hospital outpatient visits in the transition season is significantly more sensitive than in hot or cool seasons. The concentrations of SO_2, NO_2, $PM_{2.5}$ and PM_{10} were higher in the cool season, medium in the transition season, and lower in the hot season (Fig. 2). Associations between ambient air pollution and daily total non-pathogen respiratory outpatient visits were strongest during the transition season: the effect estimates were 2–6 times higher than in all seasons. The pattern of exposure to ambient air pollution in children may change from season to season [29]. Because of low temperatures, high air pollutant concentrations, and the use of central heating systems in the winter, residents generally stay indoors and close their windows. Similarly, high temperatures and the widespread use of air conditioning forces individuals to enter rooms and close windows. Thus, the exposure dose may

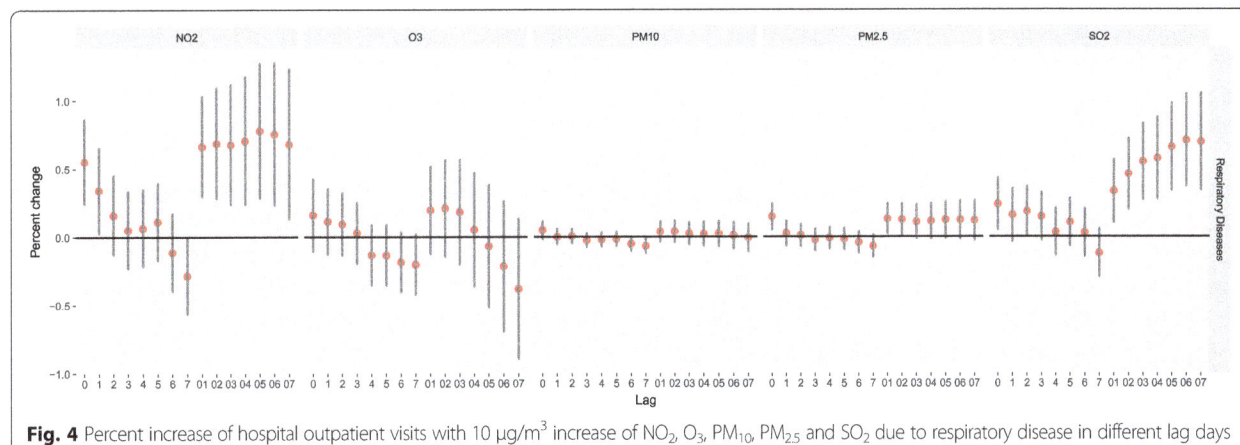

Fig. 4 Percent increase of hospital outpatient visits with 10 µg/m³ increase of NO_2, O_3, PM_{10}, $PM_{2.5}$ and SO_2 due to respiratory disease in different lag days

Table 4 Percent change (mean and 95% confidence intervals) of daily total respiratory outpatients associated with10ug/m^3 increase of pollutant concentrations in single and two-pollutant models

Pollutants	Two-pollutant models	Estimates
NO$_2$	Without adjustment	**0.66 (0.30,1.03)****
	Adjusted for O$_3$	**0.73 (0.35, 1.11)****
O$_3$	Without adjustment	0.20(−0.12, 0.51)
	Adjusted for SO$_2$	0.29(−0.03, 0.61)
	Adjusted for PM$_{2.5}$	0.24(−0.08, 0.56)
	Adjusted for PM$_{10}$	0.21(−0.11, 0.53)
	Adjusted for NO$_2$	0.31(−0.01, 0.63)
PM$_{10}$	Without adjustment	0.04(−0.04, 0.11)
	Adjusted for O$_3$	0.04(−0.03, 0.11)
PM$_{2.5}$	Without adjustment	**0.13 (0.02, 0.24)***
	Adjusted for O$_3$	**0.14 (0.03, 0.25)***
SO$_2$	Without adjustment	**0.33 (0.10, 0.56)***
	Adjusted for O$_3$	**0.37 (0.14,0.61)***
	Adjusted for PM$_{2.5}$	**0.26 (0.01, 0.53)***

Two-day moving average (lag01) concentrations of pollutants were used.
*$p < 0.05$, **$p < 0.001$

be reduced in the cool or hot seasons. One study reported that the indoor /outdoor ratio of air pollutant concentration in Beijing (China) is 0.5 and 0.7 in the cool and hot seasons, respectively (data not shown). In contrast, the climate is more pleasant in the transition season; children's outdoor activities and time with open windows in homes would be increased; therefore, exposure to ambient air pollution would likely be higher.

Previous studies have reported that the health effects of air pollution on infants and young children may be greater than in adults [30–32]. However, we found a very interesting phenomenon in our study: the effect estimate increases with age in children. Considering the differences in activity range and air pollution patterns among children of different age groups, our results may be easier to understand. Children 0–3 years of age need adult supervision and their activities are mainly indoor; consequently, their exposure to ambient air pollution is the least. Kindergarten (4–6 years) can offer a wide range of free activities, meanwhile the children are compliant and follow teachers' recommendations to stay indoors when the air quality is inadequate. Children 7–14 years of age engage in the highest activities but have a weak awareness of self-protection, therefore, exposure dose may increase with age. Although the exact air pollution exposure dose to children of different ages remains unclear, this phenomenon provides new insights into research investigating the adverse health effects of air pollution on children, and warrants careful future study.

Another important finding from our study was that pollutant states may contribute to seasonal differences.

Effect estimates of gaseous pollutants (SO$_2$, NO$_2$ and O$_3$) with total respiratory outpatient visits in the hot season were higher than those in the cool season, while the PM pollutants (PM$_{2.5}$ and PM$_{10}$) had lower estimates in the hot season than that in the cool season. That may be attributed to the constituents of the complex mix of PM$_{2.5}$ and PM$_{10}$, which may vary by season. The exact PM$_{2.5}$ compositional difference in different seasons is currently under investigation.

The varying magnitude of misclassifications of clinical diagnosis and ICD-10 codes may have introduced bias. To mitigate this bias, one ICD-10 code rematch and validate mechanism was introduced in our research. While these diagnoses made by physicians may not be accurate and completely consistent. Further studies are needed to validate these diagnoses.

Our research had limitations. First, we collected only three years' of data for the association analysis between air pollution and children respiratory outpatient visits; the GAM model, therefore, may have some instability [33]. Second, as in many previous time-series studies, we used available ambient monitoring data to assess the children's exposure to air pollutants. As a result, several issues may have arisen, given that ambient monitoring results differ from a child's exposure level to air pollutants [33, 34]. Data for the assessment of weather conditions was retrieved entirely from one monitoring station. Measurement error may have substantial implications for interpreting epidemiological studies on air pollution. Third, we evaluated the association of five air pollutants with seven different hospital outpatient outcomes. In addition, moderate-to-high correlation between PM pollution and gaseous pollutants in a selected city limited our ability to separate the independent effect for each pollutant.

Conclusions

Our findings suggest that ambient air pollutants were associated with child respiratory outpatient visits, especially for pneumonia (ICD-10 code J18), other acute lower respiratory infections (ICD-10 code J20-J21), and other diseases of upper respiratory tract (ICD-10 code J30-J39). Furthermore, our results suggest that the effect estimates in the transition season were stronger than in cold or hot seasons, and that the estimates increase with age in children. To protect the health of children, local authorities should take more measures to control air pollutant emissions.

Acknowledgements
We appreciate the Children's Hospital of Hebei Province for providing the data.

Funding

The study was supported by the National Natural Science Foundation of China (21677136), the Ph.D. Research Project of Xinxiang Medical University (XYBSKYZZ201804), Key scientific research projects in universities of Henan province (19B330004) and Peak Subject Project of Public Health in Xinxiang Medical University.

Authors' contributions

JS initiated the idea for the study and was the main supervisor, helped in writing and editing the manuscript. YL acquired the air pollution data and the meteorological data. LZ acquired the health data. ML cleaned the data, analyzed the data and prepared the initial draft. PX and YL supervised data analysis, provided statistical consultation and edited the final manuscript. DX provided scientific advice for air pollution and edited the final article. WW provided scientific and methodology consultation, edited the final manuscript. All authors read and approved the final manuscript.

Competing interests

The authors declare that they have no competing interests.

Author details

[1]School of Public Health, Xinxiang Medical University, Xinxiang 453003, China. [2]Henan International Collaborative Laboratory for Health Effects and Intervention of Air Pollution, Xinxiang 453003, China. [3]Xinxiang Medical University, Xinxiang 453003, China. [4]Hebei Chest Hospital, Shijiazhuang 050041, China. [5]National Institute of Environmental Health, Chinese Center for Disease Control and Prevention, Beijing 100021, China.

References

1. Vidale S, Campana C. Ambient air pollution and cardiovascular diseases: from bench to bedside. Eur J Prev Cardiol. 2018;25(8):818–25.
2. Requia WJ, Adams MD, Arain A, Papatheodorou S, Koutrakis P, Mahmoud M. Global Association of air Pollution and Cardiorespiratory Diseases: a systematic review, meta-analysis, and investigation of modifier variables. Am J Public Health. 2018;108(S2):S123–30.
3. Landrigan PJ. Air pollution and health. The Lancet Public health. 2017;2(1):e4–5.
4. Hadley MB, Vedanthan R, Fuster V. Air pollution and cardiovascular disease: a window of opportunity. Nat Rev Cardiol. 2018;15(4):193–4.
5. Mihaltan F, Deleanu O, Nemes R, Ulmeanu R. Air pollution and respiratory diseases - a problematic risk factor. Pneumologia. 2016;65(3):122–5.
6. Mendola P. Air pollution - who is at risk? Paediatr Perinat Epidemiol. 2017; 31(5):435–7.
7. Loomis D, Grosse Y, Lauby-Secretan B, El Ghissassi F, Bouvard V, Benbrahim-Tallaa L, Guha N, Baan R, Mattock H, Straif K, et al. The carcinogenicity of outdoor air pollution. The Lancet Oncology. 2013;14(13):1262–3.
8. Rodriguez-Villamizar LA, Magico A, Osornio-Vargas A, Rowe BH. The effects of outdoor air pollution on the respiratory health of Canadian children: a systematic review of epidemiological studies. Can Respir J. 2015;22(5):282–92.
9. Collaborators GBDRF: Global, regional, and national comparative risk assessment of 79 behavioural, environmental and occupational, and metabolic risks or clusters of risks, 1990-2015: a systematic analysis for the global burden of disease study 2015. Lancet 2016, 388(10053):1659–1724.
10. Cohen AJ, Brauer M, Burnett R, Anderson HR, Frostad J, Estep K, Balakrishnan K, Brunekreef B, Dandona L, Dandona R, et al. Estimates and 25-year trends of the global burden of disease attributable to ambient air pollution: an analysis of data from the global burden of diseases study 2015. Lancet. 2017;389(10082):1907–18.
11. Lelieveld J, Evans JS, Fnais M, Giannadaki D, Pozzer A. The contribution of outdoor air pollution sources to premature mortality on a global scale. Nature. 2015;525(7569):367–71.
12. Huang RJ, Zhang Y, Bozzetti C, Ho KF, Cao JJ, Han Y, Daellenbach KR, Slowik JG, Platt SM, Canonaco F, et al. High secondary aerosol contribution to particulate pollution during haze events in China. Nature. 2014;514(7521): 218 22.
13. Song J, Zheng L, Lu M, Gui L, Xu D, Wu W, Liu Y. Acute effects of ambient particulate matter pollution on hospital admissions for mental and behavioral disorders: a time-series study in Shijiazhuang, China. Sci Total Environ. 2018;636:205–11.
14. Goldizen FC, Sly PD, Knibbs LD. Respiratory effects of air pollution on children. Pediatr Pulmonol. 2016;51(1):94–108.
15. Friedrich MJ. UNICEF reports on the impact of air pollution on children. Jama. 2017;317(3):246.
16. Nhung NTT, Schindler C, Dien TM, Probst-Hensch N, Perez L, Kunzli N. Acute effects of ambient air pollution on lower respiratory infections in Hanoi children: an eight-year time series study. Environ Int. 2018;110:139–48.
17. Hua J, Yin Y, Peng L, Du L, Geng F, Zhu L. Acute effects of black carbon and PM(2).(5) on children asthma admissions: a time-series study in a Chinese city. Sci Total Environ. 2014;481:433–8.
18. Zheng PW, Wang JB, Zhang ZY, Shen P, Chai PF, Li D, Jin MJ, Tang ML, Lu HC, Lin HB, et al. Air pollution and hospital visits for acute upper and lower respiratory infections among children in Ningbo, China: a time-series analysis. Environ Sci Pollut Res Int. 2017;24(23):18860–9.
19. Liu Y, Hao S, Song J, Zhou L, Liu J, Wang Q, Yuan D. Xu D: [development of a method for cleaning outpatient data rapidly and generating statistical reports automatically to the analysis of time series on the air pollution and disease]. Wei sheng yan jiu = Journal of hygiene research. 2016;45(4):624–30.
20. Yang C, Chen A, Chen R, Qi Y, Ye J, Li S, Li W, Liang Z, Liang Q, Guo D, et al. Acute effect of ambient air pollution on heart failure in Guangzhou, China. Int J Cardiol. 2014;177(2):436–41.
21. Chen R, Yin P, Meng X, Liu C, Wang L, Xu X, Ross JA, Tse LA, Zhao Z, Kan H, et al. Fine particulate air pollution and daily mortality. A Nationwide analysis in 272 Chinese cities. Am J Respir Crit Care Med. 2017;196(1):73–81.
22. Li H, Chen R, Meng X, Zhao Z, Cai J, Wang C, Yang C, Kan H. Short-term exposure to ambient air pollution and coronary heart disease mortality in 8 Chinese cities. Int J Cardiol. 2015;197:265–70.
23. Zeka A, Zanobetti A, Schwartz J. Individual-level modifiers of the effects of particulate matter on daily mortality. Am J Epidemiol. 2006;163(9):849–59.
24. Wang Yiyi ZY, Lin Huang, Zhang Hongliang, Wang Changhui, Hu Jianlin: Associations between daily outpatient visits for respiratory diseases and ambient fine particulate matter and ozone levels in shanghai, China. Environ Pollut 2018, 240:754–763.
25. Gouveia N, Corrallo FP, Leon ACP, Junger W, Freitas CU. Air pollution and hospitalizations in the largest Brazilian metropolis. Revista de saude publica. 2017;51:117.
26. Mo Z, Fu Q, Zhang L, Lyu D, Mao G, Wu L, Xu P, Wang Z, Pan X, Chen Z, et al. Acute effects of air pollution on respiratory disease mortalities and outpatients in southeastern China. Sci Rep. 2018;8(1):3461.
27. Samoli E, touloumi G, Zanobetti A, Le TA, Schindler C, Atkinson R, Vonk J, Rossi G, Saez M, Rabczenko D, Schwartz J, Katsouyanni K. Investigating the dose-response relation between air pollution and total mortality in the APHEA-2 multicity project. Occup Environ Med. 2003;60:977–82.
28. Lee JY, Kim H. Ambient air pollution-induced health risk for children worldwide. The Lancet Planetary health. 2018;2(7):e285–6.
29. Chen R, Cai J, Meng X, Kim H, Honda Y, Guo YL, Samoli E, Yang X, Kan H. Ozone and daily mortality rate in 21 cities of East Asia: how does season modify the association? Am J Epidemiol. 2014;180(7):729–36.
30. Li D, Wang JB, Zhang ZY, Shen P, Zheng PW, Jin MJ, Lu HC, Lin HB, Chen K. Effects of air pollution on hospital visits for pneumonia in children: a two-year analysis from China. Environ Sci Pollut Res Int. 2018;25(10):10049–57.
31. Orellano P, Quaranta N, Reynoso J, Balbi B, Vasquez J. Effect of outdoor air pollution on asthma exacerbations in children and adults: systematic review and multilevel meta-analysis. PLoS One. 2017;12(3):e0174050.
32. Rey-Ares L, Irazola V, Althabe F, Sobrino E, Mazzoni A, Seron P, Lanas F, Calandreli M, Rubinstein A. Lower tract respiratory infection in children younger than 5 years of age and adverse pregnancy outcomes related to household air pollution in Bariloche (Argentina) and Temuco (Chile). Indoor Air. 2016;26(6):964–75.
33. Strickland MJ, Gass KM, Goldman GT, Mulholland JA. Effects of ambient air pollution measurement error on health effect estimates in time-series studies: a simulation-based analysis. Journal of exposure science & environmental epidemiology. 2015;25(2):160–6.
34. Goldman GT, Mulholland JA, Russell AG, Strickland MJ, Klein M, Waller LA, Tolbert PE. Impact of exposure measurement error in air pollution epidemiology: effect of error type in time-series studies. Environmental health : a global access science source. 2011;10:61.

21

The effect of body position on pulmonary function

Shikma Katz[1,3†], Nissim Arish[2,4†], Ariel Rokach[2,4*], Yacov Zaltzman[1] and Esther-Lee Marcus[1,4]

Abstract

Background: Pulmonary function tests (PFTs) are routinely performed in the upright position due to measurement devices and patient comfort. This systematic review investigated the influence of body position on lung function in healthy persons and specific patient groups.

Methods: A search to identify English-language papers published from 1/1998–12/2017 was conducted using MEDLINE and Google Scholar with key words: body position, lung function, lung mechanics, lung volume, position change, positioning, posture, pulmonary function testing, sitting, standing, supine, ventilation, and ventilatory change. Studies that were quasi-experimental, pre-post intervention; compared ≥2 positions, including sitting or standing; and assessed lung function in non-mechanically ventilated subjects aged ≥18 years were included. Primary outcome measures were forced expiratory volume in 1 s (FEV1), forced vital capacity (FVC, FEV1/FVC), vital capacity (VC), functional residual capacity (FRC), maximal expiratory pressure (PEmax), maximal inspiratory pressure (PImax), peak expiratory flow (PEF), total lung capacity (TLC), residual volume (RV), and diffusing capacity of the lungs for carbon monoxide (DLCO). Standing, sitting, supine, and right- and left-side lying positions were studied.

Results: Forty-three studies met inclusion criteria. The study populations included healthy subjects (29 studies), lung disease (nine), heart disease (four), spinal cord injury (SCI, seven), neuromuscular diseases (three), and obesity (four). In most studies involving healthy subjects or patients with lung, heart, neuromuscular disease, or obesity, FEV1, FVC, FRC, PEmax, PImax, and/or PEF values were higher in more erect positions. For subjects with tetraplegic SCI, FVC and FEV1 were higher in supine vs. sitting. In healthy subjects, DLCO was higher in the supine vs. sitting, and in sitting vs. side-lying positions. In patients with chronic heart failure, the effect of position on DLCO varied.

Conclusions: Body position influences the results of PFTs, but the optimal position and magnitude of the benefit varies between study populations. PFTs are routinely performed in the sitting position. We recommend the supine position should be considered in addition to sitting for PFTs in patients with SCI and neuromuscular disease. When treating patients with heart, lung, SCI, neuromuscular disease, or obesity, one should take into consideration that pulmonary physiology and function are influenced by body position.

Keywords: Body position, Lung volume, Physical therapy, Positioning, Posture, Pulmonary function, Sitting, Supine, Standing

Background

Pulmonary function tests (PFTs) provide objective, quantifiable measures of lung function. They are used to evaluate and monitor diseases that affect heart and lung function, to monitor the effects of environmental, occupational, and drug exposures, to assess risks of surgery, and to assist in evaluations performed before employment or for insurance purposes. Spirometric examination is the most common form of PFT [1]. According to ATS/ERS guidelines, PFTs may be performed either in the sitting or standing position, and the position should be recorded on the report. Sitting is preferable for safety reasons to avoid falling due to syncope [2], and might also be more convenient because of the measurement devices and patient comfort. However, people who

* Correspondence: rokach.ariel@gmail.com

†Shikma Katz and Nissim Arish contributed equally to this work.
2Pulmonary Institute, Shaare Zedek Medical Center, POB 3235, Jerusalem, Israel
4Hebrew University-Hadassah Faculty of Medicine, Jerusalem, Israel
Full list of author information is available at the end of the article

suffer from neuromuscular disease, morbid obesity, and other conditions may find it difficult to sit or stand during this test, which may influence their results.

One of the main goals of positioning, and specifically the use of upright positions, is to improve lung function in patients with respiratory disorders, heart failure, neuromuscular disease, spinal cord injury (SCI), and obesity, and in the past 20 years, various studies regarding the influence of body position on respiratory mechanics and/or function have been published. However, we did not find a systematic review that integrates findings from studies involving non-mechanically ventilated adults to derive clinical implications for respiratory care and pulmonary function test (PFT) execution.

We aimed to systematically review studies that evaluated the effect of body position on lung function in healthy subjects and non-mechanically ventilated patients with lung disease, heart disease, SCI, neuromuscular disease, and obesity.

Methods

Two researchers (SK., E-LM.) searched MEDLINE and Google Scholar for studies published from January 1998–December 2017 using the key words body position, lung function, lung mechanics, lung volumes, position change, positioning, posture, PFTs, sitting, standing, supine, ventilation, and ventilatory change, in various combinations. Each search term combination included at least one key word related to pulmonary function and at least one related to body position. The year 1998 was chosen as the beginning point due to the publication of the seminal study by Meysman and Vincken [3]. A total of 972 abstracts identified in the search were screened by the same two researchers, and full text of 151 potentially relevant articles was obtained. The full texts were evaluated and

categorized, and 108 articles not fulfilling the inclusion criteria were excluded (Fig. 1).

Articles were included if they met the following criteria: (1) Quasi-experimental, pre-post intervention. (2) Two or more body positions compared, including at least the sitting or standing position. (3) Outcome measures included assessment of lung function by forced vital capacity (FVC), forced expiratory volume in 1 s (FEV1), FEV1/FVC, vital capacity (VC), functional residual capacity (FRC), maximal expiratory pressure (PEmax), maximal inspiratory pressure (PImax), peak expiratory flow (PEF), total lung capacity (TLC), residual volume (RV), or diffusing capacity of the lungs for carbon monoxide (DLCO). (4) Study population of non-mechanically ventilated subjects. (5) Participants aged ≥18 years. (6) English language. Studies assessing lung function using other criteria and those without statistical comparisons of lung function in different positions, those enrolling individuals < 18 years or on mechanical ventilation, published conference abstracts, and systematic reviews were excluded.

Positions studied

1. Standing – unsupported active standing
2. Sitting – sitting on a chair or wheelchair with the backrest at 90° and all limbs supported
3. Supine – lying flat on the back
4. Right-side lying (RSL) – lying straight on the right side
5. Left-side lying (LSL) – lying straight on the left side

Outcome measures and defined thresholds for clinical significance

1. FVC – forced vital capacity

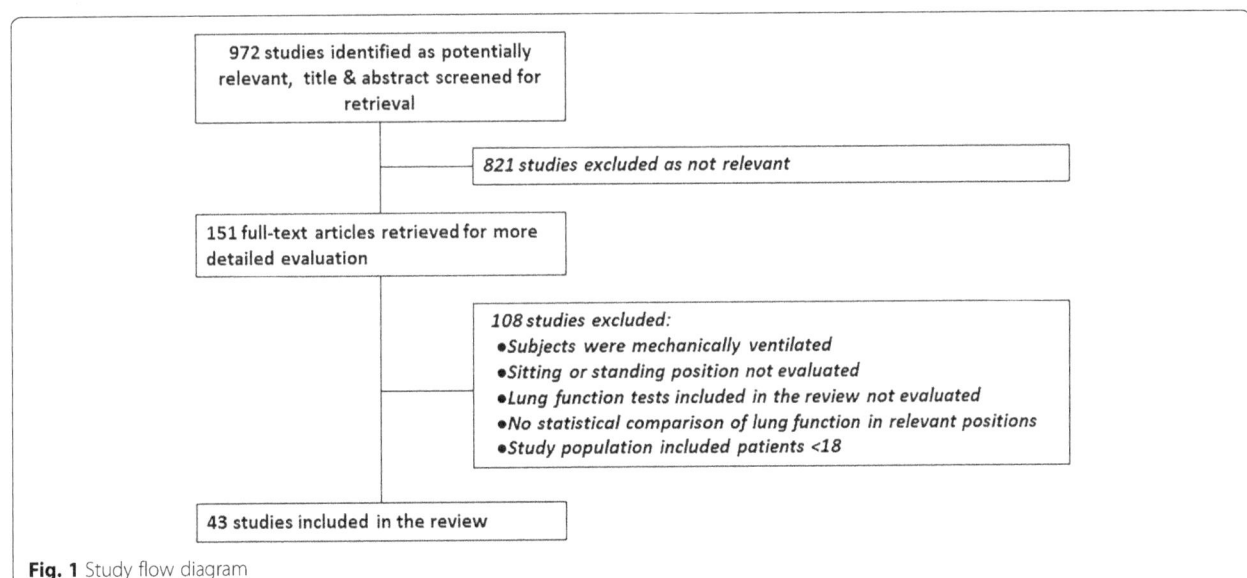

Fig. 1 Study flow diagram

- Change of 200 ml or 12% from baseline values in FVC [4]
2. FEV1– forced expiratory volume in 1 s
    - Change of 200 ml or 12% from baseline values in FEV1 [4]
3. FEV1/FVC – forced expiratory volume in 1 s divided by forced vital capacity
    - FEV1/FVC < 0.7 is defined as obstructive disease
4. VC – vital capacity
5. FRC – functional residual capacity
    - Change > 10% [5]
6. TLC – total lung capacity
    - Change > 10% [5]
7. RV – residual volume
8. Maximal expiratory pressure (PEmax)
    - Change ≥24 cmH2O [6–8]
9. Maximal inspiratory pressure (PImax)
    - Change ≤ – 13 cmH2O [6–8]
10. Peak expiratory flow (PEF)
    - Change > 10% or 60 L/min [9, 10]
11. Diffusing capacity of the lungs for carbon monoxide (DLCO)
    - Change ≥10% in DLCO [11, 12]

Two experienced pulmonologists (NA, AR) reviewed the included studies in consensus to identify statistically significant and clinically important differences in pulmonary function. Results from articles included in the review were evaluated by all authors and categorized by study population, body positions studied, and outcome measures. Data from included studies was extracted by four authors (NA, AR, SK, E-LM.) independently and in consultation when questions arose. The review was performed according to the PRISMA guidelines [13].

Although these are not interventional studies, strictly speaking, we have chosen to assess them as "before and after intervention," wherein the posture/position change is the maneuver of interest. Level of evidence was assessed according to the American Academy of Neurology (AAN) Classification of Evidence for therapeutic intervention [14]. Risk of bias was assessed according to the Quality Assessment Tool for Before-After (Pre-Post) Studies with No Control Group developed by the National Heart, Lung and Blood Institute (NHLBI) of the US National Institutes of Health (NIH) [15]. This tool is comprised of 12 questions assessing various aspects of the quality of the study. Two authors (E-LM, SK) independently scored each study using the technique from Kunstler et al. [16]. Differences were resolved in consensus, in consultation with a third author (YZ). The risk of bias was categorized as low (score 76–100%), moderate (26–75%) or high (0–25%).

Results

Studies included in the review

A total of 43 studies fully met inclusion criteria and were included in the review (Fig. 1). All studies used either consecutive, convenience, or volunteer sampling to enroll healthy individuals or subjects with various medical conditions. All studies provide Class III level of evidence.

The protocols and level of bias in the various studies are shown in Table 1 and Additional file 1: Table S1. Risk of bias was assessed as moderate in 41 studies and low in two. Quality issues were primarily related to sampling techniques for enrolling study participants. All studies used non-random sampling. Some studies investigating healthy subjects included convenience samples of young participants, mainly students. Only 7/43 studies reported sample size calculations required to reach statistical power. In addition, the details of the intervention protocol were not clearly reported in some studies (Table 1) and due to the nature of the study assessors could not be blinded to patient position or outcomes from previous tests.

A summary of study characteristics, including the positions studied, outcome measures, and main results according to the study population, is shown in Table 2. Out of 43 studies, 29 included healthy subjects, nine included patients with lung disease, four included patients with heart disease, seven included patients with SCI, three included patients with neuromuscular diseases, and four included patients with obesity. Additional file 2: Table S2 summarizes only the statistically significant findings for each relevant outcome variable, according to position, for each of the populations studied.

FVC

The association between FVC and body position in healthy subjects was investigated in 13 studies [3, 17–28]. There was a clinical and statistically significant increase in FVC in sitting vs. supine positions [3, 18, 22–27], in sitting vs. RSL and LSL [3, 21], standing vs. supine [19, 23], and standing vs. RSL and LSL [19]. In a smaller number of studies there was no change between standing and sitting [19], sitting and supine [17, 21, 28] or sitting and RSL or LSL [21], and one study [22] found a decrease in FVC from sitting to standing that was statistically but not clinically significant. Thus, in the majority of studies the more upright position was associated with increased FVC.

Four studies included subjects with lung disease [29–32]. Among asthmatic patients in one study FVC increased significantly from supine to standing [30]; however, there was no significant difference between standing and sitting or between sitting and supine, RSL, or LSL. Another study reported a statistically and

Table 1 Study protocols

1st Author (year)	Procedure	Posture and Test Randomization	Adjustment period to posture prior to measurement	Risk of Bias
Antunes (2016) [45]	Mini Wright® (Clement Clarke International Ltd. Edinburgh Way Harlow, Essex, UK) peak flow meter portable device with a disposable mouthpiece	Random position order	1 min	Moderate
Badr (2002) [46]	Pressure manometer, vitalograph (Compact, Vitalograph Ltd., Buckingham, UK)	Random position order Random test order (PEF and PEmax) Subjects instructed on equipment use, practiced before test	5 min	Low
Baydur (2001) [35]	Spirometry	Random position order	N/A	Moderate
Ben-Dov (2009) [17]	Spirometry	N/A	N/A	Moderate
Benedik (2009) [52]	Helium dilution	First position always sitting	5 min	Moderate
Ceridon (2011) [18]	Spirometry, DLCO measured by rebreathe technique	N/A	30 min supine position prior to test Time prior to seated measurement not mentioned	Moderate
Chang (2005) [53]	Spirometry, FRC measured using helium dilution	First position always supine	5 min	Moderate
Costa (2015) [54]	Mouth pressure meter	Random position order	10 min	Moderate
De (2012) [29]	Spirometry	First position was always sitting	N/A	Moderate
Elkins (2005) [47]	Pressure manometer, spirometry - mass flow sensor	Random position and test order (PEF, PEmax) Subjects instructed on equipment use, practiced before test	5 min	Low
Faggiano (1998) [58]	Single breath technique using a Medical Graphics PF/DX module (Medical Graphics St. Paul, Minn, USA) for determining DLCO	Random position order	10 min	Moderate
Ganapathi (2015) [19]	Digital spirometry (BIOPAC System Inc. Goleta, California, USA)	N/A	N/A	Moderate
Gianinis (2013) [48]	Portable peak expiratory flow-device	Random position order	N/A	Moderate
Kim (2012) [36]	Spirometry	N/A	N/A	Moderate
Linn (2000) [33]	Spirometry	Random position order	N/A	Moderate
Manning (1999) [20]	Spirometry, single breath for determining DLCO	Two protocols (Session A & B). First chosen at random then alternated for successive subjects. First position always sitting.	15 min	Moderate
McCoy (2010) [49]	Peak flow meter	Random position order. Subjects instructed on equipment use, practiced before test	N/A	Moderate
Melam (2014) [30]	Spirometry (Excel/PC-based pulmonary function tests)	Random position order	N/A	Moderate
Meysman (1998) [3]	Spirometry, peak flow meter	Random position order	10 min	Moderate
Miccinilli (2016) [40]	Spirometry	N/A	N/A	Moderate
Mohammed (2017) [31]	Spirometry	Order of positions always standing, sitting, supine, lateral decubitus	N/A	Moderate
Myint (2017) [42]	Spirometry	Order of positions was standing, sitting, supine	N/A	Moderate
Naitoh (2014) [39]	Spirometry, breath dynamometer (Chest Co. Ltd)	First position always sitting	N/A	Moderate

Table 1 Study protocols (Continued)

1st Author (year)	Procedure	Posture and Test Randomization	Adjustment period to posture prior to measurement	Risk of Bias
Ogiwara (2002) [55]	Vitalpower KH-101 (Chest M.I. Inc., Japan)	Random position order	10 min	Moderate
Ottaviano (2016) [50]	Peak flow meter	Random position order	N/A	Moderate
Palermo (2005) [21]	Spirometry, DLCO measured by a single breath technique	Random position order	15 min	Moderate
Park (2010) [34]	Spirometry	N/A	N/A	Moderate
Patel (2015) [22]	Spirometry	First position always sitting	N/A	Moderate
Peces-Barba (2004) [56]	Single breath technique, rebreathing technique for determining DLCO	N/A	3–5 min	Moderate
Poussel (2014) [38]	Spirometry	Random position order	N/A	Moderate
Razi (2007) [32]	Spirometry	Alternately sitting, standing	N/A 15 min between positions	Moderate
Roychowdhury (2011) [44]	Spirometry	N/A	N/A 5 min rest between positions	Moderate
Saxena (2006) [23]	Spirometry	N/A	N/A	Moderate
Sebbane (2015) [41]	Spirometry, multiple breath helium dilution method	First position always sitting	N/A	Moderate
Stewart (2000) [24]	Single breath method for determining DLCO	N/A, 72 h between positions	15 min	Moderate
Terson de Paleville (2014) [37]	Spirometry, MP45–36-350 differential pressure transducer Validyne Engineering, (Northridge Ca, USA)	First position always sitting	30 min	Moderate
Terzano (2009) [57]	Single breath DLCO technique	Random position order	At least 15 min	Moderate
Tsubaki (2009) [28]	Micro RPM 01 (Micro Medical, UK), spirometry	Random position order	N/A	Moderate
Varrato (2001) [25]	Spirometry	N/A	N/A	Moderate
Vilke (2000) [26]	Spirometry	First position always supine/prone	N/A	Moderate
Wallace (2013) [51]	Peak flow meter	Random position order	N/A	Moderate
Watson (2005) [43]	Multi-breath helium dilution, spirometry	N/A	N/A	Moderate
Yap (2000) [27]	Spirometry, FRC was measured using helium dilution	First position always sitting	5 min	Moderate

Risk of bias was assessed using the Quality Assessment Tool for Before-After (Pre-Post) Studies with No Control Group [15, 16]
DLCO Diffusing capacity of the lungs for carbon monoxide, *FRC* Functional residual capacity
N/A Not available, not reported in the study

clinically significant increase in FVC in standing vs. sitting, supine, RSL, and LSL and in sitting vs. supine, RSL and LSL [31]. Among obese asthmatic patients [32], and among patients with chronic obstructive pulmonary disease (COPD) [29], no difference was found in FVC between standing and sitting.

Three studies included subjects with congestive heart failure (CHF) [18, 21, 27]. In one study, FVC was reported 200 ml higher in sitting vs. RSL and LSL [21], and in the other two studies FVC was higher in sitting vs. supine by 350–400 ml, which has clinical significance [18, 27].

Six studies included patients with SCI [17, 33–37]. The effect of body position on FVC depends on the level and extent of injury. Among those with cervical SCI, FVC was higher in the supine vs. sitting position [17, 33, 34]. Other studies [35–37] did not find significant differences in FVC for patients with SCI in a pooled group of all levels of injury for these positions. However, in patients with cervical SCI, as well as those with thoracic injury in one study [36], there was an increased FVC in the supine vs. sitting, while in those with thoracic or lumbar injury FVC was higher in the sitting position [37]. The differences did not always reach statistical

Table 2 Summary of study characteristics according to study population

1st Author (Year)	No of Participants	Age (Years)	Population	Positions	Pulmonary Function	Main Findings
Meysman (1998) [3]	31	25.6 ± 3.8	Healthy	Sitting Supine RSL LSL	PEF, FVC, FEV1, PImax, PEmax	FVC, FEV1, PEF: sitting>supine; LSL, RSL, PImax: sitting>supine; PEmax: p > 0.05 between positions
Manning (1999) [20]	19	62.8 ± 6.8	Healthy older adults	Sitting LSL RSL	FVC, FEV1 DLCO/VA	FVC, FEV1: sitting>RSL & LSL; DLCO/VA: p > 0.05 between positions
Vilke (2000) [26]	20	Range 18–50	Healthy males	Sitting Supine	FVC, FEV1	FVC, FEV1: sitting>supine
Stewart (2000) [24]	10	22.3 ± 2.4	Healthy males	Sitting Supine	FVC, VC, FEV1, FEV1/FVC, PEF, DLCO	FVC, PEF: sitting>supine; DLCO: sitting< supine; FEV1, VC, FEV1/FVC: p > 0.05 between positions
Yap (2000) [27]	10	62.2 ± 1.2 Mean ± SE	Healthy	Sitting Supine	FVC, FEV1, FEV1/FVC, FRC	FVC, FEV1, FRC: sitting>supine; FEV1/FVC: p > 0.05 between positions
Varrato (2001) [25]	15	Mean 41	Healthy	Sitting Supine	FVC	FVC: sitting>supine
Badr (2002) [46]	25	34.0 ± 14.9	Healthy	Standing Sitting Supine RSL	PEmax, PEF	PEmax: standing>other positions; PEmax: sitting>supine & RSL; PEF: standing>other positions
Ogiwara (2002) [55]	20	Mean 22.8 ± 2.1 Range 21–28	Healthy	Sitting Supine RSL LSL	PEmax, PImax	PEmax, PImax: p > 0.05 between positions
Peces-Barba (2004) [56]	14	37.5 ± 11.5	Healthy	Sitting Supine	DLCO	DLCO: sitting<supine
Chang (2005) [53]	20	28.3 ± 4.8	Healthy males	Standing Supine	FRC	FRC: standing>supine
Palermo (2005) [21]	14	61 ± 8	Healthy	Sitting Supine LSL RSL	FEV1, FVC, VC, DLCO	FEV1, FVC, VC: p > 0.05 between positions; DLCO: sitting>LSL & RSL
Watson (2005) [43]	5	Mean 57	Healthy	Sitting Supine	TLC, VC, RV, FRC	TLC, VC, RV: p > 0.05 between positions; FRC sitting>supine
Saxena (2006) [23]	80	Males 21.3 ± 1.5 Females 19.6 ± 1.3	Healthy	Standing Sitting Supine	FEV1, FVC, FEV1/FVC, PEF	FEV1, FVC, PEF: standing>supine; FEV1/FVC: sitting>supine
Ben-Dov (2009) [17]	7	44 ± 10	Healthy	Sitting Supine	FVC	FVC: p > 0.05 between positions
Terzano (2009) [57]	10	59.0 ± 9.3	Healthy	Standing Sitting Supine	DLCO	DLCO: p > 0.05 between positions
Tsubaki (2009) [28]	15	22.7 ± 2.3	Healthy females	Sitting Supine	FVC, FEV1, FEV1/FVC, VC, PImax, PEmax	FEV1/FVC: sitting>supine; FVC, FEV1, VC, PImax, PEmax: p > 0.05 between positions
McCoy (2010) [49]	182	23.5 ± 2.5 (healthy and asthmatic patients)	Healthy	Standing, Sitting	PEF	PEF: p > 0.05 between positions
Ceridon (2011) [18]	12	63 ± 9	Healthy	Sitting Supine	FVC, FEV1, FEV1/FVC, DLCO	FVC, FEV1, DLCO: sitting>supine; FEV1/FVC: p > 0.05 between positions
Roychowdhury (2011) [44]	100	Range 19–22	Healthy	Sitting Supine	VC	VC: supine>sitting in females; VC: p > 0.05 between positions in males

Table 2 Summary of study characteristics according to study population (Continued)

1st Author (Year)	No of Participants	Age (Years)	Population	Positions	Pulmonary Function	Main Findings
Gianinis (2013) [48]	30	22.2 ± 2.4	Healthy	Sitting Supine RSL LSL	PEF	PEF: sitting>supine & RSL
Wallace (2013) [51]	94	23.9 ± 3.7	Healthy	Standing Sitting	PEF	PEF: standing>sitting
Naitoh (2014) [39]	20	28 ± 1.4	Healthy	Sitting Supine	FEV1,VC PEmax, PImax	FEV1, VC: sitting>supine PEmax, PImax: p > 0.05 between positions
Costa (2015) [54]	63	19.7 ± 1.5	Healthy	Sitting Supine	PImax, PEmax	PImax, PEmax: sitting>supine
Ganapathi (2015) [19]	20	Range 18–25	Healthy	Standing Sitting Supine RSL LSL	FVC, FEV1, FEV1/FVC	FVC, FEV1, FEV1/FVC: standing>supine, RSL& LSL FEV1: standing>sitting sitting>RSL FEV1/FVC: sitting>LSL
Patel (2015) [22]	45	Median 21 Range 19–23	Healthy	Standing, Sitting Supine	FVC, FEV1, PEF	FVC, FEV1, PEF: sitting>standing FVC, FEV1, PEF: sitting>supine
Antunes (2016) [45]	30	22.7 ± 2.4	Healthy	Sitting Supine	PEF	PEF: sitting>supine
Miccinili (2016) [40]	20	33.6 ± 10.5	Healthy	Sitting Supine	VC, FEV1	VC, FEV1: p > 0.05 between positions
Ottaviano (2016) [50]	76	40 ± 16	Healthy	Standing Sitting	PEF	PEF: standing>sitting
Myint (2017) [42]	15	22.6 ± 2.0	Healthy	Standing, Sitting Supine	FEV1/FVC	FEV1/FVC: p > 0.05 between positions
Badr (2002) [46]	11	66.8 ± 12.6	Chronic airflow limitation	Standing Sitting Supine RSL	PEmax, PEF	PEmax: standing>supine & RSL, PEmax: sitting>supine & RSL PEF: standing>sitting, supine, RSL
Elkins (2005) [47]	20	29 ± 8	Adult cystic fibrosis	Standing Sitting Supine RSL	PEmax, PEF	PEmax: standing & sitting>RSL PEF: standing>supine & RSL
Razi (2007) [32]	49	42.6 ± 11.8	Obesity, asthma (Mean BMI 36±5)	Standing Sitting	FVC, FEV1, FEV1/FVC	FVC, FEV1, FEV1/FVC: p > 0.05 between positions
Terzano (2009) [57]	30 Mild 10 Moderate-severe 10 Very severe 10	Mild 57.3 ± 8.6 Moderate-severe 59.8 ± 9.1 Very severe 63.7 ± 5.5	COPD	Standing Sitting Supine	DLCO	DLCO: p > 0.05 between positions
McCoy (2010) [49]	29	23.5 ± 2.5 (Healthy and asthmatic patients)	Asthma	Standing Sitting	PEF	PEF: p > 0.05 between positions
De (2012) [29]	75	61.2 ± 9.2	COPD	Standing Sitting	FVC, FEV1	FVC, FEV1: p > 0.05 between positions
Melam (2014) [30]	30	34.3 ± 3.7	Asthma	Standing, Sitting Supine	FVC, FEV1	FVC, FEV1: standing>supine
Mohammed (2017) [31]	20	39.2 ± 8.0	Asthma	Standing Sitting Supine RSL LSL	FVC, FEV1, PEF	FVC, FEV1, PEF: standing>supine, RSL, LSL FVC, FEV1: standing>sitting
Myint (2017) [42]	15	22.3 ± 2.0	Asthma	Standing	FEV1/FVC	FEV1/FVC: p > 0.05 between positions

Table 2 Summary of study characteristics according to study population (Continued)

1st Author (Year)	No of Participants	Age (Years)	Population	Positions	Pulmonary Function	Main Findings
Faggiano (1998) [58]	32	59 ± 10	CHF, males	Sitting Supine	DLCO	DLCO: $p > 0.05$ between positions; ↓DLCO in sitting in a subgroup of patients with decrease in mean pulmonary arterial pressure in this position; ↑DLCO in sitting in a subgroup of patients with increase in mean pulmonary arterial pressure in this position
Yap (2000) [27]	10	61.4 ± 2.0 *Mean±SE*	CHF	Sitting Supine	FEV1, FVC, FEV1/FVC, VC, FRC	FVC, FEV1 VC: sitting>supine FEV1/FVC, FRC: $p > 0.05$ between positions
Palermo (2005) [21]	14	62 ± 8	CHF	Sitting Supine LSL RSL	FEV1, FVC, VC, DLCO	FEV1, FVC: sitting>RSL & LSL DLCO: sitting>RSL &LSL VC: $p > 0.05$ between positions
Ceridon (2011) [18]	24	65 ± 8	CHF	Sitting Supine	FEV1, FVC, FEV1/FVC, DLCO	FEV1, FVC: sitting>supine FEV1/FVC: $p > 0.05$ between positions DLCO: $p > 0.05$ between positions
Linn (2000) [33]	222 *Tetraplegia 98 Paraplegia 124*	40 ± 11	SCI	Sitting Supine	FVC, FEV1, PEF	FVC, FEV1, PEF: sitting<supine in complete tetraplegia FVC, FEV1, PEF: $p > 0.05$ between positions in paraplegia
Baydur (2001) [35]	74 *C3-7 injury tetraplegia 31 T—L4 injury paraplegia 43*	40 ± 12	SCI	Sitting Supine	FVC, FEV1	FVC, FEV1: $p > 0.05$ between positions
Ben Dov (2009) [17]	12	42 ± 11	Neurologically stable *C5-8 tetraplegia*	Sitting Supine	FVC	FVC: sitting<supine
Park (2010) [34]	43	35.0 ± 12.6	SCI *C6-C8*	Sitting Supine	FVC	FVC: sitting<supine
Kim (2012) [36]	45 *Cervical 15 Thoracic 13 Lumbar 17*	Cervical 43.2 ± 1.3 Thoracic 49.8 ± 4.9 Lumbar 52.2 ± 4.4	SCI	Sitting Supine	FVC, FEV1	FVC, FEV1: $p > 0.05$ between positions within cervical/thoracic/lumbar subgroups FVC, FEV1: sitting<supine in cervical and thoracic injury FVC, FEV1: sitting>supine in lumbar injury Statistically significant difference in the effect of position between cervical/thoracic/lumbar subgroups
Terson de Paleville (2014) [37]	27 *Complete motor injury 13 Incomplete motor injury 14 Cervical 15, Thoracic 12*	40 ± 14	SCI	Sitting Supine	FVC, FEV1, PEmax, PImax	FVC, FEV1: $p > 0.05$ between positions for all patients together FVC: sitting<supine in cervical/complete motor injury FVC: sitting>supine in thoracic incomplete motor injury FEV1 sitting> supine in incomplete motor injury FEV1: sitting>supine in thoracic incomplete motor injury PEmax: sitting>supine all patients PEmax: sitting>supine in complete motor injury PEmax: sitting>supine in cervical incomplete motor injury

Table 2 Summary of study characteristics according to study population (*Continued*)

1st Author (Year)	No of Participants	Age (Years)	Population	Positions	Pulmonary Function	Main Findings
Miccinilli (2016) [40]	20 *C3–7 tetraplegia 9; T1–8 paraplegia 11*	Tetraplegia 29.4 ± 10.5 Paraplegia 36.6 ± 10.3	SCI	Sitting Supine	VC, FEV1	Plmax: $p > 0.05$ between positions for all patients together Plmax: sitting>supine in thoracic complete motor injury VC, FEV1: sitting<supine
Varrato (2001) [25]	38	61	ALS	Sitting Supine	FVC	FVC: sitting>supine
Park (2010) [34]	45	54.4 ± 11.1	ALS	Sitting Supine	FVC	FVC: sitting>supine
Poussel (2014) [38]	58	42.6 ± 12.9	Myotonic dystrophy	Sitting Supine	FVC, FEV1	FVC, FEV1: sitting>supine
Watson (2005) [43]	10	49 ± 6 *Mean ± SE*	Obesity Mean BMI 44±3 *Mean ±SE*	Sitting Supine	TLC, VC, RV, FRC,	TLC, VC, RV, FRC: $p > 0.05$ between positions
Razi (2007) [32]	51	39.86 ± 10.1	Obesity *Mean BMI 36.7±4.1*	Standing Sitting	FVC, FEV1, FEV1/FVC	FVC, FEV1, FEV1/FVC: $p > 0.05$ between positions
Benedik (2009) [52]	32	Range 18–75	Healthy, mild-moderate obesity *Mean BMI 32.7±3.5*	Sitting Supine	FRC	FRC: sitting>supine
Sebbane (2015) [41]	12	44 ± 14	Morbid obesity *Mean BMI 45±5* S/P bariatric surgery *Mean BMI 31 ± 5*	Sitting Supine	TLC, RV, VC, FRC, FEV1	FEV1: sitting>supine in morbid obesity TLC, RV, FRC, VC: $p > 0.05$ between positions in morbid obesity FRC, FEV1: sitting>supine in s/p bariatric surgery TLC, RV, VC: $p > 0.05$ between positions in s/p bariatric surgery

Values are mean ± S.D. unless specified other

ALS Amyotrophic lateral sclerosis, *BMI* Body mass index, *CHF* Congestive heart failure, *COPD* Chronic obstructive pulmonary disease, *DLCO* Diffusing capacity of the lungs for carbon monoxide, *DLCO/VA* Diffusing capacity of the lung for carbon monoxide divided by alveolar volume, *FEV1* Forced expiratory flow in 1 s, *FRC* Functional residual capacity, *FVC* Forced vital capacity, *LSL* Left side lying, *PEF* Peak expiratory flow, *PEmax* Maximal expiratory pressure, *PImax* Maximal inspiratory pressure, *RSL* Right side lying, *RV* Residual volume, *SCI* Spinal cord injury, *S/P* Status post, *TLC* Total lung capacity, *VC* Vital capacity

significance. Nevertheless, it is important to note that in these debilitated patients with SCI, even a small change in FVC is probably clinically significant.

Three studies evaluated patients with neuromuscular diseases [25, 34, 38]. In patients with myotonic dystrophy and in those with amyotrophic lateral sclerosis (ALS), there was a clinically and statistically significant decrease in FVC from sitting to supine [25, 34, 38]. In subjects with obesity (mean BMI 36.7) no significant difference was reported between standing and sitting [32].

FEV1

In healthy subjects, FEV1 was reported to be higher in sitting vs. supine [3, 18, 22, 23, 26, 27, 39], in sitting vs. RSL and LSL [3, 19, 20], in standing vs. sitting [23], and in standing vs. sitting, supine, RSL, and LSL [19]. However, other studies [21, 24, 28, 40] did not find significant difference for FEV1 between sitting and supine, RSL, and LSL. One study [22] reported a decrease of 120 ml in FEV1 from sitting to standing, which is statistically but not clinically significant.

Among asthmatic patients, FEV1 was higher in the standing vs. supine position, a statistically and clinically significant change; however, there was no significant difference between sitting vs. supine, RSL, and LSL positions [30]. Another study in asthmatic patients reported FEV1 to be higher in standing vs. sitting, supine, RSL, and LSL, and in sitting vs. supine, RSL and LSL [31]. Among obese asthmatic patients and those with COPD, there was no significant difference in FEV1 between standing and sitting [29, 32].

In subjects with CHF, one study found a statistically and clinically significant increase in FEV1 in sitting vs. RSL and LSL, but no difference between sitting and supine [21], while two other studies reported higher FEV1 in sitting vs. supine [18, 27].

In patients with SCI, FEV1 was recently reported to increase from sitting to supine [40]; however, other studies found that the effect of position on FEV1 in those with SCI depends on the level and extent of injury. In one study among all subjects with SCI, FEV1 was not significantly influenced by moving from sitting to supine [35], but patients with cervical injuries showed a tendency for increased FEV1 in the supine vs. sitting position while those with thoracic injuries tended towards increased FEV1 in the sitting position. Along the same vein, another study [36] found an increase is FEV1 in the sitting vs. the supine position in patients with lumbar injury while FEV1 was higher in the supine position for those with cervical spine or thoracic injuries. Although the differences between positions were not statistically significant, the effect of level of injury was statistically and clinically significant.

In another study [33], FEV1 was higher in supine vs. sitting in patients with complete tetraplegia, while in patients with incomplete injury there was no significant difference between positions. Another group [37] reported no significant change in FEV1 between the sitting and supine positions for a pooled group of patients with SCI, but in the subgroup of patients with incomplete motor injury and in those with incomplete thoracic motor injury there was a decrease in the supine position.

In patients with myotonic dystrophy, FEV1 decreased from sitting to supine [38]. Among those with obesity, FEV1 was higher in sitting vs. supine both before and after bariatric surgery [41]. In another study among obese patients, there was no difference in FEV1 between standing and sitting [32].

FEV1/FVC

Seven studies compared FEV1/FVC for different body positions in healthy subjects [18, 19, 23, 24, 27, 28, 42]. In several studies, FEV1/FVC was reported to be higher in sitting vs. supine [23, 28], in sitting vs. LSL [19], and in standing vs. supine, RSL, and LSL [19]; however, FEV1/FVC was > 70% in all body positions so the difference was not clinically significant. Other studies found no difference between sitting and supine [18, 24, 27] or standing, sitting, and supine [42].

Among subjects with asthma, CHF, and obesity no statistically significant difference in FEV1/FVC was found between the different body postures [18, 27, 32, 42].

Vital capacity

The effect of body position on vital capacity was evaluated in six studies of healthy subjects [21, 24, 28, 39, 43, 44]. In most studies no difference was reported between sitting and supine [21, 24, 28, 43] or between sitting and RSL or LSL [21]. One study [39] found that VC was higher in the sitting vs. supine position. However, another study [44] found that VC was higher in the supine vs. sitting position, but only in females.

In patients with CHF, VC was reported to be higher in sitting vs. supine in one study [27] while another study found no statistically significant difference between these positions [21]. In patients with spinal cord injury, VC was higher in the supine vs. sitting position [40]. In subjects with obesity, no difference in VC was reported between the sitting and supine positions [41, 43].

PEF

PEF in different body positions was evaluated in 13 studies [3, 22–24, 31, 33, 45–51]. Eight studies evaluated only healthy adults [3, 22–24, 45, 48, 50, 51], three evaluated healthy subjects and patients with COPD or asthma [31, 46, 49], one included adult cystic fibrosis patients [47], and one included subjects with SCI [33].

Nine studies that compared standing or sitting positions vs. supine or RSL and LSL found higher PEF in standing and sitting [3, 22–24, 31, 45–48]. Three of six studies comparing the standing and sitting positions found higher PEF in standing [46, 50, 51] and one reported higher PEF in sitting [22]. However, it is most likely that none of the differences reported in PEF are clinically significant. In SCI patients with complete tetraplegia PEF was found to be 12% higher in the supine vs. sitting position [33].

FRC

FRC was evaluated using helium dilution in five studies [27, 41, 43, 52, 53]. Among healthy subjects, FRC was higher in standing [53] and in sitting [27, 43] vs. supine, with the differences reaching statistical and clinical significance. However, the difference in sitting vs. supine was not significant among patients with obesity (mean BMI 44–45) [41, 43] or CHF [27], and was higher in sitting vs. supine in patients after bariatric surgery (mean BMI 31) [41]. Another study [52] involving subjects with mild-to-moderate obesity (mean BMI 32), reported that FRC was significantly higher both statistically and clinically in sitting vs. supine.

Total lung capacity

Two studies that evaluated TLC using helium dilution in healthy subjects [43] and in subjects with obesity [41, 43] found no statistically significant difference between the sitting and supine positions.

Residual volume

Two studies that evaluated RV using helium dilution in healthy subjects [43] and those with obesity [41, 43] found no statistically significant difference between sitting and supine.

PEmax

Six studies investigated the association between body position and PEmax in healthy subjects [3, 28, 39, 46, 54, 55]. PEmax was higher in standing vs. supine, in standing vs. sitting and RSL, in sitting vs. supine [54], and in sitting vs. supine and RSL [46]; however, the differences reported in those studies were not clinically significant. Other studies found no difference in PEmax between sitting and supine [28, 39], or between sitting, supine, RSL, and LSL [3, 55].

In COPD patients, PEmax was higher in standing or sitting vs. supine or RSL [46], and was higher in standing and sitting vs. RSL in patients with cystic fibrosis [47]. The differences were not clinically significant.

In subjects with SCI, PEmax was significantly higher in sitting vs. supine for all subjects, and for patients with motor complete injury or incomplete cervical motor injury [37].

PImax

In healthy subjects, PImax was improved in sitting vs. supine in two studies [3, 54]. However, other studies found no difference in PImax in sitting vs. supine [28, 39, 55], or sitting vs. RSL and LSL [3, 55]. In subjects with chronic SCI, no significant change was seen in PImax between sitting and supine, with the exception of a subgroup of patients with complete thoracic motor paresis where there was statistically and clinically significant improvement in sitting [37].

DLCO

Seven studies evaluated the effect of body position on diffusion capacity; six included healthy subjects [18, 20, 21, 24, 56, 57], three included patients with CHF [18, 21, 58], and one included COPD patients [57].

Among healthy subjects, two studies [24, 56] found statistically and clinically significant improvement in DLCO in supine vs. sitting and one [57] found a trend towards increased DLCO in supine vs. sitting, however this difference did not reach statistical significance. One study [18] found DLCO to be higher in the sitting vs. supine positions while another study found no difference in DLCO between these positions [21]. One study [21] reported higher DLCO in sitting vs. side lying while another study [20] found no difference between these positions. In COPD patients, no statistically significant change in DLCO was found between the sitting and the supine position [57].

Three studies investigated diffusion capacity in patients with CHF [18, 21, 58]. One study [58] found that postural changes from the supine to sitting positions induced different responses in diffusion capacity. In some patients diffusion capacity improved in the sitting position and others showed no change or a decline. On the average no statistically significant difference was found between the two positions. The authors attributed the difference in responses to variations in pulmonary circulation pressures. Another study [18] found no significant difference in diffusion capacity between the sitting and the supine positions. Side-lying was reported to reduce DLCO in comparison to sitting in the third study [21].

Discussion

Most studies in this systematic review of 43 papers evaluating the effect of body position on pulmonary function found that pulmonary function improved with more erect posture in both healthy subjects and those with lung disease, heart disease, neuromuscular diseases, and obesity. In patients with SCI, the effect is more complex and depends on the severity and level of injury. In contrast, diffusion capacity, as assessed by DLCO, increases in the supine position in healthy subjects while the effect in CHF patients is thought to depend upon pulmonary circulation pressure.

Decreased FVC in more recumbent positions may reflect both increased thoracic blood volume due to gravitational facilitation of venous return, which is more important in patients with heart failure, as well as cephalic displacement of the diaphragm due to abdominal pressure in the recumbent positions, which is more important in obese subjects [59]. In side-lying positions, even though only the dependent hemi-diaphragm is displaced, the effect on FVC appears to be similar to that observed in a supine position [59]. Other factors that may contribute to lower FVC values in side-lying positions include increased airway resistance and decreased lung compliance secondary to anatomical differences between the left and right lungs, as well as shifting of the mediastinal structures [20].

FEV1 was also higher in erect positions. Recumbent positions limit expiratory volumes and flow, which may reflect an increase in airway resistance, a decrease in elastic recoil of the lung, or decreased mechanical advantage of forced expiration, presumably affecting the large airways [20]. In asthmatic patients the increase in FVC while standing might be due to the increased diameter of the airways in this position [30].

In patients with CHF the lungs are stiff and heavy, and the heart is large and heavy, increasing the negative effects of lung-heart interdependence [60]. As cardiac dimension increases, lung volume, mechanical function, and diffusion capacity decrease [61, 62]; thus, the heart weighs on the diaphragm while sitting and on one of the lungs while in a side-lying position. This influences the ability of the lungs to expand laterally but allows the diaphragm to descend and the lungs to expand inferiorly. In side-lying positions, the heart weighs on one lung, compressing both the airways and lung parenchyma, leading to a reduction in FEV1 and FVC due to airway compression [21]. Both elastic (reduced lung compliance) and resistive loads are simultaneously increased in the supine position in CHF patients [63].

Changes in FVC from the sitting to supine positions may reflect diaphragm strength/paralysis. FVC is thus an important clinical tool for assessment of diaphragmatic weakness in patients with neuromuscular diseases [64]. In patients with ALS, supine FVC is a test of diaphragmatic weakness [65] that predicts orthopnea [25] and prognosis for survival [66, 67]. The American Academy of Neurology has concluded that in ALS patients, supine FVC is probably more effective than erect FVC in detecting diaphragm weakness and correlates better with symptoms of hypoventilation [68].

In patients with cervical SCI (tetraplegia), FVC and FEV1 increase in the supine vs. sitting position. The diaphragm increases its inspiratory excursion in the supine position because its muscle fibers are longer at end expiration, and they operate at a more effective point of their length-tension curve [69–71]. This mechanism is especially important in patients for whom the diaphragm is the main muscle for breathing, since their intercostal and abdominal muscles are inactive due to SCI.

FRC was reported to increase in upright positions in healthy subjects [27, 43, 53] and in patients with mild-to-moderate obesity [41, 52]. Changing from a supine to an upright position increases FRC due to reduced pulmonary blood volume and the descent of the diaphragm. This may change the point in which tidal breathing occurs in the volume-pressure curve, which leads to increased lung compliance, and thus an identical pressure change would produce a greater inspired volume if there is no change in respiratory drive [53]. However, among patients with CHF, no difference in FRC between sitting and supine was reported [27]. In heart failure, reduction in lung compliance in the supine position might reduce the passive change in lung volume, but FRC may be sustained above relaxation volume by an adjustment in respiratory muscle or glottal activity [27]. Among patients with obesity the sitting FRC was less than in healthy subjects but there was no further decrease in the supine position [43].

PEF, PEmax, and PImax were found to increase in upright positions in healthy subjects [3, 23, 24, 46, 48, 50, 51] and in those with lung diseases [31, 46, 47]. This may be related to changes in lung volumes with positions.

Standing and sitting have been shown to lead to the highest lung volumes [72, 73]. At higher lung volumes the elastic recoil of the lungs and the chest wall is greater. In addition, the expiratory muscles are at a more optimal region of the length-tension curve and thus are capable of generating higher intrathoracic pressure, potentially generating higher expiratory pressures and pushing air through narrow airways at high speed, which results in higher PEmax, PEF, and FEV1. As lung volumes decrease, muscle length becomes less optimal, which results in lower PEmax in sitting, compared to the standing position, and even lower in more recumbent positions. The change in PEmax influences PEF [46].

When standing, gravity pulls the mediastinal and abdominal structures down, creating more space in the thoracic cavity, which allows further expansion of the lungs and greater lung volumes [74]. This, along with the decrease in compression on the lung bases, allows alveoli to recruit and increases lung compliance. The inspiratory muscles can expand even more, which allows the diaphragm to continue contracting downwards, thus increasing lung volumes [46].

Sitting often leads to the somewhat reduced lung volumes compared with standing. This can be explained by several mechanisms. First, in sitting, abdominal organs are higher, interfering with diaphragmatic motion, thus enabling smaller inspiration. Second, the abdominal muscles are in a less optimal point in the length-tension curve, since the combination of hip flexion and higher position of the abdominal contents exert upward pressure. Third, the back of the chair may limit thoracic expansion. These three factors explain a slightly lower PEmax and PEF in sitting vs. standing [46].

Diaphragmatic strength is negatively affected by the supine position, and intrathoracic blood volume is increased. These factors lead to decreased PEmax and PEF in the supine position [3].

In side-lying positions (RSL or LSL), when the bed is flat, the abdominal contents fall forward. The dependent hemi-diaphragm is stretched to a good length for tension generation, while the nondependent hemi-diaphragm is more flattened. Changes in lung volumes may thus balance themselves out due to a better diaphragmatic contraction but decreased space in the thorax [46].

The decreased PImax observed in the supine position could be related to diaphragm overload by abdominal content displacement during maximal inspiratory effort, which could offset improved diaphragm position on the length-tension curve. In addition, the length of all other inspiratory muscles may become less optimal in supine position [75].

In patients with cervical spinal cord injury and high tetraplegia, PEF was found to be higher in the supine vs. sitting position [33] corresponding to the increase in FVC and FEV1 in the supine position.

In healthy subjects, most studies showed an increase in DLCO in supine vs. sitting [24, 56, 57]. This improvement is attributed to the moderate increase in alveolar blood volume in the supine position due to recruitment of lung capillary bed on transition from upright to supine. Age may attenuate this increase [76]. This may explain why a study that included participants with a mean age of 61 [21] found no difference in DLCO between sitting and supine.

In side-lying positions, the heart weighs on one lung, compressing both airways and lung parenchyma, reducing alveolar blood volume, and causing ventilation/ perfusion mismatch. Those effects caused reduction of diffusion capacity in the side-lying positions [21].

In COPD patients, there was no change in DLCO between sitting and supine [57]. This might be related to reduced FVC and alveolar damage in these patients. These effects might have negative impact on diffusion capacity, opposing the positive effect of the increase in blood volume in the alveoli [57].

In patients with CHF, different patterns of the effect of posture on DLCO were observed [58]. The change in DLCO was probably related to the change in alveolar blood volume, most likely due to differences in pulmonary artery pressure and heart dimensions [58].

Limitations of the study

There are a few limitations to this review. First, the level of evidence of the studies is relatively low. However, in this type of research, due to the nature of the populations studied and the interventions applied, it is impossible to perform a randomized control study. Second, most studies were performed on a small number of subjects and all studies used either consecutive, convenience, or volunteer sampling. The review included only adult subjects and it is therefore not possible to generalize the results to children and adolescents. Finally, research protocols varied between studies and detailed information about protocols were often missing. Patient cooperation during lung function testing strongly influences results. This may explain contradictory results obtained in some cases. Studies that included subjects older than 60 years did not mention the cognitive function of participants, a factor that may influence patient cooperation.

Further research in this field is needed, including studies designed to evaluate lung function in a larger number of healthy participants as well as in individuals with a variety of medical conditions. There is also a need to use a standardized protocol including randomization of postures and times between tests (e.g. for wash-out of inhaled gasses or redistribution of blood volume) in different positions to enable a better comparison of outcomes.

Conclusions

When performing pulmonary function tests, body position plays a role in its influence over test results. As seen in this review, a change in body position may have varying implications depending on the patient populations. American Thoracic Society (ATS) guidelines [2] recommend performing PFTs in the sitting or standing position, but the sitting position is usually preferred. The norms of those functions according to gender and age were established from tests performed in this position. This review suggests that for most of the subjects this is the preferred position for the test; however, clinicians should consider performing PFTs in other positions in selected patients. In patients with SCI, testing also in the supine position may provide important information. In patients with neuromuscular disorders, performing PFTs in the supine position may help to assess diaphragmatic function.

Positioning plays an important role in maximizing respiratory function when treating patients with various problems and diseases and it is important to know the implications of each position on the respiratory system of a specific patient. Understanding the influence of body position can give healthcare professionals better knowledge of optimal positions for patients with different diseases.

Additional files

Additional file 1: Table S1. Scoring for papers included in the systematic review based on the Quality Assessment Tool for Before-After (Pre-Post) Studies with No Control Group of the National Heart, Lung and Blood Institute [3, 15–31, 33–58]. (DOCX 63 kb)

Additional file 2: Table S2. Statistically significant differences in pulmonary function between the various body positions [3, 17–28, 30, 31, 33, 34, 37–41, 43–48, 50–54, 56]. (DOCX 104 kb)

Acknowledgements

The authors wish to thank Prof. Ora Paltiel, a specialist in Internal Medicine, Hematology, and Oncology who also holds a doctorate in Epidemiology and Biostatistics, for her invaluable assistance in selecting the optimal tools for assessment of the quality of evidence and potential for bias of studies included in this systematic review.
The authors wish to thank Shifra Fraifeld, a medical center-based medical writer and editor, for her editorial contribution during manuscript preparation.

Authors' contributions

SK, E-LM, NA, AR contributed to the study concept and design. SK, E-LM, NA, AR, YZ contributed to data acquisition and analysis, and interpretation of the data. The primary literature search was conducted by SK and E-LM. SK and E-LM drafted the manuscript. SK, E-LM, NA, AR, YZ critically reviewed and revised the manuscript for intellectual content. All authors reviewed the final version of the manuscript prior to submission and all accept responsibility for the integrity of the research process and findings. All authors read and approved the final manuscript.

Competing interests

The authors declare that they have no competing interests.

Author details

[1]Chronic Ventilator-Dependent Division, Herzog Medical Center, POB 3900, Jerusalem, Israel. [2]Pulmonary Institute, Shaare Zedek Medical Center, POB 3235, Jerusalem, Israel. [3]Recanati School for Community Health Professions, Faculty of Health Sciences, Ben Gurion University of the Negev, Beer Sheva, Israel. [4]Hebrew University-Hadassah Faculty of Medicine, Jerusalem, Israel.

References

1. Crapo RO. Pulmonary-function testing. N Engl J Med. 1994;331(1):25–30.
2. Miller MR, Crapo R, Hankinson J, et al. General considerations for lung function testing. Eur Respir J. 2005;26(1):153–61.
3. Meysman M, Vincken W. Effect of body posture on spirometric values and upper airway obstruction indices derived from the flow-volume loop in young nonobese subjects. Chest. 1998;114(4):1042–7.
4. Pellegrino R, Viegi G, Brusasco V, et al. Interpretative strategies for lung function tests. Eur Respir J. 2005;26(5):948–68.
5. Wanger J, Clausen JL, Coates A, et al. Standardisation of the measurement of lung volumes. Eur Respir J. 2005;26(3):511–22.
6. Goswami R, Guleria R, Gupta AK, et al. Prevalence of diaphragmatic muscle weakness and dyspnoea in Graves' disease and their reversibility with carbimazole therapy. Eur J Endocrinol. 2002;147(3):299–303.
7. Keenan SP, Alexander D, Road JD, Ryan CF, Oger J, Wilcox PG. Ventilatory muscle strength and endurance in myasthenia gravis. Eur Respir J. 1995;8(7): 1130–5.
8. Nava S, Crotti P, Gurrieri G, Fracchia C, Rampulla C. Effect of a beta 2-agonist (broxaterol) on respiratory muscle strength and endurance in patients with COPD with irreversible airway obstruction. Chest. 1992; 101(1):133–40.
9. Quanjer PH, Lebowitz MD, Gregg I, Miller MR, Pedersen OF. Peak expiratory flow: conclusions and recommendations of a working Party of the European Respiratory Society. Eur Respir J Suppl. 1997;24:2s–8s.
10. Global initiative for asthma (GINA): Global strategy for asthma management and prevention (2018 update). 2018. file:///C:/Users/owner/Downloads/wms-GINA-2018-report-V1.3–002.pdf. Accessed 29 May 2018.
11. Graham BL, Brusasco V, Burgos F, et al. 2017 ERS/ATS standards for single-breath carbon monoxide uptake in the lung. Eur Respir J. 2017;49(1). https://doi.org/10.1183/13993003.00016-2016.
12. Hathaway EH, Tashkin DP, Simmons MS. Intraindividual variability in serial measurements of DLCO and alveolar volume over one year in eight healthy subjects using three independent measuring systems. Am Rev Respir Dis. 1989;140(6):1818–22.
13. Moher D, Liberati A, Tetzlaff J, Altman DG, PRISMA Group. Preferred reporting items for systematic reviews and meta-analyses: the PRISMA statement. PLoS Med. 2009;6(7):e1000097.
14. Gronseth GS, Woodroffe LM, Getchuis TSD. Clinical practice guideline process manual. 2011. http://tools.aan.com/globals/axon/assets/9023.pdf. Accessed 29 May 2018.
15. Quality assessment tool for before-after (pre-post) studies with no control group. 2014. https://www.nhlbi.nih.gov/health-topics/study-quality-assessment-tools. Accessed 12 Aug 2018.
16. Kunstler BE, Cook JL, Freene N, et al. Physiotherapist-led physical activity interventions are efficacious at increasing physical activity levels: a systematic review and meta-analysis. Clin J Sport Med. 2018;28(3):304–15.
17. Ben-Dov I, Zlobinski R, Segel MJ, Gaides M, Shulimzon T, Zeilig G. Ventilatory response to hypercapnia in C(5-8) chronic tetraplegia: the effect of posture. Arch Phys Med Rehabil. 2009;90(8):1414–7.
18. Ceridon ML, Morris NR, Olson TP, Lalande S, Johnson BD. Effect of supine posture on airway blood flow and pulmonary function in stable heart failure. Respir Physiol Neurobiol. 2011;178(2):269–74.
19. Ganapathi LV, Vinoth S. The estimation of pulmonary functions in various body postures in normal subjects. Int J Advances Med. 2015;2(3):250–4 http://www.ijmedicine.com/index.php/ijam/article/view/360. Accessed 29 May 2018.
20. Manning F, Dean E, Ross J, Abboud RT. Effects of side lying on lung function in older individuals. Phys Ther. 1999;79(5):456–66.
21. Palermo P, Cattadori G, Bussotti M, Apostolo A, Contini M, Agostoni P. Lateral decubitus position generates discomfort and worsens lung function in chronic heart failure. Chest. 2005;128(3):1511–6.
22. Patel AK, Thakar HM. Spirometric values in sitting, standing, and supine position. Lung Pulm Resp Res. 2015;2(1):00026 http://medcraveonline.com/JLPRR/JLPRR-02-00026.php. Accessed 29 May 2018.
23. Saxena J, Gupta S, Saxena S. A study of change of posture on the pulmonary function tests : can it help COPD patients? Indian J Community Health. 2006;18(1):10–2. http://www.iapsmupuk.org/journal/index.php/IJCH/article/view/108. Accessed 29 May 2018.
24. Stewart IB, Potts JE, McKenzie DC, Coutts KD. Effect of body position on measurements of diffusion capacity after exercise. Br J Sports Med. 2000; 34(6):440–4.
25. Varrato J, Siderowf A, Damiano P, Gregory S, Feinberg D, McCluskey L. Postural change of forced vital capacity predicts some respiratory symptoms in ALS. Neurology. 2001;57(2):357–9.
26. Vilke GM, Chan TC, Neuman T, Clausen JL. Spirometry in normal subjects in sitting, prone, and supine positions. Respir Care. 2000;45(4):407–10.
27. Yap JC, Moore DM, Cleland JG, Pride NB. Effect of supine posture on respiratory mechanics in chronic left ventricular failure. Am J Respir Crit Care Med. 2000;162(4 Pt 1):1285–91.
28. Tsubaki A, Deguchi S, Yoneda Y. Influence of posture on respiratory function and respiratory muscle strength in normal subjects. J Phys Ther Sci. 2009;21(1):71–4 https://www.jstage.jst.go.jp/article/jpts/21/1/21_1_71/_article. Accessed 29 May 2018.
29. De S. Comparison of spirometric values in sitting versus standing position among patients with obstructive lung function. Indian J Allergy Asthma Immunol. 2012;26(2):86–8 http://medind.nic.in/iac/t12/i2/iact12i2p86.pdf. Accessed 29 May 2018.
30. Melam GR, Buragadda S, Alhusaini A, Alghamdi MA, Alghamdi MS, Kaushal P. Effect of different positions on FVC and FEV1 measurements of asthmatic patients. J Phys Ther Sci. 2014;26(4):591–3.
31. Mohammed J, Abdulateef A, Shittu A, Sumaila FG. Effect of different body positioning on lung function variables among patients with bronchial asthma. Arch Physiother Global Res. 2017;21(3):7–12. http://apgr.wssp.edu.pl/wp-content/uploads/2017/12/APGR-21-3-A.pdf. Accessed 29 May 2018.

32. Razi E, Moosavi GA. The effect of positions on spirometric values in obese asthmatic patients. Iran J Allergy Asthma Immunol. 2007;6(3):151–4.

33. Linn WS, Adkins RH, Gong H Jr, Waters RL. Pulmonary function in chronic spinal cord injury: a cross-sectional survey of 222 southern California adult outpatients. Arch Phys Med Rehabil. 2000;81(6):757–63.

34. Park JH, Kang SW, Lee SC, Choi WA, Kim DH. How respiratory muscle strength correlates with cough capacity in patients with respiratory muscle weakness. Yonsei Med J. 2010;51(3):392–7.

35. Baydur A, Adkins RH, Milic-Emili J. Lung mechanics in individuals with spinal cord injury: effects of injury level and posture. J Appl Physiol. 2001;90(2):405–11.

36. Kim M-K, Hwangbo G. The effect of position on measured lung function in patients with spinal cord injury. J Physical Therapy Sci. 2012;24(8):655–7 https://www.jstage.jst.go.jp/article/jpts/24/8/24_JPTS-2012-029/_article. Accessed 29 May 2018.

37. Terson de Paleville DG, Sayenko DG, Aslan SC, Folz RJ, McKay WB, Ovechkin AV. Respiratory motor function in seated and supine positions in individuals with chronic spinal cord injury. Respir Physiol Neurobiol. 2014;203:9–14.

38. Poussel M, Kaminsky P, Renaud P, Laroppe J, Pruna L, Chenuel B. Supine changes in lung function correlate with chronic respiratory failure in myotonic dystrophy patients. Respir Physiol Neurobiol. 2014;193:43–51.

39. Naitoh S, Tomita K, Sakai K, Yamasaki A, Kawasaki Y, Shimizu E. The effect of body position on pulmonary function, chest wall motion, and discomfort in young healthy participants. J Manipulative Physiol Ther. 2014;37(9):719–25.

40. Miccinilli S, Morrone M, Bastianini F, et al. Optoelectronic plethysmography to evaluate the effect of posture on breathing kinematics in spinal cord injury: a cross sectional study. Eur J Phys Rehabil Med. 2016;52(1):36–47.

41. Sebbane M, El Kamel M, Millot A, et al. Effect of weight loss on postural changes in pulmonary function in obese dubjects: a longitudinal study. Respir Care. 2015;60(7):992–9.

42. Myint WW, Htay MNN, Soe HHK, et al. Effect of body positions on lungs volume in asthmatic patients: a cross-sectinal study. J Adv Med Pharma Sci. 2017;13(4):1–6 http://www.journalrepository.org/media/journals/JAMPS_36/2017/Jun/Myint1342017JAMPS33901.pdf. Accessed 29 May 2018.

43. Watson RA, Pride NB. Postural changes in lung volumes and respiratory resistance in subjects with obesity. J Appl Physiol (1985). 2005;98(2):512–7.

44. Roychowdhury P, Pramanik T, Prajapati R, Pandit R, Singh S. In health--vital capacity is maximum in supine position. Nepal Med Coll J. 2011;13(2):131–2.

45. Antunes BO, de Souza HC, Gianinis HH, Passarelli-Amaro RC, Tambascio J, Gastaldi AC. Peak expiratory flow in healthy, young, non-active subjects in seated, supine, and prone postures. Physiother Theory Pract. 2016;32(6):489–93.

46. Badr C, Elkins MR, Ellis ER. The effect of body position on maximal expiratory pressure and flow. Aust J Physiother. 2002;48(2):95–102.

47. Elkins MR, Alison JA, Bye PT. Effect of body position on maximal expiratory pressure and flow in adults with cystic fibrosis. Pediatr Pulmonol. 2005;40(5):385–91.

48. Gianinis HH, Antunes BO, Passarelli RC, Souza HC, Gastaldi AC. Effects of dorsal and lateral decubitus on peak expiratory flow in healthy subjects. Braz J Phys Ther. 2013;17(5):435–41.

49. McCoy EK, Thomas JL, Sowell RS, et al. An evaluation of peak expiratory flow monitoring: a comparison of sitting versus standing measurements. J Am Board Fam Med. 2010;23(2):166–70.

50. Ottaviano G, Scadding GK, Iacono V, Scarpa B, Martini A, Lund VJ. Peak nasal inspiratory flow and peak expiratory flow. Upright and sitting values in an adult population. Rhinology. 2016;54(2):160–3.

51. Wallace JL, George CM, Tolley EA, et al. Peak expiratory flow in bed? A comparison of 3 positions. Respir Care. 2013;58(3):494–7.

52. Benedik PS, Baun MM, Keus L, et al. Effects of body position on resting lung volume in overweight and mildly to moderately obese subjects. Respir Care. 2009;54(3):334–9.

53. Chang AT, Boots RJ, Brown MG, Paratz JD, Hodges PW. Ventilatory changes following head-up tilt and standing in healthy subjects. Eur J Appl Physiol. 2005;95(5–6):409–17.

54. Costa R, Almeida N, Ribeiro F. Body position influences the maximum inspiratory and expiratory mouth pressures of young healthy subjects. Physiotherapy. 2015;101(2):239–41.

55. Ogiwara S, Miyachi T. Effect of posture on ventilatory muscle strength. J Phys Ther Sci. 2002;14(1):1–5. https://www.jstage.jst.go.jp/article/jpts/14/1/14_1_1/_pdf/-char/en. Accessed 29 May 2018.

56. Peces-Barba G, Rodriguez-Nieto MJ, Verbanck S, Paiva M, Gonzalez-Mangado N. Lower pulmonary diffusing capacity in the prone vs. supine posture. J Appl Physiol (1985). 2004;96(5):1937–42.

57. Terzano C, Conti V, Petroianni A, Ceccarelli D, De Vito C, Villari P. Effect of postural variations on carbon monoxide diffusing capacity in healthy subjects and patients with chronic obstructive pulmonary disease. Respiration. 2009;77(1):51–7.

58. Faggiano P, D'Aloia A, Simoni P, et al. Effects of body position on the carbon monoxide diffusing capacity in patients with chronic heart failure: relation to hemodynamic changes. Cardiology. 1998;89(1):1–7.

59. Behrakis PK, Baydur A, Jaeger MJ, Milic-Emili J. Lung mechanics in sitting and horizontal body positions. Chest. 1983;83(4):643–6.

60. Agostoni PG, Marenzi GC, Sganzerla P, et al. Lung-heart interaction as a substrate for the improvement in exercise capacity after body fluid volume depletion in moderate congestive heart failure. Am J Cardiol. 1995;76(11):793–8.

61. Agostoni PG, Cattadori G, Guazzi M, Palermo P, Bussotti M, Marenzi G. Cardiomegaly as a possible cause of lung dysfunction in patients with heart failure. Am Heart J. 2000;140(5):e24.

62. Hosenpud JD, Stibolt TA, Atwal K, Shelley D. Abnormal pulmonary function specifically related to congestive heart failure: comparison of patients before and after cardiac transplantation. Am J Med. 1990;88(5):493–6.

63. Nava S, Larovere MT, Fanfulla F, Navalesi P, Delmastro M, Mortara A. Orthopnea and inspiratory effort in chronic heart failure patients. Respir Med. 2003;97(6):647–53.

64. Fromageot C, Lofaso F, Annane D, et al. Supine fall in lung volumes in the assessment of diaphragmatic weakness in neuromuscular disorders. Arch Phys Med Rehabil. 2001;82(1):123–8.

65. Lechtzin N, Wiener CM, Shade DM, Clawson L, Diette GB. Spirometry in the supine position improves the detection of diaphragmatic weakness in patients with amyotrophic lateral sclerosis. Chest. 2002;121(2):436–42.

66. Baumann F, Henderson RD, Morrison SC, et al. Use of respiratory function tests to predict survival in amyotrophic lateral sclerosis. Amyotroph Lateral Scler. 2010;11(1–2):194–202.

67. Schmidt EP, Drachman DB, Wiener CM, Clawson L, Kimball R, Lechtzin N. Pulmonary predictors of survival in amyotrophic lateral sclerosis: use in clinical trial design. Muscle Nerve. 2006;33(1):127–32.

68. Miller RG, Jackson CE, Kasarskis EJ, et al. Practice parameter update: the care of the patient with amyotrophic lateral sclerosis: drug, nutritional, and respiratory therapies (an evidence-based review): report of the quality standards Subcommittee of the American Academy of Neurology. Neurology. 2009;73(15):1218–26.

69. Fugl-Meyer AR. Effects of respiratory muscle paralysis in tetraplegic and paraplegic patients. Scand J Rehabil Med. 1971;3(4):141–50.

70. Fugl-Meyer AR, Grimby G. Respiration in tetraplegia and in hemiplegia: a review. Int Rehabil Med. 1984;6(4):186–90.

71. Huldtgren AC, Fugl-Meyer AR, Jonasson E, Bake B. Ventilatory dysfunction and respiratory rehabilitation in post-traumatic quadriplegia. Eur J Respir Dis. 1980;61(6):347–56.

72. Wade OL, Gilson JC. The effect of posture on diaphragmatic movement and vital capacity in normal subjects with a note on spirometry as an aid in determining radiological chest volumes. Thorax. 1951;6(2):103–26.

73. Moreno F, Lyons HA. Effect of body posture on lung volumes. J Appl Physiol. 1961;16:27–9.

74. Castile R, Mead J, Jackson A, Wohl ME, Stokes D. Effects of posture on flow-volume curve configuration in normal humans. J Appl Physiol Respir Environ Exerc Physiol. 1982;53(5):1175–83.

75. Segizbaeva MO, Pogodin MA, Aleksandrova NP. Effects of body positions on respiratory muscle activation during maximal inspiratory maneuvers. Adv Exp Med Biol. 2013;756:355–63.

76. Chang SC, Chang HI, Liu SY, Shiao GM, Perng RP. Effects of body position and age on membrane diffusing capacity and pulmonary capillary blood volume. Chest. 1992;102(1):139–42.

22

Inhibition of Shp2 ameliorates monocrotaline-induced pulmonary arterial hypertension in rats

Yusheng Cheng[1,2†], Min Yu[2†], Jian Xu[2], Mengyu He[2], Hong Wang[2], Hui Kong[2*] and Weiping Xie[2*]

Abstract

Background: Src homology 2 containing protein tyrosine phosphatase (PTP) 2 (Shp2) is a typical tyrosine phosphatase interacting with receptor tyrosine kinase to regulate multiple signaling pathways in diverse pathological processes. Here, we will investigate the effect of Shp2 inhibition on pulmonary arterial hypertension (PAH) in a rat model and its potential cellular and molecular mechanisms underlying.

Methods: Monocrotaline (MCT)-induced PAH rat model was used in this study. Phps-1, a highly selective inhibitor for Shp2, was administered from 21 days to 35 days after MCT single-injection. Microcatheter method was applied to detected hemodynamic parameters. Histological methods were used to determine PVR changes in PAH rats. Moreover, cultured pulmonary artery smooth muscle cells (PASMCs) treated by platelet-derived growth factor (PDGF) with or without Phps-1 was used to investigate the potential cellular and molecular mechanisms underlying in vitro.

Results: Inhibition of Shp2 significantly attenuated MCT-induced increases of mean pulmonary arterial pressure (mPAP), right ventricular systolic pressure (RVSP) and right ventricular hypertrophy (RVH) in rats. Shp2 inhibition effectively decreased thickening of pulmonary artery media and cardiomyocyte hypertrophy as well as perivascular and myocardial fibrosis in MCT-treated rats. Moreover, Shp2 inhibition ameliorated muscularization of pulmonary arterioles in MCT-induced PAH rats. Shp2 inhibition significantly reduced platelet-derived growth factor (PDGF)-triggered proliferation and migration of human pulmonary artery smooth muscle cells (PASMCs), which might be attributed to the inactivations of Akt and Stat3 pathways.

Conclusions: Shp2 contributes to the development of PAH in rats, which might be a potential target for the treatment of PAH.

Keywords: Shp2, Pulmonary vascular remodeling, Pulmonary hypertension

Background

Pulmonary arterial hypertension (PAH) is a life-threatening disorder, characterized by progressive pulmonary vascular remodeling (PVR) leading to increased pulmonary vascular resistance, right heart failure and ultimately premature death [1]. Recent findings have suggested that abnormal vasoconstriction, vascular inflammation and remodeling, endothelial dysfunction and thrombotic arteriopathy are typical features of PAH [2]. By far, PVR, mainly caused by aberrant proliferation of pulmonary vascular cells and abnormal formation of extracellular matrix, have been recognized as the pathological features of PAH [3].

Although considerable advances have been made in treating PAH during the past decades, mortality in patients with PAH remains high [4]. One major reason is that recent available medications mainly tackle the pulmonary artery endothelial dysfunction and leave the vascular remodeling suboptimally inhibited [5]. Currently, pulmonary arterial smooth muscle cells (PASMCs) with apoptosis-resistant phenotype are well accepted as one major contributor for PVR changes in

* Correspondence: konghui@njmu.edu.cn; wpxie@njmu.edu.cn
†Yusheng Cheng and Ming Yu contributed equally to this work.
²Department of Respiratory and Critical Care Medicine, the First Affiliated Hospital of Nanjing Medical University, 300 Guangzhou Road, Nanjing 210029, Jiangsu, China
Full list of author information is available at the end of the article

PAH [2]. Thus, PASMCs is recognized as a promising target for intervention of PAH [6]. Platelet-derived growth factor (PDGF) is an important growth factor for proliferation and migration of PASMCs through activating receptor tyrosine kinases, which increases significantly and promotes PVR in patients with PAH [3]. Several clinical trials targeting PDGF signaling have been carried out to treat patients with PAH. For example, Imatinib and PK10453, two novel PDGF receptor tyrosine kinase inhibitors, are found to improve PVR efficiently [7, 8]. In this context, receptor tyrosine kinases provide new strategies for improving PAH [9, 10].

Src homology 2 containing protein tyrosine phosphatase (PTP)-2 (Shp2) is a member of the non-receptor protein tyrosine phosphates family, which has drawn growing attentions in recent years for its interaction with receptor tyrosine kinase to regulate multiple signaling pathways linked with cellular development and diverse pathological processes [11]. Shp2 is widely expressed in different tissues and enhances the migration of aortic vascular smooth muscle cells (SMCs) isolated from adult rats [12, 13]. Moreover, Shp2 promotes the activation of receptor protein tyrosine kinase of PDGF receptor β (PDGFR β) signal pathway in SMCs [14]. Interestingly, Shp2 is found to be a target of miR-204 and sustains proliferation and anti-apoptotic feature of PASMCs in PAH [15]. However, there is no data to elucidate whether Shp2 contributes to PVR changes in PAH. In this study, we investigated the effects of Shp2 inhibition on PAH in rats and its potential cellular and molecular mechanisms underlying.

Methods

Experimental animals

This study was approved by the animal ethical and welfare committee of Nanjing Medical University (Approval No. 1601271). Male Sprague-Dawley (SD) rats (weight between 200 and 250 g, 5–7 weeks age) were purchased from Bikai experiment animals center (Shanghai, China). All the animals were housed in climate-controlled conditions with 12 h light and 12 h dark cycle and had free access to chow and water for 5 days. Monocrotaline (MCT)-induced PAH rat model was used in this study. Rats were subcutaneously injected with a single dose of MCT (40 mg/kg, Sigma, St, Louis, MO). The dosage of MCT used in this study was determined by our pre-experiment work to reduce high mortality of rats after MCT administration. Twenty one days after MCT administration, rats were then intraperitoneally injected with Phps-1 (1 mg/kg, Sigma, St, Louis, MO) (a highly selective inhibitor for Shp2) or a vehicle every other day. At the end of 35 days, all rats were examined.

Hemodynamic analysis

Thirty-five days after a single injection of MCT, all rats were anaesthetised by an intramuscular injection of a cocktail of ketamine (90 mg/kg) and xylazine (10 mg/kg). The internal jugular vein was exposed by a 2–3 cm incision over the right ventral neck area. A polyethylene catheter connected to a pressure transducer was inserted into the right external jugular vein and threaded into the right ventricle, and then into right ventricular and pulmonary artery to measure systolic pressure (RVSP) and mean pulmonary artrial pressure (mPAP). Another catheter was inserted into left carotid artery to measure systemic arterial pressure (SAP) by a polygraph system (MP100, BIOPAC System, Inc., Santa Barbara, CA, USA). After homodynamic measurements, all anaesthetised rats were euthanized by exsanguination.

Histological analysis

Right ventricle and distal lungs of rats removed en bloc were fixed in 4% paraformaldehyde, and then sectioned at 5-μm for subsequntly stainings. Hematoxylin and eosin staining was used to determine cardiomyocyte hypertrophy and pulmonary artery media thickness (PAWT). More than 20 images of distal pulmonary arterioles per rat (diameter between 30 and 100 μm) were captured using a microscopic digital camera and analysis program (Becton Dickinson). The PAWT is defined as the distance between inner and outer elastic lamina. Vessel external diameter (ED) was determined. The relative PAMT (%) was calculated as $100 \times 2PAMT/ED$. Cardiomyocyte hypertrophy was determined by cross sectional area (CSA) of cardiomyocyte. Moreover, sectioned lung tissues and myocardial tissues were stained with Masson's trichrome staining which indicated the scales of collagen deposition, and the results were assessed by Image J software. Right ventricular hypertrophy (RVH) was presented as the ratio of right ventricle (RV) weight/ Left ventricle (LV) + septum (S) weight [16].

Cell culture and reagents

PASMCs and cell culture medium components were obtained from ScienCell Research Laboratories (San Diego, CA), and used according to the manufacturer's instructions. Briefly, PASMCs were maintained in smooth muscle cell medium (SMCM) supplemented with 2% fetal bovine serum (FBS), 1% penicillin / streptomycin and 1% mixed growth factors at 5% CO_2 and 37 °C. The cells were starved for 24 h in SMCM with serum and growth factors free before subsequent experiments. Platelet derived growth factor (PDGF)-BB was obtained from Roche Group (Roche, USA).

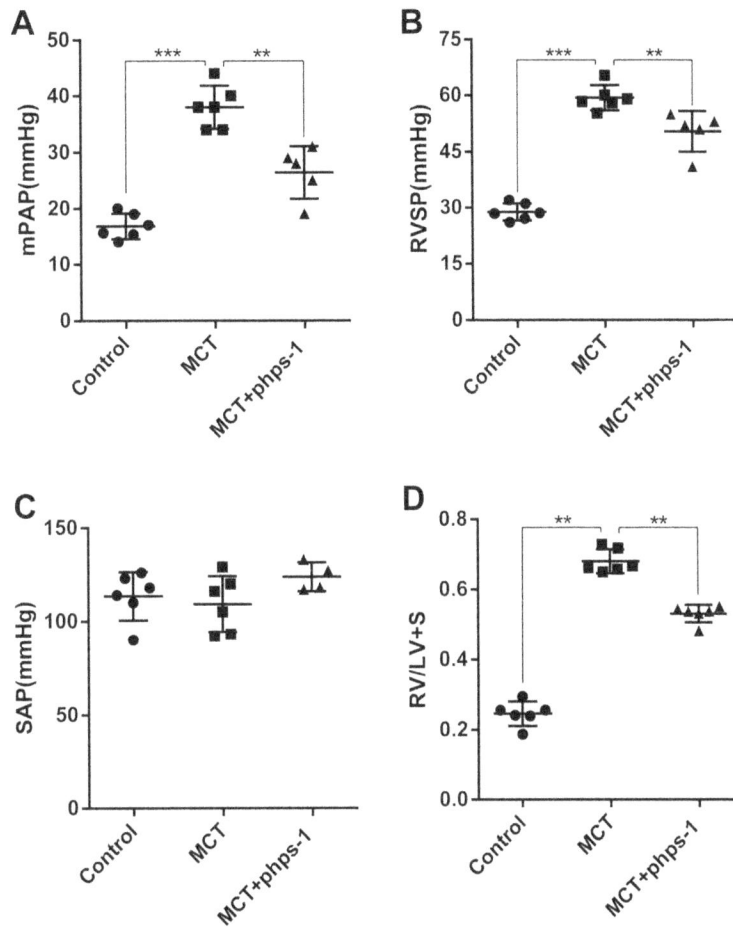

Fig. 1 Shp2 inhibition improves mPAP, RVSP and RVH, without affecting SAP in MCT-induced PAH rats. **a** Phps-1 inhibited MCT- induced increases of mPAP and RVSP **b** ($n = 6$ for Control or MCT group, $n = 5$ for MCT + Phps-1group) without affecting SAP **c** ($n = 6$ for Control or MCT group, $n = 4$ for MCT + Phps-1 group). **d** Phps-1 suppressed MCT- induced increase of RVH, as indicated by RV/LV + S ($n = 6$ for each group). Data was presented as means ± standard deviation (SD), ** $P < 0.01$ and *** $P < 0.001$

Immunofluorescent assay

Fresh lung tissues were embedded in OCT compound (Sakura Finetek, Torrance, CA, USA) and frozen in a dry-ice acetone bath. Seven-μm sectioned tissues were kept at − 80 °C until analysis. Tissue sections were incubated for 24 h at 4 °C with rabbit monoclonal anti-α-smooth muscle actin (α-SMA) antibody (1: 200, Abcam, USA) along with mouse monoclonal anti-CD31 antibody (2 μg/ml,Abcam, USA). After washes, sections were incubated with Alexa Fluor 488 goat anti-mouse IgG (Invitrogen, Molecular Probes, Carlsbad, CA, USA; 1:1000) and Alexa Fluor 594 goat anti-rabbit IgG (Invitrogen; 1:1000) at room temperature for 1 h. The immunolabeled frozen sections were detected with Pannoramic Viewer (3DHISTECH 1.15.3). At least 60–80 distal pulmonary arterioles per rat were assessed. The muscularization of distal pulmonary arterioles was determined by calculating the percent of arteries that were fully, partially and not muscularuized.

Cell proliferation assay

Cell counting kit-8 method was used to determine PASMCs cell proliferation as described previously [17]. Briefly, PASMCs at 10,000 cells each well were planted into 96-well plates in 100 μl of culture medium and incubated with different treatment for 24 h. After treatment, 10 μl of CCK-8 reagent (Dojindo Molecular Technologies, Kumamoto, Japan) was added to each well 4 h before the end of incubation. The optical density value (OD) of each sample was measured at a wavelength of 450 nm on a microplate reader (Thermo Scientific, CA, USA). The results of cell viability measurement were expressed as the absorbance at OD 450.

Transwell migration assay

Migration of PASMCs was determined by Transwell assay, as described previously [18]. Shortly, 50,000 cells were seeded on the top of each polycarbonate filter with 8-μm pores (Corning) in 0.1 ml of basal medium, and

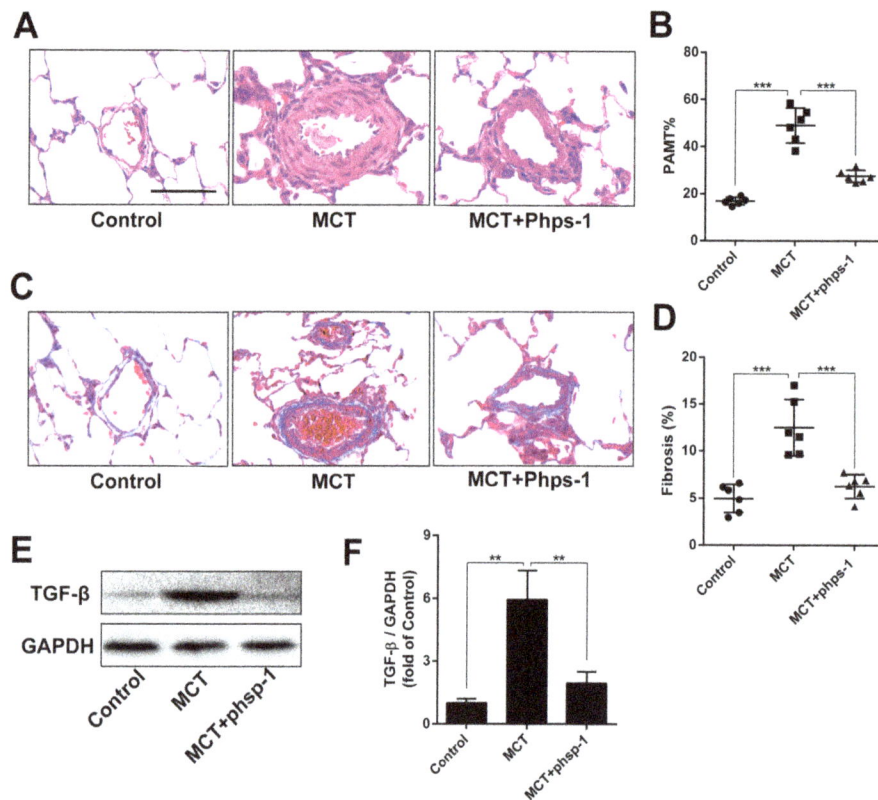

Fig. 2 Shp2 inhibition attenuates MCT-induced thickening of PAMT and perivascular fibrosis. **a** Representative images of hematoxylin and eosin staining for PAMT, Scale bar = 30 μm. **b** Quantification of PMWT ($n = 6$ for each group). **c** Representative images of Masson's trichrome staining for detecting perivascular fibrosis (blue), Scale bar = 30 μm. **d** Hemi-quantification of perivascular fibrosis ($n = 6$ for each group). **e** and **f** Phps-1 reversed MCT-induced overexpression of TGF-β in lungs ($n = 3$). Data was presented as means ± standard deviation (SD), ** $P < 0.01$ and *** $P < 0.001$

then stimulated by PDGF (20 ng/ml) with or without Phps-1 (20 μM) for 12 h. Following exposure, the cells were fixed in 4% paraformaldehyde for 30 min and stained with 5% crystal violet (Beytime, China) for 30 min. Unmigrated cells were then scraped off the top of the filter. For each filter, at least five randomly chosen fields were imaged to obtain a total cell count.

Western blotting analyses

Isolated lungs tissues or PASMCs were lysed in RIPA Lysis Buffer (Pierce Inc.) supplemented with 1% protease inhibitor cocktail (Roche) and 1 mM phenylmethylsulfonyl fluoride (PMSF). Serum-starve PASMCs were stimulated by PDGF (20 ng/ml) for 15 min with or without Phps-1 (20 μM) pre-treatment for 30 min. And then, proteins were detected by western blotting method. Lysates were centrifuged at 12,000 rpm at 4 °C for 15 min, and supernatants were collected for subsequent western blot analysis. Protein samples were separated on a SDS-PAGE gel and polyvinylidene fluoride membranes. Next, the membranes were blocked with 5% non-fat milk powder in Tris-buffered saline containing 0.1% Tween 20 for 1 h at room temperature, and then, the

membranes were probed overnight at 4 °C with primary antibody: phospho-Shp2 (Santa Cruz, CA, USA), Shp2 (Santa Cruz, CA, USA), Akt (Cell Signaling Technology, Danvers, USA), phospho-Akt (p-Akt) (Cell Signaling Technology, Danvers, USA), transforming growth factor-β (TGF-β) (Cell Signaling Technology, Danvers, USA), phospho-Stat3 (Cell Signaling Technology, Danvers, USA), Stat3 (Cell Signaling Technology, Danvers, USA). Then, the blot was incubated with the appropriate horseradish-peroxidase (HRP)-conjugated rabbit IgG (Santa Cruz, CA, USA) or HRP-conjugated goat IgG as a secondary antibody (Santa Cruz, CA, USA). The signals were visualized using an enhanced chemilu-minescence (ECL) reagent kit (Thermo fisher scientific, Waltham, USA), and analyzed with Bio-Rad Gel Doc/Chemi Doc Imaging System and Image J software..

Statistics

All values are presented as means ± standard deviation (SD). Data were analyzed using GraphPad prism 6.0. Comparisons were made using one-way analysis of variance (ANOVA) with Bonferroni multiple comparisons test. Statistical significance was defined as $P < 0.05$.

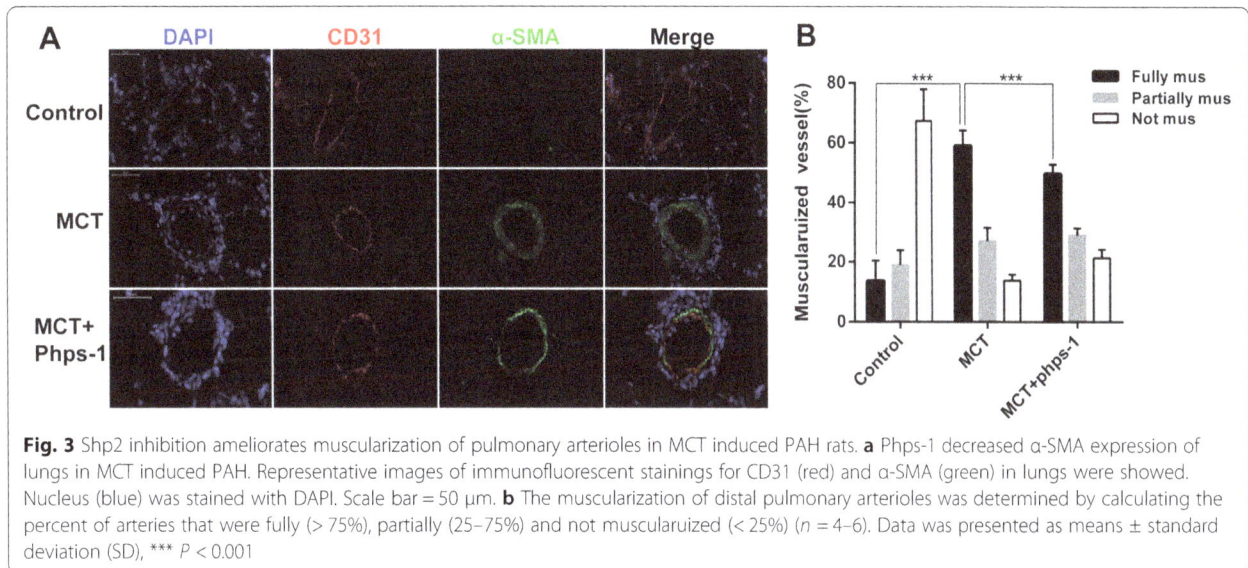

Fig. 3 Shp2 inhibition ameliorates muscularization of pulmonary arterioles in MCT induced PAH rats. **a** Phps-1 decreased α-SMA expression of lungs in MCT induced PAH. Representative images of immunofluorescent stainings for CD31 (red) and α-SMA (green) in lungs were showed. Nucleus (blue) was stained with DAPI. Scale bar = 50 μm. **b** The muscularization of distal pulmonary arterioles was determined by calculating the percent of arteries that were fully (> 75%), partially (25–75%) and not muscularuized (< 25%) (n = 4–6). Data was presented as means ± standard deviation (SD), *** P < 0.001

Results

Shp2 inhibition improves mPAP, RVSP and RVH in MCT-induced PAH rats

In PAH rat, curatively treated with Shp2 inhibitor Phps-1markedly decreased MCT-induced elevation in mPAP (Fig. 1a) as well as RVSP (Fig. 1b). However, the Phps-1 had not significant effect on SAP (Fig. 1c). Similarly, Phps-1 partially reversed MCT induced increase of RVH, as indicated by weight ratio of RV/ (LV + S) (Fig. 1d). Thus,

Shp2 inhibition effectively reduced mPAP, RVSP and RVH in MCT-induced PAH rats.

Shp2 inhibition attenuates MCT-induced thickening of PAMT and perivascular fibrosis

As shown in Fig. 2a and b, the PAMT was significantly thickened in MCT-induced PAH rats, which was alleviated by Phps-1 treatment. Masson's trichrome staining showed that Phps-1 reversed MCT-induced perivascular

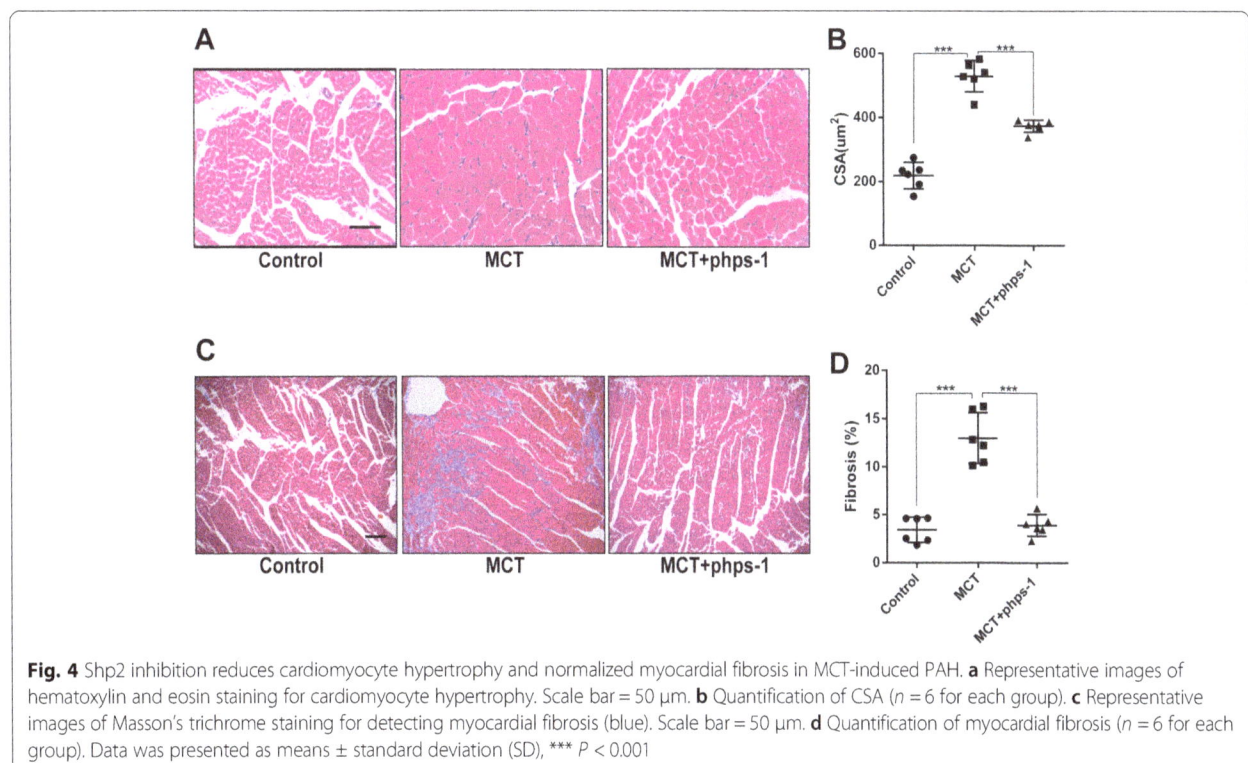

Fig. 4 Shp2 inhibition reduces cardiomyocyte hypertrophy and normalized myocardial fibrosis in MCT-induced PAH. **a** Representative images of hematoxylin and eosin staining for cardiomyocyte hypertrophy. Scale bar = 50 μm. **b** Quantification of CSA (n = 6 for each group). **c** Representative images of Masson's trichrome staining for detecting myocardial fibrosis (blue). Scale bar = 50 μm. **d** Quantification of myocardial fibrosis (n = 6 for each group). Data was presented as means ± standard deviation (SD), *** P < 0.001

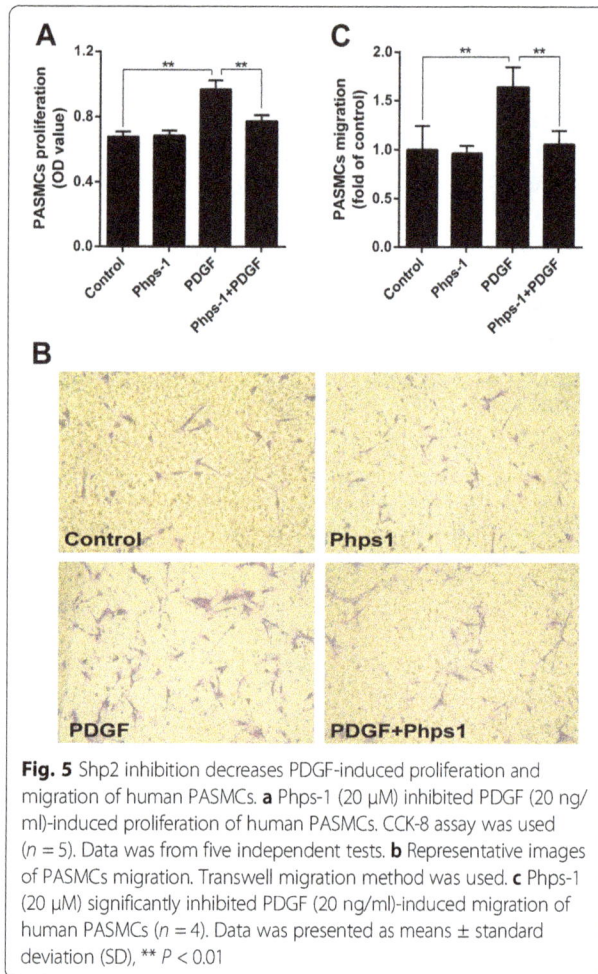

Fig. 5 Shp2 inhibition decreases PDGF-induced proliferation and migration of human PASMCs. **a** Phps-1 (20 μM) inhibited PDGF (20 ng/ml)-induced proliferation of human PASMCs. CCK-8 assay was used ($n = 5$). Data was from five independent tests. **b** Representative images of PASMCs migration. Transwell migration method was used. **c** Phps-1 (20 μM) significantly inhibited PDGF (20 ng/ml)-induced migration of human PASMCs ($n = 4$). Data was presented as means ± standard deviation (SD), ** $P < 0.01$

fibrosis (Fig. 2c and d). Moreover, Phps-1 significantly inhibited MCT-induced overexpression of TGF-β in lung tissues (Fig. 2e and f). Therefore, inhibition of Shp2 significantly improved thickening of PAMT and perivascular fibrosis in MCT-induced PAH rats.

Shp2 inhibition ameliorates muscularization of pulmonary arterioles in rats

The muscularization of pulmonary arterioles was evaluated by immunofluorence of smooth muscle cell marker α-SMA. As shown in Fig. 3a, α-SMA was over-expressed in PAH group compared to control group, which was remarkably inhibited by the treatment of Phps-1. Statistical analysis indicated that Phps-1 treatment significantly decreased portion of fully muscularized pulmonary arteries induced by MCT (Fig. 3b).

Shp2 inhibition reduces cardiomyocyte hypertrophy and myocardial fibrosis in MCT- induced PAH rats

Persistent elevated pulmonary arterial pressure could lead to cardiomyocyte hypertrophy and fibrosis in PAH. CSA of cardiomyocyte analysis based on hematoxylin and eosin

staining showed that Phps-1 significantly suppressed MCT-induced cardiomyocyte hypertrophy (Fig. 4a and b). Morever, semiquantitative analysis of myocardial fibrosis by Masson's trichrome staining demonstrated that Phps-1 reversed myocardial fibrosis in MCT-induced PAH rats (Fig. 4c and d).

Shp2 inhibition decreases PDGF-induced proliferation and migration of PASMCs

PDGF is a key growth factor promoting the proliferation and migration of PASMCs in the development of PAH. In cultured human PASMCs, suppressing the activation of Shp2 by selective inhibitor Phps-1 blocked PDGF-stimulated cells proliferation (Fig. 5a). Additionally, transwell assay showed that Phps-1 efficiently inhibited PDGF-induced migration of PASMCs (Fig. 5b and c).

Shp2 inhibition blocks PDGF-stimulated activations of Akt and Stat3 signaling

As shown in Fig. 6, PDGF dramatically activated Shp2 by enhancing the phosphorylation of Shp2. Akt and Stat3 are two important kinases involved in PDGF receptor signal transduction. As expected, PDGF also induced potent phosphorylation of Akt and Stat3 in cultured human PASMCs. However, these stimulant effects of PDGF on phosphorylation of Shp2, as well as Akt and Stat3 were effectively blocked by Phps-1 (Fig. 6).

Discussion

The main findings of this study suggest that Shp2 is an important contributor to the development of PAH. Pharmacological inhibition of Shp2 by its highly selective inhibitor Phps-1 markedly decreased MCT-induced elevation of mPAP and RVSP, as well as MCT-induced PVR, including decreasing PAMT, suppressing perivascular collagen deposit and ameliorating muscularization of distal pulmonary arterioles. In addition, data from in vitro studies suggests that Akt and Stat3 pathways are involved in the beneficial effects of Shp2 inhibition on PDGF-induced proliferation and migration of human PASMCs.

Currently, several tyrosine kinase inhibitors for improving remodeling pulmonary vascular in PAH have been investigated [19]. For example, Imatinib, a potent receptor tyrosine kinase inhibitor for treatment of chronic myeloid leukemia, was found to effectively reverse PVR in animal models of PAH and improved the hemodynamics and exercise capacity in PAH patients [20, 21]. Sorafenib, a mutikinase inhibitor of tyrosine kinases as well as serine-threonine kinases, prevented PVR and improved cardiac functions in experimental model of pulmonary hypertension [22]. Therefore, receptor tyrosine kinases provide promising new targets for

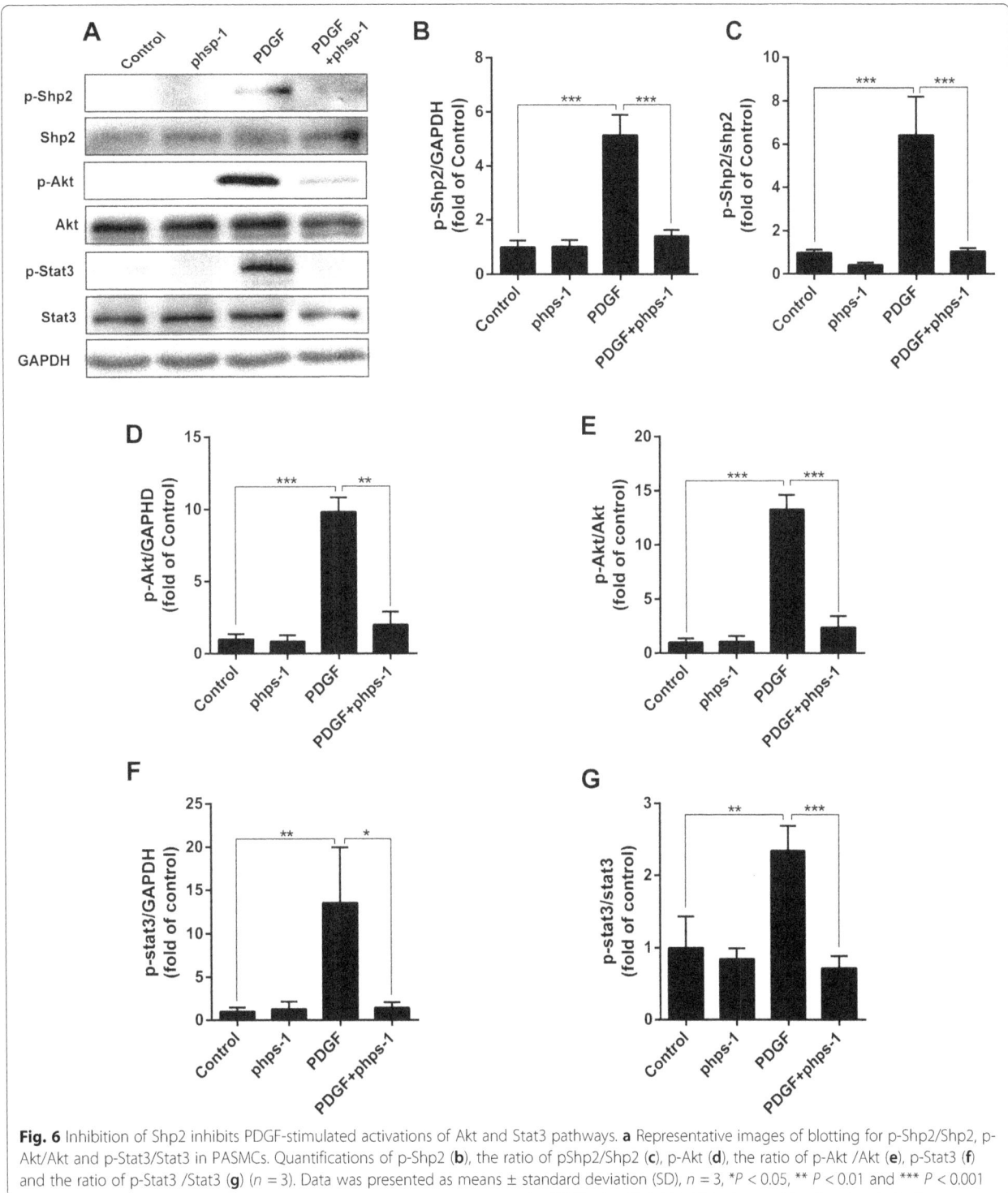

Fig. 6 Inhibition of Shp2 inhibits PDGF-stimulated activations of Akt and Stat3 pathways. **a** Representative images of blotting for p-Shp2/Shp2, p-Akt/Akt and p-Stat3/Stat3 in PASMCs. Quantifications of p-Shp2 (**b**), the ratio of pShp2/Shp2 (**c**), p-Akt (**d**), the ratio of p-Akt /Akt (**e**), p-Stat3 (**f**) and the ratio of p-Stat3 /Stat3 (**g**) ($n = 3$). Data was presented as means ± standard deviation (SD), $n = 3$, *$P < 0.05$, ** $P < 0.01$ and *** $P < 0.001$

improving PAH. As a key mediator for several receptor tyrosine kinases and SRC-family kinases, Shp2 regulates signal transduction of diverse growth factors and hormones relating to fundamental cellular function [23–25]. Phps-1 is found to be a highly selective inhibitor for Shp2, which binds the catalytic site of Shp2 and blocks

Shp2-dependent signaling [26]. For example, Phps-1 effectively inhibits TGF-β1-induced epithelial-mesenchymal transition in lung epithelial A549 cells [27]. Additionally, Phps-1 is reported to alleviate airway inflammation and airway hyper-responsiveness in allergic mice [28]. Of note, the beneficial effect of tyrosine kinase antagonist in PAH was accompanied by dose-dependent decreases in SAP [29]. As a typical tyrosine phosphatase, Shp2 interacts with tyrosine kinase to regulate proliferation and migration of smooth muscle cells [11]. Thus, theoretically, Shp2 inhibition might influence SAP in PAH. However, in our study, Phps-1 improved mPAP, RVSP and RVH in MCT-induced PAH rats with no significant effect on SAP. This may be attributed to limited dosage of Phps-1 used in the present study. Moreover, this result also suggests Phps-1 may have tissue-selective distribution in pulmonary circulation rather than systemic circulation. Improvement of PVR is one of major goals of current medications for PAH, which delays increases of pulmonary arterial pressure and right heart afterload and decreases mortality of PAH ultimately [5]. In the present study, inhibition of Shp2 effectively reduced increases of PAMT and perivascular fibrosis in PAH rat lungs. Moreover, Shp2 inhibition ameliorated pulmonary arterioles muscularization in rats. Therefore, inhibition of Shp2 effectively inhibited PVR in MCT-induced PAH rats.

Myocardial hypertrophy and fibrosis caused by pressure-overload of RV results in dysfunction of RV in PAH. [30]. In this study, we revealed that inhibition of Shp2 suppressed myocardial hypertrophy and reversed myocardial fibrosis in MCT-induced PAH rats. So far, dysfunction of Shp2 has been demonstrated to cause disorders of myocardium structure and function. Loss-of-function mutations in PTPN11 gene, which encodes the Shp2, leads to congenital heart disease and adult-onset heart hypertrophy [31]. Hypertrophic cardiomyopathy caused by Shp2 dysfunction is mediated by aberrant activation of Akt, focal adhesion kinase and mammalian target of rapamycin. Inhibition of Shp2 remarkably prevents heart hypertrophy [32]. In summary, Shp2 contributes to maladaptive remodeling of RV in MCT-induced PAH rats.

PDGF is an important growth factor in the development of PAH, stimulating proliferation of PASMCs by activating Stat3 and Akt signal pathways [33, 34]. In the present study, inhibition of Shp2 significantly inhibited PDGF-stimulated proliferation and migration of human PASMCs. It is reported that Shp2 is necessary for the activation of Akt pathway in vascular smooth muscle cell hypertrophy [35]. Meanwhile, Shp2 promotes PDGF-stimulated Akt activation in fibroblasts [23]. In this study, we found inhibition of Shp2 effectively blocked PDGF-induced activations of Akt and Stat3 in PASMCs. Thus, Akt and Stat3 pathways are involved in the beneficial effects of Shp2 inhibition on PDGF-induced proliferation and migration of human PASMCs.

However, there are several limitations in this study. First, it did not clarify whether inhibition of Shp2 could modulate other growth factors including basic fibroblast growth factor (FGF), insulin-like growth factor-1 (IGF-1)

and epidermal growth factor (EGF) in spite of Shp2 inhibition significantly decreased TGF-β expression in MCT-induced PAH rat lungs. Those growth factors are reported to associate with the development of PVR [36–39]. Second, the effect of Shp2 on fibroblast cells is not investigated. However, Shp2 inactivation markedly decreased peri-vascular cells proliferations in lungs of PAH (data not shown). Finally, the mechanisms of Shp2 regulating PVR remain to be further fully investigated.

Conclusions

Our findings demonstrated that inhibition of Shp2 ameliorates MCT-induced PAH in rats, which might be a potential target for the treatment of PAH.

Acknowledgements
We gratefully acknowledge the critical revision of Professor Zhangjian Huang.

Funding
The design of the study and collection, analysis, and interpretation of data were supported by Anhui Provincial Key projects of Natural Science Foundation for Colleges and Universities (KJ2017A264) and Key projects of Wannan Medical College (KY22340150). Manuscript writing and revision was supported by the National Natural Science Foundation of China (NSFC) (81273571).

Authors' contributions
CY, YM, XJ, HM, WH, KH and XW contributed to the concept and design, analysis and interpretation as well as manuscript drafting. All authors read and approved the final manuscript.

Competing interests
The authors declare that they have no competing interests.

Author details
[1]Department of Respiratory and Critical Care Medicine, Yijishan Hospital of Wannan Medical College, 2 Zeshan West Road, Wuhu 241001, Anhui, China. [2]Department of Respiratory and Critical Care Medicine, the First Affiliated Hospital of Nanjing Medical University, 300 Guangzhou Road, Nanjing 210029, Jiangsu, China.

References
1. Hadri L, Kratlian RG, Benard L, Maron BA, Dorfmuller P, Ladage D, Guignabert C, Ishikawa K, Aguero J, Ibanez B, et al. Therapeutic efficacy of AAV1.SERCA2a in monocrotaline-induced pulmonary arterial hypertension. Circulation. 2013;128(2):512–23.
2. McLaughlin VV, Shah SJ, Souza R, Humbert M. Management of pulmonary arterial hypertension. J Am Coll Cardiol. 2015;65(18):1976–97.
3. Perros F, Montani D, Dorfmuller P, Durand-Gasselin I, Tcherakian C, Le Pavec J, Mazmanian M, Fadel E, Mussot S, Mercier O, et al. Platelet-derived growth factor expression and function in idiopathic pulmonary arterial hypertension. Am J Respir Crit Care Med. 2008;178(1):81–8.
4. Galie N, Humbert M, Vachiery JL, Gibbs S, Lang I, Torbicki A, Simonneau G, Peacock A, Vonk Noordegraaf A, Beghetti M, et al. 2015 ESC/ERS Guidelines for the diagnosis and treatment of pulmonary hypertension: The Joint Task Force for the Diagnosis and Treatment of Pulmonary Hypertension of the European Society of Cardiology (ESC) and the European Respiratory Society (ERS): Endorsed by: Association for European Paediatric and Congenital Cardiology (AEPC), International Society for Heart and Lung Transplantation (ISHLT). Eur Heart J. 2016; 37(1):67–119.

5. Antoniu SA. Targeting PDGF pathway in pulmonary arterial hypertension. Expert Opin Ther Targets. 2012;16(11):1055–63.

6. Wang R, Zhou SJ, Zeng DS, Xu R, Fei LM, Zhu QQ, Zhang Y, Sun GY. Plasmid-based short hairpin RNA against connective tissue growth factor attenuated monocrotaline-induced pulmonary vascular remodeling in rats. Gene Ther. 2014;21(11):931–7.

7. Takahashi J, Orcholski M, Yuan K, de Jesus Perez V. PDGF-dependent beta-catenin activation is associated with abnormal pulmonary artery smooth muscle cell proliferation in pulmonary arterial hypertension. FEBS Lett. 2016; 590(1):101–9.

8. Medarametla V, Festin S, Sugarragchaa C, Eng A, Naqwi A, Wiedmann T, Zisman LS. PK10453, a nonselective platelet-derived growth factor receptor inhibitor, prevents the progression of pulmonary arterial hypertension. Pulm Circ. 2014;4(1):82–102.

9. Barst RJ. PDGF signaling in pulmonary arterial hypertension. J Clin Invest. 2005;115(10):2691–4.

10. Ten Freyhaus H, Berghausen EM, Janssen W, Leuchs M, Zierden M, Murmann K, Klinke A, Vantler M, Caglayan E, Kramer T, et al. Genetic ablation of PDGF-dependent signaling pathways abolishes vascular remodeling and experimental pulmonary hypertension. Arterioscler Thromb Vasc Biol. 2015;35(5):1236–45.

11. Kandadi MR, Stratton MS, Ren J. The role of Src homology 2 containing protein tyrosine phosphatase 2 in vascular smooth muscle cell migration and proliferation. Acta Pharmacol Sin. 2010;31(10):1277–83.

12. Adachi M, Iwaki H, Shindoh M, Akao Y, Hachiya T, Ikeda M, Hinoda Y, Imai K. Predominant expression of the src homology 2-containing tyrosine phosphatase protein SHP2 in vascular smooth muscle cells. Virchows Arch. 1997;430(4):321–5.

13. Dixit M, Zhuang D, Ceacareanu B, Hassid A. Treatment with insulin uncovers the motogenic capacity of nitric oxide in aortic smooth muscle cells: dependence on Gab1 and Gab1-SHP2 association. Circ Res. 2003;93(10): e113–23.

14. Wu JH, Goswami R, Cai X, Exum ST, Huang X, Zhang L, Brian L, Premont RT, Peppel K, Freedman NJ. Regulation of the platelet-derived growth factor receptor-beta by G protein-coupled receptor kinase-5 in vascular smooth muscle cells involves the phosphatase Shp2. J Biol Chem. 2006;281(49): 37758–72.

15. Courboulin A, Paulin R, Giguere NJ, Saksouk N, Perreault T, Meloche J, Paquet ER, Biardel S, Provencher S, Cote J, et al. Role for miR-204 in human pulmonary arterial hypertension. J Exp Med. 2011;208(3):535–48.

16. Huertas A, Tu L, Thuillet R, Le Hiress M, Phan C, Ricard N, Nadaud S, Fadel E, Humbert M, Guignabert C. Leptin signalling system as a target for pulmonary arterial hypertension therapy. Eur Respir J. 2015;45(4): 1066–80.

17. Sun K, Xue H, Wang H, Wang Q, Zuo XR, Xie WP, Wang H. The effects of siRNA against RPL22 on ET-1-induced proliferation of human pulmonary arterial smooth muscle cells. Int J Mol Med. 2012;30(2):351–7.

18. Leggett K, Maylor J, Undem C, Lai N, Lu W, Schweitzer K, King LS, Myers AC, Sylvester JT, Sidhaye V, Shimoda LA. Hypoxia-induced migration in pulmonary arterial smooth muscle cells requires calcium-dependent upregulation of aquaporin 1. Am J Phys Lung Cell Mol Phys. 2012;303(4):L343–53.

19. Sakao S, Tatsumi K. Vascular remodeling in pulmonary arterial hypertension: multiple cancer-like pathways and possible treatment modalities. Int J Cardiol. 2011;147(1):4–12.

20. Castagnetti F, Di Raimondo F, De Vivo A, Spitaleri A, Gugliotta G, Fabbiano F, Capodanno I, Mannina D, Salvucci M, Antolino A, et al. A population-based study of chronic myeloid leukemia patients treated with imatinib in first line. Am J Hematol. 2017;92(1):82–7.

21. Ciuclan L, Hussey MJ, Burton V, Good R, Duggan N, Beach S, Jones P, Fox R, Clay I, Bonneau O, et al. Imatinib attenuates hypoxia-induced pulmonary arterial hypertension pathology via reduction in 5-hydroxytryptamine through inhibition of tryptophan hydroxylase 1 expression. Am J Respir Crit Care Med. 2013;187(1):78–89.

22. Klein M, Schermuly RT, Ellinghaus P, Milting H, Riedl B, Nikolova S, Pullamsetti SS, Weissmann N, Dony E, Savai R, et al. Combined tyrosine and serine/threonine kinase inhibition by sorafenib prevents progression of experimental pulmonary hypertension and myocardial remodeling. Circulation. 2008;118(20):2081 90.

23. Tajan M, de Rocca SA, Valet P, Edouard T, Yart A. SHP2 sails from physiology to pathology. Eur J Med Genet. 2015;58(10):509–25.

24. Furcht CM, Munoz Rojas AR, Nihalani D, Lazzara MJ. Diminished functional role and altered localization of SHP2 in non-small cell lung cancer cells with EGFR-activating mutations. Oncogene. 2013;32(18):2346–55.

25. Sausgruber N, Coissieux MM, Britschgi A, Wyckoff J, Aceto N, Leroy C, Stadler MB, Voshol H, Bonenfant D, Bentires-Alj M. Tyrosine phosphatase SHP2 increases cell motility in triple-negative breast cancer through the activation of SRC-family kinases. Oncogene. 2015;34(17):2272–4.

26. Hellmuth K, Grosskopf S, Lum CT, Wurtele M, Roder N, von Kries JP, Rosario M, Rademann J, Birchmeier W. Specific inhibitors of the protein tyrosine phosphatase Shp2 identified by high-throughput docking. Proc Natl Acad Sci U S A. 2008;105(20):7275–80.

27. Li S, Wang L, Zhao Q, Liu Y, He L, Xu Q, Sun X, Teng L, Cheng H, Ke Y. SHP2 positively regulates TGFbeta1-induced epithelial-mesenchymal transition modulated by its novel interacting protein Hook1. J Biol Chem. 2014; 289(49):34152–60.

28. Xia LX, Hua W, Jin Y, Tian BP, Qiu ZW, Zhang C, Che LQ, Zhou HB, Wu YF, Huang HQ, et al. Eosinophil differentiation in the bone marrow is promoted by protein tyrosine phosphatase SHP2. Cell Death Dis. 2016;7:e2175.

29. Pankey EA, Thammasiboon S, Lasker GF, Baber S, Lasky JA, Kadowitz PJ. Imatinib attenuates monocrotaline pulmonary hypertension and has potent vasodilator activity in pulmonary and systemic vascular beds in the rat. Am J Physiol Heart Circ Physiol. 2013;305(9):H1288–96.

30. Vonk-Noordegraaf A, Haddad F, Chin KM, Forfia PR, Kawut SM, Lumens J, Naeije R, Newman J, Oudiz RJ, Provencher S, et al. Right heart adaptation to pulmonary arterial hypertension: physiology and pathobiology. J Am Coll Cardiol. 2013;62(25 Suppl):D22–33.

31. Lauriol J, Cabrera JR, Roy A, Keith K, Hough SM, Damilano F, Wang B, Segarra GC, Flessa ME, Miller LE, et al. Developmental SHP2 dysfunction underlies cardiac hypertrophy in Noonan syndrome with multiple lentigines. J Clin Invest. 2016;126(8):2989–3005.

32. Schramm C, Edwards MA, Krenz M. New approaches to prevent LEOPARD syndrome-associated cardiac hypertrophy by specifically targeting Shp2-dependent signaling. J Biol Chem. 2013;288(25):18335–44.

33. Li MX, Jiang DQ, Wang Y, Chen QZ, Ma YJ, Yu SS, Wang Y. Signal mechanisms of vascular remodeling in the development of pulmonary arterial hypertension. J Cardiovasc Pharmacol. 2016;67(2):182–90.

34. Schermuly RT, Dony E, Ghofrani HA, Pullamsetti S, Savai R, Roth M, Sydykov A, Lai YJ, Weissmann N, Seeger W, Grimminger F. Reversal of experimental pulmonary hypertension by PDGF inhibition. J Clin Invest. 2005;115(10):2811–21.

35. Haider UG, Roos TU, Kontaridis MI, Neel BG, Sorescu D, Griendling KK, Vollmar AM, Dirsch VM. Resveratrol inhibits angiotensin II- and epidermal growth factor-mediated Akt activation: role of Gab1 and Shp2. Mol Pharmacol. 2005;68(1):41–8.

36. Dahal BK, Cornitescu T, Tretyn A, Pullamsetti SS, Kosanovic D, Dumitrascu R, Ghofrani HA, Weissmann N, Voswinckel R, Banat GA, et al. Role of epidermal growth factor inhibition in experimental pulmonary hypertension. Am J Respir Crit Care Med. 2010;181(2):158–67.

37. Liu Y, Cao Y, Sun S, Zhu J, Gao S, Pang J, Zhu D, Sun Z. Transforming growth factor-beta1 upregulation triggers pulmonary artery smooth muscle cell proliferation and apoptosis imbalance in rats with hypoxic pulmonary hypertension via the PTEN/AKT pathways. Int J Biochem Cell Biol. 2016;77(Pt A):141–54.

38. Sun M, Ramchandran R, Chen J, Yang Q, Raj JU. Smooth muscle insulin-like growth Factor-1 mediates hypoxia-induced pulmonary hypertension in neonatal mice. Am J Respir Cell Mol Biol. 2016;55(6):779–91.

39. Zhou S, Li M, Zeng D, Sun G, Zhou J, Wang R. Effects of basic fibroblast growth factor and cyclin D1 on cigarette smoke-induced pulmonary vascular remodeling in rats. Exp Ther Med. 2015;9(1):33–8.

23

Circulating serotonin levels in COPD patients: a pilot study

Pietro Pirina[1,2]* (iD), Elisabetta Zinellu[1], Panagiotis Paliogiannis[3], Alessandro G. Fois[2], Viviana Marras[2], Salvatore Sotgia[3], Ciriaco Carru[3] and Angelo Zinellu[3]

Abstract

Background: Chronic obstructive pulmonary disease (COPD) is a major and increasing global health problem. Serotonin is a neurotransmitter that participates in several pulmonary functions and it has been involved in oxidative stress, which plays essential roles in the pathogenesis of COPD. The current study aimed at establishing the levels of circulating serotonin in COPD, and investigating eventual relations between serotonin and oxidative stress markers.

Methods: Whole blood serotonin was assessed in 43 consecutive patients with stable COPD and in 43 age and sex-matched healthy controls.

Results: Serotonin blood levels were significantly higher in COPD patients than in controls (median 0.81 μmol/L, IQR: 0.61–4.02 vs 0.65 μmol/L, IQR: 0.53–1.39, $p = 0.02$). The univariate logistic regression analysis evidenced that serotonin levels are independently associated with presence of COPD (crude OR = 7.29, 95% CI: 1.296–41.05, $p = 0.003$) and such an association was confirmed also after adjusting for several confounders (OR 21.92, 95% CI 2.02–237.83; $p = 0.011$).

Conclusions: Our study showed higher levels of circulating serotonin in COPD and an inverse correlation with the worsening of airway obstruction. Future studies are necessary to investigate the clinical utility of this finding.

Keywords: COPD, Oxidative stress, Serotonin, Markers

Background

COPD is an increasing global health problem that nowadays represents the third leading cause of death in the world [1, 2]. It is a chronic progressive disease characterized by a not fully reversible airflow limitation, associated with a chronic inflammation of the lungs and small airways [3, 4]. Although cigarette smoking represents the most known risk factor, in-door and out-door pollution, second-hand smoking and genetic conditions, such as α_1 antitrypsin deficiency, are considered important additional risk factors [5–7]. The noxious compounds present in cigarette smoke and in environmental pollution, trigger the inflammatory response of the airways and the lungs in susceptible subjects,

causing epithelial injury with subsequent production of reactive oxygen species (ROS) [8, 9]. The increased amount of oxidants together with the depletion of antioxidant defenses, results in oxidative stress. It is now recognized that oxidative stress is involved in the pathogenesis of COPD [9, 10] and, in this regard, several biomarkers have been evaluated [11].

Serotonin (5-hydroxytyptamine, 5-HT) is a ubiquitous neurotransmitter that plays important roles in pulmonary functions, being involved in the modulation of respiratory rhythm and in pulmonary vasoconstriction [12, 13]. Furthermore, serotonin has been implicated in the pathogenesis of some of the main comorbidities of COPD, like depression [14, 15] despite the relation between serotonin, COPD and depression is still to be verified.

Moreover, serotonin has been reported to induce oxidative stress via monoamine oxidase-dependent pathway in human heart valves [16] and in mesenchymal

* Correspondence: pirina@uniss.it
[1]Department of Respiratory Diseases, University Hospital Sassari (AOU), Sassari, Italy
[2]Department of Clinical and Experimental Medicine, University of Sassari, Sassari, Italy
Full list of author information is available at the end of the article

stem cells [17] indicating that serotonin metabolism may be involved in oxidative stress. Its role in the genesis and maintenance of oxidative stress in COPD patients is not well-established. In this pilot study we focused on the assessment of blood serotonin levels in COPD patients compared to healthy controls and in relation to airway obstruction severity; we have also evaluated potential associations between serotonin and oxidative stress markers, like thiobarbituric acid reactive substances (TBARS) and protein sulfhydryl groups (PSH), which have been demonstrated in previous studies to be altered in patients with COPD [18, 19].

Methods

Subjects

This case–control pilot study involved 43 consecutive patients with stable COPD (mean age 74.8 ± 5.9 years, range 52–85 years), treated at the Respiratory Unit of the University of Sassari.

The diagnosis of COPD was made in accordance with the Global Initiative for Chronic Obstructive Lung Disease criteria [20]. The patients enrolled did not have a previous diagnosis of COPD and they were not under treatment with long- or short-acting β-agonists, or long-acting muscarinic antagonists, as well as with inhaled corticosteroids at least within 4 weeks prior to enrollment. Each patient performed respiratory function tests and underwent physical examination, blood tests and chest radiographs. The functional diagnosis of COPD was based on the presence of not fully reversible airflow limitation, defined by a post-bronchodilator ratio of forced expiratory volume in 1 s to forced vital capacity (FEV1/FVC) < 70% of the predicted value [4]. In order to collect demographic and clinical data, including smoking history and information about occupational and/or in-door and out-door pollutants exposure, a structured questionnaire was administered. In particular, patients who were never smokers, had been exposed to other COPD risk factors: half of them were women exposed to second-hand smoke, three of them had worked as miners and therefore exposed to silica powders and two of them had been exposed to indoor pollutants (biomass heating, etc).

A group of 43 age- and sex-matched healthy controls, with no medical history, was also included. Subjects with severe concomitant diseases, such as heart diseases, kidney and liver diseases, systemic inflammatory diseases, patients with severe COPD and patients with a history of asthma and atopic diseases, were excluded from the study. The study was approved by the Institutional Local Ethics Committee (Azienda Sanitaria Locale n°1 di Sassari (Italy) (prot. 2175/CE del 21/04/2015). The subjects who decided to participate, signed a written informed consent before enrollment.

Biochemical analysis

The levels of serotonin in whole blood of COPD subjects and healthy controls were determined according to a method previously described [21]. The inter-assay CV was < 8%. The oxidative stress indices TBARS and PSH were measured as previously reported [22, 23]. TBARS assay was employed to measure malondialdehyde (MDA) and other aldehydes produced by lipid peroxidation induced by reactive oxygen species. TBARS were determined by measuring the absorbance at 535 nm after reaction with thiobarbituric acid. A calibration curve was obtained using MDA as reference standard. Plasma PSH determination was performed by spectrophotometry with 5,5′-dithiobis-2-nitrobenzoic acid (DTNB) as titrating agent by measuring the absorbance of conjugate at 405 nm. Concentration in samples was determined from a GSH standard curve. ROS can oxidize protein SH to disulfide or sulfenic acid, leading to a reduction in –SH groups.

Statistical analysis

The results are expressed as mean (mean ± SD) or median values (median and IQR). The distribution of variables was evaluated by means of Shapiro-Wilk test. The statistical comparisons between groups were assessed by means of unpaired Student's t-test or Mann-Whitney rank sum test, as appropriate. Correlations between variables were estimated using Spearman's or Pearson's correlation, as appropriate. In order to verify the presence of association between variables potentially implicated in disease development, logistic regression analysis was performed. Receiver operating characteristics (ROC) curve analysis was used to test the ability of serotonin to predict COPD, alone and in combination with TBARS and PSH. ROC curves were obtained with calculation of the area under the curve (AUC). Optimal cut-off maximizing sensitivity and specificity was selected according to the Youden Index.

Statistical analyses were performed using MedCalc for Windows, version 15.4 64 bit (MedCalc Software, Ostend, Belgium) and SPSS for Windows, version 14.0 32 bit (IBM Corporation; Armonk, NY, USA).

Results

Table 1 reports the demographic and clinical characteristics in controls and COPD patients. As expected, COPD patients showed a reduced FEV_1 and FEV_1/FVC ratio. There were no between-group differences in smoking status or BMI. Serotonin blood levels were significantly higher in COPD patients (median 0.81 μmol/L, IQR: 0.61–4.02) than in controls (median 0.65 μmol/L, IQR: 0.53–1.39), $p = 0.02$ (Fig. 1). As previously reported TBARS concentrations significantly increased, and PSH

Table 1 Clinical and functional parameters of healthy subjects and COPD patients

	Controls (n = 43)	COPD (n = 43)
Age (years)	73 ± 7	75 ± 6
Gender (F/M)	9/34	9/34
BMI (kg/m^2)	26 ± 4	27 ± 4
Never smoked	14 (33%)	10 (23%)
Current smokers	3 (7%)	3 (7%)
Ex smokers	26 (60)	30 (70%)
FEV1 (L)	2.8 ± 0.6	2.0 ± 0.6**
FEV1 (% predicted)	112 ± 14	80 ± 18**
FVC (L)	3.4 ± 0.7	2.9 ± 0.8*
FVC (% predicted)	108 ± 15	88 ± 15**
FEV1/FVC	80.4 ± 3.9	66.6 ± 4.8**
RV (L)	2.0 ± 0.5	3.4 ± 0.9**
RV (% predicted)	105 ± 12	137 ± 32**
TLC (L)	6.0 ± 1.1	6.4 ± 1.1
TLC (% predicted)	107 ± 10	108 ± 14
RV/TLC (%)	32 ± 3	53 ± 9**

FEV1 Forced Expiratory Volume in the 1st second, *FVC* Forced Vital Capacity, *FEV1/FVC* Tiffeneau index (calculated as LLN)
*$p < 0.01$, **$p < 0.001$ obtained by Student's t-test

concentrations significantly decreased, according to COPD presence [18]. However, no significant correlations were observed between serotonin blood levels and oxidative stress indices. As reported in Fig. 2, Spearman's correlations in the whole study population indicated that serotonin blood values are inversely associated with FEV$_1$ (rho = − 0.25, $p = 0.023$) and FVC

(rho = − 0.26, $p = 0.017$). Table 2 summarizes the results of the univariate logistic regression analysis, which evidenced that serotonin levels were independently associated with presence of COPD (crude OR = 7.29, 95% CI: 1.296–41.05, $p = 0.003$). This association remained significant also after adjusting for age, gender, BMI, smoking status, and oxidative stress indices (OR 21.92, 95% CI 2.02–237.83; $p = 0.011$).

ROC curve analysis was performed to evaluate the sensitivity, specificity, and diagnostic accuracy of serum serotonin levels alone, or in combination with PSH and TBARS, in distinguishing COPD from healthy subjects (Fig. 3 and Table 3). Serotonin alone, with a cut-off of 0.78 μmol/L discriminated COPD from controls with 53.5% sensitivity and 74.4% specificity (AUC = 0.647, 95% CI 0.537–0.747, $p = 0.014$). Serotonin in combination with PSH and TBARS produced the best result, with an AUC of 0.830 (95% CI 0.733–0.902, $p < 0.0001$), sensitivity 76.7% and specificity 74.4%. Pairwise comparison of ROC curves indicated that the combination of serotonin, PSH and TBARS yield a significant increase in AUC (+ 0.183, $p = 0.0035$) compared to AUC obtained with serotonin alone.

Discussion

Serotonin is a biogenic amine known for its role as a neurotransmitter. It is synthesized from L-tryptophan within the central nervous system (CNS), where it is stored in the presynaptic neurons. Serotonin synthesis outside the CNS is limited to enterochromaffin cells, while platelets take up serotonin from plasma representing a further major storing site for serotonin [24]. The main metabolic pathway of serotonin is the

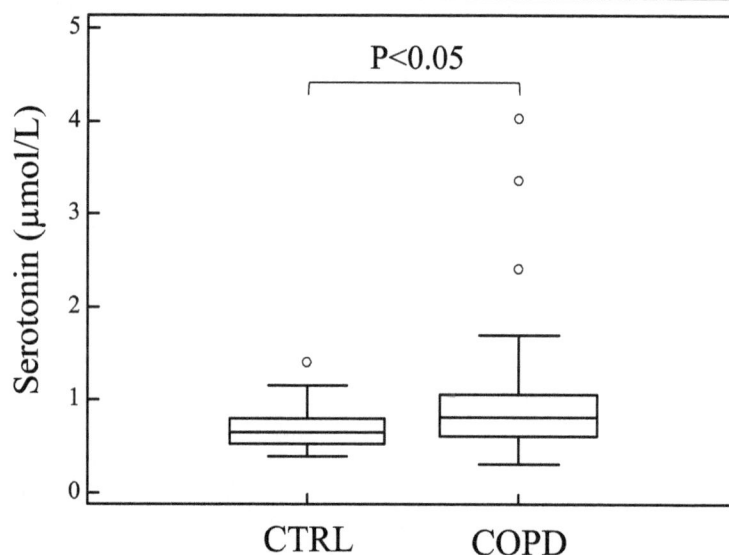

Fig. 1 Blood levels of serotonin in healthy subjects (n = 43) and in the totality of COPD patients (n = 43). The central horizontal line on each box represents the median, the ends of the boxes are 25 and 75 percentiles and the error bars 5 and 95%. *P*-values derived from Student's t-test

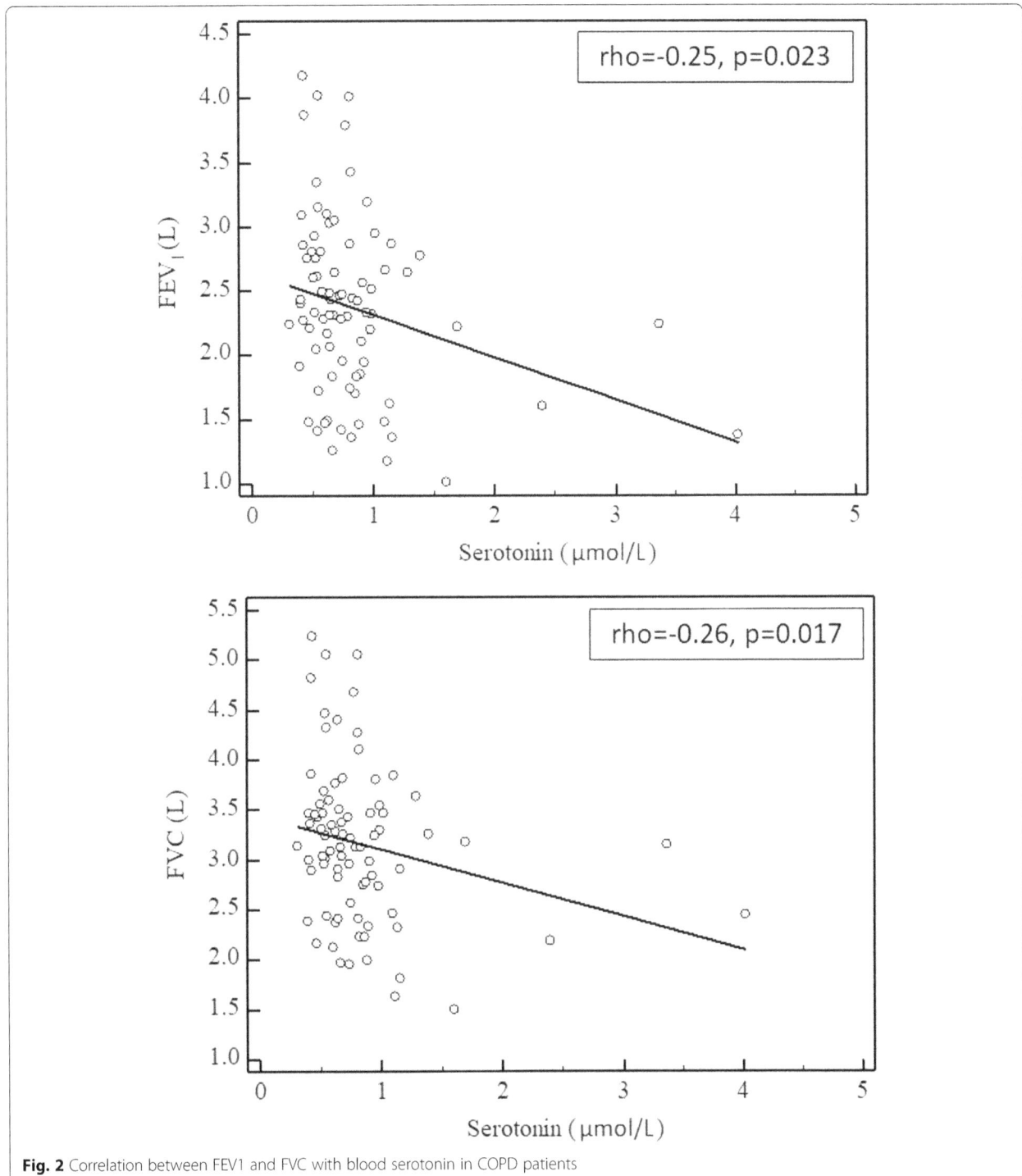

Fig. 2 Correlation between FEV1 and FVC with blood serotonin in COPD patients

metabolism by monoamine oxidase (MAO) that cataly-
ses the oxidative deamination of the amine substrate,
with production of its aldehyde intermediate and
hydrogen peroxide as a by-product. The aldehyde intermediate is then rapidly oxidized by aldehyde dehydrogenase to 5-hydroxyindoleacetic acid [24, 25].

It is known that lung represent an important site in
which removal and metabolism of serotonin take

place [26]. The ability of the endothelial cells of the
lungs to metabolise amines may be reduced in disease
states, and this could explain their increased levels in
the circulation. Elevated circulating levels of serotonin
have been reported in respiratory diseases such as
asthma [27] and lung cancer [28]. COPD has also
been associated with a variation of a transporter gene
involved in serotonin re-uptake [29] and metabolites

Table 2 Predicting factors for chronic obstructive pulmonary disease

Factor	Univariate analysis			Multivariate analysis		
	Crude OR	95%CI	p-value	OR	95%CI	p-value
Age	1.035	0.967–1.109	0.749	0.998	0.917–1.088	0.978
Gender	1.000	0.368–2.720	0.061	1.567	0.341–7.203	0.563
BMI	1.076	0.953–1.216	0.692	1.108	0.942–1.303	0.217
Smoking status	1.404	0.551–3.581	1.000	0.516	0.144–1.854	0.319
PSH	0.427	0.258–0.705	0.0001	0.289	0.144–0.580	0.0005
TBARS	1.816	1.053–3.131	0.02	2.947	1.322–6.570	0.008
Serotonin	7.294	1.296–41.05	0.003	21.92	2.02–237.83	0.011

BMI body mass index, *PSH* protein sulfhydryl groups, *TBARS* thiobarbituric acid reactive substances, *OR* odds ratio, *CI* confidence interval

of the serotonin pathway have been associated with adverse outcome in exacerbated COPD [30]. Furthermore, it is now recognized that oxidative stress is involved in the pathogenesis of COPD [9, 10] and it has been reported that serotonin induces oxidative stress via MAO-dependent pathway in human heart valves [16] and in mesenchymal stem cells [17]. Moreover, it has been described that cigarette smoke, a major COPD risk factor, inhibit MAO in different species in vitro [31]. Such evidences suggest that serotonin may play relevant roles in the pathogenesis of COPD.

Our study has evidenced a significant increase in serotonin levels in COPD patients compared to controls. Spearman's correlations indicated that blood serotonin values are inversely associated with FEV1 and FVC, to confirm an association of serotonin levels not only with the presence of COPD, but also with the severity of airway obstruction. The univariate logistic regression analysis has shown that serotonin levels were independently associated with presence of COPD also after adjusting for age, gender, BMI, smoking status, and oxidative stress indices.

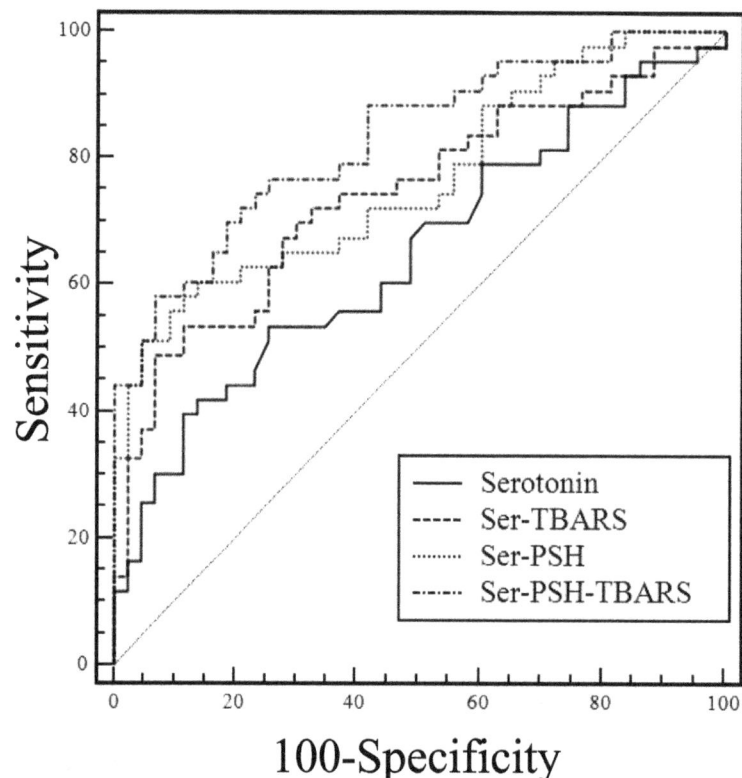

Fig. 3 The area under receiver operating characteristic curves of serotonin

Table 3 Prognostic accuracy of serotonin alone or in combination with TBARS and MDA

Marker	AUC	95%CI	p value	Cut-off	Sensib	Specif
Serotonin	0.647	0.537–0.747	0.014	> 0.780	53.5%	74.4%
Ser-TBARS	0.741	0.635–0.829	< 0.0001	> 0.543	53.5%	88.4%
Ser-PSH	0.764	0.660–0.849	< 0.0001	> 0.569	60.5%	86.1%
Ser-PSH-TBARS	0.830	0.733–0.902	< 0.0001	> 0.460	76.7%	74.4%

PSH protein sulfhydryl groups, *TBARS* thiobarbituric acid reactive substances, *MDA* malondialdehyde, *AUC* area under the curve, *CI* confidence interval

Lau et al. [32], investigated the role of serotonin in the pathogenesis of COPD and found higher levels of circulating serotonin in patients compared to healthy controls. Unlike us, they examined only male COPD subjects who were significantly older than controls, and found a positive correlation between serotonin levels and age in pathological subjects. Moreover, in their analysis they prevalently included moderate to very severe COPD cases, finding no differences in serotonin levels according to disease progression. In our study, we confirmed the presence of higher blood serotonin levels in COPD compared to age- and sex-matched controls. As opposed to the study of Lau et al., our patients had a mild-moderate degree of airway obstruction (FEV1 > 50%). From this point of view these patients can be considered in the early phase of the disease. In fact, they were all newly diagnosed patients who had not yet started a treatment. These data support the hypothesis that serotonin could be a predictive marker of the onset of COPD. Moreover, the inverse correlation that we found between serotonin levels and FEV1 and FVC, suggests a relation of this molecule with the worsening of airway obstruction.

The ROC curve analysis for serotonin significantly discriminate patients with COPD from those without COPD and showed that the diagnostic accuracy is higher when serotonin is combined with TBARS and PSH. In particular, the triple combination of serotonin, TBARS and PSH increased significantly the AUC of the ROC curve. Although it is an interesting result, its clinical validity and usefulness needs to be further investigated. Moreover, Spearman's correlation analysis failed to find a relationship between serotonin and oxidative stress biomarkers. This could be due to the low number of subjects involved, in particular to the absence of severe COPD subjects. The small number of cases, and the lack of advanced stage COPD patients represent the main limitations of our work. On the other hand, our study is the first to investigate blood serotonin levels in a cohort of early COPD cases and has several strengths, like its prospective case-match design, the accurate statistical analysis, and the research of associations with other well-established biomarkers of oxidative stress.

Conclusions

Our study confirms literature data showing an involvement of serotonin in the pathogenesis of COPD, demonstrating a statistically significant increase of circulating serotonin levels in an early phase of the disease, and a relation with the worsening of the airway obstruction. Given the need of biomarkers useful to detect and monitor COPD and its response to treatments, this seems to be a promising result that need to be further investigated.

Acknowledgements
Not applicable.

Funding
This research did not receive any specific grant from funding agencies in the public, commercial, or not-for-profit sectors.

Authors' contributions
PP1 participated in the design of the study and drafted the manuscript. EZ helped to draft the manuscript and contributed to the biochemical analysis. PP2 and AGF helped to draft the manuscript. VM and SS contributed to the biochemical analysis. CC contributed to the statistical analysis. AZ conceived and designed the study, was responsible for data extraction and performed statistical analysis. All authors have critically revised the manuscript and have approved the final version.

Competing interests
The author Pietro Pirina is currently acting as an Associate Editor for BMC Pulmonary Medicine. All other authors declare that they have no competing interests.

Author details
[1]Department of Respiratory Diseases, University Hospital Sassari (AOU), Sassari, Italy. [2]Department of Clinical and Experimental Medicine, University of Sassari, Sassari, Italy. [3]Department of Biomedical Sciences, University of Sassari, Sassari, Italy.

References
1. López-Campos JL, Tan W, Soriano JB. Global burden of COPD. Respirology. 2016;21(1):14–23.
2. Lozano R, Naghavi M, Foreman K, Lim S, Shibuya K, Aboyans V, Abraham J, Adair T, Aggarwal R, Ahn SY, Alvarado M, Anderson HR, Anderson LM, Andrews KG, Atkinson C, et al. Global and regional mortality from 235 causes of death for 20 age groups in 1990 and 2010: a systematic analysis for the Global Burden of Disease Study 2010. Lancet. 2012;380(9859):2095–128.
3. Decramer M, Janssens W, Miravitlles M. Chronic obstructive pulmonary disease. Lancet. 2012;379:1341–51.
4. Vogelmeier CF, Criner GJ, Martinez FJ, Anzueto A, Barnes PJ, Bourbeau J, Celli BR, Chen R, Decramer M, Fabbri LM, Frith P, Halpin DM, López Varela MV, Nishimura M, Roche N, Rodriguez-Roisin R, Sin DD, Singh D, Stockley R, Vestbo J, Wedzicha JA, Agusti A. Global Strategy for the Diagnosis, Management, and Prevention of Chronic Obstructive Lung Disease 2017 Report: GOLD Executive Summary. Eur Respir J. 2017;49(3). https://doi.org/10.1183/13993003.00214-2017.
5. Mannino DM, Buist AS. Global burden of COPD: risk factors, prevalence, and future trends. Lancet. 2007;370:765–73.
6. Eisner MD, Anthonisen N, Coultas D, Kuenzli N, Perez-Padilla R, Postma D, Romieu I, Silverman EK, Balmes JR, Committee on Nonsmoking COPD, Environmental and Occupational Health Assembly. An official American Thoracic Society public policy statement: novel risk factors and the global

burden of chronic obstructive pulmonary disease. Am J Respir Crit Care Med. 2010;182:693–718.

7. Gooptu B, Ekeowa UI, Lomas DA. Mechanisms of emphysema in alpha1-antitrypsin deficiency: molecular and cellular insights. Eur Respir J. 2009;34:475–88.

8. Larsson K. Aspects on pathophysiological mechanisms in COPD. J Intern Med. 2007;262(3):311–40.

9. Kirkham PA, Barnes PJ. Oxidative stress in COPD. Chest. 2013;144(1):266–73.

10. Santus P, Corsico A, Solidoro P, Braido F, Di Marco F, Scichilone N. Oxidative stress and respiratory system: pharmacological and clinical reappraisal of N-acetylcysteine. COPD. 2014;11(6):705–17.

11. Zinellu E, Zinellu A, Fois AG, Carru C, Pirina P. Circulating biomarkers of oxidative stress in chronic obstructive pulmonary disease: a systematic review. Respir Res. 2016;17(1):150.

12. Hilaire G, Voituron N, Menuet C, Ichiyama RM, Subramanian HH, Dutschmann M. The role of serotonin in respiratory function and dysfunction. Respir Physiol Neurobiol. 2010;174(1–2):76–88.

13. Morecroft I, Loughlin L, Nilsen M, Colston J, Dempsie Y, Sheward J, Harmar A, MacLean MR. Functional interactions between 5-hydroxytryptamine receptors and the serotonin transporter in pulmonary arteries. J Pharmacol Exp Ther. 2005;313(2):539–48.

14. Blier P, El Mansari M. Serotonin and beyond: therapeutics for major depression. Philos Trans R Soc Lond Ser B Biol Sci. 2013;368(1615):20120536.

15. Yohannes AM, Alexopoulos GS. Depression and anxiety in patients with COPD. Eur Respir Rev. 2014;23(133):345–9.

16. Peña-Silva RA, Miller JD, Chu Y, Heistad DD. Serotonin produces monoamine oxidase-dependent oxidative stress in human heart valves. Am J Physiol Heart Circ Physiol. 2009;297(4):H1354–60.

17. Trouche E, Mias C, Seguelas MH, Ordener C, Cussac D, Parini A. Characterization of monoamine oxidases in mesenchymal stem cells: role in hydrogen peroxide generation and serotonin-dependent apoptosis. Stem Cells Dev. 2010;19(10):1571–8.

18. Zinellu A, Fois AG, Sotgia S, Sotgiu E, Zinellu E, Bifulco F, Mangoni AA, Pirina P, Carru C. Arginines plasma concentration and oxidative stress in mild to moderate COPD. PLoS One. 2016;11(8):e0160237.

19. Zinellu A, Fois AG, Sotgia S, Zinellu E, Bifulco F, Pintus G, Mangoni AA, Carru C, Pirina P. Plasma protein thiols: an early marker of oxidative stress in asthma and chronic obstructive pulmonary disease. Eur J Clin Investig. 2016; 46(2):181–8.

20. Global Strategy for the Diagnosis, Management, and Prevention of Chronic Obstructive Lung Disease 2017 Report. GOLD Executive Summary. Am J Respir Crit Care Med. 2017;195(5):557–82.

21. Zinellu A, Sotgia S, Deiana L, Carru C. Reverse injection capillary electrophoresis UV detection for serotonin quantification in human whole blood. J Chromatogr B Anal Technol Biomed Life Sci. 2012;895–896:182–5.

22. Esterbauer H, Cheeseman KH. Determination of aldehydic lipid peroxidation products: malonaldehyde and 4-hydroxynonenal. Methods Enzymol. 1990; 186:407–21.

23. Ellman GL. Tissue sulfhydryl groups. Arch Biochem Biophys. 1959;82(1):70–7.

24. Mohammad-Zadeh LF, Moses L, Gwaltney-Brant SM. Serotonin: a review. J Vet Pharmacol Ther. 2008;31(3):187–99.

25. Lewis A, Miller JH, Lea RA. Monoamine oxidase and tobacco dependence. Neurotoxicology. 2007;28(1):182–95.

26. Block ER, Stalcup SA. Metabolic functions of the lung. Of what clinical relevance? Chest. 1982;81(2):215–23.

27. Lechin F, van der Dijs B, Orozco B, Lechin M, Lechin AE. Increased levels of free serotonin in plasma of symptomatic asthmatic patients. Ann Allergy Asthma Immunol. 1996;77(3):245–53.

28. Takahashi C, Goto E, Taira S, Kataoka N, Nishihara M, Katsumata T, Goto I, Takiuchi H. Serotonin syndrome in a patient with small cell lung cancer. Gan To Kagaku Ryoho. 2013;40(8):1059–61.

29. Ishii T, Wakabayashi R, Kurosaki H, Gemma A, Kida K. Association of serotonin transporter gene variation with smoking, chronic obstructive pulmonary disease, and its depressive symptoms. J Hum Genet. 2011;56(1):41–6.

30. Meier MA, Ottiger M, Vögeli A, Steuer C, Bernasconi L, Thomann R, Christ-Crain M, Henzen C, Hoess C, Zimmerli W, Huber A, Mueller B, Schuetz P. Activation of the serotonin pathway is associated with poor outcome in COPD exacerbation: results of a long-term cohort study. Lung. 2017;195(3):303–11.

31. Khalil AA, Davies B, Castagnoli N Jr. Isolation and characterization of a monoamine oxidase B selective inhibitor from tobacco smoke. Bioorg Med Chem. 2006;14:3392–8.

32. Lau WK, Chan-Yeung MM, Yip BH, Cheung AH, Ip MS, Mak JC, COPD Study Group of the Hong Kong Thoracic Society. The role of circulating serotonin in the development of chronic obstructive pulmonary disease. PLoS One. 2012;7(2):e31617.

24

Efficacy of regional arterial embolization before pleuropulmonary resection in 32 patients with tuberculosis-destroyed lung

Gang Chen, Fang-Ming Zhong* ⓘ, Xu-Dong Xu, Guo-Can Yu and Peng-Fei Zhu

Abstract

Background: Treatment of tuberculous-destroyed lung (TDL) with pleuropulmonary resection is challenging. Pulmonary hemorrhage is a frequent complication of this surgical procedure. Continuous efforts have been made to investigate clinical procedures that may reduce intraoperative bleeding effectively. In this study, we evaluated the feasibility and safety of regional arterial embolization before pleuropulmonary resection in patients with TDL.

Methods: The clinical data of 32 patients with TDL were retrospectively reviewed and analyzed. These patients were admitted to the hospital between July 2009 and November 2016. All of the patients had moderate to massive hemoptysis and received regional arterial embolization in affected areas. Then, these patients underwent pleuropulmonary resection within 1 week to 2 months after embolization.

Results: The results showed that 25 patients (78.1%) had bronchial artery, and all patients had non-bronchial systemic artery found in affected areas. Mild to moderate chest pain was reported in 6 patients, and fever was reported in 2 patients. Intraoperative blood loss during pleuropulmonary resection in patients who had received preoperative regional arterial embolization was 625.6 ± 352.6 ml. Duration of the operation was 120.3 ± 75.2 min. Bronchopleural fistulae and empyema were found in 3 cases (9.4%).

Conclusion: Performance of regional arterial embolization before pleuropulmonary resection offers a safe and feasible option that reduces intraoperative blood loss and shortens operative time in patients with TDL.

Keywords: Tuberculous destroyed lung, Pleuropulmonary resection, Regional arterial embolization

Impact statement

Performance of regional arterial embolization before pleuropulmonary resection appeared to be a safe and feasible option that reduced intraoperative bleeding volume and shortened duration of operation in patients with TDL.

Background

Tuberculosis (TB) may cause extensive destruction of the lung and compromise lung function. Pathological changes such as extensive fibrosis, bronchial stenosis, and bronchiectasis are commonly observed in the TB-destroyed lung (TDL) [1]. Erosion of a pulmonary

* Correspondence: fangming574330@163.com
Department of Thoracic Surgery, Tuberculosis Surgery, Hangzhou Red Cross Hospital, No. 208 Huancheng East Road, Xiacheng District, Hangzhou 310003, Zhejiang, China

artery branch due to TDL can cause bleeding, resulting in gas exchange disorder or sometimes a life-threatening situation [2]. Management options of TDL include the use of anti-TB agents (for active-TB cases), antibiotics (for inactive-TB cases), or surgical intervention. Unfortunately, the prevalence of multidrug resistance (MDR) is high [3]. Bronchial artery embolization (BAE) works in some patients, but a high recurrence rate prevents its widespread application in clinical practice [4]. In the light of this, surgical resection is an option for consideration.

The most common surgical procedure for patients with TDL is pleuropulmonary resection [2, 5–7]. TDL affected areas are usually extensive with severe adhesions. In addition, they are accompanied with recurrent infections, abundant collateral circulation, and hemorrhage. Complications are likely to occur during the procedure of separation in conventional pleuropulmonary resection of TDL. Homeostasis is difficult to maintain during the operation [8]. To minimize the complication rate, reducing intraoperative blood loss is an important factor to consider. Recently, our hospital has adopted a procedure of regional arterial embolization in combination with pleuropulmonary resection, in order to reduce intraoperative and postoperative bleeding. Thirty-two TDL patients with massive hemoptysis received regional arterial embolization before pleuropulmonary resection between July 2009 and November 2015. We retrospectively analyzed these cases and evaluated the efficacy of regional arterial embolization in combination with pleuropulmonary resection. The results may provide insight into the development of new treatment options for patients with TDL.

Methods
Baseline information
A total of 32 patients with TDL were included in this study. The disease duration ranged from 30 to 240 months, with a mean of 56.7 months. All patients received a standard or other non-standard preoperative anti-tuberculosis therapy. Demographics (gender and age), disease duration, location of the destroyed lung and indications are shown in Table 1. Tuberculosis was diagnosed by pathological or etiological examination. The diagnostic criteria included: 1) positive acid-fast bacilli in respiratory specimens (e.g. sputum, bronchoscopy lavage fluid, surgically resected lung tissue) by smear or culture; 2) PCR-positive for *Mycobacterium*

Table 1 Demographics, indications and locations of destroyed lung in patients

Clinical features	Results
Demographics	
Gender	
Male (n)	21(65.6%)
Female (n)	11(34.4%)
Age (years)	
Range	25–69
Mean ± SD	37.8 ± 11.2
Duration of disease (month)	
Mean ± SD	56.7 ± 26.5
Locations of destroyed lung (n)	
Unilateral lung	20(62.5%)
Single upper lobe	9(28.1%)
Middle or lower lobe	3(9.4%)
Indications (n)	
Hemoptysis	32(100%)
Continuously positive smear	9(28.1%)
Pulmonary aspergillosis	13(40.6%)

tuberculosis RNA in respiratory specimens; 3) caseating granuloma found in the histopathological examination of surgically resected lung tissue. The ethics review board of Hangzhou Red Cross Hospital approved this study. Surgeons, who had legal eligibility for interventional treatment and extensive experience in tuberculosis thoracic surgery, conducted all interventional procedures and operations.

Criteria for diagnosis and inclusion
We defined patients with TDL as those presenting with a destroyed lung with a history of tuberculosis (diagnosed by physician with proof of positive smears/cultures). Computed tomography (CT) scan was performed to examine the lesions of parenchymal destruction. All patients included in this study fulfilled the eligibility criteria. The inclusion criteria were as follows: (a) TDL affected areas in at least one lung lobe; (b) history of moderate to massive hemoptysis (amount of hemoptysis was greater than 100 mL within 24 h); (c) repeated episodes of cough or hemoptysis after conventional treatment (e.g. first-line/second-line anti-tuberculosis drugs, intravenous and oral hemostatic drugs, vascular embolization). Exclusion criteria were as follows: (a) incomplete clinical information; (b) history of thoracic surgery; (c) active tuberculosis without standardized anti-tuberculosis medical treatment; (d) uncontrolled concomitant diseases such as heart failure, asthma, idiopathic pulmonary fibrosis, and malignant tumor.

Preoperative preparation
All patients received CT scan, bronchoscopy, routine blood test, heart and lung function tests, sputum TB smear/culture, and drug sensitivity test before the surgery.

Preoperative fiberoptic bronchoscopy was used to confirm absence of active endobronchial tuberculosis in all cases. Patients received standard anti-tuberculosis treatment for at least 6 months. Thereafter, patients who still had acid-fast bacilli-positive sputum smear were given second-line anti-tuberculosis treatment (sodium aminosalicylate, amikacin, ethionamide and levofloxacin) for at least 3 months. Those with signs of pulmonary aspergillosis in radiological images received preoperative itraconazole or voriconazole for at least 1 month.

Arterial supply of lesions was preliminarily identified by multislice spiral CT (MSCT). Then, embolization of regional systemic arteries was performed at the interventional center. Finally, pleuropulmonary resection was performed in the operation room within 1 week to 2 months.

All patients were followed up for 6 to 48 months, and reports of complications were collected during outpatient visits or subsequent readmission.

Regional arterial embolization

Arterial supply to the affected areas was examined by MSCT. A transfemoral artery puncture was next made. Cordis 4F/5F C2 or VER135 angiographic catheter, Merit Meastro 28MC24130SN microcatheter were used in the surgery. Digital subtraction images were taken after injection of iodinated contrast agent. Particle embolization was performed as distal as possible in order to avoid embolization of adjacent spinal arteries. A mixture of 500–700 m Particle Embolic Agent (PVA) or gelatin sponge particles and the diluted contrast agent were used as the embolic material for peripheral arteries. Short acting embolic agents such as gelatin sponge were used in the surgical areas, and permanent embolic agents such as PVA were used in areas out of the planned surgical site. Gelatin sponge was used as an embolic material for main vessels. Blood supply to the main bronchus area was preserved. Lastly, the catheters were removed and the puncture sites were pressurized for hemostasis. The duration of embolization ranged from 30 min to 120 min, with a mean of 45 min. If postoperative complications occurred, treatment was given immediately to relieve the symptoms.

Pleuropulmonary resection

Patients were placed in the contralateral decubitus position and underwent general anesthesia. Incisions of 5–10 cm were made at the 4th or 5th intercostal space between the mid-axillary lines, and separations were performed. If possible, the pulmonary hilum was treated with priority, as it may reduce the amount of bleeding during the operation. When it is difficult to separate the pulmonary vessels, a direct incision of the pericardial sac may be made. The bronchial stump was sutured with an automatic suturing device,then with a 3–0 free suture. Argon knife treatment was usedfor the bleeding wound. After a complete hemostasis was reached, thoracic cavity was repeatedly flushed with warm saline. Thoracic cavity was closedwith standard procedure.

Statistical analysis

Data were shown as mean ± standard deviation (SD). All data were analyzed by SPSS 23.0 statistical software packages.

Results

The results of interventional angiography showed that 25 cases (78.1%) had bronchial artery, with pathological changes, in the affected areas. The non-bronchial systemic artery (NBSA) was noted in all patients: 26 cases (81.3%) with posterior intercostal arteries, 5 cases (15.6%) with internal thoracic arteries, 11 cases (34.4%) with external thoracic arteries, 9 cases (28.1%) with subclavian arteries, and 8 cases (25.0%) with inferior phrenic arteries.

Of the 32 patients, 20 patients received pleuropneumonectomy, 12 patients received pleurolobectomy (upper lobe resection in 7 cases, lower lobe resection in 3 cases, upper lobe resection and segmentectomy in 2 cases). After preoperative regional arterial embolization, the estimated intraoperative blood loss was 625.6 ± 352.6 mL, and the operative time was 120.3 ± 75.2 min. Six patients received 3–5 h of postoperative mechanical ventilation in the ICU.

All the regional arterial embolization and pleuropulmonary resections were successfully completed. All cases were diagnosed with pulmonary tuberculosis. No death was reported.

Complications of the interventional therapy were reported in 8 cases. These included 6 cases of mild to moderate thoracodynia, which were relieved after treatment with non-steroidal analgesics and 2 cases of fever, which were relieved after treatment with antibiotics and antipyretic. Renal failure, paralysis and other complications were not observed.

Postoperative complications were found in 6 cases. These included 3 cases (9.37%) of persistent pulmonary air leak, of which 2 cases fully recovered by continuous suction drainage, and 1 case was treated with open thoracic drainage after 6 months (the patient underwent continuous closed chest drainage 6 months after surgery, and pneumothorax was still observed). Postoperative empyema occurred in 3 cases, immediately after surgery in 2 cases, and 1 month postoperatively in 1 case. All of them were cured by continuous thoracic drainage. Safety follow-up was performed for all the 32 patients (range, 6 to 48 months; median, 30 months). Among these patients, five were MDR or mono-resistant, in which 1 was H resistant, 2 were HR resistant, 1 was HRS resistant, and 1 was HRES resistant (H: isoniazid; R: rifampicin; E: ethambutol; S: streptomycin). Chest roentgenogram and sputum bacteriological investigations were conducted in the follow-up visits. The sputum negative conversion rate and the clinical cure rate were 100%.

Discussion

Tuberculosis can cause extensive destruction of the lung. Expansion ofblood vessels may occur after repeated infections, and pulmonary hemorrhage is a frequent complication of conventional pleuropulmonary resection of TDL. Duan et al. suggested that intraoperative blood loss over 1000 mL and operative time more than 4 h are two important risk factors of postoperative complications [8]. Bai et al. reported a group of 172 patients of TDL, who received surgical treatment, and the operative blood loss reached 1240.0 ± 1122.5 mL [9], suggesting that the intraoperative blood loss was generally large in TDL patients. Therefore, the control of blood loss is important for the success of pleuropulmonary resection of TDL.

In the present study, we found that mediastinal pleural adhesion was relatively loose even though the pleural cavity had dense adhesions. Therefore, we mostly isolated mediastinal adhesions with priority to facilitate exposure and separation of pulmonary vessels. The probability of upper lobe damage was high, which occurred in 29 cases (90.6%) in our study. Adhesion at the upper portion of the pleural cavity was difficult to separate, because of the combined thoracic constriction deformity. In addition, the abnormal blood vessels at the pleural adhesions were very dense; therefore, wound bleeding occurred frequently when the pleura was separated. In our operations, the 4th intercostal approach was taken if the major lesion was in the upper lobe. Vats were used to enlarge the field of vision if necessary. Pale ischemic changes were found in many wounds during the operations. After pre-embolization of regional blood vessels, wound bleeding was significantly reduced during the separation of pleural adhesions. Overall, the arterial embolization procedure appeared to reduce the risk of bleeding, and the duration of operation was shortened in subsequent separation and resection of the lesion.

NBSA may be more likely to occur in patients with hemoptysis caused by tuberculosis. Jiang et al. reported that hemoptysis in more than half of different cases was related to NBSA [10]. Adhesions formed among the lung, intercostal, subclavian, and the parietal pleura. Repeated infections lead to regional vasodilatation, and collateral circulation becomes more abundant (Fig. 1). In our study, all patients were complicated with NBSA blood supply; 26 cases (81.3%) had posterior intercostal arteries, 5 cases (15.6%) had internal thoracic arteries, 11 cases (34.4%) had external thoracic arteries, 9 cases (28.1%) had subclavian arteries, and 8 cases (25.0%) had inferior phrenic arteries. These types of artery supply caused operative challenges, including increased intraoperative bleeding and longer duration of operation.

CT angiography (CTA) is an effective method for accurate evaluation of blood vessel responsible for hemoptysis. It has a high sensitivity for diagnosis of pathological artery [11]. Dual arterial CTA of the bronchial artery and non-bronchial artery can provide better preoperative

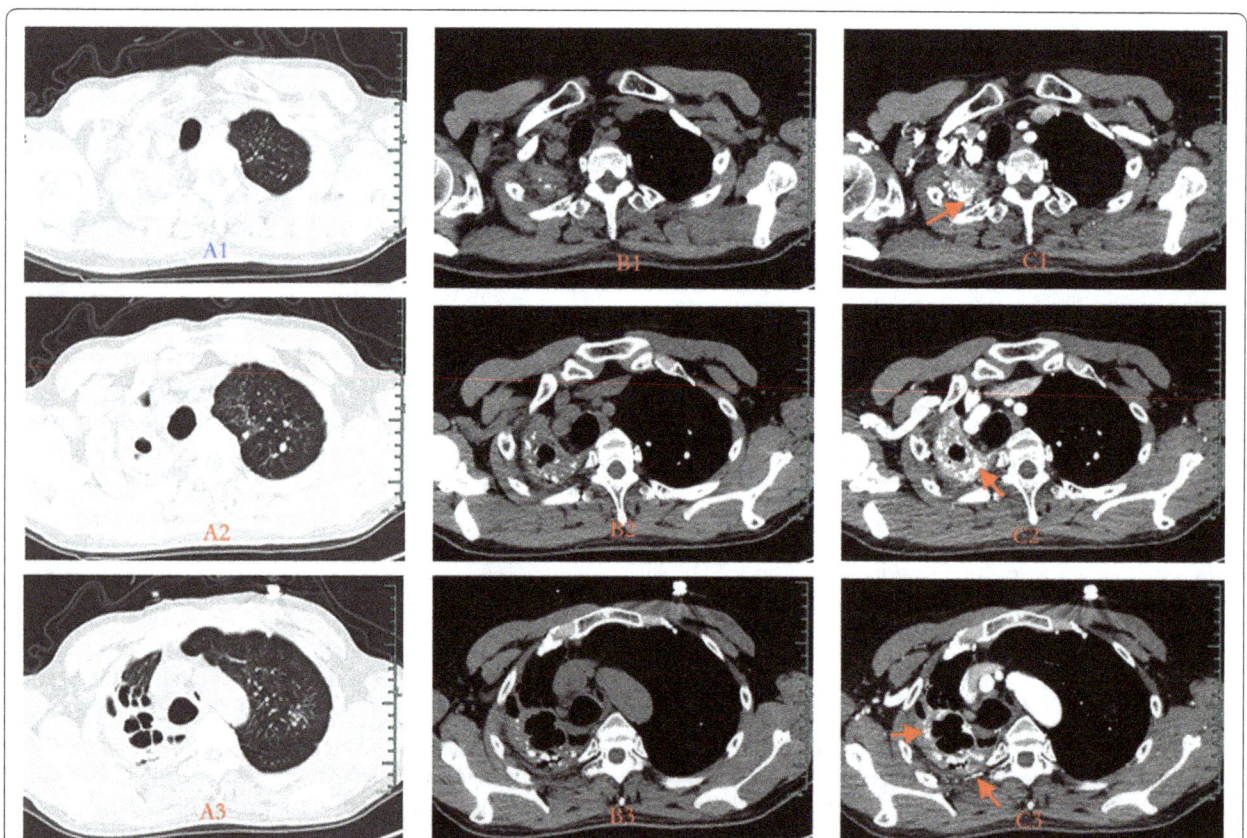

Fig. 1 MSCT images taken before regional arterial embolization (male, 58 years old, repeated episodes of hemoptysis for more than 2 years; after two intervention treatments, hemoptysis was still observed, the largest amount of hemoptysis was 500 mL): vascular enhanced CT showed an increased supply of blood at the pleura

Efficacy of regional arterial embolization before pleuropulmonary resection in 32 patients...

203

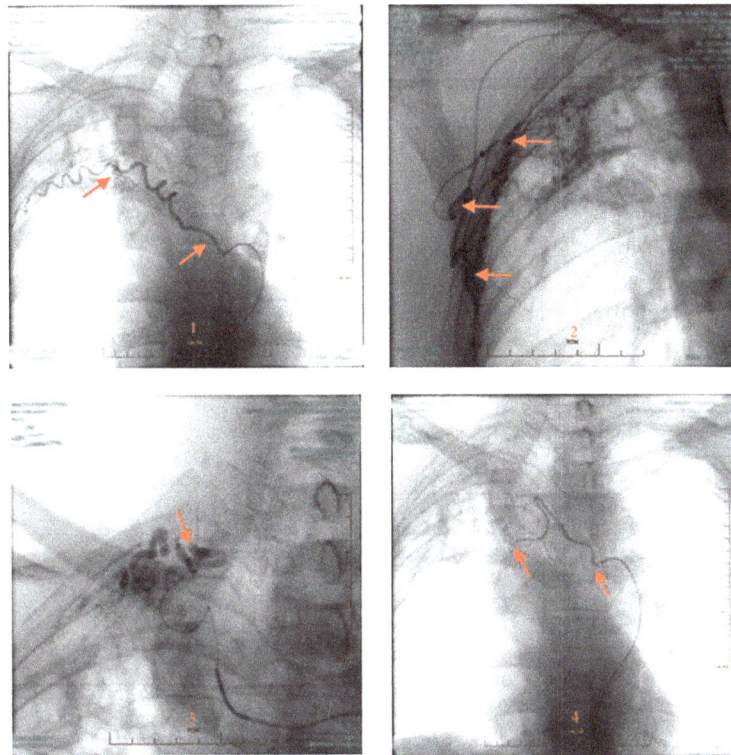

Fig. 2 Parts of pathologic arteries in the lesion of TDLs, which were found in the course of interventional therapy (the same case as Fig. 1). 1: pathological posterior intercostal artery; 2: pathological external thoracic artery; 3: pathological subclavian artery; 4: pathological bronchial artery

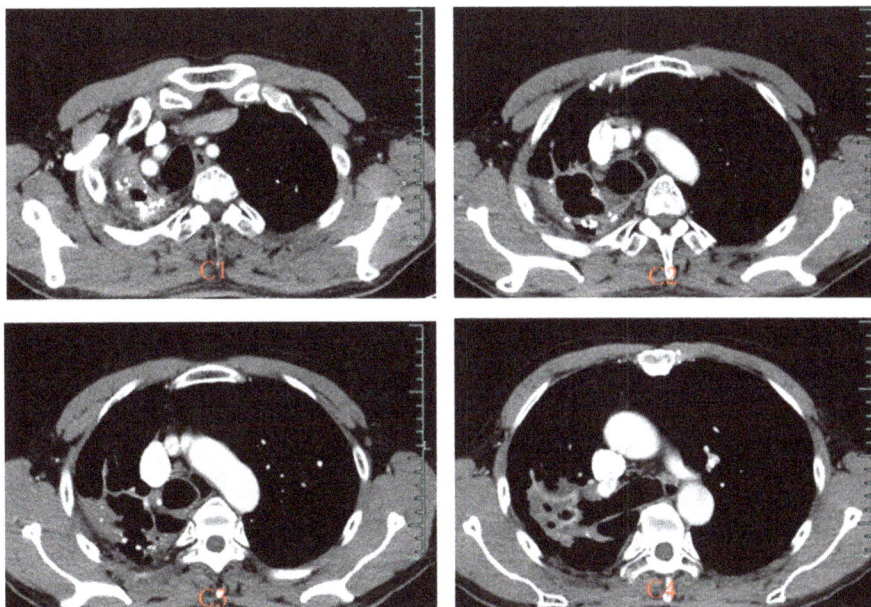

Fig. 3 CT images taken 1 month after regional arterial embolization. (The same case as in Fig. 1):vascular enhanced CT showed a marked reduction in blood supply at the pleura, compared with the time before embolization

guidance for percutaneous catheter embolization [12]. In particular, it helps to avoid missing the observation of arteries such as the subclavian artery and the internal thoracic artery. In our department, dual arterial CTA of the BA and the NBSA were arranged to fully assess the distribution of the system arteries in the affected areas. Therefore, the target blood vessel was found and embolized by injecting embolic agents under DSA guidance (Fig. 2). After vascular embolization, abnormal blood vessels at the pleural adhesions were markedly reduced (Fig. 3). Pre-embolization appeared to provide good surgical conditions for subsequent pleuropulmonary resection. It is important to emphasize that the effect of preoperative arterial embolization in the surgical area is temporary. Short acting embolic agents such as gelatin sponge were used, and the vessels in the main bronchus area were preserved. As a result, the blood supply to the bronchial stump was not affected, and the risk of postoperative pleural fistula was minimized. Lastly, vascular embolization should not be too thorough; operation that may damage ectopic vessels should be avoided. Complications such as spinal cord injury and transient dysphagia were not observed in our study.

Conclusions

The current study has its limitation, for example the sample size was small, and prospective studies are needed to confirm the findings. In addition, patients with TDL without massive hemoptysis were not included because of treatment indications or ethical reasons. In summary, the findings of the current study suggested that regional arterial embolization before pleuropulmonary resection for TDL may reduce the risk of pleuropulmonary resection, shorten the operation time, and reduce postoperative complications. Further study is warranted to investigate if this treatment can be widely adopted in clinical settings for patients with TDL.

Authors' contributions
GC and FZ contributed to the conception and design of the study; XX and GYcontributed to the acquisition of data; PZ performed the experiments; XX contributed to the analysis of data; GC wrote the manuscript; all authors reviewed and approved the final version of the manuscript.

Competing interests
The authors declare that they have no competing interests.

References

1. Rhee CK, Yoo KH, Lee JH, Park MJ, Kim WJ, Park YB, et al. Clinical characteristics of patients with tuberculosis-destroyed lung. Int J Tuberc Lung Dis. 2013;17:67–75.
2. Patel R, Singh A, Mathur RM, Sisodiya A. Emergency pneumonectomy: a life-saving measure for severe recurrent hemoptysis in tuberculosis cavitary lesion. Case Rep Pulmonol. 2015;2015:897896.
3. Cai BY, Chu NH, Kang WL. An analysis on drug-resistance status and clinical characteristics in 115 tuberculosis cases with collapsed lung. Chin J Antituberculosis. 2012;34:380–3.
4. Kim SW, Lee SJ, Ryu YJ, Lee JH, Chang JH, Shim SS, et al. Prognosis and predictors of rebleeding after bronchial artery embolization in patients with active or inactive pulmonary tuberculosis. Lung. 2015;193:575–81.
5. Issoufou I, Sani R, Belliraj L, Ammor FZ, Moussa Ounteini A, Ghalimi J, et al. Pneumonectomy for tuberculosis destroyed lung: A series of 26 operated cases. Revue De Pneumologie Clinique. 2016;72:288–92.
6. Subotic D, Yablonskiy P, Sulis G, Cordos I, Petrov D, Centis R, et al. Surgery and pleuro-pulmonary tuberculosis: a scientific literature review. J Thorac Dis. 2016;8:E474–85.
7. Huang CL, Zhang W, Ni ZY, Zuo T, Zhou M, Xu J, et al. Efficacy of video-assisted thoracoscopic surgery for 29 patients with tuberculosis-destroyed lung. Int J Clin Exp Med. 2015;8:18391–8.
8. Duan L, Jiang GN, Xu XX. Total pneumonectomy in 84 cases of unilateral non tuberculous lesion of the lung. Chin J Thorac Cardiovasc Surg. 2012;28:688–9.
9. Bai L, Hong Z, Gong C, Yan D, Liang Z. Surgical treatment efficacy in 172 cases of tuberculosis-destroyed lungs. Eur J Cardiothorac Surg. 2012;41:335–40.
10. Jiang S, Zhu XH, Sun XW. Nonbronchial systemic arteries: incidence and endovascular interventional management for hemoptysis. Chin J Radiol. 2009;43:629–33.
11. Lin Y, Chen Z, Yang X, Zhong Q, Zhang H, Yang L, et al. Bronchial and non-bronchial systemic arteries: value of multidetector ct angiography in diagnosis and angiographic embolisation feasibility analysis. J Med Imaging Radiat Oncol. 2013;57:644–51.
12. Cheng Z, Shang J, Tang J, Sun Z, Chen J, Zhang L, et al. Evaluations of bronchial and nonbronchial systemic arteries in patients with hemoptysis at dual-source computed tomograph: comparison with conventional angiography. Zhonghua Yi Xue Za Zhi. 2014;94:3370–3.

25

Self-reported walking and associated factors in the Spanish population with chronic obstructive pulmonary disease

Pedro Barbolla Benito[1][*] [iD] and Germán Peces-Barba Romero[2]

Abstract

Background: The level of physical activity among individuals with chronic obstructive pulmonary disease (COPD) is associated with the disease severity and prognosis. The aim of this study was to describe the prevalence of self-reported walking at least 150 min per week and the associated factors among the Spanish population with COPD.

Methods: Analyses were based on data drawn from the 2009 European Health Interview Survey in Spain (2009 EHIS). Twenty-two thousand one hundred eighty-eight subjects participated in the survey (response rate of 96.5%). Participants were classified according to international physical activity recommendations. The prevalence of walking among participants with and without COPD (≥40 years old) was described. Univariate and multivariate logistic regression models were used to study the association of walking with socio-demographic and health outcome variables.

Results: Of the participants with COPD, 55.0% reached the minimum walking recommendations compared to 59.9% of the general population. The level of walking physical activity of the participants with COPD differed according to sex, age, educational level, area of residence, living as a couple, self-rated health status, mental health, body mass index and hospital admissions. In the multivariate analysis, being male, < 65 years old, living in an area with ≥50,000 inhabitants, no diagnosed depression or anxiety and self-reported good to very good health were factors significantly associated with walking ≥150 min per week.

Conclusions: Sex, age, area of residence, mental disorders and self-rated health are associated with weekly walking time in the Spanish population with COPD.

Keywords: Chronic obstructive pulmonary disease, Physical activity, Epidemiology, Spain

Background

Chronic obstructive pulmonary disease (COPD) is a common, preventable and treatable disease characterised by persistent respiratory symptoms and limited airflow, generally associated with exposure to harmful agents such as tobacco. The most frequent symptoms are cough, dyspnea and sputum production [1]. The prevalence of this disease in Spain is about 10% of adults aged over 40 years old, being almost three-times higher in men [2]. There are also important geographical variations in the distribution of the COPD population, as well as the diagnosis and treatment [3].

Physical inactivity is one of the main risk factors for global mortality, and is associated with the development of multiple health problems and chronic diseases [4]. The American College of Sports Medicine (ACSM) recommends physical activity equivalent to at least 150 min of moderate activity a week for healthy adults as well as for people suffering from a chronic disease [5]. However, it is documented that people with COPD usually undertake insufficient levels of physical activity [6]. As physical activity is related to relevant disease determinants including severity and prognosis, low activity levels could have an important impact in these patients [7, 8]. In addition, health outcomes such as quality of life and mental health are also associated with the level of physical activity performed by this population [9–11].

* Correspondence: jbsot.pedro@gmail.com
[1]Autonomous University of Madrid, Ciudad Universitaria de Cantoblanco, Madrid 28049, Spain
Full list of author information is available at the end of the article

Walking is the most common physical activity modality performed by the general population. Moreover, it is a low-risk and accessible activity, and is associated with multiple systemic and emotional benefits [12]. According to the ACSM, walking is classified as a moderate intensity activity and is suitable to achieve the minimum physical activity recommendations [5].

Recent Spanish research has described the prevalence of different levels of walking physical activity among populations with COPD. The authors have also observed that lower self-reported walking times are related to worse markers of disease severity in COPD, such as BODE index, dyspnea score, CAT score, Global Initiative for Chronic Obstructive Lung Disease (GOLD) classification or COPD exacerbations. [13]. However, to the best of our knowledge, no studies have focused on the association of walking recommendations with socio-demographic and health determinants in a representative sample of the Spanish population with COPD. The objective of this study was twofold: [1] to describe the prevalence of weekly walking recommendations in people with and without COPD in Spain; and [2] to study the association between walking recommendations with socio-demographic variables, self-rated health status and mental health in a representative sample of the Spanish population with COPD.

Methods

This descriptive study was based on data drawn from the 2009 European Health Interview Survey (EHIS) of the Spanish population. The survey was carried out by the National Institute of Statistics (NIE). The 2009 EHIS was a face-to-face interview survey, conducted between April 2009 and March 2010.

The study was carried out in all Spanish provinces. The survey used a three-stage sampling approach with stratification of the first-stage units, which represented the census section. The second-stage units involved the main family dwellings. Finally, an adult aged 16 years or older was selected to be interviewed within each household. Finally 22,188 subjects participated in the survey. The final response rate was 96.5% of the theoretical sample (n = 23,004) to be representative of the Spanish population. Other details of the survey can be found on the website of the NIE [14]. As this research was carried out using a publicly available and anonymised database, it was not necessary to obtain ethical approval to carry out the study.

Socio-demographic characteristics, body mass index and hospital admissions

The socio-demographic characteristics assessed were sex, age (40–64 years or ≥ 65 years), educational level (no studies completed, primary studies completed or secondary studies completed or over), living as a couple (yes or no)

and the number of inhabitants in their area of residence (< 50,000 or ≥ 50,000 inhabitants). The body mass index (BMI) was calculated from the self-reported height and weight. Those participants with a BMI ≥30 $kg.m^{-2}$ were considered "obese". Participants were classified according to their smoking status as either "smokers" or "non-smokers". Hospital admissions were assessed based on the question "have you been admitted at least 1 night in the last 12 months", to which participants answered "no" or "yes".

Walking physical activity

The level of physical activity was obtained from the total time spent undertaking walking activity per week. The EHIS used the International Physical Activity Questionnaire-Short Form (IPAQ-SF), which aims to measure the total physical activity (work-related, transport-related and health-enhancing physical activity). The participants answered the questions: "during the last 7 days, on how many days did you walk for at least 10 minutes at a time?"; and "How much time did you usually spend walking on one of those". The subjects were classified according to the minimum physical activity recommendations as either < 150 min per week or ≥ 150 min per week. The participants were also classified in relation to their level of physical activity as either low (< 150 min per week), moderate (≥150 to 299 min per week) or high (≥300 min per week). In both cases, the participants were classified according to the physical activity guidelines [5].

Chronic obstructive pulmonary disease and comorbidities

The respondent was considered to have COPD when he or she answered affirmatively to the question "has a doctor told you that you suffer from chronic bronchitis, emphysema or COPD". The chronic comorbidities included in the study were asthma, coronary heart disease, myocardial infarction, arthritis, cancer, diabetes, stroke and liver dysfunction. The participants were classified as having "none", "one" or "two or more" of these comorbidities.

Self-rated health and mental health

Self-rated health (SRH) was assessed based on the question "how would you describe your health status in general". The five possible answers, scored on a scale ranging from 1 "very good" to 5 "very bad", were grouped into three categories: good to very good, regular, and bad to very bad. The presence of mental disorders was assessed based on the questions "has a doctor told you that you suffer from chronic depression" and "has a doctor told you that you suffer from suffer from chronic anxiety". Those who answered affirmatively to one or both of these questions were considered to suffer from a mental illness.

Table 1 Subjects characteristics with and without COPD in the 2009 EHIS

Variable	COPD (N/%)	No COPD (N/%)	p
Sex			
Males	530 (51%)	5709 (47%)	0.012
Females	508 (49%)	6443 (53%)	
Age group			
40–64	467 (45%)	8366 (68.8%)	< 0.001
≥ 65	571 (55%)	3785 (31.2%)	
Living as a couple			
Yes	707 (68.2%)	8933 (73.6%)	< 0.001
Educational level			
No studies	90 (8.7%)	392 (3.2%)	< 0.001
Primary studies	326 (31.5%)	2086 (17.2%)	
Secondary studies	619 (59.8%)	9657 (79.6%)	
Area of residence			
< 50.000	512 (49.3%)	5725 (47.1%)	0.171
≥ 50.000	526 (50.7%)	6426 (52.9%)	
Smoking status			
Yes	227 (24.1%)	2954 (25.6%)	0.313
BMI (cat.)			
< 30 kg.m^{-2}	658 (70.8%)	9153 (80.7%)	< 0.001
≥ 30 kg.m^{-2}	271 (29.2%)	2190 (19.3%)	
Comorbidities			
None	265 (25.6%)	7909 (65.3%)	< 0.001
1	379 (36.7%)	2985 (24.6%)	
≥ 2	391 (37.8%)	1226 (10.1%)	
Self-rated health			
Very good/good	315 (30.4%)	7929 (65.2%)	< 0.001
Fair	401 (38.6%)	3016 (24.8%)	
Bad/Very bad	322 (31.0%)	1206 (9.9%)	
Mental illness			
Yes	278 (27.0%)	1555 (12.8%)	< 0.001
Hospital admission			
Yes	234 (22.6%)	1122 (9.2%)	< 0.001
OVERALL	1038 (7.9%)	12,151 (92.1%)	

Chi-square test statistical significance (p-value < 0.05)

Statistical analysis

All data were weighted according to the EHIS sample design. The sample characteristics of participants with and without COPD were described as the weighted sample size and percentage (%). The same was done for participants with COPD according to the minimum recommendations for physical activity. The prevalence of individuals who met physical activity recommendations between the COPD and non-COPD groups was compared using the chi-square test and logistic regression tests,

adjusted for sex and age group. The level of physical activity in the COPD group was described for all variables. Weighted bivariable and multivariable logistic regression models were used to estimate the association between the minimum walking recommendations (≥150 min per week) and the rest of the variables in participants with COPD. Firstly, bivariable logistic regression models were used to study the role of each variable. Secondly, a multivariable regression model was performed with all the variables whose role was identified to be statistically significant in the bivariable models. All statistical analyses were performed using the IBM SPSS statistical package (version 20; IBM Corp. Armonk, NY). A p-value of < 0.05 was considered statistically significant.

Results

The total number of subjects aged 40 years and older included in the study was 13,199 (6956 females and 6243 males). The prevalence of self-reported COPD was 7.9% (95% CI [7.4, 8.3]). The prevalence of COPD among participants aged 40–64 years was 5.3% (95% CI [4.8, 5.8]) and 13.1% (95% CI [12.1, 14.1]) in those older than 65 years ($p < 0.001$).

Table 1 shows the distribution of participants with and without COPD according to their socio-demographic characteristics and health determinants. Participants with COPD had a significantly lower level of education, higher prevalence of comorbidities, obesity and mental illness, and worse SRH. There were also significant differences in sex, age, living as a couple, and hospital admissions.

Table 2 shows the proportion of participants with and without COPD that undertook walking according to the physical activity recommendations. The prevalence of individuals who met walking recommendations (≥150 min per week) in the COPD group was 55% (95% CI [51.9, 58.1]) compared to 59.9% (95% CI [59.0, 60.8]) in the group without COPD ($p = 0.002$ for the chi-square test and $p = 0.011$ for the adjusted logistic regression). The

Table 2 Prevalence of adherence to walking recommendations (≥ 150 min per week) in COPD and non-COPD

Variables	COPD	No COPD	p
	% (95% C.I.)	% (95% C.I.)	
Sex			
Males	60.3 (56.1–64.6)	63.3 (62.1–64.6)	0.058[a]
Females	49.4 (45.0–53.9)	56.9 (55.6–58.1)*	0.030[a]
Age group			
40–64	62.5 (58.0–67.0)	61.4 (60.3–62.4)	0.623[b]
≥ 65	49.0 (44.8–53.1)	56.7 (55.1–58.3)*	< 0.001[b]
OVERALL	55.0 (51.9–58.1)	59.9 (59.0–60.8)*	0.011[c]

95% CI 95% Confidence Interval; *Statistical significance (p-value < 0.05) for chi-square test; [a]p for the logistic regression adjusted by age group; [b]p for the logistic regression adjusted by sex; [c]p for the logistic regression adjusted by age group and sex

percentage of people with COPD who declared that they did not walk for at least 10 min in a row on any day of the week was 31.2% compared to 23.1% of the general population (Fig. 1).

Table 3 shows the prevalence of self-reported walking (< 150 min per week or ≥ 150 min per week) in participants with COPD according to socio-demographic characteristics and health determinants. Figure 2 shows the level of physical activity (low, moderate and high level of walking activity) in participants with COPD according to the study variables. Those COPD participants aged 65 years and older, those with a lower educational level, those who did not live as a couple and those who lived in areas with < 50,000 inhabitants seem to be less active. In addition, a higher prevalence of low walking levels was observed among those suffering from another physical or mental disease, obese participants and those with worse SRH. People who had to be hospitalised at least once over the last 12 months for any reason also tended to be less active.

Table 4 shows the association between walking and socio-demographic variables and health determinants in participants with COPD, analysed using bivariable and multivariable logistic regression models. In the bivariable analysis, walking ≥150 min per week was significantly associated with all study variables except for smoking status. In the multivariable analysis, sex, age, place of residence, mental illness and SRH were independently and significantly associated with minimum physical activity recommendations.

Discussion

In this study, being ≥65 years old was associated with less walking in people with COPD. The level of walking physical activity is associated with socio-demographic characteristics and the health status of people with COPD. In addition, the factors independently associated with reaching the minimum recommendations of physical activity (≥150 min walking per week) were sex, age, place of residence, better SRH and a lower prevalence of mental illnesses such as depression or anxiety.

In the present study, the differences observed in the level of physical activity among participants with and without COPD were rather low when compared to previous studies [15]. Two possible explanations are: firstly, participants of our study were drawn from a general representative sample of the Spanish adult population, therefore, they were not necessarily healthy, and secondly, we have only studied walking and we have not included other modalities of physical activity. Our results show that 55% of participants with COPD reported walking ≥150 min per week. This percentage is similar to that reported in previous studies in which 52% of patients with COPD met walking physical activity recommendations. [16], although somewhat higher than that obtained by Pitta et al. who observed that only 30% of patients with COPD reach ACSM walking recommendations [6]. However, two recent multicentre studies conducted in different Spanish populations with COPD have reported that the prevalence of low level of PA, defined as a walking time of > 30 min/day, was observed in a relatively low number of participants (86 and 85%, respectively) [11, 13]. These differences may be due to characteristics of the participants with COPD, the lack of physician confirmed diagnosis of COPD in our study and the location of the sample.

In our study population, the socio-demographic factors that were independently associated with physical activity recommendations were sex, age and the number of inhabitants in their area of residence. The association between the level of physical activity with age and sex is consistent with the literature. Younger adult population, particularly males, were more likely to achieve higher levels of physical activity [17]. However, in the INSEPOC study in Spain, no significant differences were observed in the total daily walking time between men and women with COPD [18]. Sex differences in self-reporting walking in our study should be interpreted carefully since the prevalence of COPD in female in the EHIS is usually higher than the prevalence reported by national and multi-centre epidemiological studies [2, 13, 15, 18].

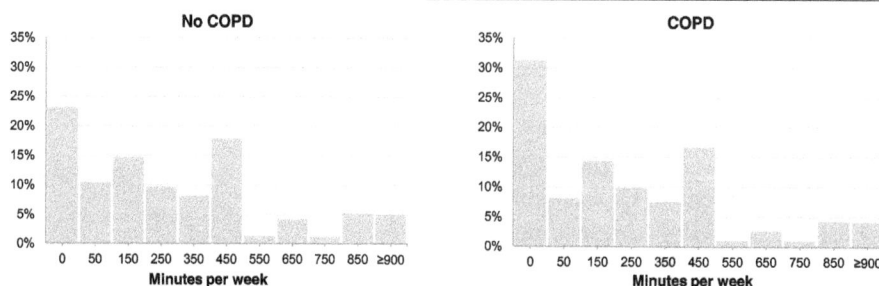

Fig. 1 Distribution (%) of the participants with and without COPD according to the total walking time (minutes per week). Abbreviations: COPD, Chronic Obstructive Pulmonary Disease

Table 3 Prevalence of self-reported walking (< 150 min per week or ≥ 150 min per week) in participants with COPD according to socio-demographic characteristics and health determinants

Variables	< 150 min/week (N/%)	≥150 min/week (N/%)	p
Sex			
Males	202 (44.8%)	308 (55.9%)	0.001
Females	249 (55.2%)	244 (44.1%)	
Age group			
40–64	167 (37.0%)	279 (50.6%)	< 0.001
≥ 65	284 (63.0%)	273 (49.4%)	
Living as a couple			
Yes	282 (62.4%)	401 (72.7%)	< 0.001
Educational level			
No studies	57 (12.7%)	32 (5.8%)	< 0.001
Primary studies	162 (35.9%)	161 (29.2%)	
Secondary studies	232 (51.5%)	358 (65.0%)	
Area of residence			
< 50.000	250 (55.4%)	252 (45.7%)	0.002
≥ 50.000	202 (44.6%)	300 (54.3%)	
Smoking status			
Yes	90 (23.2%)	128 (24.5%)	0.655
Comorbidities			
None	87 (19.3%)	169 (30.7%)	< 0.001
1	159 (35.2%)	203 (36.6%)	
≥ 2	205 (45.5%)	178 (32.3%)	
BMI (cat.)			
< 30 kg.m^{-2}	251 (65.6%)	439 (74.9%)	0.002
≥ 30 kg.m^{-2}	132 (34.4%)	112 (25.1%)	
Mental illness			
Yes	156 (35.1%)	130 (20.3%)	< 0.001
Self-rated health			
Very good/good	96 (43.7%)	209 (37.9%)	< 0.001
Fair	159 (35.1%)	225 (40.8%)	
Bad/Very bad	197 (43.7%)	117 (21.2%)	
Hospital admission			
Yes	127 (28.1%)	102 (18.4%)	< 0.001

Chi-square test statistical significance (p-value < 0.05)

Previous studies have shown that both younger and adult populations living in larger cities tend to be more physically active [19, 20]. Moreover, people living in smaller towns declare more environmental barriers, such us the lack of sidewalks, street lights, and difficulty in accessing facilities [19], which has been shown to play an important role in the level of physical activity of the population [21]. One study carried out in the city of Barcelona observed that two-thirds of daily walking trips exceeded 10 min [22]. These findings could help explain the results observed in the present study. Nevertheless, we were unable to find enough relevant studies in the literature to compare to our results. Our findings and the lack of information in the current literature highlight the need for future studies focusing on the role of environmental, geographic and social barriers in the level of physical activity in people with COPD.

Regular walking for at least 10 min every day in the COPD population could be a critical factor associated with mental and cognitive health status [23]. A recent study in Spain observed a clear relationship between walking less than 30 min a day and depression and a poorer quality of life in a group of patients with COPD. These researchers considered both quality of life and depression, which are both potential independent predictors of the level of physical activity of people suffering from this disease [11]. In the present study, participants who reached the minimum weekly recommendations for walking physical activity declared a better self-rated health status and lower prevalence of depression and anxiety. It has also been observed that the longer a person with COPD walks per day the lower the probability of suffering from depression [24]. However, it should be noted that our study did not take into account several relevant clinical determinants such as the BODE index, which has been shown to be closely related to depression in people with COPD [25].

We also observed that people who were admitted to hospital at least once during the past year for any reason tended to be less active. In addition, the bivariable analysis showed that hospital admission is inversely associated with self-reported walking recommendations. However, in the multivariable analysis this association was not statistically significant. Even so, previous epidemiological studies have shown a clear association between any type of regular physical activity and a lower risk of hospital admission due to exacerbated illness in this group of patients [8, 26].

Limitations and strengths

Our results need to be interpreted within the context of the study's limitations. The main limitation of the present study is related to its cross-sectional design, which prevented us from establishing any causal relationship. Another limitation is related to the way the information was obtained. The socio-demographic characteristics and factors associated with COPD were self-reported and, therefore, subject to bias and erroneous classification. However, this is compensated for by the high number of participants that are included in this type of health survey, which are periodically carried out. Moreover, the diagnosis of COPD was based on unvalidated self-reports, without having taken into account the results of a pulmonary function test, which may

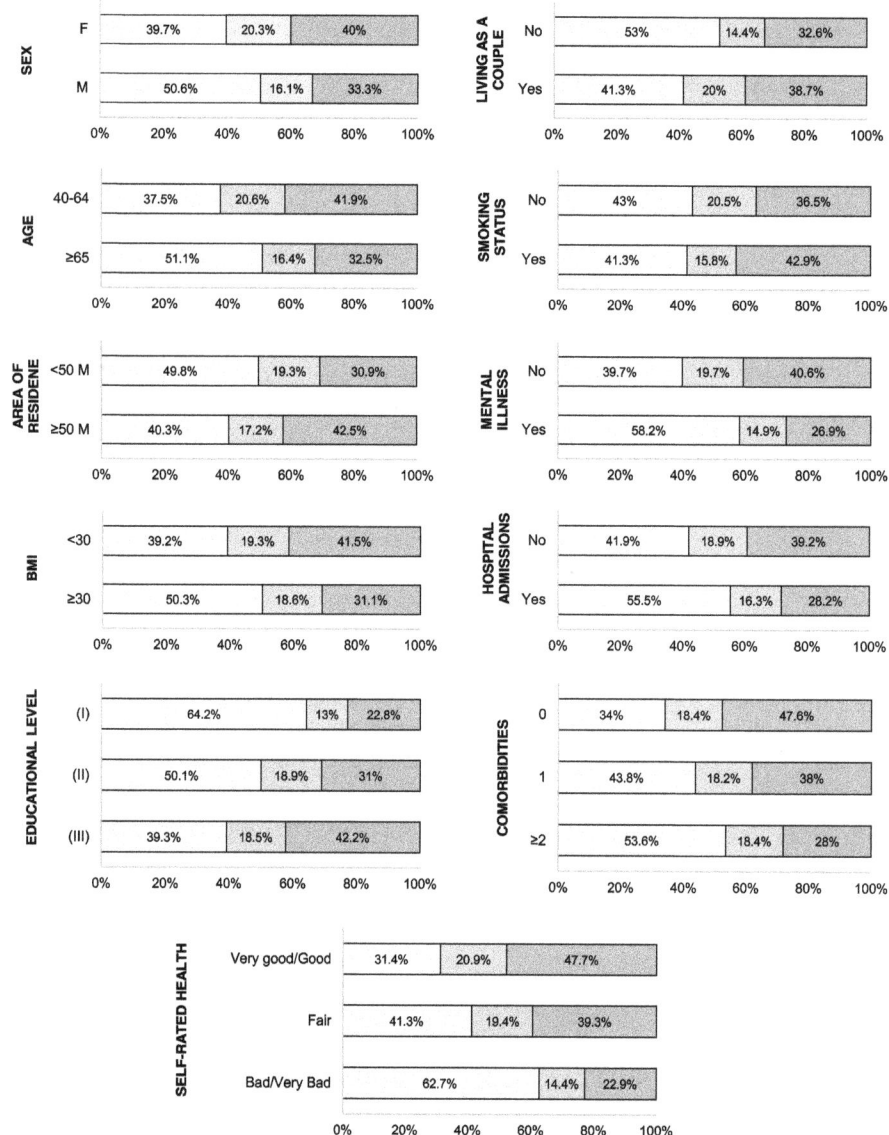

Fig. 2 Percentage of people with COPD who report walking < 150 min per week (■), 150 to 299 min per week (■), ≥300 min per week (■) according to the sociodemographic variables, health status and metal health. Abbreviations: M, male; F, female; A. Residence: area of residence, M: thousand; (I), no studies; (II), primary studies completed; (III), secondary studies completed or over; BMI, Body Mass Index, < 30 kg.m^{-2} and ≥ 30 kg.m^{-2}

represent a bias related to the true prevalence of COPD within the population. Relevant clinical determinants of the disease, such as the BODE index, exacerbations, dyspnea or GOLD classification, which have been shown to be associated with the level of physical activity, could not be obtained from the 2009 EHIS [13]. However, this format has been previously used by other authors to study several aspects related to this disease in Spain, and reasonable reliability has been previously observed [27, 28].

Finally, the survey used the International Physical Activity Questionnaire-Short Form (IPAQ-SF) to assess physical activity, which could incorrectly estimate the real level of physical activity [29]. Moreover, some authors have demonstrated that the intensity of walking in in patients with moderate-to-very severe COPD does not reach the level of moderate physical activity [30]. It is well known that physical activity assessed from self-reported data is not as accurate as other objective assessment tools such as pedometers or accelerometers [31]. In addition, this questionnaire assessed physical activity as both walking for transportation and for leisure. Physical activity as leisure time has a positive association with perceived quality of life, while walking for transportation is inversely associated with quality of life [32]. Nevertheless, its validity and reliability are acceptable for

Table 4 Bivariable and multivariable logistic regression analysis for socio-demographic characteristics and health determinants in participants with COPD according to the walking recommendations (≥ 150 min per week)

Variables	≥ 150 min per week			
	Unajusted OR[a] 95% CI	p	Ajusted OR[b] 95% CI	p
Sex				
Females	1		1	
Males	1.56 (1.21–2.00)	< 0.05	1.49 (1.10–2.01)	< 0.05
Age group				
40–64	1		1	
≥ 65	0.58 (0.45–0.74)	< 0.05	0.69 (0.50–0.95)	< 0.05
Living as couple				
No	1		1	
Yes	1.61 (1.23–2.10)	< 0.05	1.18 (0.85–1.61)	NS
Educational level				
No studies	1		1	
Primary studies	1.78 (1.10–2.89)	< 0.05	1.79 (0.98–3.25)	NS
Secondary studies	2.77 (1.74–4.40)	< 0.05	1.72 (0.95–3.11)	NS
Area of residence				
< 50.000	1		1	
≥ 50.000	1.47 (1.15–1.89)	< 0.05	1.42 (1.07–1.88)	< 0.05
Smoking status				
No	1		–	–
Yes	1.07 (0.79–1.46)	NS	–	–
BMI (cat.)				
< 30 kg.m^{-2}	1		1	
≥ 30 kg.m^{-2}	0.64 (0.48–0.85)	< 0.05	0.75 (0.55–1.03)	NS
Comorbidities				
None	1		1	
1	0.66 (0.47–0.92)	< 0.05	0.89 (0.61–1.29)	NS
≥ 2	0.45 (0.32–0.62)	< 0.05	1.02 (0.67–1.54)	NS
Mental illness				
No	1		1	
Yes	0.47 (0.36–0.63)	< 0.05	0.68 (0.48–0.96)	< 0.05
Self-rated health				
Very good/good	1		1	
Fair	0.65 (0.47–0.89)	< 0.05	1.01 (0.70–1.47)	NS
Bad/Very bad	0.27 (0.20–0.38)	< 0.05	0.49 (0.32–0.75)	< 0.05
Hospital admission				
No	1		1	
Yes	0.58 (0.43–0.78)	< 0.05	0.76 (0.54–1.07)	NS

OR Odds Ratio, *95% CI* Confidence Interval, *NS* No Significant; [a]unadjusted OR: bivariable analysis; [b]adjusted OR: multivariable model adjusted for all variables with a statistically significant role in the univariate analysis; Statistical significance (*p*-value < 0.05)

studies with very large samples because objective measurements are not easy to take in representative surveys at a national level due to the high economic cost [33].

The strengths of this study include the sample size and country representativeness, meaning that the results can be generalised for the entire adult Spanish population with the same characteristics.

Conclusions

To sum up, this study provides additional evidence that people with COPD undertake less self-reported walking activity than the general population in Spain, mainly in older participants. In addition, socio-demographic and health outcomes such as sex, age, area of residence, mental illness and self-rated health status are associated with self-reported weekly walking time recommendations in COPD participants.

Future large, prospective, population-wide studies are required to further explore the temporality of the associations observed between walking and socio-demographic and health outcomes in this investigation.

Acknowledgements
Not applicable.

Funding
None.

Authors' contributions
PBB and GPBR conceived the research question and designed the study. PBB performed the statistical analyses. PBB and GPBR interpreted the results and wrote the first draft of the manuscript. Both authors reviewed and approved the final version of the manuscript.

Competing interests
The authors declare that they have no competing interests.

Author details
[1]Autonomous University of Madrid, Ciudad Universitaria de Cantoblanco, Madrid 28049, Spain. [2]Department of Pneumology IIS-Fundación Jiménez Díaz, Center for Biomedical Research in the Network, Respiratory Diseases (Spanish acronym CIBERES), Calle de Melchor Fernández Almagro, 3, Madrid 28029, Spain.

References
1. Vogelmeier CF, Criner GJ, Martinez FJ, Anzueto A, Barnes PJ, Bourbeau J, et al. Global strategy for the diagnosis, management and prevention of chronic obstructive lung disease 2017 report. Am J Respir Crit Care Med. 2017;195:557–82.
2. Miravitlles M, Soriano JB, Garcia-Rio F, Munoz L, Duran-Tauleria E, Sanchez G, et al. Prevalence of COPD in Spain: impact of undiagnosed COPD on quality of life and daily life activities. Thorax. 2009;64:863–8.
3. Soriano JB, Miravitlles M, Borderías L, Duran-Tauleria E, Río FG, Martínez J, et al. Geographical variations in the prevalence of COPD in Spain: relationship to smoking, death rates and other determining factors. Arch Bronconeumol. 2010;46:522–30.

4. Warburton DE, Nicol CW, Bredin SS. Health benefits of physical activity: the evidence. CMAJ. 2006;174:801–9.

5. Haskell WL, Lee I, Pate RR, Powell KE, Blair SN, Franklin BA, et al. Physical activity and public health: updated recommendation for adults from the American College of Sports Medicine and the American Heart Association. Circulation. 2007;116:1081–93.

6. Pitta F, Troosters T, Spruit MA, Probst VS, Decramer M, Gosselink R. Characteristics of physical activities in daily life in chronic obstructive pulmonary disease. Am J Respir Crit Care Med. 2005;171:972–7.

7. Waschki B, Kirsten A, Holz O, Müller K, Meyer T, Watz H, et al. Physical activity is the strongest predictor of all-cause mortality in patients with COPD: a prospective cohort study. Chest. 2011;140:331–42.

8. Vaes AW, Garcia-Aymerich J, Marott JL, Benet M, Groenen MT, Schnohr P, et al. Changes in physical activity and all-cause mortality in COPD. Eur Respir J. 2014;44:1199–209.

9. Bossenbroek L, de Greef MH, Wempe JB, Krijnen WP, ten Hacken NH. Daily physical activity in patients with chronic obstructive pulmonary disease: a systematic review. COPD. 2011;8:306–19.

10. Katz P, Chen H, Omachi TA, Gregorich SE, Julian L, Cisternas M, et al. The role of physical inactivity in increasing disability among older adults with obstructive airway disease. J Cardiopulm Rehabil Prev. 2011;31:193–7.

11. Miravitlles M, Cantoni J, Naberan K. Factors associated with a low level of physical activity in patients with chronic obstructive pulmonary disease. Lung. 2014;192:259–65.

12. Davison RR, Grant S. Is walking sufficient exercise for health? Sports Med. 1993;16:369–73.

13. Ramon MA, Esquinas C, Barrecheguren M, Pleguezuelos E, Molina J, Quintano JA, et al. Self-reported daily walking time in COPD: relationship with relevant clinical and functional characteristics. Int J COPD. 2017;12:1173–81.

14. Encuesta Europea de Salud en España 2009 [http://www.ine.es/dyngs/INEbase/es/categoria.htm?c=Estadistica_P&cid=1254735573175].

15. Vorrink SN, Kort HS, Troosters T, Lammers JJ. Level of daily physical activity in individuals with COPD compared with healthy controls. Respir Res. 2011;12:33.

16. Pitta F, Troosters T, Probst VS, Lucas S, Decramer M, Gosselink R. Possíveis conseqüências de não se atingir a mínima atividade física diária recomendada em pacientes com doença pulmonar obstrutiva cronica estável. J Bras Pneumol. 2006;32:301–8.

17. Bamana A, Tessier S, Vuillemin A. Association of perceived environment with meeting public health recommendations for physical activity in seven European countries. J Public Health. 2008;30:274–81.

18. Naberan K, Azpeitia Á, Cantoni J, Miravitlles M. Impairment of quality of life in women with chronic obstructive pulmonary disease. Respir Med. 2012;106:367–73.

19. Badland H, Schofield G. Understanding the relationship between town size and physical activity levels: a population study. Health Place. 2006;12:538–46.

20. Lasheras L, Aznar S, Merino B, López EG. Factors associated with physical activity among Spanish youth through the National Health Survey. Prev Med. 2001;32:455–64.

21. Giles-Corti B, Broomhall MH, Knuiman M, Collins C, Douglas K, Ng K, et al. Increasing walking: how important is distance to, attractiveness, and size of public open space? Am J Prev Med. 2005;28:169–76.

22. Marquet O, Miralles-Guasch C. The walkable city and the importance of the proximity environments for Barcelona's everyday mobility. Cities. 2015;42:258–66.

23. Shiue I. Daily walking >10 min could improve mental health in people with historical cardiovascular disease or COPD: Scottish health survey, 2012. Int J Cardiol. 2015;179:375–7.

24. Miravitlles M, Molina J, Quintano JA, Campuzano A, Pérez J, Roncero C, et al. Factors associated with depression and severe depression in patients with COPD. Respir Med. 2014;108:1615–25.

25. González-Gutiérrez MV, Velázquez JG, García CM, Maldonado FC, Jiménez FJG, Vargas FG. Predictive model for anxiety and depression in Spanish patients with stable chronic obstructive pulmonary disease. Arch Bronconeumol. 2016;52:151–7.

26. Garcia-Aymerich J, Lange P, Benet M, Schnohr P, Anto JM. Regular physical activity reduces hospital admission and mortality in chronic obstructive pulmonary disease: a population based cohort study. Thorax. 2006;61:772–8.

27. Rodríguez-Rodríguez P, Jiménez-García R, Hernández-Barrera V, Carrasco-Garrido P, Puente-Maestu L, de Miguel-Díez J. Prevalence of physical disability in patients with chronic obstructive pulmonary disease and associated risk factors. COPD. 2013;10:611–7.

28. De Miguel Díez J, García RJ, Barrera VH, Maestu LP, Del Cura González MI, Bailón MM, et al. Trends in self-rated health status and health services use in COPD patients (2006–2012). A Spanish population-based survey. Lung. 2015;193:53–62.

29. Lee PH, Macfarlane DJ, Lam T, Stewart SM. Validity of the international physical activity questionnaire short form (IPAQ-SF): a systematic review. Int J Behav Nutr Phys Act. 2011;8:115.

30. Vitorasso R, Camillo CA, Cavalheri V, Aparecida Hernandes N, Cortez Verceze A, Sant'Anna T, et al. Is walking in daily life a moderate intensity activity in patients with chronic obstructive pulmonary disease? Eur J Phys Rehabil Med. 2012;48:587–92.

31. Harris TJ, Owen CG, Victor CR, Adams R, Ekelund U, Cook DG. A comparison of questionnaire, accelerometer, and pedometer: measures in older people. Med Sci Sports Exerc. 2009;41:1392–402.

32. Jurakić D, Pedišić Ž, Greblo Z. Physical activity in different domains and health-related quality of life: a population-based study. Qual Life Res. 2010;19:1303–9.

33. Van der Ploeg HP, Tudor-Locke C, Marshall AL, Craig C, Hagströmer M, Sjöström M, et al. Reliability and validity of the international physical activity questionnaire for assessing walking. Res Q Exerc Sport. 2010;81:97–101.

26

EGFR mutation status in Tunisian non-small-cell lung cancer patients evaluated by mutation-specific immunohistochemistry

Zohra Mraihi[1*] (iD), Jihen Ben Amar[2], Hend Bouacha[2], Soumaya Rammeh[3] and Lamia Hila[1*]

Abstract

Background: Screening mutations in epidermal growth factor receptor (EGFR) to analyze non-small-cell lung cancer (NSCLC) profile is the criterion to choose the best therapeutic strategy.
New Oncology guidelines recommend EGFR mutation analysis before prescribing tyrosine kinase inhibitors (TKIs) treatment.
Majority of lung cancer patients are diagnosed at advanced stages and generally only small biopsies materials are available for diagnostic and molecular characterization. The aim of this first work is to screen EGFR mutation status in Tunisian NSCLC by mutation-specific immunohistochemistry (IHC) and molecular biology, to estimate the relevance of proposing TKIs as a new therapeutic line.

Methods: E746-A750 deletion and L858R mutations were screened in 50 unselected NSCLC formalin-fixed paraffin-embedded (FFPE) tissue samples. Mutation expression by IHC was evaluated by intensity and percentage of staining and correlated to patients' data. DNA was extracted and EGFR mutations were analyzed by Sanger sequencing. Positive and negative controls were included for EGFR mutations in order to support the results.

Results: Among our patients (48 men and 2 women) all adenocarcinoma (confirmed by histology and IHC with TTF1/Napsin A), 94% were smokers exceeding the tobacco risk threshold (at least 25 pack-years) and the women were none. 44% had EGFR mutation by IHC: 26% had simple mutation and 18% had concurrent mutation. All mutated cases were smokers except a woman who was none. Concurrent mutations patients exceeded 40 pack-years. 91.4% of IHC results were validated by molecular analysis (100% of negative and 85% of positive cases) showing either T > G (exon 21) or 2235–2249 del (exon 19).

Conclusions: These preliminary results confirm the usefulness of IHC to detect EGFR mutations but the frequency of concurrent mutations doesn't appear in favor of EGFR TKIs treatment. In fact, literature reports a significantly worse response compared to those with single mutation when treated by TKIs.

Keywords: EGFR, Non-small-cell lung cancer, Mutation-specific immunohistochemistry, Targeted therapy

Background

Lung cancer is a major cause of cancer-related mortality worldwide and is expected to remain a major health problem with increasing cases [1]. It is the leading reason of cancer death among men and the second in women, after breast cancer in the world [2]. In Tunisia, the lung is the main cancerous localization for male and

an increasing incidence is observed with significant loss of life years in men (nearly a third of years of life lost) [3]. In 2015, World Health Organization (WHO) proposed new criteria for diagnosis and subclassification of lung cancer. These new guidelines were developed because two thirds of lung cancer diagnosis, presenting in advanced stages, are often established on small biopsy and cytology specimens [4–7].

This classification is not very different from historical one, since it also divides lung cancer in two groups: small and non-small-cell lung cancer (SCLC and

---

* Correspondence: zohra_mraihi@yahoo.fr; lamia_hila@yahoo.fr
[1]Genetic Department, Faculté de Médecine de Tunis, Université de Tunis El Manar, Tunis, Tunisia
Full list of author information is available at the end of the article

NSCLC). The latter including: adenocarcinoma (ADC), squamous cell carcinoma (SCC), large cell carcinomas (LC), sarcomatoid carcinomas and mixed. Up to 85% of reported lung cancers are NSCLC. ADC accounts for more than 50% of these cases [8, 9].

One advance in cancer treatment is personalized medicine, where therapeutic is based on histology and genetic characteristics of each tumor. Last years, molecular mechanisms involved in lung cancer became better known and current treatments are now oriented toward efficient molecular-targeted therapies to improve pejorative prognosis [7, 10, 11].

Detection of driver mutations in NSCLC transformed thoracic oncology introducing oral small molecule tyrosine kinase inhibitors (TKIs) targeting specific EGFR mutations. EGFR mutations lead to strongest response to TKIs such as gefitinib [12, 13] and erlotinib [14]. Thus, evaluation of EGFR mutation status is important before undertaking therapy decision in advanced NSCLC. Hence, the importance, for pathologists to classify NSCLC into specific subtypes for determining eligibility to molecular testing and therapeutic strategies [9, 11, 15].

In Tunisia, in daily practice, we investigate only EGFR expression by classic IHC (total EGFR antibody). In the present study, we aimed to evaluate, for the first time in Tunisia, the use of EGFR mutation-specific antibodies for immunohistochemical (IHC) screening in NSCLC patients by comparing it with molecular analysis. IHC allows simultaneous analysis of level proteins expression and molecular characterization of tumor for specific molecular alterations and isn't dependent on percentage of tumor cells in the sample unlike molecular tests, high costing and missing sensitivity as DNA is mainly obtained from FFPE tissues known to give poor quality DNA for sequencing [15, 16]. This study will evaluate IHC as a recourse analysis when molecular analysis is not possible and especially for small biopsies.

Methods

Study design

This retrospective study, which obtained ethical agreement, initially enrolled 50 unselected patients, 2 women and 48 men, from January 2010 to December 2014. Patients' selection was based on the clinical diagnosis of NSCLC and clinical informations were obtained for each patient from the medical record database of Pneumology Department of EPS Charles Nicolle at Tunis. The study was done blindly without knowing histologic analysis results.

FFPE biopsies were collected from the tissue bank of Pathological Anatomy and Cytology Department. All cases were confirmed as NSCLC, by an experienced pathologist, based on hematoxylin and eosin (HE) staining according to the WHO criteria [7].

Lung biopsies collected were small but FFPE tissue sections analyzed by IHC presented at least 20% of tumor cells. The two most frequent mutations, E746-A750 del and L858R substitution respectively in exon 19 and 21 were screened.

Immunohistochemical analysis

Histological classification and immunohistochemical staining were realized, for the 50 cases, upon 3 μm FFPE sections HE stained after deparaffinization with xylene and rehydration through a graded series of ethanol concentrations.

For each patient, two slides were labeled, with antibody and protocol-specific bar codes, and loaded into a Benchmark GX (Ventana Medical Systems Inc) automated stainer. Slides were treated with Standard Cell Conditioning 1 (Ventana Medical Systems Inc) for 60 min. We used E746-A750 del (SP111) Rabbit Monoclonal Primary Antibody (ref 790–4650) and L858R (SP125) Rabbit Monoclonal Primary Antibody (ref 790–4649) from Ventana Medical Systems Inc.

Immunoreactivity was revealed with ultraView Universal DAB detection kit (Ventana Medical Systems Inc). The slides were counterstained with hematoxylin and bluing reagent for 4 min each. Positive and negative controls were run simultaneously. Negative control staining was performed by omitting the primary antibody and positive using lung adenocarcinoma known to express EGFR mutations.

Each slide was examined and scored, based on intensity and percentage of staining, independently by two pathologists based which were blinded to patients'clinicopathological and molecular data. In case of discordance, final result was done after approval of both.

Scoring methodology

Immunoreactivity or IHC staining was scored according to the H-score (Histo-score) criteria, which assess the percentage (P) of positive cells (0–100%) multiplied by staining intensity (I) (0, no staining; 1, soft; 2, moderate; 3, strong; 4, very dark).

Final score varying from 0 to 400, [H = 1 x (% cells 1+) + 2 x (% cells 2+) + 3 x (% cells 3+) + 4 x (% cells 4+)] was calculated for each patient by two readers using the score with the maximum value [17].

Molecular analysis

In order to confirm the molecular status of the analyzed cases by IHC, we perform molecular analysis, for both positive and negative cases, by Sanger sequencing to detect EGFR mutations. 15 cases were excluded from the molecular analysis, since there were no available residual FFPE tumor tissue samples. Indeed our work was retrospective and ethically we don't have the right to exhaust the biopsies of patients.

Samples of DNA with known molecular status were analyzed in this study as controls: normal and EGFR mutation-positive presenting deletion in exon 19 and L858R point mutation in exon 21 (wild-type and mutated DNA cell lines: NCI-A549, NCI-H-1650 and NCI-H-1975, from Procell). DNA samples from 10 EGFR mutation-negative tumor lung tissue specimens, also negative by IHC, were enrolled in order to support our conclusions. DNA extraction was done using QIAamp DNA FFPE Tissue kit was used (Qiagen) according to the manufacturer's protocol. The PCR was performed for the 2 exons 19 and 21 with specific primers [11, 17].

25 µL PCR reaction mixtures contain 100 ng DNA and 1.25 units Taq Polymerase. Amplification was done as follows: 33 cycles at 95 °C for 30s, 65 °C for 30s and 72 °C for 45 s followed by 7 min extension at 72 °C. EGFR gene was amplified by polymerase chain reaction using specific primers and DNA sequencing was performed using the ABI 3710 Genetic Analyzer (Applied Biosystems).

Results

Patients' characteristics

Our cases included 48 men and 2 women, with a median age of 59.9 years (range 41–81 years). 3 never smokers and 47 former/current smokers. Histological analysis (TTF1 + Napsin A) revealed only ADC cases. Percentage of tumor cells was variable, but all had at least 20% and 74% of whom more than 30%.

Stage at the time of diagnosis was determined according to the tumor, node and metastasis (TNM) staging system: 37 patients were classified at stage IV, while 13 at IIIa or IIIb. Characteristics of patients are shown in Table 1. Metastases were present in 34.2% of the cases (bone, cerebral, hepatic ...). Most patients were treated with chemotherapy or surgery. No one benefited from targeted therapy. At the time of writing, 10 patients died (20%).

Survival estimation could only be achieved at 24 months, with a follow-up time from 1 to 24 months because of long time of medical care patients left to private sector. Overall survival was 6 months. Better survival was observed in patients aged less than 60 years.

EGFR mutation-specific antibody IHC staining

Expression of E746-A750 del and L858R was evaluated in all 50 patients by IHC. The staining intensity was scored: blue: score 0, light brown: score 1, medium brown: score 2, dark brown: score 3 and very dark brown: score 4 (Fig. 1). Antibodies have distinct immunoreactivity for plasma membrane and cytoplasm of tumor cells. Cells showing membranous / cytoplasmic staining alone or in association were considered as positive and scored (Fig. 2).

Table 1 Patients' characteristics ($n = 50$)

Characteristics	n
Total	50
Age (year)	
Median	59,9
Range	41–81
Sex	
Male	48
Female	2
Smoking history	
Never-smoker	3
Former/current smoker	47
pTNM stage[a]	
IV	37
IIIa or IIIb	13
Type of treatment	
Surgery	4
Chemotherapy	21
Radiotherapy	3
Combined[b]	5
Transferred to private sector	17
Deceased cases	10

pTNM pathologic tumor-node-metastasis
[a]TNM classification 7th edition
[b]chemotherapy+radiotherapy

Immunoscoring

Amount of EGFR mutations was determined, for all patients, by calculating H-score, which evaluate heterogeneity of staining, based on estimation of staining area (%) per each intensity, since lung tumors are known to have heterogeneous mutational status.

Patients with only staining intensity 0 and 1+ were considered as negative for EGFR overexpression. The final H-score ranged from [0–240].

22/50 (44%) harbored an EGFR mutation by IHC and therefore 28 cases were negative.

26% (13/22) patients had simple mutation: 9 cases E746-A750 del and 4 cases L858R.

18% (9/22) patients had concurrent mutations E746-A750 del and L858R. 88.9% (8/9) of them were men. Only a woman who was non-smoker, stage IIIb had concurrent mutation.

67% (6/9) of patients, with concurrent exon 19 and 21 mutations, were at stage IV. 100% of men with concurrent mutation were smokers, 67% of whom were current and exceeding the risk threshold of lung cancer (at least 25 pack-years). Among former smokers, all exceeded 40 pack-years with variable consumption periods.

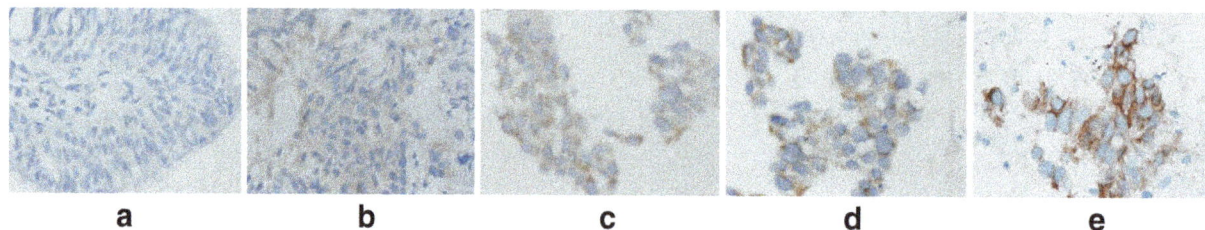

Fig. 1 Immunostaining of tumor specimens with mutation-specific antibodies illustrating the scale of intensity of staining (original magnification, 40×); **a**: score 0; **b**: score 1; **c**: score 2; **d**: score 3 and **e**: score 4

Molecular analysis

EGFR mutation detection was performed by PCR followed by Sanger sequencing for 35 patients (20 positive and 15 negative IHC cases) for which we could obtain DNA. Mutations were confirmed by sequencing for 17 of 20 positive cases by IHC (2 of the 22 positive IHC cases were not tested since we could not obtain DNA). 8 were concurrent and 9 simple mutations (7 had E746-A750 del and 2 had L858R mutation). One case of the concurrent mutations by IHC was only confirmed for a simple mutation (E746-A750 del). The most frequent EGFR mutation was E746-A750 del for exon 19 harboring 2235–2249 del 15 bp. For L858R mutated cases, 2573 T > G point mutation in exon 21 was detected (Fig. 3).

Correlation IHC/molecular analysis

For the confirmed cases by molecular analysis (17 positive and 15 negative), the final H-score ranged from [50–240]: for simple mutation from [60–200] and for concurrent from [70–240]. IHC results were not confirmed by molecular analysis in 15% (3/20) of cases harboring an H-score less than 50. Then, they can be considered as false positive cases.

Majority of confirmed cases had H-score greater than 100 and 55% of concurrent mutations harbored for both a score superior to 110.

It is important to take in account the percentage of cells for each staining intensity (0 to 4+). All our IHC positive cases confirmed by sequencing presented a mix of staining intensity.

88.9% (8/9) of concurrent mutations and 72.7% (8/11) of simple mutations detected by IHC were confirmed, since 2 samples were not analyzed by sanger. Only one concurrent mutation was not confirmed and was classified as simple (E746-A750 del).

Sensitivity and specificity of IHC-based method

In the nonmalignant tissues included in patient biopsies, no mutations of EGFR were observed both by IHC and sequencing. All negative EGFR IHC cases tested (15 cases) were confirmed by molecular analysis, after Sanger sequencing, and mutations were confirmed for 85% (17/20) of cases positive by IHC.

Sensitivity of IHC technique to detect EGFR mutation status compared to molecular analysis is concordant for 85% considering only positive cases by IHC and rise to 91.4% when we include negative IHC cases tested (32/35). Specificity to detect EGFR mutations by IHC was 100%: all IHC negative tissues from our patients tested (15 cases were we could obtain DNA) were confirmed by molecular analysis.

Discussion

WHO Classification, 2015 of Lung Tumors, updated the diagnostic criteria in all lung cancer specialties: clinical, epidemiology, radiology, genetics, histology, cytology, IHC and molecular analysis [7].

Development of IHC provided better classification and reclassification of specific entities. Publications focused on the possibility of detecting mutated protein such as EGFR, BRAF... directly on lung cancer tissue by

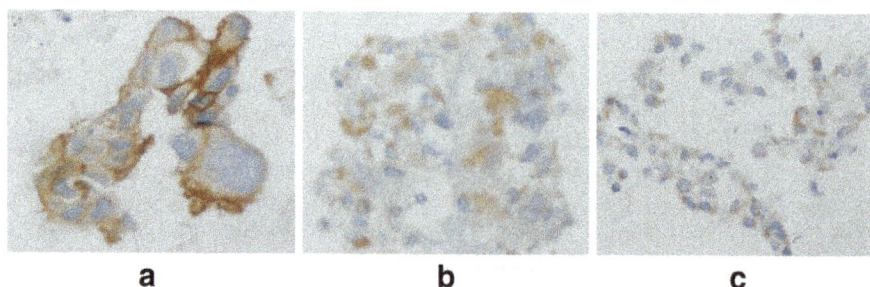

Fig. 2 Membranous (**a**) / cytoplasmic (**b**) and mixte staining (**c**) (Original magnification, 40×)

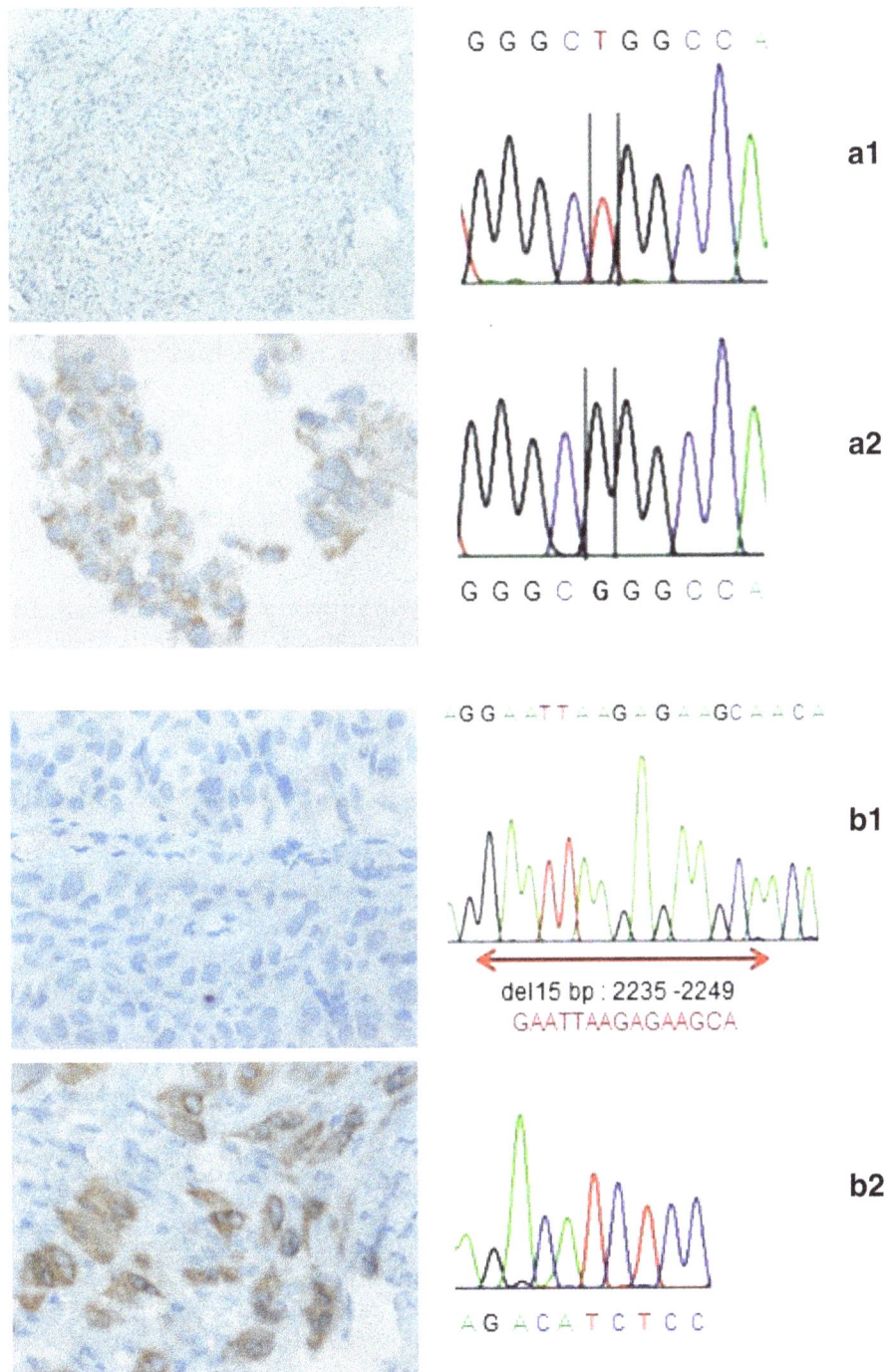

Fig. 3 Concordance analysis IHC and DNA sequencing: *L858R*: **a1** (Patient 7): Left -- > negative IHC (Original magnification, 10×) / Right -- > normal electropherogram. **a2** (Patient 19): Left -- > positive IHC (Original magnification, 40×) Right -- > 2573 T > G point mutation in exon 21. *E746-A750*: **b1** (Patient 44): Left -- > negative IHC (Original magnification, 40×) Right -- > normal electropherogram. **b2** (Patient 33): Left -- > positive IHC (Original magnification, 40×) / Right -- > 2235–2249 del 15 bp

mutation-specific IHC with 92% of sensitivity which is comparable to DNA sequencing [15, 18].

But, there is a substantial need of data from several regions of the world, notably Africa, due to a lack of mutation testing. This is also the case in Tunisia.

We report the first Tunisian study carried out in 50 patients, enrolled from January 2010 to December 2014, by mutation-specific IHC to detect the most frequently EGFR mutations (exon 19 E746-A750 del and exon 21 L858R substitution), in FFPE tissues from small lung biopsies. Our patients were unselected, contrary to majority of works, analyzing EGFR mutations, done in patients with advanced stage or failing treatments (surgical or first-line chemotherapy).

Histological results (TTF-1/Napsin A) were consistent with ADC. 74% of them were at stage IV (Table 1). These results are concordant with literature.

A variable expression level of mutant EGFR proteins by immunoscoring was observed in the same tissue for all patients, indicating intratumoral heterogeneity. This observation is in line with literature which provides that abundance of EGFR mutation differs within each tissue [11]. For this purpose, we used H-score which takes in account this heterogeneity. There are two methods for immunoscoring, automated and manual, and two types of score, Q and H. We choose to use manual method to calculate H-score, although it is more difficult to compute, because Q-score ignores variable intensity of staining.

44% of our patients showed at least one EGFR mutation by IHC. This is concordant with the average mutation rate in many regions of Asia (Japan, Malaysia, Singapore,...). It is higher than overall Europe (15%), but similar to Germany and Turkey (up to 41%), noting that the number of studies by country remains relatively low [19–21].

Mutations average is variable for each study and each country. This variation can be explained by ethnicity which was not examined in most reported publications.

We choose to detect the most common NSCLC associated EGFR mutations, E746-A750 del and L858R, because they account together for 86 to 90% of total EGFR mutations (45% for E746-A750 del and 40–45% for L858R) [11, 17, 21–23].

Our result was based on H-score. IHC was considered positive, only for cases harboring high staining intensity (2+, 3+ and 4+). Patients with only 1+ were considered as negative for EGFR overexpression.

Among our mutated patients by IHC, we found 26% simple and 18% concurrent mutations. The most frequent mutation was in exon 19, 36% of our cases harboring E746-A750 del.

26% presented a substitution L858R in exon 21.

IHC results were confirmed in 91.4% of cases by molecular analysis. This is in accordance with literature [19].

IHC can be considered as an efficient specific tool to precise mutational status of patients.

Specificity to detect EGFR mutations was 100%. The relevance of sequencing has been validated by the use of negative and positive controls (cell lines).

Mutations types observed in Tunisian population are concordant with Indian and Moroccan studies which report E746-A750 del, as the most frequent mutation [19, 24].

18% of our patients harbored concurrent mutations by IHC. 88.9% of them were confirmed by sequencing. This result is little bit higher compared to literature

(2.1 to 14%) [25–28]. This may be a Tunisian specificity, perhaps in relation with high frequency of smokers, noting that most studies enrolled Asian patients [20]. The only African study in literature is from Morocco and didn't report concurrent mutations [24].

ADC histology and smoking history are the only significant independent predictors of EGFR mutation status [29].

Concurrent mutations were found in 43.7% of mutated men, all smokers exceeding 40 pack-years, and in one non-smoker woman. These profile and prevalence are not contradictory with literature. Although most studies reported a higher prevalence in non-smoker ADC women, in the PIONEER study more than 50% of patients with EGFR mutations were not non-smoker women [20, 25–30].

These results support EGFR mutation testing for all NSCLC patients.

In Tunisia, there are 1.7 million of smokers, aged from 10 to 70 years causing 10,000 cases of death each year (Plan for control of cancer in Tunisia 2015–2019). Tunisia is considered by WHO the most tobacco-consuming Arab country (35% of population).The latest statistical data highlights that most lung cancers are due to smoking in Tunisia and according to National Consumption Institute of Tunisia, most smokers consume smuggled cigarettes of poor quality, for economic reasons, multiplying by 11 the carcinogenic risk [31, 32].

Our results support this fact and pinpoint the pressing need for health authorities to inform and educate people relating to harmful effects of tobacco, focusing on primary prevention to discourage young people from taking up this practice but also supporting those wishing to stop smoking.

Actually in Tunisia, chemotherapy is the primary treatment for NSCLC. Our aim was to estimate the relevance of proposing TKIs for our patients as a new therapeutic line since patients harboring activating EGFR mutations can benefit from treatment with molecules like gefitinib and erlotinib [26, 30].

These preliminary results (majority of smokers and rate of concurrent mutations) don't appear to support the use of TKIs for NSCLC in Tunisia, since smoking cigarettes (≥ 30 pack-years) is a negative predictive factor for TKIs treatment and the non-smoking mutated patients have the highest benefit from it [33, 34].

As well concurrent mutations lead to a worse response to TKIs treatment compared to single mutations (38% versus 89%, $p < 0.001$; ORR = 23.8%) [25, 26].

Only Zhang reported a better response in patients with co- mutations, treated with gefitinib or erlotinib, this contrary result may be explained by the small number of patients (3) treated [27].

Identifying subgroups of patients responding poorly to TKIs treatment may improve patients' management [29].

Mechanisms of low response rate to TKIs are not clear, they may result from molecular conformation changes of EGFR tyrosine kinase domain caused by concurrent mutations [30].

To conclude, the good concordance between EGFR IHC and molecular sequencing data encourages the use of EGFR mutation-specific IHC as an easy and quick EGFR status "screening" approach. A negative IHC result is confident for the absence of EGFR mutation thus avoiding molecular analysis. By contrast, IHC positivity further requires gene sequencing to definitively assess the presence of EGFR mutation avoiding false positive cases.

In addition, although in the awareness of possible false positive, a relevant application of mutation-specific IHC is a better management of small size and/or low content tumor cells samples. It will avoid a second biopsy to obtain supplementary tissues to identify mutations especially for advanced cancer or tumor with limited cells [23]. Indeed, in daily practice, we are often confronted with little biopsies which will be included in paraffin for pathological analyzes. The latter will generally give small quantities with poor quality DNA, not always making molecular studies possible.

Conclusion

There is a great need for further investigations to confirm the real contribution of EGFR mutation in lung cancer worldwide.

In Tunisia, this is the first report, which despite the small number of patients, gives a good concordance between molecular and IHC results, emphasizing the interest of setting up targeted IHC, in daily practice, to explore EGFR mutations in small biopsies of lung cancer but should be expanded to clarify relevance of TKIs treatment.

Authors' contributions
ZM and LH designed the study, analyzed the data, wrote and revised the manuscript. JBA and HB contributed with patient recruitment and clinical data and SR contributed with pathological data and participates to the IHC analysis. All authors approved the final version.

Competing interests
The authors declare that they have no competing interests.

Author details
[1]Genetic Department, Faculté de Médecine de Tunis, Université de Tunis El Manar, Tunis, Tunisia. [2]Pulmonary Department, EPS Charles Nicolle, Faculté de Médecine de Tunis, Université de Tunis El Manar, Tunis, Tunisia. [3]Pathological Anatomy and Cytology Department, EPS Charles Nicolle, Faculté de Médecine de Tunis, Université de Tunis El Manar, Tunis, Tunisia.

References
1. Siegel RL, Miller KD, Jemal A. Cancer statistics, 2016. CA Cancer J Clin. 2016;66:7–30.
2. Torre LA, Siegel RL, Jemal A. Lung Cancer statistics. Adv Exp Med Biol. 2016; 893:1 19.
3. Lazaar-Ben Gobrane H, Hajjem S, Aounallah-Skhiri H, Achour N, Hsairi M. Mortality from cancer in Tunisia: calculating years of life lost. Santé publique. 2011;23:31–40.
4. Travis WD, Brambilla E, Noguchi M, et al. The new IASLC/ATS/ERS international multidisciplinary lung adenocarcinoma classification. J Thoracic Oncol. 2011;6:244–85.
5. Lindeman NI, Cagle PT, Beasley MB, Chitale DA, Dacic S, Giaccone G, Jenkins RB, Kwiatkowski DJ, Saldivar JS, Squire J, Thunnissen E, Ladanyi M. Molecular testing guideline for selection of lung cancer patients for EGFR and ALK tyrosine kinase inhibitors: guideline from the College of American Pathologists, International Association for the Study of Lung Cancer, and Association for Molecular Pathology. J Thorac Oncol. 2013;8:823–59.
6. Leighl NB, Rekhtman N, Biermann WA, Huang J, Mino-Kenudson M, Ramalingam SS, West H, Whitlock S, Somerfield MR. Molecular testing for selection of patients with lung cancer for epidermal growth factor receptor and anaplastic lymphoma kinase tyrosine kinase inhibitors: American Society of Clinical Oncology endorsement of the College of American Pathologists/international association for the study of lung cancer/ association for molecular pathology guideline. J Clin Oncol. 2014;32:3673–9.
7. Travis WD, Brambilla E, Nicholson AG, Yatabe Y, Austin JHM, Beasley MB, Chirieac LR, Dacic S, Duhig E, Flieder DB, Geisinger K, Hirsch FR, Ishikawa Y, Kerr KM, Noguchi M, Pelosi G, Powell CA, Tsao MS, Wistuba I. The 2015 World Health Organization classification of lung tumors. Impact of genetic, clinical and radiologic advances since the 2004 classification. J Thorac Oncol. 2015;10:1243–60.
8. Zugazagoitia J, Enguita AB, Nuñez JA, Iglesias L, Ponce S. The new IASLC/ ATS/ERS lung adenocarcinoma classification from a clinical perspective: current concepts and future prospects. J Thorac Dis. 2014;6:526–36.
9. Petersen I, Warth A. Lung cancer: developments, concepts, and specific aspects of the new WHO classification. J Cancer Res Clin Oncol. 2016; 142:895–904.
10. Ilie M, Long E, Hofman V, Dadone B, Marquette CH, Mouroux J, Vignaud JM, Begueret H, Merlio JP, Capper D, von Deimling A, Emile JF, Hofman P. Diagnostic value of immunohistochemistry for the detection of the BRAFV600E mutation in primary lung adenocarcinoma Caucasian patients. Ann Oncol. 2013;24:742–8.
11. Zhao J, Wang X, Xue L, Xu N, Ye X, Zeng H, Lu S, Huang J, Akesu S, Xu C, He D, Tan Y, Hong Q, Wang Q, Zhu G, Hou Y, Zhang X. The use of mutation-specific antibodies in predicting the effect of EGFR-TKIs in patients with non-small-cell lung cancer. J Cancer Res Clin Oncol. 2014;140:849–57.
12. Lynch TJ, Bell DW, Sordella R, Gurubhagavatula S, Okimoto RA, Brannigan BW, Harris PL, Haserlat SM, Supko JG, Haluska FG, Louis DN, Christiani DC, Settleman J, Haber DA. Activating mutations in the epidermal growth factor receptor underlying responsiveness of non–small-cell lung Cancer to Gefitinib. N Engl J Med. 2004;350:2129–39.
13. Paez JG, Jänne PA, Lee JC, Tracy S, Greulich H, Gabriel S, Herman P, Kaye FJ, Lindeman N, Boggon TJ, Naoki K, Sasaki H, Fujii Y, Eck MJ, Sellers WR, Johnson BE, Meyerson M. EGFR mutations in lung cancer: correlation with clinical response to gefitinib therapy. Science. 2004;304:1497–500.
14. Pao W, Miller V, Zakowski M, Doherty J, Politi K, Sarkaria I, Singh B, Heelan R, Rusch V, Fulton L, Mardis E, Kupfer D, Wilson R, Kris M, Varmus H. EGF receptor gene mutations are common in lung cancers from "never smokers" and are associated with sensitivity of tumors to gefitinib and erlotinib. Proc Natl Acad Sci. 2004;101:13306–11.
15. Yu J, Kane S, Wu J, Benedettini E, Li D, Reeves C, Innocenti G, Wetzel R, Crosby K, Becker A, Ferrante M, Cheung WC, Hong X, Chirieac LR, Sholl LM, Haack H, Smith BL, Polakiewicz RD, Tan Y, Gu TL, Loda M, Zhou X, Comb MJ. Mutation-specific antibodies for the detection of EGFR mutations in non-small-cell lung cancer. Clin Cancer Res. 2009;15:3023–8.
16. Xiong Y, Bai Y, Leong N, Laughlin TS, Rothberg PG, Xu H, Nong L, Zhao J, Dong Y, Li T. Immunohistochemical detection of mutations in the epidermal growth factor receptor gene in lung adenocarcinomas using mutation-specific antibodies. Diagn Pathol. 2013;8:2.
17. Kato Y, Peled N, Wynes MW, Yoshida K, Pardo M, Mascaux C, Ohira T, Tsuboi M, Matsubayashi J, Nagao T, Ikeda N, Hirsch FR. Novel epidermal growth factor receptor mutation-specific antibodies for non-small cell lung Cancer immunohistochemistry as a possible screening method for epidermal growth factor receptor mutations. J Thorac Oncol. 2010;5:1551–8.
18. Piton N, Borrini F, Bolognese A, Lamy A, Sabourin JC. KRAS and BRAF mutation detection: is immunohistochemistry a possible alternative to molecular biology in colorectal Cancer? Gastroenterol Res Pract. 2015;2015:753903.

19. Jain D, Iqbal S, Walia R, Malik P, Cyriac S, Mathur SR, Sharma MC, Madan K, Mohan A, Bhalla A, Pathy S, Kumar L, Guleria R. Evaluation of epidermal growth factor receptor mutations based on mutation specific immunohistochemistry in non-small cell lung cancer: a preliminary study. Indian J Med Res. 2016;143(3):308–14.

20. Midha A, Dearden S, McCormack R. EGFR mutation incidence in non-small-cell lung cancer of adenocarcinoma histology: a systematic review and global map by ethnicity (mutMapII). Am J Cancer Res. 2015;5(9):2892–911.

21. Prabhakar CN. Epidermal growth factor receptor in non-small cell lung cancer. Transl Lung Cancer Res. 2015;4:110–8.

22. Fan X, Liu B, Xu H, Yu B, Shi S, Zhang J, Wang X, Wang J, Lu Z, Ma H, Zhou X. Immunostaining with EGFR mutation-specific antibodies: a reliable screening method for lung adenocarcinomas harboring EGFR mutation in biopsy and resection samples. Hum Pathol. 2013;44:1499–507.

23. Kim CH, Kim SH, Park SY, Yoo J, Kim SK, Kim HK. Identification of EGFR mutations by immunohistochemistry with EGFR mutation-specific antibodies in biopsy and resection specimens from pulmonary adenocarcinoma. Cancer Res Treat. 2015;47:653–60.

24. Errihani H, Inrhaoun H, Boukir A, Kettani F, Gamra L, Mestari A, Jabri L, Bensouda Y, Mrabti H, Elghissassi I. Frequency and type of epidermal growth factor receptor mutations in Moroccan patients with lung adenocarcinoma. J Thorac Oncol. 2013;8:1212–4.

25. Wei Z, An T, Wang Z, Chen K, Bai H, Zhu G, Duan J, Wu M, Yang L, Zhuo M, Wang Y, Liu X, Wang J. Patients harboring epidermal growth factor receptor (EGFR) double mutations had a lower objective response rate than those with a single mutation in non-small cell lung cancer when treated with EGFR-tyrosine kinase inhibitors. Thorac Cancer. 2014;5:126–32.

26. Barnet MB, O'Toole S, Horvath LG, Selinger C, Yu B, Chin Ng C, Boyer M, Cooper WA, Kao S. EGFR-co-mutated advanced NSCLC and response to EGFR tyrosine kinase inhibitors. J Thorac Oncol. 2017;12:585–90.

27. Zhang GC, Lin JY, Wang Z, Zhou Q, Xu CR, Zhu JQ, Wang K, Yang XN, Chen G, Yang JJ, Huang YJ, Liao RQ, Wu YL. Epidermal growth factor receptor double activating mutations involving both exons 19 and 21 exist in Chinese non-small cell lung Cancer patients. Clin Oncol. 2007;19:499–506.

28. Kobayashi S, Canepa HM, Bailey AS, Nakayama S, Yamaguchi N, Goldstein MA, Huberman MS, Costa DB. Compound EGFR mutations and response to EGFR tyrosine kinase inhibitors. J Thorac Oncol. 2013;8:118–22.

29. Tanaka T, Matsuoka M, Sutani A, Gemma A, Maemondo M, Inoue A, Okinaga S, Nagashima M, Oizumi S, Uematsu K, Nagai Y, Moriyama G, Miyazawa H, Ikebuchi K, Morita S, Kobayashi K, Hagiwara K. Frequency of and variables associated with the EGFR mutation and its subtypes. Int J Cancer. 2010;126:651–5.

30. Shigematsu H, Lin L, Takahashi T, Nomura M, Suzuki M, Wistuba II, Fong KM, Lee H, Toyooka S, Shimizu N, Fujisawa T, Feng Z, Roth JA, Herz J, Minna JD, Gazdar AF. Clinical and biological features associated with epidermal growth factor receptor gene mutations in lung cancers. J Natl Cancer Inst. 2005;97:339–46.

31. The global tobacco crisis - World Health Organization (2008). Available at: http://www.who.int/tobacco/mpower/mpower_report_tobacco_crisis_2008.pdf. Accessed 17 Mar 2017.

32. Plan pour la lutte contre le cancer en Tunisie 2015–2019. République Tunisienne - Ministère de la santé. Available at: http://www.iccp-portal.org/system/files/plans/Plan_pour_la_lutte_contre_le_cancer_2015-2019_Tunisie.pdf. Accessed 17 Mar 2017.

33. Kim MH, Kim HR, Cho BC, Bae MK, Kim EY, Lee CH, Lee JS, Kang DR, Kim JH. Impact of cigarette smoking on response to epidermal growth factor receptor (EGFR)-tyrosine kinase inhibitors in lung adenocarcinoma with activating EGFR mutations. Lung Cancer. 2014;84:196–202.

34. Zhang Y, Kang S, Fang W, Hong S, Liang W, Yan Y, Qin T, Tang Y, Sheng J, Zhang L. Impact of smoking status on EGFR-TKI efficacy for advanced non small-cell lung Cancer in EGFR mutants: a meta-analysis. Clin Lung Cancer. 2015;16:144–51.

27

The influence of anemia on one-year exacerbation rate of patients with COPD-PH

Wei Xiong[1,2], Mei Xu[3], Bigyan Pudasaini[2], Xuejun Guo[1] and Jinming Liu[2*]

Abstract

Background: Anemia is prevalent not only in COPD but also in pulmonary hypertension. We postulated that anemia may have certain prognostic value in COPD concomitant with PH due to COPD (COPD-PH).

Methods: We performed a 12-month prospective investigation to follow up COPD patients with or without PH assessed by right heart catheterization. Eligible patients were enrolled, stratified into COPD-PH-anemia group ($n = 40$), COPD-PH group ($n = 42$), COPD-anemia group ($n = 48$), and COPD group($n = 50$), and then followed up for 12 months.

Results: After the follow-up, for both of the actual variation value and variation rate, the increase of NT-pro BNP ($P<0.001$; $P = 0.03$) and CAT score ($P = 0.001$; 0.002), as well as the decrease of PaO_2 ($P = 0.03$; 0.086) and Peak VO_2 ($P = 0.021$; 0.009) in COPD-PH-anemia group were highest among four groups. The cumulative one-year survival rates were similar among four groups ($P = 0.434$). The cumulative exacerbation-free rate was lowest in COPD-PH-anemia group among four groups ($P<0.001$). Hemoglobin was an independent promoting factor for the probability of hospitalization due to exacerbation $\geq$ 1/year in patients with COPD-PH-anemia [HR 3.121(2.325–5.981); $P<0.001$].

Conclusions: Anemia is a promoting factor for the worsening of exercise capacity, deterioration of hypoxemia, declining of life quality, and aggravation of exacerbations in patients with COPD-PH-anemia, by contrast with COPD-PH, COPD-anemia, and COPD.

Keywords: COPD, Pulmonary hypertension, Anemia, Prognosis, Hemoglobin

Background

Chronic obstructive pulmonary disease (COPD) has become the third leading cause of death worldwide and is projected to be the disease with the seventh greatest burden worldwide in 2030. It is a major chronic cause of morbidity and mortality all over the world. Many patients suffer from this disease for many years, and die prematurely due to itself or its complications [1–3].

Pulmonary hypertension (PH) is a pathophysiological disorder involving multiple clinical disciplines, which majorly include multiple cardiovascular and respiratory diseases [4]. It may develop in the advanced stage of COPD and is basically due to hypoxic vasoconstriction of pulmonary capillaries, eventually leading to structural changes which include intimal hyperplasia and the consequent smooth muscle hypertrophy [5–7]. Once PH develops in patients with COPD, what may follow are the deteriorated exercise capacity, worsened hypoxemia and shortened survival [8–10].

In patients with COPD, systemic inflammatory mediators may contribute to skeletal muscular atrophy or cachexia, and initiate or aggravate anemia [11], meanwhile, anemia is common in patients with PH and may be associated with reduced exercise capacity, and with a higher mortality [12–16]. Therefore, since anemia had been evident to be prevalent in both COPD and PH, we wondered how the prognostic role anemia was in PH due to COPD. For patients with COPD related PH, there are many shared prognostic factors between COPD and PH, such as DLcO, 6MWD, PaO_2, mMRC score and peak VO_2 which all decline worse than in either of COPD or PH alone providing the inter-related basis for the assessment of COPD-PH. To date, no existing studies have concerned this subject. Therefore, this study was

* Correspondence: jinmingliu2013@126.com
Xuejun Guo and Jinming Liu are joint corresponding authors
[2]Department of Cardiopulmonary Circulation, Shanghai Pulmonary Hospital, Tongji University School of Medicine, Shanghai, China
Full list of author information is available at the end of the article

designed to explore the potential prognostic value of anemia in PH due to COPD.

Methods

Study design

We performed a 12-month prospective study to investigate the role of anemia in COPD concomitant with PH. All eligible patients were screened out according to inclusion and exclusion criteria and then stratified into COPD-PH-anemia group, COPD-PH group, COPD-anemia group, and COPD group, to be followed up for 12 months. Variables encompassing routine blood test (RBT), COPD assessment test (CAT), pulmonary function test (PFT), cardiopulmonary exercise test (CPET), 6 min walk distance (6MWD), and arterial blood gas analysis (ABGA) were assessed at the baseline and the endpoint. Cumulative exacerbation counting and all-cause mortality were documented during the follow-up. All relevant variables were compared amongst the four groups after the finish of follow-up. During the enrollment of the patients, we equalized the variables of factors which might impact the prognosis to the maximum extent except for hemoglobin. Since our subjects were primarily patients with COPD, so we focused mainly on the equalization of GOLD stage, AE history, and co-morbidities. Meanwhile, we eliminated the difference of therapies by standardizing the treatment according to the guidelines. This protocol was approved by the institutional review board of Shanghai Pulmonary Hospital. Written informed consent was obtained from all patients.

Study population

All eligible patients were enrolled from a cohort of patients with COPD with or without PH assessed by right heart catheterization (RHC) between 2013 and 2016 of the department of cardiopulmonary circulation of Shanghai Pulmonary Hospital Tongji University, due to at least one of the following reasons: 1) episodes of RV failure or suspected PH by echocardiographic findings; 2) suspected PAH or CTEPH; 3) candidates for lung transplantation or lung volume reduction.

Eligible patients were enrolled according to the inclusion criteria and the exclusion criteria. Inclusion criteria: 1) age ≥ 40 yrs.; 2) a diagnosis of COPD at all stages/groups, defined as an FEV_1: FVC ratio of less than 0.70 after bronchodilator use plus respiratory symptoms, a history of exposure to risk factors (e.g., smoking, air pollution, biomass combustion), or both, measured 20 min after the inhalation of 400 µg of albuterol (Ventolin, Glaxo Wellcome) [11]; 3) a diagnosis with PH on the presence of mean pulmonary arterial pressure (mPAP) ≥ 25 mmHg and pulmonary artery wedge pressure (PAWP) ≤ 18 mmHg in RHC or an exclusion of PH by mPAP< 25 mmHg in RHC [4]; 4) with or without a

diagnosis of anemia defined as a hemoglobin concentration of < 13 g/dL for males and 12 g/dL⁻for females [17]. Exclusion criteria: 1) a diagnosis of other chronic pulmonary diseases including, asthma or asthma-COPD overlap (ACO), bronchiectasis, tuberculosis, obliterative bronchiolitis, diffuse panbronchiolitis, interstitial lung disease, or combined pulmonary fibrosis and emphysema; 2) a diagnosis of PH in Group 1, Group 2, Group 4, or Group 5 according to the classifications in 2015 ESC/ERS guidelines [4]; 3) patients with hematological diseases including secondary anemia such as anemia due to cancer or immunological diseases or hemorrhage, or receive regimens which affect hemoglobin except for anti-anemia therapy; 4) patients who lived on plateau all the time; 5) patients who were lost to follow-up or who did not comply with COPD-related or PH-related treatments.

Assessments

We performed the assessments encompassing several aspects which were exercise capacity, hypoxemia, life quality, acute exacerbation and all-cause mortality. The detailed variables we focused were hemoglobin, carboxyhemoglobin, methemoglobin in RBT, PaO_2 in ABGA, FEV_1 of the predicted value in PFT, peak VO_2 in CPET, CAT score, NT-pro BNP and 6MWD. All assessments were performed when patients were at their stable status. In case of patients happened to be in an exacerbated state at the moment of assessment, the evaluation would be postponed till patients recovered from exacerbations. Exacerbation was defined as an acute worsening of respiratory symptoms that result in additional therapy [18, 19]. At the end of each month during the follow-up, study personnel determined the patients' status including exacerbations, hospitalizations due to exacerbations, and survival status in the previous month by telephone contact.

Statistical analysis

According to the prevalence of COPD (11.7%), the anemia prevalence in COPD (12.3–23%), and the prevalence of PH in COPD (50–90%), to ensure the 95% confidential interval, we estimated we at least needed to measure in total of 159 cases of COPD patients, in which at least 82 cases of COPD-anemia in total, 75 cases of COPD-PH in total, and at least 36 cases of COPD-PH-anemia.

Measurement data was presented as mean ± standard deviation or median with interquartile range according to their distribution. Categorical data was presented as frequencies and percentages. Exacerbation-free rates and survival rates at different time-points were estimated by means of Kaplan−Meier method, and any differences between groups were evaluated with a stratified log-rank test. The multiple testing among all groups was conducted by using ANOVA with Bonferroni correction.

The change of patients' variables between the baseline and the study completion was calculated: change = (variable at completion- variable at baseline); the change rate was calculated: change rate = (variable at completion-variable at baseline)/variable at baseline. Cox regression analysis was performed to assess the correlation between variables and the probability of hospitalizations due to exacerbations ≥ 1 time per year. A p-value < 0.05 was defined as being of statistical significance.

Results
Demographics and characteristics of the patients
This investigation was launched in January, 2016, and finished in December, 2017, following the finish of follow-up of the last enrolled patient. After the exclusion of 10 cases with at least one of the following diagnoses of asthma, bronchiectasis, tuberculosis, obliterative bronchiolitis, diffuse panbronchiolitis, interstitial lung disease, or combined pulmonary fibrosis and emphysema, 6 cases with a diagnosis of PH in Group 1, Group 2, Group 4, or Group 5, and 3 cases with hematological diseases, or receive regimens which affect hemoglobin except for anti-anemia therapy, amongst 207 cases, finally, a total of 188 eligible patients were screened out to access to the follow-up program. Then after the loss of 8 cases to the follow-up, in the end, 180 cases entered into the final full analysis set. Throughout all of them, the cases in COPD-PH-anemia group, COPD-PH group, COPD-anemia group, and COPD group were 40, 42, 48, and 50, respectively. The overall mean age and male/female sex ratio of all eligible patients were 66.1 years and

131/49, respectively. No statistical difference was found among four groups in regard to age, sex ratio, smoking history, AE history, FEV_1, GOLD stages, and COPD groups ($P > 0.05$ for all comparisons), except for BMI ($P = 0.025$), mPAP ($P = 0.016$), 6MWD ($P = 0.003$), NT-pro BNP ($P<0.001$), PaO_2 ($P = 0.006$), peak VO_2($P = 0.018$) and hemoglobin ($P = 0.036$) at the baseline. By means of a routine blood test, among 88 cases with anemia, 45 cases were identified to be normocytic anemia, 33 cases were microcytic anemia, and 10 cases were macrocytic anemia. Demographics and characteristics of the patients at the baseline were summarized in Table 1. LTOT was prescribed according to patients' indication before and during the study period. No statistical difference regarding LTOT was found among four groups ($P = 0.085$).

Comparison of variation of variables between the baseline and the endpoint among four groups
The results demonstrated that no statistical difference were found regarding the FEV_1 among four groups in both aspects of actual variation value and variation rate ($P = 0.057;0.062$). Except the variation rates of PaO_2 were similar among four groups($P = 0.086$), no matter regarding actual variation value or variation rate, the increase of NT-pro BNP ($P<0.001;P = 0.03$) and CAT score ($P = 0.001;0.002$) in COPD-PH-anemia group were significantly highest among four groups, whereas the decrease of PaO_2 ($P = 0.03;0.086$) and Peak VO_2 ($P = 0.021;0.009$) in COPD-PH-anemia group were significantly highest among four groups (Table 2).

Table 1 Demographics and characteristics of all the patients at the baseline

Variables	COPD-PH-anemia ($n = 40$)	COPD-PH ($n = 42$)	COPD-anemia ($n = 48$)	COPD ($n = 50$)	P value
Age-yrs	65.9 ± 5.3	68.7 ± 8.1	62.6 ± 6.7	67.2 ± 7.5	0.587
Sex (M/F)-%	75.0/25.0	71.4/28.6	68.8/31.2	76.0/24.0	0.661
BMI-kg/m^2	18.5 ± 5.8	21.6 ± 6.2	22.4 ± 4.7	25.1 ± 7.1	0.025
Smoking history (Y/N)-%	90.0/10.0	88.1/11.9	85.4/14.6	86.0/14.0	0.549
FEV_1 of predicted value-%	40.7 ± 25.9	43.8 ± 19.6	47.7 ± 22.6	42.3 ± 17.8	0.383
AE history- no.	2.8 ± 1.5	2.5 ± 2.3	2.6 ± 1.7	2.2 ± 1.8	0.446
GOLD (I/II/III/IV)-%	0/7.5/47.5/45.0	0/11.9/45.2/42.9	0/8.3/41.7/50.0	0/10.0/43.1/46.9	0.125
Group (A/B/C/D)-%	0/12.5/40.0/47.5	0/14.3/47.6/38.1	0/14.6/43.8/41.6	0/16.0/40.0/44.0	0.374
mPAP-mmHg	33.8 ± 18.5	30.2 ± 22.6	20.6 ± 15.3	18.9 ± 25.4	0.016
CAT score-points	23.5 ± 10.2	16.9 ± 13.8	22.2 ± 8.6	18.7 ± 15.1	0.186
6MWD-m	298.9 ± 183.4	353.6 ± 164.7	382.1 ± 173.7	452.3 ± 152.2	0.003
NT-pro BNP-ng/L	1608.2 ± 679.8	1344.9 ± 852.4	556.7 ± 391.1	374.6 ± 421.0	<0.001
PaO_2-mmHg	45.3 ± 13.8	50.7 ± 18.1	55.6 ± 16.4	65.7 ± 17.2	0.006
Peak VO_2-ml/min/kg	13.9 ± 5.7	15.2 ± 7.3	18.5 ± 6.2	22.2 ± 8.1	0.018
Hemoglobin-g/dL^{-1}	9.4 ± 5.5	14.2 ± 6.7	10.7 ± 8.3	13.8 ± 4.9	0.036

Note: *COPD* chronic obstructive pulmonary disease, *PH* pulmonary hypertension, *BMI* body mass index, *FEV$_1$* forced expiatory volume in 1 s, *AE* acute exacerbation, *GOLD* global Initiative for Chronic Obstructive lung Disease, *mPAP* mean pulmonary arterial pressure, *CAT* COPD assessment test, *6MWD* 6-min walking distance, *NT-proBNP* N-terminal pro-brain natriuretic peptide, *PaO$_2$* arterial blood oxygen tension, *Peak VO$_2$* peak oxygen consumption

Table 2 Comparison of the change and changing rate of patients' variables between the baseline and the endpoint among four groups

Variables	COPD-PH-anemia (n = 40)	COPD-PH (n = 42)	COPD-anemia (n = 48)	COPD (n = 50)	P value
FEV₁-% (%)	−8.8 ± 3.6(− 10.1 ± 5.3)	−8.5 ± 6.4(− 10.6 ± 4.6)	− 7.2 ± 5.1(− 8.3 ± 7.2)	−7.6 ± 4.2(−9.1 ± 4.8)	0.057(0.062)
CAT score-points (%)	12.6 ± 5.8(23.7 ± 15.1)	6.5 ± 3.7(19.2 ± 12.4)	6.6 ± 4.0(22.3 ± 10.6)	4.7 ± 3.2(20.1 ± 8.8)	0.001(0.002)
6MWD-m (%)	−59.5 ± 45.6(− 32.2 ± 18.8)	−34.3 ± 41.2(− 26.5 ± 14.3)	−28.4 ± 40.1(− 20.5 ± 16.2)	− 19.7 ± 38.3(− 16.5 ± 12.3)	0.007(0.01)
NT-pro BNP- ng/L (%)	597.1 ± 154.4(31.3 ± 20.4)	466.8 ± 191.0(25.5 ± 22.3)	125.7 ± 112.1(19.5 ± 17.2)	133.6 ± 108.5(15.2 ± 13.3)	<0.001(0.03)
PaO₂-mmHg (%)	−10.7 ± 5.8(− 10.9 ± 8.6)	−7.6 ± 5.3(− 11.7 ± 7.0)	−6.6 ± 5.4(−8.8 ± 7.5)	− 4.9 ± 4.5(− 7.9 ± 7.2)	0.03(0.086)
Peak VO₂-ml/min/kg (%)	−3.5 ± 1.6(− 32.4 ± 10.3)	−2.8 ± 1.9(− 25.5 ± 13.6)	−2.4 ± 2.1(− 17.7 ± 8.8)	−1.8 ± 1.4(− 10.3 ± 11.7)	0.021(0.009)

Note: *FEV₁* forced expiatory volume in 1 s, *CAT* COPD assessment test, *6MWD* 6-min walking distance, *NT-proBNP* N-terminal pro-brain natriuretic peptide, *PaO₂* arterial blood oxygen tension, *Peak VO₂* peak oxygen consumption

Comparison of cumulative overall survival, exacerbation-free rate amongst four groups

At the end of the follow-up, the cumulative overall mortality were 19 cases, in which 7cases were in COPD-PH-anemia group, 5 cases were in COPD-PH group, 4 cases were in COPD-anemia group, and 3cases were in COPD group(*P* = 0.096). Among all the deceased, 10 patients died of respiratory failure, 7 patients died of heart failure, 2 cases died of sudden death. In a Kaplan–Meier analysis, the results demonstrated that the cumulative one-year survival rates were similar amongst COPD-PH-anemia group, COPD-PH group, COPD-anemia group, and COPD group (*P* = 0.434) (Fig. 1.) Throughout the whole process of follow-up, the mean annual exacerbations or hospitalizations counting per patient were 3.5 and 1.8 times in COPD-PH-anemia group, 2.6 and 1.7 times in COPD-PH group, 2.4 and 1.3 times in COPD-anemia group, as well as 1.8 and 0.8 times in COPD group, respectively (*P* = 0.005; *P* = 0.018). At the end of the follow-up, the cases with at least one exacerbation or one hospitalization were 118(65.6%) and 66 (36.7%) cases, respectively. The prevalence of exacerbations or hospitalizations were 35(87.5%) and 16(40.0%) in COPD-PH-anemia group, 28(66.7%) and 15(35.7%) in COPD-PH group, 30(62.5%) and 12(25.0%) in COPD-anemia group, as well as 25 (50%) and 10(20.0%) in COPD group [*P* = 0.033(*P*<0.001); *P* = 0.065(*P* = 0.005)]. In a Kaplan–Meier analysis, the results demonstrated that the cumulative exacerbation-free proportion was lowest in COPD-PH-anemia group, and highest in COPD group, whereas no statistical difference was found between COPD-PH group and COPD-anemia group(*P*<0.001) (Fig. 2.).

Correlation between risk factors and exacerbations in each group by multivariate regression analysis

After an univariate analysis between risk factors and the development of hospitalizations due to exacerbations ≧ 1/ year, then adjusting for age, sex, smoking history and BMI, a multivariate analysis demonstrated that, for patients with COPD-PH-anemia, along with per decrease of 1 g/dL⁻¹ of

hemoglobin, the hazard ratio of hospitalizations ≧ 1/year was 3.121, being similar with some variables such as AE history and COPD groups. Also in a multivariate regression analysis between dyshemoglobins which were carboxyhemoglobin as well as methemoglobin and the risk for hospitalizations ≧ 1/year, the results showed that only carboxyhemoglobin was positively correlated with the development of hospitalizations ≧ 1/year especially in COPD-PH-anemia group (Table 3.)

Discussion

In consideration of anemia may have certain prognostic value in patients with pulmonary hypertension due to COPD, whereas little of them was known quoad hoc, thus we performed this study. In this study, we found that, among COPD-PH-anemia group, COPD-PH group, COPD-anemia group, and COPD group, the patients in COPD-PH-anemia group had the most deterioration in exercise capacity, hypoxemia, life quality, and highest risk of acute exacerbations, except for the similar overall survival rates among all groups, in a 12-month interval.

To our best knowledge, no existing comparable study is eligible to be the contrast with this study, therefore, what we can discuss hereby is this investigation exclusively. Since PH is also a concomitant co-morbidity just like anemia, we primarily regarded the subjects as COPD patients, then as PH or not. In order to present the the impact of anemia on COPD-PH to the maximum extent, we set up not only COPD-PH, but also COPD-anemia and COPD as control. Besides the information of impact of anemia on COPD-PH, we could also obtain the information regarding the different impact of anemia on COPD-PH and COPD, respectively, by contrast with sole COPD. It cannot be denied that secondary polycythemia is a common phenomenon in patients with COPD just like anemia, in other words, the two pathophysiologic processes may potentially happen in patients with COPD simultaneously, especially in early stage of COPD. Therefore, since the basic hemoglobin level of COPD may be higher than that of normal person, we adopted the diagnostic criteria of WHO for anemia which are

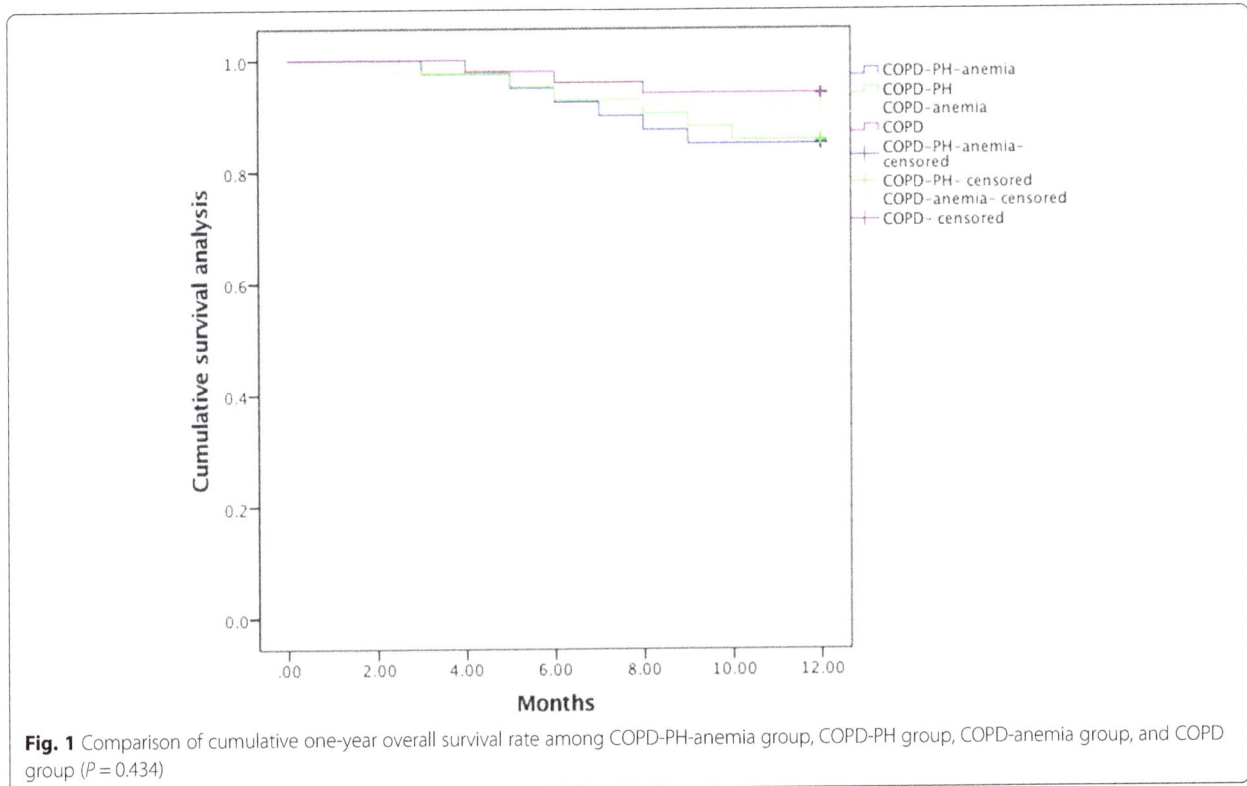

Fig. 1 Comparison of cumulative one-year overall survival rate among COPD-PH-anemia group, COPD-PH group, COPD-anemia group, and COPD group ($P = 0.434$)

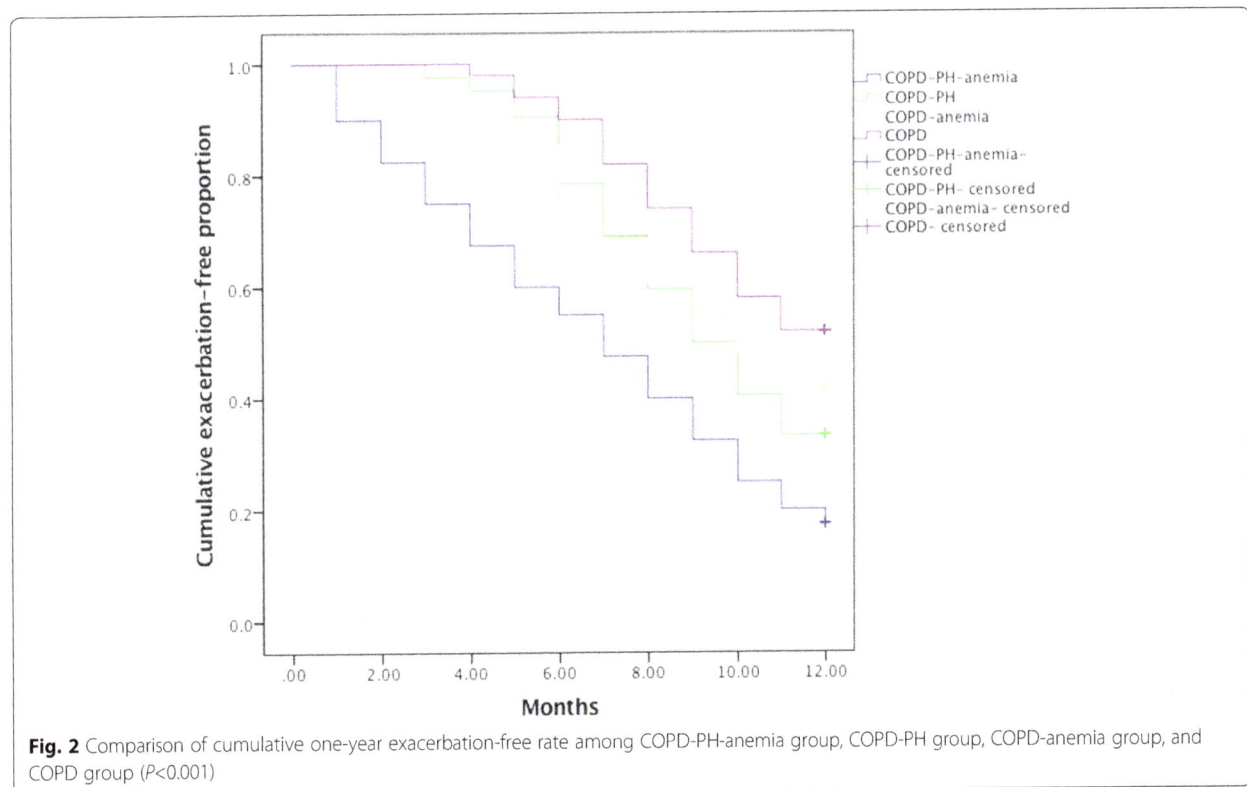

Fig. 2 Comparison of cumulative one-year exacerbation-free rate among COPD-PH-anemia group, COPD-PH group, COPD-anemia group, and COPD group ($P<0.001$)

Table 3 Correlation between risk factors and the probability of hospitalizations ≧ 1/year in each group by multivariate regression analysis

Variables	COPD-PH-anemia (n = 40)	COPD-PH (n = 42)	COPD-anemia (n = 48)	COPD (n = 50)
	HR (95%CI), P value	HR (95%CI), P value	HR (95%CI), P value	HR (95%CI), P value
FEV_1-per decrease of 10%	2.565(1.225–3.764) 0.003	2.439(1.219–3.664) 0.002	2.108(1.321–4.214) 0.005	1.884(0.871–3.265) 0.003
AE history-per increase of 1 time	3.338(1.532–4.698) <0.001	3.157(1.339–5.310)< 0.001	2.541(1.210–4.311)0.001	2.226(1.722–3.827)0.001
GOLD-per progression of 1 stage	2.765(1.555–3.827)0.008	2.672(1.246–3.981)0.005	2.519(1.433–3.646)0.001	1.987(0.592–3.218)0.037
Group-per progression of 1 level	3.102(1.426–3.223) <0.001	2.453(1.002–3.528)0.002	2.313(1.038–3.297)0.004	2.124(0.762–3.281)0.014
PaO_2-per decrease of 10 mmHg	2.384(1.542–3.456)0.02	2.176(1.256–3.642)0.006	2.987(1.777–3.562)0.007	1.733(0.888–3.213)0.028
Peak VO_2-per decrease of 10 ml/min/kg	2.182(1.214–3.628)0.003	2.815(1.118–3.823)0.033	2.143(1.143–3.427)0.004	2.054(1.076–3.665)0.029
6MWD-per decrease of 100 m	1.676(0.662–3.186)0.036	1.501(0.855–3.222)0.044	1.453(0.337–3.212)0.038	1.222(0.443–3.251)0.057
Hemoglobin -per decrease of 1 g/dL^{-1}	3.121(2.325–5.981) <0.001	1(reference)	2.756(1.985–3.784) <0.001	1(reference)
Carboxyhemoglobin-per increase of 0.1 g/dL^{-1}	2.838(1.698–5.210)0.001	2.663(1.520–3.228)0.001	2.437(1.265–3.884)0.001	1.688(1.104–3.651)0.002

Note: *COPD* chronic obstructive pulmonary disease, *PH* pulmonary hypertension, *FEV*$_1$ forced expiatory volume in 1 s, *AE* acute exacerbation, *GOLD* global Initiative for Chronic Obstructive lung Disease, *PaO*$_2$ arterial blood oxygen tension, *Peak VO*$_2$ peak oxygen consumption, *6MWD* 6-min walking distance

< 13 g/dL for males and < 12 g/dL for females, respectively, instead of the criteria of anemia in China which are <12 g/l for male and <11 g/l for female, respectively, to eliminate the potential confounding of secondary polycythemia.

To start with, except for hemoglobin which was predetermined to be different among four groups, the demographics showed that no statistical difference was found in regard to age, sex ratio, smoking history, AE history, FEV_1, GOLD stages, and COPD groups, suggesting the homogeneity was considerable at least from the perspective of COPD, among all eligible patients at the baseline. Nevertheless, some variables such as mPAP, 6MWD, NT-pro BNP, PaO_2, and peak VO_2 were heterogenous among all eligible patients at the baseline partially attributable to the role of PH. Interestingly, the BMI in COPD-PH-anemia group was lowest among four groups suggesting anemia may interrelate with nutritional status. It is noteworthy that the cause of anemia was majorly due to normocytic type which conformed to the characteristics of COPD [11]. As for microcytic type being the second major cause, we believe it is related to PH [12–16].

After the follow-up, the results showed no dramatic variation regarding the FEV_1 which is a COPD-related variable concerning airflow limitation, whereas the variations of NT-pro BNP, CAT score, PaO_2 and Peak VO_2 were significant among four groups in which the COPD-PH-anemia group had the worst deterioration. This indicated that, anemia impacted more seriously on patients with COPD-PH than on mere COPD, encompassing the perspectives of life quality, ventricular dysfunction, and hypoxemia especially whilst exercise, except for airflow limitation. On account of the

impairment of oxygen-transporting function in anemia, patients with COPD-PH-anemia are naturally more liable to develop ingravescent fatigue, heart failure and hypoxemia rather than airflow limitation, by contrast with either COPD-PH or COPD.

The next comparison of cumulative overall survival showed no difference of cumulative one-year survival rates among four groups. This could be interpreted as that anemia makes no difference on the survival of patients with COPD-PH or COPD for at least 1 year. By contrast, in the study of Pernille et al., anemia could be used to predict mortality. In view of Pernille's study was a five-year retrospective review, while ours was a one-year prospective investigation, the investigating period in this study may be too limited to uncover the difference of mortality among different groups [20].

In the study of Pernille, et al., low level of hemoglobin are frequent in COPD patients with acute exacerbations [20]. In our study, the comparison of exacerbations demonstrated that COPD-PH-anemia group had the most mean annual exacerbations or hospitalizations counting, the highest prevalent rate of exacerbations or hospitalizations, and lowest cumulative exacerbation-free rate among patients among four groups. It means that, by contrast with simple COPD, anemic COPD, or simple COPD-PH, COPD-PH-anemia has the highest risk for developing an exacerbation. It is believed that, by deteriorating life quality, ventricular dysfunction, and hypoxemia, anemia contributes to the aggravation of exacerbations.

The last correlation analysis between risk factors and hospitalizations showed that, being similar with some exacerbation-related classical predictors in COPD such as AE history and COPD groups [11], hemoglobin was an independently contributing factor for the probability of hospitalizations $\geq$ 1/year in COPD patients especially patients with COPD-PH-anemia. Decremental hemoglobin is a promoting factor for the incremental exacerbations or hospitalizations. By the way, we also performed a correlation analysis between some dyshemoglobins which were carboxyhemoglobin as well as methemoglobin and hospitalizations. The results demonstrated that carboxyhemoglobin was positively correlated with the development of hospitalizations $\geq$ 1/year in all four groups especially in COPD-PH-anemia group rather than methemoglobin. Likewise, in the study of Yasuda et al., the carboxyhemoglobin level at exacerbations were significantly higher than those at stable stage, the increased arterial carboxyhemoglobin was correlated to the severity of COPD resulting from systemic inflammation and reactive oxygen species [21].

Some systematic inflammatory diseases such as connective tissue disease are frequently concomitant with anemia of chronic disease through the mechanism of the production of inflammatory mediators damaging the generation of erythrocytes. Likewise, COPD which is one of systematic inflammatory diseases is generally concomitant with the elevation of IL-1, IL-6 and TNF-a level in circulation inducing the development of anemia [22]. Some studies demonstrated that anemia was closely related to C reactive protein which is an inflammatory biomarker [23, 24]. Besides, inflammatory mediators may also result in skeletal muscular atrophy and cachexia further deteriorating anemia [11]. On the other hand, patients with pulmonary hypertension commonly develop right ventricular dysfunction in which 15% are concomitant with anemia [25–28]. Its mechanism is due to the release of inflammatory mediators whilst heart failure, the activation of renin-angiotensin system [28]. All these may explain the impressive prevalence of anemia in COPD-PH.

The clinical implications of this study are considered to be the following: first, the results of our study may urge clinicians to be aware of the serious prevalence of anemia in COPD patients concomitant with PH; second, clinician could be vigilant about the severely adverse impact of anemia on the prognosis of COPD-PH in order to inform patients' family members timely and take action in advance; third, under some circumstances in which a dilemma exists in the assessment of prognosis, anemia could be an eligible weight which can be taken into account.

The strength of this study consisted in: first, the eligible patients being studied all underwent RHC which is the only gold standard for the diagnosis of PH to date, to ascertain wether they had PH or not, ensuring the eligibility of PH-negative COPD controls; second, we compared the longitudinal variation and variation rate between the baseline and the endpoint instead of comparing the variables at the endpoint, to reflect the time-dependent impact that anemia would result in. Nevertheless, several limitations existed in this study. First, the sample size was not very large due to the nature of prospective investigation. A large-scale study is warranted in the future. Second, obviously we have no comments to make on the potential difference of overall survival amongst different groups beyond one-year follow-up which might be too short to show the discrepancy. The last but not least, in view of the patients being reviewed in this study were all Chinese patients, the results of this study may not be applicable for other races.

Conclusions

In summary, in this study, we may draw a conclusion that anemia is a promoting factor for worse deterioration of exercise capacity, deterioration of hypoxemia, declining of life quality, as well as aggravation of exacerbations or hospitalizations in patients with COPD-PH-anemia, by contrast with patients with COPD-PH, COPD-anemia, or COPD.

Acknowledgements

We sincerely thank Dr. Lan Wang, Dr. Jian Guo, Dr. Sugang Gong, Dr. Jing He, Dr. Qinhua Zhao, Dr. Rong Jiang, Dr. Cijun Luo, Dr. Hongling Qiu, Dr. Wenhui Wu, Dr. Minqi Liu, Dr. Tianxiang Chen, Dr. Xingxing Sun, and Dr. Chuanyu Wang of Department of Cardiopulmonary Circulation, Shanghai Pulmonary Hospital, Tongji University School of Medicine, Shanghai, China, for their assistance in this study.

Funding

This work was supported by the following funds: The Program of Shanghai Natural Science Foundation (16ZR1429000); the Program of Development Center for Medical Science and Technology, National Health and Family Planning Commission of the People's Republic of China (ZX-01-C2016144)

Authors' contributions

WX conceived of the study, and participated in its design, performance, statistics, coordination, drafting and revising of the manuscript. MX conceived of the study, and participated in its design, statistics, coordination, drafting and revising of the manuscript. XJG conceived of the study, and participated in its design, statistics, coordination, and revising of the manuscript. BP participated in its design, statistics, performance, coordination, drafting and revising of the manuscript. JML conceived of the study, and participated in its design, coordination and revising of the manuscript. All authors read and approved the final manuscript.

Competing interests

The authors declare that they have no competing interests.

Author details

[1]Department of Respiratory Medicine, Xinhua Hospital, Shanghai Jiaotong University School of Medicine, No. 1665, Kongjiang Road, Yangpu District, Shanghai 200092, People's Republic of China. [2]Department of Cardiopulmonary Circulation, Shanghai Pulmonary Hospital, Tongji University School of Medicine, Shanghai, China. [3]Department of Pediatrics, Dinghai Community Health Service Center, Tongji University School of Medicine, Shanghai, China;Department of Pediatrics, Kongjiang Hospital, Yangpu District, Shanghai, China.

References

1. Lozano R, Naghavi M, Foreman K, et al. Global and regional mortality from 235 causes of death for 20 age groups in 1990 and 2010: a systematic analysis for the global burden of disease study 2010. Lancet. 2012;380:2095–128.
2. Yang G, Wang Y, Zeng Y, et al. Rapid health transition in China, 1990-2010: findings from the global burden of disease study 2010. Lancet. 2013;381: 1987–2015.
3. Mathers CD, Loncar D. Projections of global mortality and burden of disease from 2002 to 2030. PLoS Med. 2006;3(11):e442.
4. Galiè N, Humbert M, Vachiery J-L, et al. 2015 ESC/ERS guidelines for the diagnosis and treatment of pulmonary hypertension. Eur Respir J. 2015;46:879–82.
5. Sakao S, Voelkel NF, Tatsumi K. The vascular bed in COPD: pulmonary hypertension and pulmonary vascular alterations. Eur Respir Rev. 2014; 23(133):350–5.
6. Peinado VI, Pizarro S, Barbera JA. Pulmonary vascular involvement in COPD. Chest. 2008;134(4):808–14.
7. Wells JM, Washko GR, Han MK, et al. Pulmonary arterial enlargement and acute exacerbations of COPD. N Engl J Med. 2012;367(10):913–21.
8. Oswald-Mammosser M, Weitzenblum E, Quoix E, et al. Prognostic factors in COPD patients receiving long-term oxygen therapy. Importance of pulmonary artery pressure. Chest. 1995;107:1193–8.
9. Kessler R, Faller M, Weitzenblum E, et al. "Natural history" of pulmonary hypertension in a series of 131 patients with chronic obstructive lung disease. Am J Respir Crit Care Med. 2001;164:219–24.
10. Lettieri CJ, Nathan SD, Barnett SD, et al. Prevalence and outcomes of pulmonary arterial hypertension in advanced idiopathic pulmonary fibrosis. Chest. 2006;129:746–52.
11. Global Strategy for the Diagnosis, Management and Prevention of COPD, Global Initiative for Chronic Obstructive Lung Disease (GOLD). Publication list; 2017. http://goldcopd.org/gold-2017-global-strategy-diagnosis-management-prevention-copd/.
12. Ruiter G, Lankhorst S, Boonstra A, et al. Iron deficiency is common in idiopathic pulmonary arterial hypertension. Eur Respir J. 2011;37:1386–91.
13. Ruiter G, Lanser IJ, de Man FS, et al. Iron deficiency in systemic sclerosis patients with and without pulmonary hypertension. Rheumatology (Oxford). 2014;53:285–92.
14. Broberg CS, Bax BE, Okonko DO, et al. Blood viscosity and its relationship to iron deficiency, symptoms, and exercise capacity in adults with cyanotic congenital heart disease. J Am Coll Cardiol. 2006;48:356–65.
15. Rhodes CJ, Howard LS, Busbridge M, et al. Iron deficiency and raised hepcidin in idiopathic pulmonary arterial hypertension clinical prevalence, outcomes, and mechanistic insights. J Am Coll Cardiol. 2011;58:300–9.
16. Van De Bruaene A, Delcroix M, Pasquet A, et al. Iron deficiency is associated with adverse outcome in Eisenmenger patients. Eur Heart J. 2011;32:2790–9.
17. World Health Organization. Iron deficiency anemia. assessment, prevention, and control. A guide for programme managers. Geneva: WHO; 2001.
18. Wedzicha JA, Seemungal TA. COPD exacerbations: defining their cause and prevention. Lancet. 2007;370(9589):786–96.
19. Seemungal TA, Donaldson GC, Paul EA, et al. Effect of exacerbation on quality of life in patients with chronic obstructive pulmonary disease. Am J Respir Crit Care Med. 1998;157(5Pt1):1418–22.
20. Pernille A, Petersen T, Pedersen CT, et al. Association between hemoglobin and prognosis in patients admitted to hospital for COPD. Int J COPD. 2016;11:2813–20.
21. Yasuda H, Yamaya M, Nakayama K, et al. Increased arterial carboxyhemoglobin concentrations in chronic obstructive pulmonary disease. Am J Respir Crit Care. 2005;171:1246–51.
22. Weiss G, Goodnough LT. Anemia of chronic disease. N Engl J Med. 2005; 352:1011–23.
23. John M, Hoernig S, Doehner W, et al. Anemia and inflammation in COPD. Chest. 2005;127:825–9.
24. Markoulaki D, Kostikas K, Papatheodorou G, et al. Hemoglobin, erythropoietin and systemic inflammation in exacerbations of chronic obstructive pulmonary disease. Eur J Intern Med. 2011;22:103–7.
25. Tanner H, Moschovitis G, Kuster GM, et al. The prevalence of anemia in chronic heart failure. Int J Cardiol. 2002;86:115–21.
26. Cromie N, Lee C, Struthers AD. Anaemia in chronic heart failure: what is its frequency in the UK and its underlying causes? Heart. 2002;87:377–8.
27. Ezekowitz JA, McAlister FA, Armstrong PW. Anemia is common in heart failure and is associated with poor outcomes: insights from a cohort of 12065 patients with new-onset heart failure. Circulation. 2003;107:223–5.
28. Okonko DO, Anker SD. Anemia in chronic heart failure: pathogenetic mechanisms. J Card Fail. 2004;10(Suppl. 1):S5–9.

Marked deterioration in the quality of life of patients with idiopathic pulmonary fibrosis during the last two years of life

K. Rajala[1,2]* (iD), J. T. Lehto[3], E. Sutinen[4], H. Kautiainen[5], M. Myllärniemi[6] and T. Saarto[7]

Abstract

Background: Idiopathic pulmonary fibrosis (IPF) is a chronic disease with a high symptom burden and poor survival that influences patients' health-related quality of life (HRQOL). We aimed to evaluate IPF patients' symptoms and HRQOL in a well-documented clinical cohort during their last two years of life.

Methods: In April 2015, we sent the Modified Medical Research Council Dyspnea Scale (MMRC), the modified Edmonton Symptom Assessment Scale (ESAS) and a self-rating HRQOL questionnaire (RAND-36) to 300 IPF patients, of which 247 (82%) responded. Thereafter, follow-up questionnaires were sent every six months for two years.

Results: Ninety-two patients died by August 2017. Among these patients, HRQOL was found to be considerably low already two years before death. The most prominent declines in HRQOL occurred in physical function, vitality, emotional role and social functioning ($p < 0.001$). The proportion of patients with MMRC scores ≥3 increased near death. Breathlessness and fatigue were the most severe symptoms. Symptom severity for the following symptoms increased significantly and reached the highest mean scores during the last six months of life (numeric rating scale/ standard deviation): breathlessness (7.1/2.8), tiredness (7.0/2.3), dry mouth (6.0/3.0), cough (5.8/2.9), and pain with movement (5.0/3.5).

Conclusions: To our knowledge this is the first study demonstrating, that IPF patients experience remarkably low HRQOL already two years before death, especially regarding physical role. In addition, they suffer from severe breathlessness and fatigue. Furthermore, physical, social and emotional wellbeing deteriorate, and symptom burden increases near death. Regular symptom and HRQOL measurements are essential to assess palliative care needs in patients with IPF.

Keywords: Idiopathic pulmonary fibrosis, Palliative care, Health related quality of life, Symptoms

Background

Idiopathic pulmonary fibrosis (IPF) is a chronic disease with high morbidity and poor survival [1–4]. It occurs mainly in older adults, but the etiology of this progressive disease is still unknown [1]. Although the disease trajectory of IPF is variable, for many patients with IPF, survival is worse than many common malignancies. This necessitates early integration of palliative care to improve patients' quality of life (QOL) and to relieve symptoms in addition to disease-specific pharmacological treatment and lung transplant assessment [5–9].

Existing studies have shown low health-related quality of life (HRQOL) in IPF patients. However, only few of them were prospective longitudinal studies, and most were relatively small in terms of sample size or were concentrated on pharmacological treatment [10–12]. IPF patients have been shown to suffer from lower HRQOL in real-life studies than in clinical studies [12, 13].

IPF patients suffer from many difficult symptoms, of which breathlessness and cough are the most common ones [8, 10, 14–20]. In addition, a substantial proportion of patients report anxiety, depression and pain [10, 21–26].

Dyspnea is a major contributor to HRQOL, and decreased HRQOL is associated with higher mortality [27, 28]. In a prospective Australian longitudinal registry study, impaired HRQOL was related to frequent respiratory

* Correspondence: kaisa.rajala@fimnet.fi
[1]Department of Palliative Care, Comprehensive Cancer Center,, Helsinki University Hospital, Paciuksenkatu 21, Po BOX 180, FI-00290 Helsinki, Finland
[2]Faculty of Medicine, University of Helsinki, Helsinki, Finland
Full list of author information is available at the end of the article

hospitalizations and higher mortality [27]. However, to our knowledge, no previous studies have reported changes in HRQOL and symptom burden in connection with forthcoming death.

This study aimed to investigate IPF patients' HRQOL and symptom burden during the last two years of life in a prospective longitudinal follow-up study to recognise needs for palliative care and end-of-life care planning and to characterise their symptom burden in a unique follow-up setting.

Materials and methods
Study population
The FinnishIPF study is a national prospective clinical registry of IPF patients that was established in 2012. IPF diagnosis is based on the ATS/ERS 2011/2015 criteria [1, 6]. Nearly all Finnish IPF patients are initially evaluated at public university and central hospitals. Patients from these specialist centres with informed consent are included in the FinnishIPF registry, which consists of approximately 76% of all Finnish IPF patients [2]. Currently, the registry contains data from over 700 IPF patients.

All 300 patients registered in the FinnishIPF study in April 2015 were asked to participate in this substudy by sending an informed consent form together with the questionnaires. Those who did not respond within two weeks were called and reminded. Of the 300 registered patients, 247 (82%) provided informed consent for this substudy, answered the first questionnaire and were included in this study. Subsequently, the same questionnaire was sent to the patients five times at six months intervals until August 2017.

Data collection and questionnaires
Disease and sociodemographic characteristics were collected from patient records and with a separate questionnaire (Additional file 1). These included the date of birth, sex, age, marital status, education, living conditions, physical activity level, the need for assistance in daily activities, the date of IPF diagnosis, smoking status, and comorbidities. Patients were asked the frequency of leisure time physical exercise that causes breathlessness and sweating for a minimum 30 min during the preceding six months. Death certificates were acquired from the "National Authority for Collecting and Compiling Statistics on Various Fields of Society and Economy".

The questionnaires regarding HRQOL and symptoms were the RAND 36-Item Health Survey (RAND-36), the Modified Medical Research Council Dyspnea Scale (MMRC), and the modified Edmonton Symptom Assessment Scale (ESAS).

RAND-36 [29] is a general QOL measurement tool with existing Finnish general population reference values [30].

RAND-36 is similar to the previously IPF-validated short-Form-36 [30–32]. RAND-36 is divided into eight health concepts [29, 30]. Concepts are scored on a scale from 1 to 100, where a lower score indicates a worse HRQOL during the past four weeks [29, 30]. The concepts are as follows: "general health" (five questions), "vitality" (four questions regarding energy level and tiredness), "bodily pain" (two questions), "physical functioning" (ten questions regarding the ability to take care of personal hygiene and the ability to move and exercise), "physical role" (four questions regarding role limitations due to physical health), "mental health" (five questions regarding mood, depression and anxiety), "emotional role" (three questions regarding role limitations due to emotional problems), and "social functioning" (two questions) [29, 30].

The self-rated MMRC measures the degree of disability that breathlessness causes during day-to-day activities on a scale from 0 to 4, in which 0 indicates no breathlessness except during strenuous exercise, 1 indicates shortness of breath when walking up a slight hill or hurrying on a level, 2 indicates walking slower than people of same age on a level because of breathlessness or needing to stop to for breath when walking at one's own pace on a level, 3 indicates needing to stop for breath after a few minutes when walking on a level or after walking approximately 100 m, and 4 indicates that the patient is too breathless to leave the house or is breathless when dressing or undressing [33, 34].

The ESAS is a numeric self-rating symptom-based scale that was originally developed to assess the symptoms of cancer patients [35, 36]. Different symptoms are measured on Numeric Rating Scale (NRS) from 0 (no symptoms) to 10 (the worst possible symptoms) [36–38]. In this study, we used a version including 12 symptoms (pain at rest, pain with movement, tiredness, nausea, depression, anxiety, insomnia, loss of appetite, shortness of breath, cough, constipation, dry mouth, and overall wellbeing). There is a lack of evidence to recommend cut-off points for the ESAS. However, an NRS score ≥ 4 is commonly used as a trigger for more comprehensive symptom assessment in clinical practice [39].

Statistics and ethical aspects
The study population characteristics are presented as the means with standard deviations (SD) or as counts with percentages. Patients' answers were grouped, according the time they answered from the aspect of death. The Kaplan-Meier method was used to estimate the cumulative mortality after the diagnosis. We used restricted cubic splines to detect a possible non-linear dependency. A non-linear relationship between the RAND-36 domains, symptom severity, the MMRC and time before death were assessed by using 5-knot-restricted cubic spline

random-effects regression models with appropriate distribution and link functions. Models included age and gender (only main effects) as covariates. A test of interaction between independent variables was performed through the MFPIgen command. The length of the distribution (months before death) of knots was located at the 5th, 27.5, 50th, 72.5, and 95th percentiles, which correspond to time before death of – 22, – 15, – 9, – 5 and – 1. The locations of the knots were determined by the percentiles recommended in Harrell's publication [40].The normality of the variables was tested by using the Shapiro-Wilk test. The Finnish general population values for the eight Rand-36 domains were weighted to match the gender and age distribution of the study population, statistical analysis between our population and general population was not performed [30]. The Stata 15.0 [41] statistical package was used for the analysis.

The ethics committee of Helsinki University Central Hospital approved this study (381/13/03/01/2014). The Finnish National Institute for Health and Welfare (Dnro THL/1161/5.05.01/2012) approved the screening of hospital registries for patients with IPF. All participating patients provided written informed consent to participate to this specific study.

Results

Of the 247 patients included in the study 92 (37%) died by August 2017 and were included in our follow-up cohort (Fig. 1).

The cumulative mortality of the patient cohort ($n = 92$) is presented in Fig. 2. The median overall survival was 4.4 years (IQR 3.1–5.7). Patient characteristics are shown in Table 1. A majority of the patients had comorbidities, of which cardiovascular diseases were the most common ones. None of the patients had lung cancer when entering the study, but two patients were diagnosed with lung cancer during the follow-up. Lung function measurements within the last six months of life were available in only 28 (30%) of the patients (mean FVC 2.21 (SD 0.6), 57%). Antifibrotic medication was used by 33 (35%) of the patients.

The proportion of the patients who could not perform continuous moderate intensity physical exercise for at least 30 min during the previous six months increased from 34% 18–24 months before death to 62% during the last six months of life. Six months before death, 67% of the patients reported needing assistance with their daily activities, while 18–24 months before death this proportion was 56%.

Health-related quality of life

Figure 3 shows the changes in the different dimensions of HRQOL measured with RAND-36 during two years

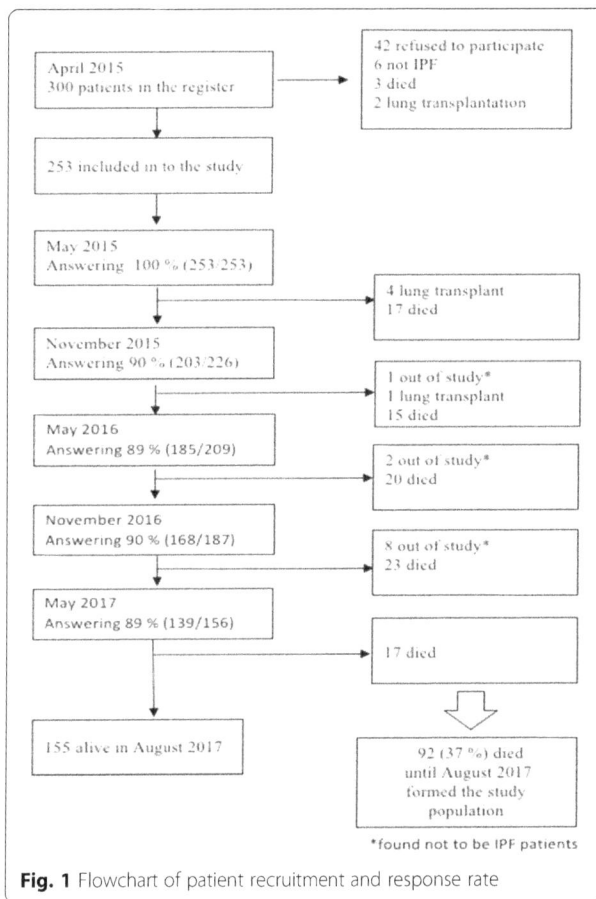

Fig. 1 Flowchart of patient recruitment and response rate

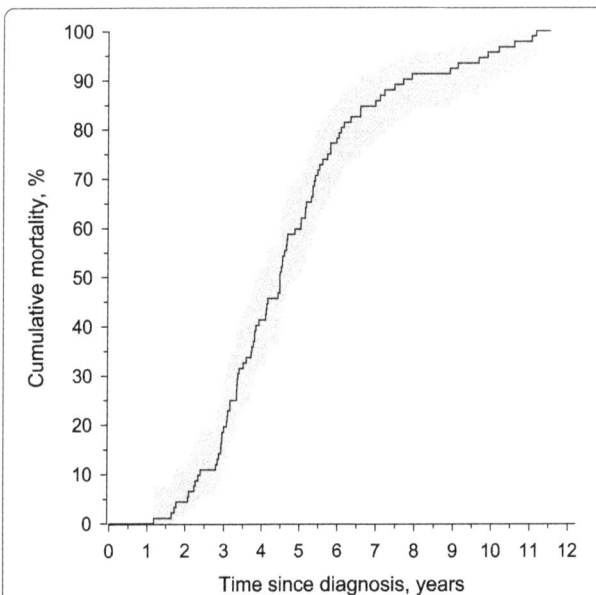

Fig. 2 Cumulative mortality after the diagnosis of IPF. Time-point of the diagnosis is marked with 0 and 95% confidence intervals with the grey area. Kaplan-Meier method was used to estimate the cumulative mortality

Table 1 Patient characteristics

Total number of patients	92
Age, mean (range)	75 (57–92)
Males n (%)	67 (73)
Duration of IPF in years, mean (SD)	3.6 (2.3)
Education in years, mean (SD)	10 (3)
Living alone, n (%)	31 (34)
Working, n (%)	4 (4)
Smoking status, n (%)[a]	
Smoker	6 (7)
Ex-smoker	50 (54)
Never-smoker	36 (39)
FVC (litres), mean (SD)[b]	2.9 (0.8)
FVC (% of predicted), mean (SD)[b]	78 (16)
Diffusion capacity, mean(SD)[c]	54 (13)
Co-morbidities[e], n (%)	
Hypertension	41 (45)
Coronary heart disease	35 (38)
Diabetes	24 (26)
Heart failure	23 (25)
COPD	20 (22)
Cancer	16 (17)
Asthma	8 (9)
No co-morbidities	13 (14)
Number of co-morbidities, median (range)	2 (0–7)
Place of death, n (%)[b]	
Hospital[d]	62 (67)
Home	19 (22)
Nursing home	4 (5)
Hospice	3 (3)

[a]smoking status, forced volume vital capacity (FVC) and diffusion capacity are recorded at the time of diagnosis and other factors at the time of the first questionnaire
[b]Data missing from 4 patients; [c] data missing from 12 patients; [d]10 in intensive care unit; [e] patient-reported co-morbidities

before death. The decline in HRQOL was highly significant in all dimensions except in physical role, which showed very low scores by 24 months before death.

Symptoms

The intensity change of the symptoms measured by the ESAS during the last two years of life is presented in Fig. 4. The intensity of all symptoms except pain at rest and insomnia increased significantly near death. During the last six months of life, the mean NRS scores were as follows: 7.1 (SD 2.8) for breathlessness, 7.0 (SD 2.3) for tiredness, 6.0 (SD 2.5) for wellbeing, 6.0 (SD 3.0) for dry mouth, 5.8 (SD 2.9) for cough, 5.0 (SD 3.5) for pain with movement, 3.9 (SD 3.1) for insomnia, 3.9 (SD 2.9) for

anxiety, 3.8 (SD 2.9) for depression, 3.6 (SD 3.1) for constipation, 3.4 (SD 3.3) for loss of appetite, 3.1 (SD 2.8) for pain at rest and 1.8 (SD 2.5) for nausea.

The steep change in the proportion of patients with MMRC scores ≥3 (needing to stop walking after approximately 100 m or a few minutes because of breathlessness) during the last two years of life is shown in Fig. 5.

Discussion

In this study, we demonstrate a rapidly increasing impairment in HRQOL and escalating symptom burden in IPF patients approaching death. Low HRQOL together with severe breathlessness and fatigue were detected as early as two years before death. In addition, several dimensions of HRQOL declined further and the severity of many symptoms other than dyspnea increased during the last two years of life.

In the present study, HRQOL was considerably impaired two years prior to death in IPF patients. Physical role, i.e., role limitations due to physical health, was exceptionally low, but physical functioning, vitality and general health appeared to be below the general population level as well. Similar to our findings, an Australian registry study of 516 IPF patients reported HRQOL impairments in all domains, with the lowest score in activity, i.e., activities that cause or are limited by breathlessness [27]. The importance of decreased HRQOL was further highlighted in a recent study by Furukawa et al. that demonstrated that low HRQOL was actually an independent prognostic factor [28].

Although previous studies have demonstrated low HRQOL in IPF patients [10–12], none of them focused on the HRQOL from the aspect of approaching death in a follow-up setting. The uniqueness of this study stems from the continuing follow-up until death, and the subsequent finding of a salient decline in HRQOL during the last two years of life that was intensified near death. Deterioration was identified in all domains except physical role, which was already remarkably low two years before death. The most integral impairment was in physical, social and emotional functioning and vitality. In the Australian registry study, approximately one-third (38%) of the IPF patients experienced clinically important differences in the decline of HRQOL during 12 months [27]. However, in that study, no HRQOL data was available from the period preceding death [27].

In lung cancer, functional concerns relating to physical movement or functioning predominate patients' symptom burden throughout the disease course and have a negative impact on HRQOL [42]. In addition, the severity of symptoms escalates, and the number of severe symptoms increases during the last three months of life [42–44]. A steep decline in HRQOL at the end-of-life is

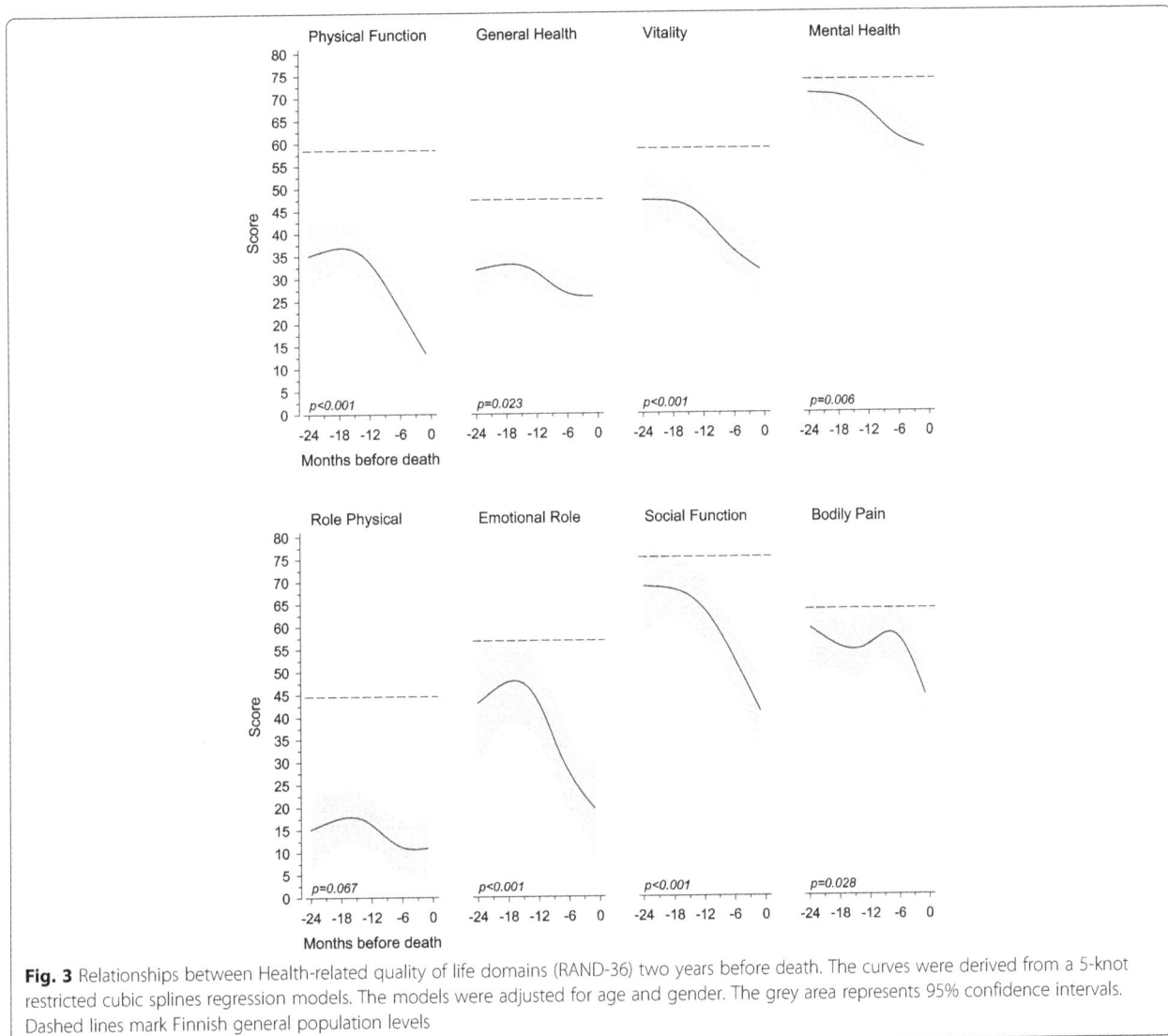

Fig. 3 Relationships between Health-related quality of life domains (RAND-36) two years before death. The curves were derived from a 5-knot restricted cubic splines regression models. The models were adjusted for age and gender. The grey area represents 95% confidence intervals. Dashed lines mark Finnish general population levels

typical in patients dying of cancer compared with other terminally ill patients [45, 46]. In COPD patients, HRQOL gradually declines over time without a steeper decline at the end-of-life [47]. Our data imply that patients with IPF experience gradual impairments in HRQOL comparable to COPD patients but suffer from a pronounced, rapid deterioration in HRQOL during the last year of life, more closely resembling the disease trajectory of cancer.

Our results corroborate earlier findings on dyspnea and cough as the most severe symptoms in IPF patients regardless of the disease phase [10, 21, 27, 48]. The intensity of dyspnea increased during the follow-up, being one of the most severe symptoms before death. In a previous IPF registry study, dyspnea yielded the strongest association with impaired HRQOL accounting for 71% of the variation in HRQOL [27]. In addition,

exertion dyspnoea measured by the MMRC has been shown to correlate to HRQOL and symptom burden [21, 49].

In addition to dyspnea, other activity-limiting symptoms such as fatigue and pain in movement were among the most severe symptoms in our study. These activity-limiting symptoms can lead to physical inactivity and functional impairment, triggering a vicious circle with worse HRQOL. The intensity of depression and anxiety were, however, relatively mild two years before death, although these symptoms increased thereafter. In a recent study, depression was an independent predictor for HRQOL impairment, although it only accounted for 3.5% of the variation, whereas dyspnea accounted for 71% [27]. Our results suggest that the relief of activity-limiting symptoms together with psychosocial support may improve HRQOL in advanced IPF.

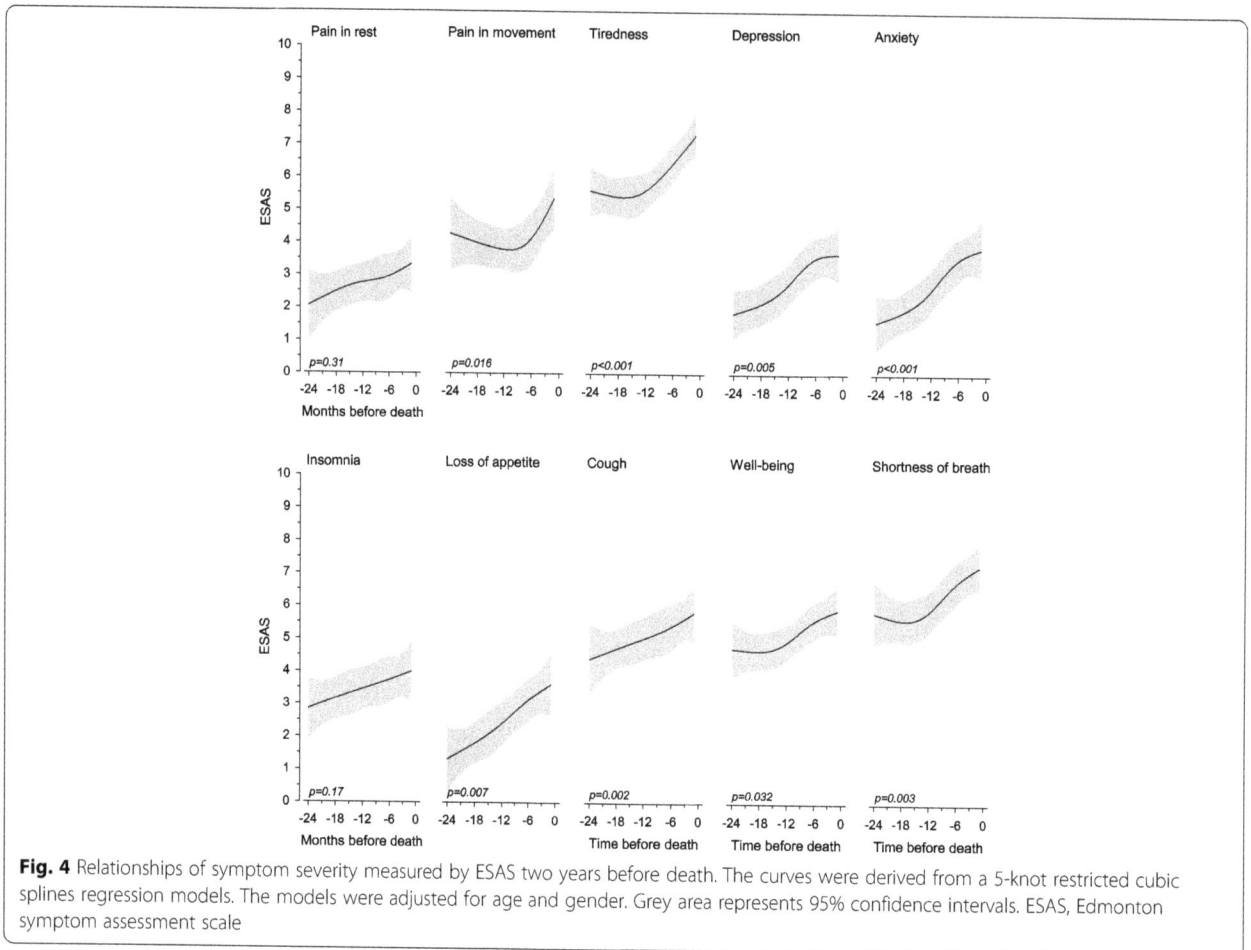

Fig. 4 Relationships of symptom severity measured by ESAS two years before death. The curves were derived from a 5-knot restricted cubic splines regression models. The models were adjusted for age and gender. Grey area represents 95% confidence intervals. ESAS, Edmonton symptom assessment scale

As discussed above, patients with advanced IPF, COPD and lung cancer suffer from a heavy symptom burden and deteriorating HRQOL. This calls for comprehensive symptom management and integrated palliative care concomitant with disease-modifying therapies [21, 27, 47, 50–52]. Early integrated palliative care for patients with lung cancer has shown substantial benefits, such as lower depression scores, higher HRQOL, better communication of end-of-life care preferences, less aggressive care at the end-of-life, and longer overall survival [51, 53]. Similarly, a randomised trial demonstrated better control of dyspnea and a survival benefit with integrated palliative care in patients with COPD and interstitial lung disease [54]. In addition to cancer patients, early integrated palliative care may reduce end-of-life acute care utilisation, and allow patients with IPF to die in their preferred locations [55–58]. Integrated palliative care in IPF patients seems to lower respiratory-related emergency room visits and hospitalisations and may allow more patients to die at home [55]. In this study, 67% of patients died in hospital and 11% in intensive care, which is in line with earlier findings, implying the

necessity of improvements in advanced care planning and palliative care of patients with IPF [55, 59]. Our results provide insight into the most important needs of end-stage IPF patients and support the use of early-integrated palliative care, which should include symptom control beyond treatment for dyspnea and psychosocial support.

The relatively small study population limits our study, as did not having systematic follow-up data on lung function, which is at least partially due to the poor conditions of many of our patients. Our study is to our knowledge first to present follow-up data of HRQOL and symptoms for over two years before death. The strength is its real-life longitudinal design, with a unique cohort of IPF patients approaching death with an outstanding response rate, particularly considering the fact that some of the patients were probably too weak to respond during their final days or weeks of life. To our knowledge, this is the first study describing comprehensive patient-reported data on the HRQOL and symptom burden of IPF patients from the perspective of approaching death.

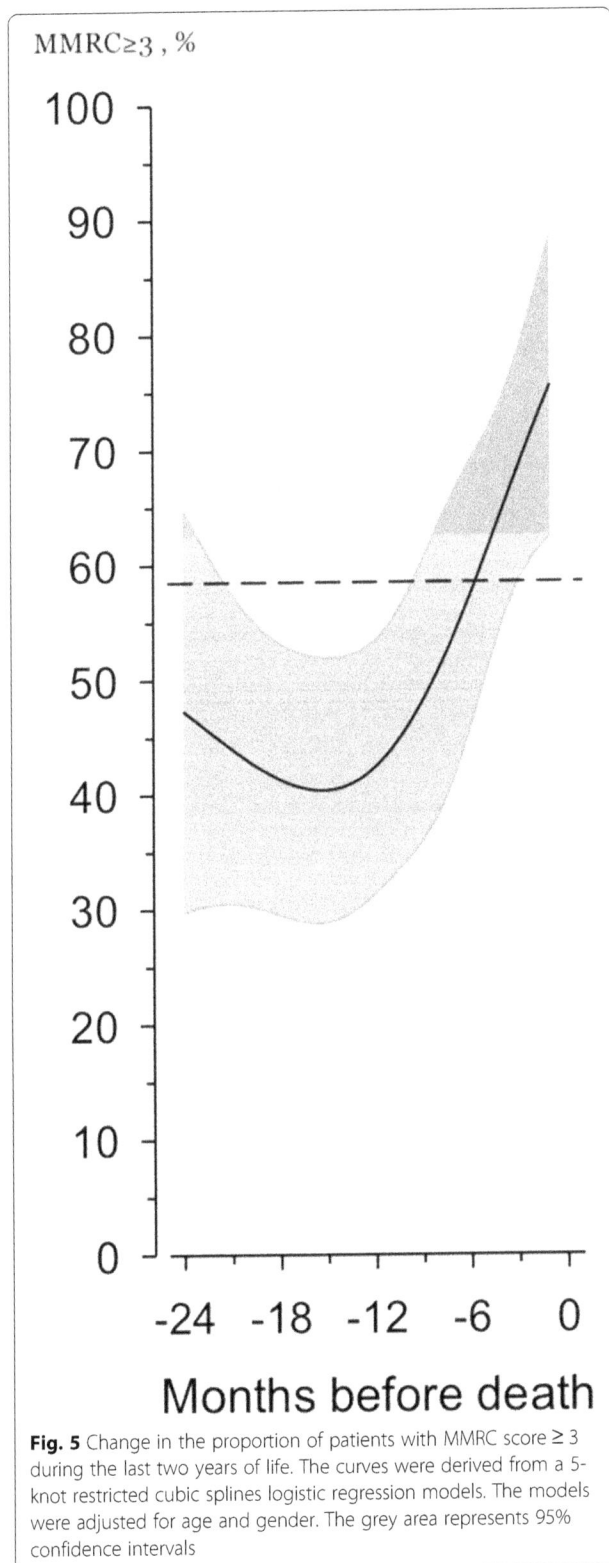

Fig. 5 Change in the proportion of patients with MMRC score ≥ 3 during the last two years of life. The curves were derived from a 5-knot restricted cubic splines logistic regression models. The models were adjusted for age and gender. The grey area represents 95% confidence intervals

Conclusion

Patients with IPF suffer from exceptionally low HRQOL together with severe breathlessness and fatigue already two years before death. In addition, physical and emotional wellbeing further deteriorates near death concurrently with escalating overall symptom burden. In clinical practice, structured measurements of HRQOL and symptoms are necessary to guide high-quality early-integrated palliative care and end-of-life planning in IPF patients.

Acknowledgements
We are grateful for the patients that consented in participating this study. The authors express gratitude to the participants of the FinnishIPF consortium: Kaarteenaho R, Saarelainen S, Kankaanranta H, Böök A, Salomaa ER, Kaunisto J, Hodgson U and Purokivi M. The authors are also immensely grateful to the numerous pulmonary physicians, who have contributed to the study by including patients and asking for informed consents: Vaden J, Pekonen M, Tapanainen H, Lajunen H, Saarinen A, Suuronen U, Lammi L, Lehtonen K, Männistö J, Salmi I, Torkko M, Torkko P, Erkkilä M, Andersen H, Jaakkola J, Rinne H, Alho M-L, Pietiläinen M, Toljamo T, Palomäki M, Nylund E, Ahonen E, Impola P, Saviaro S, Pusa L, Vilkman S, Ekroos H, Vuori P Hedman J, Lahti M and Mursu A.

Funding
The Academy of Finland, Sigrid Jusélius Foundation, Foundation of the Finnish Anti-Tuberculosis Association, Governmental subsidy for health sciences research have supported Lung Factor research group. Kaisa Rajala has received grants mentioned on conflicts of interest.

Authors' contributions
Study design: KR, JL, ES, TS, MM. Data Collection: KR, ES, MM. Data analysis: KR, JL, ES, TS, MM, HK. Written report: KR, JL, ES, TS, MM, HK. All authors read and approved the final manuscript. KR takes responsibility of the whole work.

Competing interests
Kaisa Rajala has received grants from Foundation of the Finnish Anti-Tuberculosis Association, Helsinki University Hospital Comprehensive Cancer Center and Väinö and Laina Kivi foundation. Other authors have no conflicts of interest affecting this work.

Author details
[1]Department of Palliative Care, Comprehensive Cancer Center,, Helsinki University Hospital, Paciuksenkatu 21, Po BOX 180, FI-00290 Helsinki, Finland. [2]Faculty of Medicine, University of Helsinki, Helsinki, Finland. [3]Department of Oncology, Palliative Care Unit, Tampere University Hospital and Faculty of Medicine and Life Sciences, University of Tampere, Tampere, Finland. [4]Faculty of Medicine, University of Helsinki, Helsinki, Finland. [5]Primary Health Care Unit, Kuopio University Hospital, Finland and Folkhälsan Research Center, Helsinki, Finland. [6]University of Helsinki and Helsinki University Hospital, Heart and Lung Center, Department of Pulmonary Medicine, Helsinki, Finland. [7]Helsinki University Hospital, Comprehensive Cancer Center, Department of Palliative Care and Faculty of Medicine, University of Helsinki, Helsinki, Finland.

References

1. Raghu G, Collard HR, Egan JJ, Martinez FJ, Behr J, Brown KK, et al. An official ATS/ERS/JRS/ALAT statement: idiopathic pulmonary fibrosis: evidence-based guidelines for diagnosis and management. Am J Respir Crit Care Med. 2011 Mar;183(6):788–824.

2. Kaunisto J, Kelloniemi K, Sutinen E, Hodgson U, Piilonen A, Kaarteenaho R, et al. Re-evaluation of diagnostic parameters is crucial for obtaining accurate data on idiopathic pulmonary fibrosis. BMC Pulm Med [Internet]. 2015;15:92 Available from: https://doi.org/10.1186/s12890-015-0074-3.

3. Richeldi L, du Bois RM, Raghu G, Azuma A, Brown KK, Costabel U, et al. Efficacy and safety of Nintedanib in idiopathic pulmonary fibrosis. N Engl J Med [Internet]. 2014;370(22):2071–82 Available from: https://www.nejm.org/doi/abs/10.1056/NEJMoa1402584.

4. King TE, Bradford WZ, Castro-Bernardini S, Fagan EA, Glaspole I, Glassberg MK, et al. A phase 3 trial of Pirfenidone in patients with idiopathic pulmonary fibrosis. N Engl J Med [Internet]. 2014;370(22):2083–92 Available from: http://www.nejm.org/doi/10.1056/NEJMoa1402582.

5. Behr J, Richeldi L. Recommendations on treatment for IPF. Respir Res [Internet]. 2013;14(Suppl. 1):S6 Available from: http://respiratory-research.com/content/14/S1/S6.

6. Raghu G, Rochwerg B, Zhang Y, Garcia CAC, Azuma A, Behr J, et al. An official ATS/ERS/JRS/ALAT clinical practice guideline: treatment of idiopathic pulmonary fibrosis: an update of the 2011 clinical practice guideline. Am J Respir Crit Care Med. 2015;192(2):e3–19.

7. Kalluri M, Richman-Eisenstat J. Early and integrated palliative care to achieve a home death in idiopathic pulmonary fibrosis. J Pain Symptom Manage [Internet]. 2017;53(6):1111–5 Available from: https://doi.org/10.1016/j.jpainsymman.2016.12.344.

8. Raghu G, Richeldi L. Current approaches to the management of idiopathic pulmonary fibrosis. Respir Med [Internet]. 2017;129:24–30 Available from: https://doi.org/10.1016/j.rmed.2017.05.017.

9. Caminati A, Cassandro R, Torre O, Harari S. Severe idiopathic pulmonary fibrosis: What can be done? Eur Respir Rev [Internet]. 2017;26(145) Available from: https://doi.org/10.1183/16000617.0047-2017.

10. Ahmadi Z, Wysham NG, Lundström S, Janson C, Currow DC, Ekström M. End-of-life care in oxygen-dependent ILD compared with lung cancer: a national population-based study. Thorax [Internet]. 2016;71(6):510–6 Available from: http://thorax.bmj.com/lookup/doi/10.1136/thoraxjnl-2015-207439.

11. Tomioka H, Imanaka K, Hashimoto K, Iwasaki H. Health-related quality of life in patients with idiopathic pulmonary fibrosis -cross-sectional and longitudinal study. Intern Med [Internet] 2007;46(18):1533–1542. Available from: http://joi.jlc.jst.go.jp/JST.JSTAGE/internalmedicine/46.6218?from=CrossRef%5Cn. http://www.ncbi.nlm.nih.gov/pubmed/17878639.

12. Richeldi L, Cottin V, du Bois RM, Selman M, Kimura T, Bailes Z, et al. Nintedanib in patients with idiopathic pulmonary fibrosis: combined evidence from the TOMORROW and INPULSIS?? trials. Respir Med. 2015;113:74–9.

13. Kreuter M, Swigris J, Pittrow D, Geier S, Klotsche J, Prasse A, et al. Health related quality of life in patients with idiopathic pulmonary fibrosis in clinical practice: insights-IPF registry. Respir Res [Internet]. 2017;18(1):139 Available from: http://respiratory-research.biomedcentral.com/articles/10.1186/s12931-017-0621-y.

14. Hubbard RB, Smith C, Le Jeune I, Gribbin J, Fogarty AW. The association between idiopathic pulmonary fibrosis and vascular disease: a population-based study. Am J Respir Crit Care Med. 2008;178(12):1257–61.

15. Kreuter M, Ehlers-Tenenbaum S, Palmowski K, Bruhwyler J, Oltmanns U, Muley T, et al. Impact of comorbidities on mortality in patients with idiopathic pulmonary fibrosis. PLoS One. 2016;11(3):1–18.

16. Hyldgaard C, Hilberg O, Bendstrup E. How does comorbidity influence survival in idiopathic pulmonary fibrosis? Respir Med [Internet]. 2014;108(4):647–53 Available from: https://doi.org/10.1016/j.rmed.2014.01.008.

17. Nathan SD, Basavaraj A, Reichner C, Shlobin OA, Ahmad S, Kiernan J, et al. Prevalence and impact of coronary artery disease in idiopathic pulmonary fibrosis. Respir Med [Internet]. 2010;104(7):1035–41 Available from: https://doi.org/10.1016/j.rmed.2010.02.008.

18. King CS, Nathan SD. Idiopathic pulmonary fibrosis: effects and optimal management of comorbidities. Lancet Respir Med. 2017;5(1):72–84.

19. Buendía-Roldán I, Mejía M, Navarro C, Selman M. Idiopathic pulmonary fibrosis: clinical behavior and aging associated comorbidities. Respir Med. 2017;129:46–52.

20. Bajwah S, Higginson IJ, Ross JR, Wells AU, Birring SS, Riley J, et al. The palliative care needs for fibrotic interstitial lung disease: a qualitative study of patients, informal caregivers and health professionals. Palliat Med [Internet]. 2013;27(9):869–76 Available from: http://www.ncbi.nlm.nih.gov/pubmed/23885010

21. Yount SE, Beaumont JL, Chen S-Y, Kaiser K, Wortman K, Van Brunt DL, et al. Health-related quality of life in patients with idiopathic pulmonary fibrosis. Lung [Internet]. 2016;194(2):227–34 Available from: http://link.springer.com/10.1007/s00408-016-9850-y.

22. Ryerson CJ, Berkeley J, Carrieri-Kohlman VL, Pantilat SZ, Landefeld CS, Collard HR. Depression and functional status are strongly associated with dyspnea in interstitial lung disease. Chest. 2011;139(3):609–16.

23. Akhtar AA, Ali MA. Smith RP. Chron Respir Dis: Depression in patients with idiopathic pulmonary fibrosis; 2013.

24. Matsuda T, Taniguchi H, Ando M, Kondoh Y, Kimura T, Kataoka K, et al. Depression is significantly associated with the health status in patients with idiopathic pulmonary fibrosis. Intern Med [Internet]. 2017;56(13):1637–44 Available from: http://www.ncbi.nlm.nih.gov/pubmed/27274328.

25. van Manen MJG, Geelhoed JJM, Tak NC, Wijsenbeek MS. Optimizing quality of life in patients with idiopathic pulmonary fibrosis. Ther Adv Respir Dis [Internet]. 2017;11(3):157–69 Available from: https://www.ncbi.nlm.nih.gov/pmc/articles/PMC5933652/.

26. Lee YJ, Choi SM, Lee YJ, Cho Y-J, Il YH, Lee J-H, et al. Clinical impact of depression and anxiety in patients with idiopathic pulmonary fibrosis. PLoS One [Internet]. 2017;12(9):e0184300 Available from: http://dx.plos.org/10.1371/journal.pone.0184300.

27. Glaspole IN, Chapman SA, Cooper WA, Ellis SJ, Goh NS, Hopkins PM, et al. Health-related quality of life in idiopathic pulmonary fibrosis: data from the Australian IPF registry. Respirology. 2017;22(5):950–6.

28. Furukawa T, Taniguchi H, Ando M, Kondoh Y, Kataoka K, Nishiyama O, et al. The St. George's Respiratory Questionnaire as a prognostic factor in IPF. Respir Res [Internet]. 2017;18(1):18 Available from: http://respiratory-research.biomedcentral.com/articles/10.1186/s12931-017-0503-3.

29. Hays RD, Morales LS. The RAND-36 measure of health-related quality of life, Ann Med [Internet]. 2001;33(5):350–7 Available from: http://www.ncbi.nlm.nih.gov/pubmed/11491194.

30. Aalto AM, Aro AR, Teperi J. RAND-36 terveyteen liittyvan elamanlaadun mittarina. Mittarin luotettavuus ja suomalaiset vaestoarvot. Stakes, Sos ja terveysalan tutkimus- ja Kehitt tutkimuksia. 1999;101:78.

31. Swigris JJ, Olson AL, Brown KK. Understanding and optimizing health-related quality of life and physical functional capacity in idiopathic pulmonary fibrosis. Patient Relat Outcome Meas [Internet]. 2016;7:29 Available from: https://www.ncbi.nlm.nih.gov/pmc/articles/PMC5519463/.

32. Swigris JJ, Brown KK, Behr J, du Bois RM, King TE, Raghu G, et al. The SF-36 and SGRQ: validity and first look at minimum important differences in IPF. Respir Med [Internet]. 2010;104(2):296–304 Available from: https://doi.org/10.1016/j.rmed.2009.09.006.

33. Mahler DA, Wells CK. Evaluation of clinical for rating dyspnea. Chest. 1988; 93:580–6.

34. Bestall JC, Paul EA, Garrod R, Garnham R, Jones PW, Wedzicha JA. Usefulness of the Medical Research Council (MRC) dyspnoea scale as a measure of disability in patients with chronic obstructive pulmonary disease. Thorax [Internet]. 1999;54(7):581–6 Available from: http://www.pubmedcentral.nih.gov/articlerender.fcgi?artid=1745516&tool=pmcentrez&rendertype=abstract.

35. Bruera E, Kuehn N, Miller MJ, Selmser P, Macmillan K. The Edmonton symptom assessment system (ESAS): a simple method for the assessment of palliative care patients. J Palliat Care. 1991;7(2):6–9.

36. Hui D, Bruera E. The Edmonton symptom assessment system 25 years later: past, present, and future developments. J Pain Symptom Manage [Internet]. 2017;53(3):630–43 Available from: https://doi.org/10.1016/j.jpainsymman.2016.10.370.

37. Chang VT, Hwang SS, Feuerman M. Validation of the Edmonton symptom assessment scale. Cancer. 2000;88(9):2164–71.

38. Hannon B, Dyck M, Pope A, Swami N, Banerjee S, Mak E, et al. Modified Edmonton symptom assessment system including constipation and sleep: validation in outpatients with cancer. J Pain Symptom Manage [Internet]. 2015; 49(5):945–52 Available from: https://doi.org/10.1016/j.jpainsymman.2014.10.013.

39. Oldenmenger WH, De Raaf PJ, De Klerk C, Van Der Rijt CCD. Cut points on 0-10 numeric rating scales for symptoms included in the Edmonton symptom assessment scale in cancer patients: a systematic review. J Pain Symptom Manage [Internet]. 2013;45(6):1083–93 Available from: https://doi.org/10.1016/j.jpainsymman.2012.06.007.

40. Harrell F. Regression modeling strategies with applications to linear models, logistic regression, and survival analysis. New York: Springer Series in Statistics; 2001.

41. StataCorp LP; Collage Station, Texas, USA; 2017.

42. LeBlanc TW, Nickolich M, Rushing CN, Samsa GP, Locke SC, Abernethy AP. What bothers lung cancer patients the most? A prospective, longitudinal electronic patient-reported outcomes study in advanced non-small cell lung cancer. Support Care Cancer. 2015;23(12):3455–63.

43. Iyer S, Taylor-Stokes G, Roughley A. Symptom burden and quality of life in advanced non-small cell lung cancer patients in France and Germany. Lung Cancer [Internet]. 2013;81(2):288–93 Available from: https://doi.org/10.1016/j.lungcan.2013.03.008.

44. Brown S, Thorpe H, Napp V, Brown J. Closeness to death and quality of life in advanced lung Cancer patients. Clin Oncol. 2007;19(5):341–8.

45. ManLois Downey MA, Ruth A, Engelberg RA. Quality-of-Life Trajectories at the End of Life: Assessments Over Time by Patients with and without Cancer. J Am Geriatr Soc. 2011;58(3):472–9.

46. Teno JM, Weitzen S, Fennell ML, Mor V. Dying trajectory in the last year of life: does Cancer trajectory fit other diseases? J Palliat Med [Internet]. 2001; 4(4):457–64 Available from: https://www.ncbi.nlm.nih.gov/pubmed/?term=teno+2001+Dying+trajectory+in+the+last+year+of+life%3A+does+Cancer+trajectory+fit+other+diseases.

47. Habraken JM, van der Wal WM, ter Riet G, Weersink EJM, Toben F, Bindels PJE. Health-related quality of life and functional status in end-stage COPD: a longitudinal study. Eur Respir J [Internet]. 2011;37(2):280–8 Available from: http://erj.ersjournals.com/cgi/doi/10.1183/09031936.00149309.

48. Behr J, Kreuter M, Hoeper MM, Wirtz H, Klotsche J, Kosche D, et al. Management of patients with idiopathic pulmonary fibrosis in clinical practice: the INSIGHTS-IPF registry. Eur Respir J [Internet]. 2015;46(1):186–96 Available from: https://doi.org/10.1183/09031936.00217614.

49. Rajala K, Lehto JT, Sutinen E, Kautiainen H, Myllärniemi M, Saarto T. mMRC dyspnoea scale indicates impaired quality of life and increased pain in patients with idiopathic pulmonary fibrosis. ERJ Open Res [Internet]. 2017; 3(4):00084–2017 Available from: http://openres.ersjournals.com/lookup/doi/10.1183/23120541.00084-2017.

50. Mohan A, Singh P, Singh S, Goyal A, Pathak A, Mohan C, et al. Quality of life in lung cancer patients: impact of baseline clinical profile and respiratory status: original article. Eur J Cancer Care (Engl). 2007;16(3):268–76.

51. Temel JS, Greer JA, Muzikansky A, Gallagher ER, Admane S, Jackson VA, et al. Early palliative Care for Patients with metastatic non–small-cell lung Cancer. N Engl J Med [Internet]. 2010;363(8):733–42 Available from: http://www.nejm.org/doi/abs/10.1056/NEJMoa1000678.

52. Rajala K, Lehto JT, Saarinen M, Sutinen E, Saarto T, Myllärniemi M. End-of-life care of patients with idiopathic pulmonary fibrosis. BMC Palliat Care [Internet]. 2016;15(1):85 Available from: http://www.ncbi.nlm.nih.gov/pubmed/27729035.

53. Temel JS, Greer JA, El-Jawahri A, Pirl WF, Park ER, Jackson VA, et al. Effects of early integrated palliative care in patients with lung and gi cancer: a randomized clinical trial. J Clin Oncol. 2017;35(8):834–41.

54. Higginson IJ, Bausewein C, Reilly CC, Gao W, Gysels M, Dzingina M, et al. An integrated palliative and respiratory care service for patients with advanced disease and refractory breathlessness: a randomised controlled trial. Lancet Respir Med [Internet]. 2014;2(12):979–87 Available from: https://doi.org/10.1016/S2213-2600(14)70226-7.

55. Kalluri M, Claveria F, Ainsley E, Haggag M, Armijo-Olivo S, Richman-Eisenstat J. Beyond Idiopathic Pulmonary Fibrosis diagnosis: Multidisciplinary care with an early integrated palliative approach is associated with a decrease in acute care utilization and hospital deaths. J Pain Symptom Manage [Internet]. 2017; Available from: http://www.ncbi.nlm.nih.gov/pubmed/29101086.

56. Bakitas MA, Tosteson TD, Li Z, Lyons KD, Hull JG, Li Z, et al. Early versus delayed initiation of concurrent palliative oncology care: patient outcomes in the ENABLE III randomized controlled trial. J Clin Oncol. 2015;33(13):1438–45.

57. Marie B, Balan S, Brokaw FC, Seville J, Jay G. The project ENABLE II randomized controlled trial to improve palliative Care for Patients with advanced Cancer. JAMA. 2009;302(7):741–9.

58. Zimmermann C, Swami N, Krzyzanowska M, Hannon B, Leighl N, Oza A, et al. Early palliative care for patients with advanced cancer: a cluster-randomised controlled trial. Lancet. 2014;383(9930):1721–30.

59. Lindell KO, Nouraie M, Klesen MJ, Klein S, Gibson KF, Kass DJ, et al. Randomised clinical trial of an early palliative care intervention (SUPPORT) for patients with idiopathic pulmonary fibrosis (IPF) and their caregivers: protocol and key design considerations. BMJ Open Respir Res [Internet]. 2018;5(1):e000272 Available from: http://bmjopenrespres.bmj.com/lookup/doi/10.1136/bmjresp-2017-000272.

Permissions

All chapters in this book were first published in PM, by BioMed Central; hereby published with permission under the Creative Commons Attribution License or equivalent. Every chapter published in this book has been scrutinized by our experts. Their significance has been extensively debated. The topics covered herein carry significant findings which will fuel the growth of the discipline. They may even be implemented as practical applications or may be referred to as a beginning point for another development.

The contributors of this book come from diverse backgrounds, making this book a truly international effort. This book will bring forth new frontiers with its revolutionizing research information and detailed analysis of the nascent developments around the world.

We would like to thank all the contributing authors for lending their expertise to make the book truly unique. They have played a crucial role in the development of this book. Without their invaluable contributions this book wouldn't have been possible. They have made vital efforts to compile up to date information on the varied aspects of this subject to make this book a valuable addition to the collection of many professionals and students.

This book was conceptualized with the vision of imparting up-to-date information and advanced data in this field. To ensure the same, a matchless editorial board was set up. Every individual on the board went through rigorous rounds of assessment to prove their worth. After which they invested a large part of their time researching and compiling the most relevant data for our readers.

The editorial board has been involved in producing this book since its inception. They have spent rigorous hours researching and exploring the diverse topics which have resulted in the successful publishing of this book. They have passed on their knowledge of decades through this book. To expedite this challenging task, the publisher supported the team at every step. A small team of assistant editors was also appointed to further simplify the editing procedure and attain best results for the readers.

Apart from the editorial board, the designing team has also invested a significant amount of their time in understanding the subject and creating the most relevant covers. They scrutinized every image to scout for the most suitable representation of the subject and create an appropriate cover for the book.

The publishing team has been an ardent support to the editorial, designing and production team. Their endless efforts to recruit the best for this project, has resulted in the accomplishment of this book. They are a veteran in the field of academics and their pool of knowledge is as vast as their experience in printing. Their expertise and guidance has proved useful at every step. Their uncompromising quality standards have made this book an exceptional effort. Their encouragement from time to time has been an inspiration for everyone.

The publisher and the editorial board hope that this book will prove to be a valuable piece of knowledge for researchers, students, practitioners and scholars across the globe.

List of Contributors

Jodie Birch
Institute of Cellular Medicine, Newcastle University, M2060 Leech Building, The Medical School, Framlington Place, Newcastle upon Tyne NE2 4HH, UK

Katy L. M. Hester and Anthony De Soyza
Institute of Cellular Medicine, Newcastle University, M2060 Leech Building, The Medical School, Framlington Place, Newcastle upon Tyne NE2 4HH, UK
Sir William Leech Centre for lung research, The Freeman Hospital, High Heaton, Newcastle upon Tyne Hospitals NHS Foundation Trust, Newcastle upon Tyne NE7 7DN, UK

Andrew J. Fisher and Paul A. Corris
Institute of Cellular Medicine, Newcastle University, M2060 Leech Building, The Medical School, Framlington Place, Newcastle upon Tyne NE2 4HH, UK Institute of Transplantation, The Freeman Hospital, High Heaton, Newcastle upon Tyne Hospitals NHS Foundation Trust, Newcastle upon Tyne NE7 7DN, UK

Syba S. Sunny
Sir William Leech Centre for lung research, The Freeman Hospital, High Heaton, Newcastle upon Tyne Hospitals NHS Foundation Trust, Newcastle upon Tyne NE7 7DN, UK

F. Kate Gould
Department of Medical Microbiology, The Freeman Hospital, High Heaton, Newcastle upon Tyne Hospitals NHS Foundation Trust, Newcastle upon Tyne NE7 7DN, UK

Gareth Parry, John H. Dark, Stephen C. Clark, Gerard Meachery and James Lordan
Institute of Transplantation, The Freeman Hospital, High Heaton, Newcastle upon Tyne Hospitals NHS Foundation Trust, Newcastle upon Tyne NE7 7DN, UK

Erica Lin
Department of Internal Medicine, 200 First St. SW, Rochester, MN 55905, USA

Andrew H. Limper and Teng Moua
Division of Pulmonary and Critical Care Medicine, Mayo Clinic, 200 First St. SW, Rochester, MN 55905, USA

Hans Hedenström and Andrei Malinovschi
Department of Medical Sciences, Clinical Physiology, Uppsala University Hospital, SE-751 85 Uppsala, Sweden

Amir Farkhooy
Department of Medical Sciences, Clinical Physiology, Uppsala University Hospital, SE-751 85 Uppsala, Sweden
Department of Medical Sciences: Respiratory, Allergy and Sleep Research, Uppsala University, Uppsala, Sweden

Christer Janson
Department of Medical Sciences: Respiratory, Allergy and Sleep Research, Uppsala University, Uppsala, Sweden

Johan Bodegård
Department of Cardiology, Oslo University Hospital, Ullevaal, Norway

Jan Erik Erikssen
Faculty of Medicine, University of Oslo, Oslo, Norway

Knut Stavem
Institute of Clinical Medicine, University of Oslo, Lørenskog, Norway
Department of Pulmonary Medicine, Medical Division, Akershus University Hospital, Lørenskog, Norway
Health Services Research Unit, Akershus University Hospital, Lørenskog, Norway

Mohammad Alsumrain and Jay H. Ryu
Division of Pulmonary and Critical Care Medicine, Gonda 18 South, Mayo Clinic, 200 First St. SW, Rochester, MN 55905, USA

Gisela Hovold, Fredrik Kahn and Lisa I. Påhlman
Department of Clinical Sciences Lund, Division of Infection Medicine, BMC B14, Lund University, Skåne University Hospital, Tornavägen 10, SE-22184 Lund, Sweden

Victoria Palmcrantz
Skåne University Hospital, Clinic of Paediatrics, Lund, Sweden

Arne Egesten
Department of Clinical Sciences Lund, Respiratory Medicine and Allergology, Lund University, Lund, Sweden

Yinfeng Kong, Zhijun Li, Tingyu Tang, Haiyan Wu, Juan Liu, Liang Gu, Tian Zhao and Qingdong Huang
Department of Respiratory Medicine in Zhejiang Hospital, 12 Lingyin Road, Xihu District, Hangzhou 310013, Zhejiang Province, China

Hong-xia Wu, Xiao-feng Xiong, Min Zhu and De-yun Cheng
Department of Respiratory and Critical Care Medicine, West China Hospital, Sichuan University, NO.37 Guoxue Alley, Chengdu 610041, Sichuan, China

Jia Wei
Department of Respiratory Medicine, Chengdu Second People's Hospital, Chengdu, China

Kai-quan Zhuo
Department of Neurosurgery, Suining Municipal Hospital of TCM, Suining, China

William D. Cornwell, Gerard J. Criner and Thomas J. Rogers
Center for Inflammation, Translational and Clinical Lung Research, Lewis Katz School of Medicine, Temple University, Philadelphia, PA 19140, USA
Department of Thoracic Medicine and Surgery, Lewis Katz School of Medicine, Temple University, Philadelphia, PA 19140, USA

Victor Kim and Marie Elena Vega
Department of Thoracic Medicine and Surgery, Lewis Katz School of Medicine, Temple University, Philadelphia, PA 19140, USA

Xiaoxuan Fan
Temple University Flow Cytometry Facility, Lewis Katz School of Medicine, Temple University, Philadelphia, PA 19140, USA

Frederick V. Ramsey
Department of Clinical Sciences, Lewis Katz School of Medicine, Temple University, Philadelphia, PA 19140, USA

Shibo Wu
Department of Respiratory Medicine, Lihuili Hospital, Ningbo Medical Center, No. 57, Xin'ning Road, Ningbo 315041, China

Kaitai Liu
Department of Radiation Oncology, Lihuili Hospital, Ningbo Medical Center, Ningbo 315041, China

Feng Ren
Department of Radiology, Lihuili Hospital, Ningbo Medical Center, Ningbo 315041, China

Dawei Zheng
Department of Thoracic Surgery, Lihuili Hospital, Ningbo Medical Center, Ningbo 315041, China

Deng Pan
Department of Diagnosis, Ningbo Diagnostic Pathology Center, No. 79, Huan'cheng Road, Ningbo 315021, China

Shilpa Dogra and Joshua Good
Faculty of Health Sciences (Kinesiology), University of Ontario Institute of Technology, 2000 Simcoe St N, Oshawa, ON L1H-7K4, Canada

Matthew P. Buman
College of Health Solutions, Arizona State University, 550 N 3rd Street, Phoenix, AZ 85004, USA

Paul A. Gardiner
Faculty of Medicine, The University of Queensland, Level 2, Building 33, Princess Alexandra Hospital, Woolloongabba, QLD 4102, Australia

Jennifer L. Copeland
Department of Kinesiology and Physical Education, University of Lethbridge, 4401 University Drive, Lethbridge, AB T1K 3M4, Canada

Michael K. Stickland
Faculty of Medicine and Dentistry, University of Alberta, and G.F. Macdonald Centre for Lung Health, 3-135 Clinical Sciences Building, 11304 - 83 Avenue, Edmonton, Alberta T6G 2J3, Canada

Bassel Mourad
Respiratory Cellular and Molecular Biology, Woolcock Institute of Medical Research, The University of Sydney, Sydney, NSW 2006, Australia
Molecular Biosciences, School of Life Sciences, University of Technology Sydney, Building 4, 15 Broadway, Ultimo, NSW 2007, Australia

Alicia B. Mitchell
Respiratory Cellular and Molecular Biology, Woolcock Institute of Medical Research, The University of Sydney, Sydney, NSW 2006, Australia
Department of Respiratory Medicine, Concord Repatriation General Hospital, Concord, NSW 2139, Australia
Molecular Biosciences, School of Life Sciences, University of Technology Sydney, Building 4, 15 Broadway, Ultimo, NSW 2007, Australia

Brian G. G. Oliver
Respiratory Cellular and Molecular Biology, Woolcock Institute of Medical Research, The University of Sydney, Sydney, NSW 2006, Australia

Molecular Biosciences, School of Life Sciences, University of Technology Sydney, Building 4, 15 Broadway, Ultimo, NSW 2007, Australia
Centre for Health Technologies, University of Technology Sydney, Sydney, NSW 2007, Australia
Emphysema Centre, Woolcock Institute of Medical Research, The University of Sydney, Sydney, NSW 2006, Australia

Lachlan Buddle
Department of Respiratory Medicine, Concord Repatriation General Hospital, Concord, NSW 2139, Australia

Matthew J. Peters and Lucy C. Morgan
Department of Respiratory Medicine, Concord Repatriation General Hospital, Concord, NSW 2139, Australia
Concord Clinical School, University of Sydney, Sydney, NSW 2006, Australia

Domenico Acanfora, Mauro Carone, Chiara Acanfora, Giuseppe Piscosquito and Marialaura Longobardi
Maugeri Scientific Clinical Institutes, SpA SB, Institute of Care and Scientific Research, Rehabilitation Institute of TeleseTerme, Benevento, Italy

Pietro Scicchitano, Annapaola Zito, Ilaria Dentamaro and Marco Matteo Ciccone
Section of Cardiovascular Diseases, Department of Emergency and Organ Transplantation, School of Medicine, University of Bari, Bari, Italy

Roberto Maestri
Maugeri Scientific Clinical Institutes, SpA SB, Institute of Care and Scientific Research, Rehabilitation Institute of Montescano, Pavia, Italy

Gerardo Casucci
San Francesco Hospital-TeleseTerme, Telese, BN, Italy

Raffaele Antonelli-Incalzi
Institute of Internal Medicine, Chair of Geriatry, Policlinico Gemelli, School of Medicine, Rome, Italy

Won-Il Choi, Hyun Jung Kim, Sun Hyo Park and Jae Seok Park
Department of Internal Medicine, Keimyung University Dongsan Hospital, Daegu 41931, Republic of Korea

Sonila Dauti
Department of Internal Medicine, Keimyung University Dongsan Hospital, Daegu 41931, Republic of Korea
Department of Allergology, Hospital Serive of Kavaje, Kavaje, Albania

Choong Won Lee
Department of Occupational and Environmental Medicine, Sungso Hospital, Andong, Republic of Korea

Sabrina Carvajalino
Fundación Santa Fé de Bogotá, Bogotá, Colombia

Carla Reigada and Miriam J. Johnson
Hull York Medical School, Hertford Building, University of Hull, Hull, UK

Mendwas Dzingina and Sabrina Bajwah
Cicely Saunders Institute, Bessemer Rd, London, UK

Fen Yang, Yuncui Wang, Hui Hu and Zhenfang Xiong
School of Nursing, Hubei University of Chinese Medicine, Wuhan, China

Chongming Yang
Research Support Center, Brigham Young University, Provo, UT, USA

Kaitlyn A. Barrow, Maria P. White, Lucille M. Rich and Maryam Naushab
Center for Immunity and Immunotherapies, Seattle Children's Research Institute, Seattle, WA, USA

Stephen R. Reeves and Jason S. Debley
Center for Immunity and Immunotherapies, Seattle Children's Research Institute, Seattle, WA, USA
Pulmonary and Sleep Medicine Division, Department of Pediatrics, University of Washington, Seattle, WA, USA

Lu Bai and Youmin Guo
Department of Radiology, Xi'an Jiaotong University Medical College First Affiliated Hospital, Xi'an, China

Xia Wei
Department of Radiology, Xi'an Jiaotong University Medical College First Affiliated Hospital, Xi'an, China
Department of Respiratory Medicine, The Ninth Hospital of Xi'an Affiliated Hospital of Xi'an Jiaotong University, Xi'an, China

Qi Ding, Jingting Ren and Jiuyun Mi
Department of Respiratory Medicine, The Ninth Hospital of Xi'an Affiliated Hospital of Xi'an Jiaotong University, Xi'an, China

Nan Yu
Department of Radiology, The Affiliated Hospital of Shaanxi University of Traditional Chinese Medicine, Xianyang, Shaanxi, China

Jianying Li
Department of Respiratory Medicine, Central Hospital of Xi'an Affiliated Hospital of Xi'an Jiaotong University, Xi'an, Shaanxi, China

Min Qi
Department of Radiology, Shaanxi Provincial People's Hospital, Xi'an, China

Zhijian Huang and Feiyu Sun
Department of Emergency, Xia'men Traditional Chinese Medicine Hospital affiliated to Beijing University of Traditional Chinese Medicine, Xia'men, Fujian, China

Wei Zhang and Jian Yang
Department of Respiratory, Jiangning Hospital affiliated to Nanjing Medical University, Nanjing, Jiangsu, China

Hongwei Zhou
Department of Intensive Care Unit, Xia'men Traditional Chinese Medicine Hospital affiliated to Beijing University of Traditional Chinese Medicine, No.1739 Xianyue Road, Xia'men 361009, Fujian, China

Seijiro Sato, Yuki Shimizu, Tatsuya Goto, Akihiko Kitahara, Terumoto Koike and Masanori Tsuchida
Division of Thoracic and Cardiovascular Surgery, Niigata University Graduate School of Medical and Dental Sciences, 1-757 Asahimachi-dori, Chuo-ku, Niigata-shi, Niigata 951-8510, Japan

Hiroyuki Ishikawa
Department of Radiology and Radiation Oncology, Niigata University Graduate School of Medical and Dental Sciences, Niigata, Japan

Takehiro Watanabe
Department of Thoracic Surgery, National Hospital Organization Nishi-Niigata Chuo National Hospital, Niigata, Japan

Pengwei Xu and Yuchun Li
School of Public Health, Xinxiang Medical University, Xinxiang 453003, China

Jie Song and Weidong Wu
School of Public Health, Xinxiang Medical University, Xinxiang 453003, China
Henan International Collaborative Laboratory for Health Effects and Intervention of Air Pollution, Xinxiang 453003, China

Mengxue Lu
Xinxiang Medical University, Xinxiang 453003, China

Liheng Zheng
Hebei Chest Hospital, Shijiazhuang 050041, China

Yue Liu and Dongqun Xu
National Institute of Environmental Health, Chinese Center for Disease Control and Prevention, Beijing 100021, China

Yacov Zaltzman
Chronic Ventilator-Dependent Division, Herzog Medical Center, Jerusalem, Israel

Shikma Katz
Chronic Ventilator-Dependent Division, Herzog Medical Center, POB 3900, Jerusalem, Israel
Recanati School for Community Health Professions, Faculty of Health Sciences, Ben Gurion University of the Negev, Beer Sheva, Israel

Esther-Lee Marcus
Chronic Ventilator-Dependent Division, Herzog Medical Center, POB 3900, Jerusalem, Israel
Hebrew University-Hadassah Faculty of Medicine, Jerusalem, Israel

Nissim Arish and Ariel Rokach
Pulmonary Institute, Shaare Zedek Medical Center, POB 3235, Jerusalem, Israel
Hebrew University-Hadassah Faculty of Medicine, Jerusalem, Israel

Yusheng Cheng
Department of Respiratory and Critical Care Medicine, Yijishan Hospital of Wannan Medical College, 2 Zeshan West Road, Wuhu 241001, Anhui, China
Department of Respiratory and Critical Care Medicine, the First Affiliated Hospital of Nanjing Medical University, 300 Guangzhou Road, Nanjing 210029, Jiangsu, China

Min Yu, Jian Xu, Mengyu He, Hong Wang, Hui Kong and Weiping Xie
Department of Respiratory and Critical Care Medicine, the First Affiliated Hospital of Nanjing Medical University, 300 Guangzhou Road, Nanjing 210029, Jiangsu, China

Elisabetta Zinellu
Department of Respiratory Diseases, University Hospital Sassari (AOU), Sassari, Italy

Pietro Pirina
Department of Respiratory Diseases, University Hospital Sassari (AOU), Sassari, Italy
Department of Clinical and Experimental Medicine, University of Sassari, Sassari, Italy

Alessandro G. Fois and Viviana Marras
Department of Clinical and Experimental Medicine, University of Sassari, Sassari, Italy

Panagiotis Paliogiannis, Salvatore Sotgia, Ciriaco Carru and Angelo Zinellu
Department of Biomedical Sciences, University of Sassari, Sassari, Italy

Gang Chen, Fang-Ming Zhong, Xu-Dong Xu, Guo-Can Yu and Peng-Fei Zhu
Department of Thoracic Surgery, Tuberculosis Surgery, Hangzhou Red Cross Hospital, No. 208 Huancheng East Road, Xiacheng District, Hangzhou 310003, Zhejiang, China

Pedro Barbolla Benito
Autonomous University of Madrid, Ciudad Universitaria de Cantoblanco, Madrid 28049, Spain

Germán Peces-Barba Romero
Department of Pneumology IIS-Fundación Jiménez Díaz, Center for Biomedical Research in the Network, Respiratory Diseases (Spanish acronym CIBERES), Calle de Melchor Fernández Almagro, 3, Madrid 28029, Spain

Zohra Mraihi and Lamia Hila
Genetic Department, Faculté de Médecine de Tunis, Université de Tunis El Manar, Tunis, Tunisia

Jihen Ben Amar and Hend Bouacha
Pulmonary Department, EPS Charles Nicolle, Faculté de Médecine de Tunis, Université de Tunis El Manar, Tunis, Tunisia

Soumaya Rammeh
Pathological Anatomy and Cytology Department, EPS Charles Nicolle, Faculté de Médecine de Tunis, Université de Tunis El Manar, Tunis, Tunisia

Xuejun Guo
Department of Respiratory Medicine, Xinhua Hospital, Shanghai Jiaotong University School of Medicine, No. 1665, Kongjiang Road, Yangpu District, Shanghai 200092, People's Republic of China

Wei Xiong
Department of Respiratory Medicine, Xinhua Hospital, Shanghai Jiaotong University School of Medicine, No. 1665, Kongjiang Road, Yangpu District, Shanghai 200092, People's Republic of China
Department of Cardiopulmonary Circulation, Shanghai Pulmonary Hospital, Tongji University School of Medicine, Shanghai, China

Bigyan Pudasaini and Jinming Liu
Department of Cardiopulmonary Circulation, Shanghai Pulmonary Hospital, Tongji University School of Medicine, Shanghai, China

Mei Xu
Department of Pediatrics, Dinghai Community Health Service Center, Tongji University School of Medicine, Shanghai, China;Department of Pediatrics, Kongjiang Hospital, Yangpu District, Shanghai, China

K. Rajala
Department of Palliative Care, Comprehensive Cancer Center, , Helsinki University Hospital, Paciuksenkatu 21, FI-00290 Helsinki, Finland
Faculty of Medicine, University of Helsinki, Helsinki, Finland

J. T. Lehto
Department of Oncology, Palliative Care Unit, Tampere University Hospital and Faculty of Medicine and Life Sciences, University of Tampere, Tampere, Finland

E. Sutinen
Faculty of Medicine, University of Helsinki, Helsinki, Finland

H. Kautiainen
Primary Health Care Unit, Kuopio University Hospital, Finland and Folkhälsan Research Center, Helsinki, Finland

M. Myllärniemi
University of Helsinki and Helsinki University Hospital, Heart and Lung Center, Department of Pulmonary Medicine, Helsinki, Finland

T. Saarto
Helsinki University Hospital, Comprehensive Cancer Center, Department of Palliative Care and Faculty of Medicine, University of Helsinki, Helsinki, Finland

Index

www.ingramcontent.com/pod-product-compliance
Lightning Source LLC
Chambersburg PA
CBHW080509200326
41458CB00012B/4139